EPIDEMIOLOGIC METHODS

SECOND EDITION

EPIDEMIOLOGIC METHODS

Studying the Occurrence of Illness

NOEL S. WEISS

THOMAS D. KOEPSELL
University of Washington

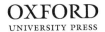

OXFORD
UNIVERSITY PRESS

OXFORD
UNIVERSITY PRESS

Oxford University Press is a department of the University of Oxford.
It furthers the University's objective of excellence in research, scholarship,
and education by publishing worldwide.

Oxford   New York
Auckland   Cape Town   Dar es Salaam   Hong Kong   Karachi
Kuala Lumpur   Madrid   Melbourne   Mexico City   Nairobi
New Delhi   Shanghai   Taipei   Toronto

With offices in
Argentina   Austria   Brazil   Chile   Czech Republic   France   Greece
Guatemala   Hungary   Italy   Japan   Poland   Portugal   Singapore
South Korea   Switzerland   Thailand   Turkey   Ukraine   Vietnam

Oxford is a registered trademark of Oxford University Press
in the UK and certain other countries.

Published in the United States of America by
Oxford University Press
198 Madison Avenue, New York, NY 10016

Library of Congress Cataloging-in-Publication Data
Weiss, Noel S., Koepsell, Thomas D., author.
Epidemiologic methods : studying the occurrence of illness / Noel S. Weiss, Thomas D. Koepsell. — Second edition.
p. ; cm.
Includes bibliographical references.
ISBN 978–0–19–531446–5 (alk. paper)
I. Weiss, Noel S., 1941– author.   II. Title.   III. Title: Epidemiologic methods.
[DNLM: 1. Epidemiologic Methods. WA 950]
RA652.4
614.4—dc23
2014001643

CONTENTS

PREFACE

Epidemiology at any given time is something more than the total of its established facts. It includes their orderly arrangement into chains of inference which extend more or less beyond the bounds of direct observation. Such of these chains as are well and truly laid guide investigation to the facts of the future.

—WADE HAMPTON FROST[1]

Between us, we have accumulated more than 60 person-years teaching courses on the principles and methods of epidemiology. We have jointly taught a two-course sequence at the University of Washington since the mid-1980s. During this time, we have listened to the reactions of many students who were being introduced to this field. One came from a woman who said she derived an almost esthetic pleasure from epidemiology: she found both efficiency and beauty in the process of taking raw observations on the occurrence of an illness in humans and weaving them into "chains of inferences" about the causes of that illness, which often had the potential to lead to prevention.

We suspect that not too many of our students would have used the word *esthetic* to describe any of their feelings about our course, even their positive feelings. (Some might have said that *anesthetic* better characterized some of the class sessions!) Nonetheless, we like to think that the first student had internalized what we were trying to convey—that the techniques of structuring observations and analyzing the information gathered (upon which so much time and effort are expended in class) are to be used to produce "...chains [that] are well and truly laid..." in the hope of guiding "investigation to the facts of the future." Having produced extensive classroom materials to achieve our goals, we felt that with a little (!) extra labor we could organize these materials into a book for other students of epidemiology.

Which students? The book is aimed at beginning and intermediate students of epidemiologic methods. It is meant to serve as an introduction to the field for people who intend to conduct epidemiologic research themselves, or who need methodological expertise to interpret and synthesize properly the results of epidemiologic research produced by others. It starts at the beginning, so to speak, but covers much of the material in more detail than would be desired by a reader who wished only to have a general appreciation of epidemiology. Those who have already taken an introductory course in epidemiology may find here a welcome review of basic concepts, as well as new, more advanced material.

A brief outline of the book may be helpful. Chapter 1 tells the story of a real disease outbreak, introducing epidemiologic concepts and designs along the way that will be covered in depth in later chapters. Chapter 2 sets forth an epidemiologic view of diseases and populations, leading into Chapters 3 and 4, on measuring disease frequency in populations. Chapter 5 paints the "big picture" of research designs in epidemiology, so that their names are familiar when used in chapters that follow. Chapters 6 and 7 highlight several specific sources of numerator and denominator data in epidemiology and provide examples of the person/place/time conceptual framework that underlies many descriptive epidemiologic studies.

As a transition into analytic epidemiology, Chapter 8 discusses the kinds of epidemiologic evidence that bear on an inference that an association may be causal. Chapter 9 also focuses on associations, describing several quantitative measures of excess risk that can be calculated from epidemiologic data. Chapter 10 introduces several quantitative techniques for assessing the reliability and validity of epidemiologic measurements and describes

---

[1] From his introduction to: *Snow J. Snow on Cholera.* New York: The Commonwealth Fund, 1936.

how measurement error affects observed associations. Chapter 11 describes what confounding is, how it is traditionally assessed, and basic methods for its control. Chapter 12 (new in this edition) discusses more advanced aspects of confounding: alternative conceptualizations, causal diagrams, multi-variable analysis, data-reduction approaches, inverse probability–weighting, instrumental variables, and time-dependent confounding.

Chapters 13–16 each focus in depth on a class of epidemiologic study designs: randomized trials, cohort studies, case-control studies, and ecologic and multi-level studies. Chapter 17 discusses the implications for epidemiologic studies of the temporal relationship between exposure and outcome. Chapter 18 describes ways in which epidemiologic studies can be designed and analyzed to enhance the likelihood that a true association is detected.

Chapters 19–21 cover methodological aspects of several key topics in epidemiology: screening for disease, short-term disease outbreaks, and evaluating the effects of societal and institutional policies on health.

As the book's title indicates, the discussion throughout focuses on the means by which epidemiologic research is conducted and interpreted, not on the substantive knowledge about specific diseases or exposures that has accumulated from specific studies.

Two things that will distinguish this book from others with similar goals are its liberal use of examples from the published medical literature, and the sets of questions that appear at the end of most chapters. Most of these questions pertain to actual published studies, our purpose being to emphasize the applicability of the principles and methods to real-life situations.

From the beginning, the book has been a joint enterprise by the two of us. Each of us drafted about half of the chapters. Noel was lead author on chapters 8–9, 11, 14–15, and 17–18; Tom was lead author on chapters 1–7, 12–13, 16, and 21. Chapters 10 and 19 were co-authored by both of us. Each of us was the primary critical reviewer of the other's draft chapters, and both of us are prepared to stand by the book as a whole. Jennifer Lloyd and Jeffrey Duchin, epidemiologists with Public Health Seattle and King County, contributed the chapter on outbreak investigation, for which we are grateful.

There being no better way of deciding the order of our names on the entire book, we agreed to alternate the order with each edition. As the result of a fateful coin flip, Tom was first author on the first edition, and Noel is now first author on the second edition.

We gratefully acknowledge helpful comments on draft chapters from several colleagues and students. Ali Rowhani-Rahbar, Peter Cummings, and Amanda Phipps kindly reviewed some of the chapters and made many useful suggestions. Several cohorts of students in our two-quarter course sequence on epidemiologic methods have used the first edition as their main textbook and provided feedback about errors and points of confusion. The second edition has benefited from their sharp eyes.

Noel S. Weiss
Thomas D. Koepsell

Introduction: An Epidemic of Blindness in Young Children

DISCOVERY

On February 14, 1941, a Boston pediatrician named Dr. Stewart Clifford was making a routine house call on one of his patients, a baby girl then about three months old. She had been born prematurely, weighing about four pounds at birth. But except for some brief early episodes of turning blue (cyanosis), she had done well during her hospital stay and had been discharged.

As Dr. Clifford examined her, he noticed something odd about the baby's eyes. Her gaze wandered aimlessly, and her eyes jerked rapidly from side to side. There were prominent gray opacities in both eyes. He was puzzled and concerned: by all appearances, the baby girl was blind.

Dr. Clifford called in Dr. Paul Chandler, a leading Boston ophthalmologist. Dr. Chandler had not seen this baby's condition before. To permit a fuller evaluation, the baby was hospitalized again and examined under anesthesia. The main abnormality (illustrated in Figure 1.1) was a gray mass of scar tissue attached to the back of the lens and covered with blood vessels. It later became clear that this tissue was all that remained of a retina that had been so badly damaged by hemorrhage and inflammation that it had delaminated from the back of the eye, become scarred and fibrous, and floated forward to affix itself to the lens. The baby girl was completely and irreversibly blind.

This first case proved not to be a bizarre, isolated occurrence. Within a week, Dr. Clifford encountered another blind infant with the same condition. Soon another consultant ophthalmologist, Dr. Theodore Terry, had gathered information on five such cases in the Boston area, whom he described in an article in the *American Journal of Ophthalmology* (Terry, 1942). Shared pathological features among these early cases led to calling the condition *retrolental*

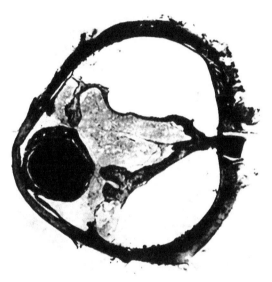

FIGURE 1.1 Cross-section of an eye showing retrolental fibroplasia.

(Reprinted courtesy of Dr. Arnall Patz)

fibroplasia (RLF), referring to proliferation of fibrous scar tissue behind the lens.

EPIDEMIC

Once Dr. Terry's description of RLF appeared in the medical literature, other physicians began to look for it and to find it. By 1945, Dr. Terry published a description of 117 cases, all but five of them in babies who had been born prematurely (Terry, 1945). Across the country, the California School for the Blind reported a sharp rise in the number of RLF cases over time among babies born in Southern California, as shown in Figure 1.2 (Silverman, 1980). Within just a few years after its discovery, RLF went from being literally unknown to being the most

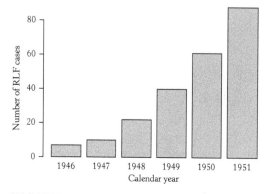

FIGURE 1.2 Number of retrolental fibroplasia (RLF) cases by calendar year in Southern California, 1946 to 1951. (Based on data from Silverman [1980])

common cause of blindness in preschool children in the United States. Worldwide, more than 10,000 babies developed the condition.

EARLY SEARCH FOR POSSIBLE CAUSES

The rapid rise in the frequency of RLF and its serious consequences led to an intensive search for a cause or causes. Early case series suggested that most children diagnosed with RLF had been born prematurely. Whether the condition was already present at birth or developed after birth remained unclear. One study that helped to clarify these issues was by Owens and Owens (1949), who performed monthly standardized eye examinations from birth to six months of age on 111 babies born at Johns Hopkins Hospital and who weighed 2,000 grams (4.4 pounds) or less at birth. To determine whether the degree of prematurity was related to risk of RLF, they grouped study babies according to birth weight, a characteristic strongly related to prematurity. All babies in the study appeared to have normal eyes at birth, but 12.1% of babies who weighed <1,360 grams at birth developed RLF, as compared to only 1.3% of babies with higher birth weight—over a ninefold difference.

In the course of the monthly eye examinations, Owens and Owens could observe the sequence of pathological events that led to RLF among babies who developed it. A typical progression was: (1) dilation of retinal vessels; (2) wild proliferation of vessels throughout the retina, even protruding into the vitreous humor; (3) retinal hemorrhage, swelling, and inflammation; and finally, (4) scarring and detachment of the retina. Still, the disease did not *always* progress inexorably to end in scarring; in some cases, it seemed to stop at earlier stages.

Both the association with prematurity and the pathological evolution of RLF suggested some possible causes. The care of premature infants had advanced in many ways during the 1940s (James and Lanman, 1976). Techniques for giving babies fluids by vein or subcutaneously had come into widespread use, providing new ways to prevent or treat dehydration and to administer medications. Several vitamin and mineral deficiencies were recognized and treated with supplements. Incubators made it easier to control temperature and humidity in the baby's local environment and offered a barrier to infection. With immature lungs, many premature babies experienced cyanosis or respiratory distress, which could be treated with supplemental oxygen piped into the incubator or delivered by nasal catheter or face mask. Penicillin offered a potent new weapon against infectious complications. These and other medical innovations had sharply increased a premature baby's chances of survival.

Improved survival of premature babies raised the possibility that RLF was a complication of prematurity that had escaped notice until a sufficient number of such babies survived long enough to develop the disease. Table 1.1 shows results from a

TABLE 1.1. SURVIVORSHIP AND OCCURRENCE OF RETROLENTAL FIBROPLASIA BY BIRTH WEIGHT AND CALENDAR YEAR—MANCHESTER, ENGLAND, 1947–1951

Birth weight	Calendar Year				
	1947	1948	1949	1950	1951
A. Number of surviving infants					
<3 lb.	4	7	9	16	13
3–3.5 lb.	11	13	18	21	22
3.5–4 lb.	31	27	30	38	30
Over 4 lb.	72	92	50	75	50
B. Number of surviving infants who developed RLF					
<3 lb.	1	0	2	5	12
3–3.5 lb.	0	0	0	2	12
3.5–4 lb.	0	0	0	2	9
Over 4 lb.	0	0	0	2	9
C. Proportion of survivors who developed RLF					
<3 lb.	0.25	0.00	0.22	0.31	0.92
3–3.5 lb.	0.00	0.00	0.00	0.10	0.55
3.5–4 lb.	0.00	0.00	0.00	0.05	0.30
Over 4 lb.	0.00	0.00	0.00	0.03	0.18

(Source: Jefferson [1952])

study by Jefferson (1952) in Manchester, England, that addressed this possibility. Panel A of the table shows the number of surviving babies in each year from 1947 to 1951, by birth weight. Panel B shows the number, and panel C the proportion, of surviving babies who developed RLF, also broken out by birth weight and year. Reading horizontally in panel A, we see that the number of survivors increased steadily over time among babies who weighed <3 pounds or 3–3.5 pounds at birth, while the time trends in babies weighing over 3.5 pounds suggest no such increase. These observations could be compatible with improving survival over time among infants with the lowest birth weights. In panel B, we also see an increasing number of babies with RLF over time in each birth weight category. This simply confirms that the RLF epidemic did not spare Manchester.

Most revealing, however, are the patterns in panel C, which shows the *proportion* of surviving babies who developed RLF, by birth weight category and year. Each proportion was computed by dividing the number of RLF cases in each year and birth weight category by the corresponding number of surviving babies. These data show that: (1) within any given year, the proportion developing RLF was generally greatest among babies with the lowest birth weight; and (2) within each birth weight category, the proportion of survivors who developed RLF increased markedly over time. This second observation is direct evidence that, at least in Manchester, the epidemic was due not just to increased survival of premature babies, but also to increased risk of developing RLF among survivors.

EARLY TREATMENTS

Early therapies for RLF sought to arrest progression of the disease through the pathological stages described earlier. It was thought that the increase in the caliber and density of blood vessels might be a response to hypoxia, to which premature infants were known to be vulnerable. A retinal disease in mice with some RLF-like features appeared to result from experimentally lowered oxygen levels (Ingalls, 1948). This line of thinking provided further impetus for liberal oxygen supplementation in premature infants, especially those with early signs of RLF.

Another approach to treatment was based on observations that some premature infants had abnormally low adrenal corticosteroid levels, and that the

pathology of RLF was reminiscent of connective-tissue diseases in adults. A group of New York–based physicians tried adrenocorticotropic hormone (ACTH) treatments for babies with early signs of RLF, hoping that it would suppress inflammation and scarring. Of 31 babies who received ACTH, 25 appeared to respond, with reversal of the early changes of RLF and preserved eyesight (Blodi *et al.*, 1951). Given the paucity of effective treatments, early reports of success with ACTH were welcome news.

Unfortunately, doubts about ACTH soon began to emerge. Some clinicians noted many disturbing treatment failures (Laupus, 1951; Pratt, 1951). They also noted that some early cases that had *not* been treated with ACTH did not progress inexorably to scarring and blindness. Thus, it was not clear how effective ACTH really was.

In an attempt to provide more convincing evidence, Reese *et al.* (1952) undertook a second study of ACTH treatment using a different research design, as diagrammed in Figure 1.3. This time the study included a second group of similar babies who did

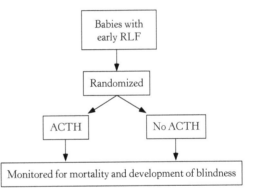

	Treatment received			
	ACTH		NO ACTH	
Outcome	NO.	%	No.	%
Deaths[a]	6/36	17%	1/49	2/5
Blindness[b]	10/30	33%	7/36	19%

[a] Published report gives only total numbers of deaths and babies, combining randomized-trial results with an rearlier, non-randomized comparison
[b] Number and % of eyes treated

FIGURE 1.3 Study design and results evaluating ACTH as treatment for early retrolental fibroplasia. (Source: Reese *et al.* [1952])

not receive ACTH. To form the ACTH and no-ACTH groups, an equal number of white marbles and blue marbles were placed in a box. Each time a new baby with early RLF was found to be eligible, a marble was removed from the box without looking at it. Its color determined whether the baby received ACTH or not. The investigators sought to keep other forms of treatment similar in both groups, and they monitored all babies with standardized eye examinations. The results yielded a rude shock: not only was progression of RLF more common in the ACTH group, but death was more frequent in that group as well, apparently due to increased risk of infection. ACTH had been found to be ineffective and even dangerous as treatment for RLF, and ACTH quickly fell out of favor.

NARROWING THE SEARCH FOR POSSIBLE CAUSES

A decade after the first cases had been reported, more than 50 factors had been suggested as possible contributors to the rising incidence of RLF (Silverman, 1980). Some factors had changed little during the period of rising RLF incidence—the gender mix of newborn babies, for example—and thus could hardly explain the epidemic. Other factors were not readily modifiable and hence offered few opportunities for prevention or treatment. Yet the remaining list of plausible and possible contributing causes was lengthy. If each factor had required a randomized trial like the ACTH study to confirm or exclude its role, the process would have been long and costly.

But in 1949, Kinsey and Zacharias showed how other research approaches could be used to narrow the field of plausible hypotheses in order to focus attention on a few main suspects. Their paper reported results from three related studies. The first involved identifying 53 babies who weighed four pounds or less at birth, who had been born at the Boston Lying-In Hospital during a ten-year study period, and who were known to have developed RLF. They were compared with a second group, of 298 babies, who also weighed four pounds or less at birth, had been born at the same hospital over the same ten-year period, but were known not to have developed RLF. The researchers then systematically reviewed the hospital records and, when necessary, interviewed mothers and pediatricians for both groups of babies. They compared prenatal factors, labor and delivery characteristics, postnatal complications, and patterns of neonatal care between the two groups. In

so doing, they investigated no fewer than 47 potential risk factors in a single study: investigating each additional factor required merely gathering another piece of information about each subject. Moreover, the information needed on the 53 RLF cases and 298 no-RLF controls concerned past events that had already occurred by the time data collection began, so the study was completed fairly quickly.

For three factors, the observed differences between groups were larger than chance alone could easily explain. Compared to controls without RLF, the RLF cases were less likely to be a first-born child, spent an average of ten more days in the newborn nursery after birth, and received supplemental oxygen for an average of nine more days. The authors noted that having spent more time in the nursery and receiving supplemental oxygen might have reflected worse general health among the cases. Many other factors proved to about equally common between RLF cases and controls, making it less likely that they were important causes of RLF.

The second study by Kinsey and Zacharias built on the observation that the number of RLF cases each year had risen sharply at the study hospital during the mid-1940s, an era when several changes had occurred in treatment patterns for premature babies. They sought to determine whether changes over time in the use of any particular treatment coincided with changes in the frequency of RLF. As shown in Figure 1.4, they identified three factors that looked suspicious: use of iron supplements ($FeSO_4$), use of water-soluble vitamins (thought to be better absorbed than the lipid-soluble vitamins previously used), and the amount of supplemental oxygen used. Of these, they considered the temporal correlations with iron and vitamins to be the most striking.

The third study reported by Kinsey and Zacharias was motivated by two other observations: first, the incidence of RLF seemed to differ considerably among babies born at different hospitals; and second, hospitals had different policies and practices about how they treated premature babies, leading to wide variation in treatment patterns. Kinsey and Zacharias reasoned that the hospital-to-hospital variation in RLF frequency and in treatment might be linked. Accordingly, they gathered data from eight urban hospitals, focusing especially on use of water-miscible vitamins and on iron supplementation in relation to RLF incidence.

As shown in Table 1.2, the Boston hospital (their own) with the highest incidence of RLF had used water-soluble vitamins and iron supplements

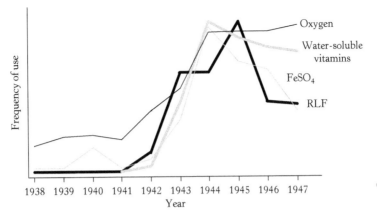

FIGURE 1.4 Trends over time in use of selected treatments and incidence of retrolental fibroplasia among babies weighing 3–4 lbs. at birth at Boston Lying-In Hospital, 1938–1947. (Source: Kinsey and Zacharias [1949])

frequently. At a hospital in New York that reported using no water-miscible vitamins and no iron, RLF had affected fewer than 1% of babies. Yet the overall pattern of variation failed to implicate one treatment over the other. Nonetheless, after reviewing these results, the investigators arranged to have use of water-soluble vitamins and iron supplements curtailed at their hospital. Unfortunately, the number of new RLF cases remained high and was apparently unaffected by the change (Kinsey and Chisholm, 1951).

On the other side of the world, an Australian pediatrician, Dr. Kate Campbell (1951), began to

suspect that the oxygen-RLF association that Kinsey and Zacharias had observed but discounted might not be simply an artifact of worse general health or of early aggressive treatment of RLF. She noted that RLF was more common in the United States than in England, where the use of supplemental oxygen was more restricted. She had also learned that clinicians in England had seen a striking increase in RLF after new, tightly sealed incubators had been installed, permitting delivery of oxygen at higher concentrations than before. Campbell conducted a small study of her own, comparing three groups of premature babies treated in the Melbourne area who had been subject to different treatment practices with regard to supplemental oxygen. Most babies treated at Institution I had been placed in a cot (incubator) that delivered oxygen at high concentration. Babies treated at Institution II wore a catheter or face mask that delivered lower inhaled oxygen concentrations. A third group of babies under private care had been treated with various oxygen delivery methods that also provided relatively low concentrations of oxygen. She found that RLF had occurred in 19% of premature babies at Institution I, compared with only 7% of the babies treated in other two settings. While acknowledging the small size of her study, she questioned in print whether oxygen supplementation might actually be causing RLF.

Other reports from around the world painted a confusing picture. At Charity Hospital in New Orleans (Exline and Harrington, 1951), no cases of RLF were found despite what was regarded as liberal use of oxygen supplementation. (It was noted later,

TABLE 1.2. TREATMENT OF BABIES WEIGHING 3–4 LBS. AT BIRTH AND INCIDENCE OF RETROLENTAL FIBROPLASIA AT EIGHT URBAN HOSPITALS

Location	Use of water-miscible vitamins	Use of iron	Incidence of RLF (%)
Boston	None	Low	0.9
Boston	High	High	20.2
Baltimore	Low	Low	1.0
New York	None	None	0.7
Cincinnati	None	High	6.8
Birmingham, England	None	Low	0.0
Providence	High	Low	5.2
Providence	None	Low	4.0

(Source: Kinsey and Zacharias [1949])

however, that incubators in the large newborn unit there were frequently opened, allowing oxygen to escape, and that oxygen levels were seldom directly measured.) Other hospitals in Oxford, England, and Paris, France, had seen no reduction in RLF after oxygen use was restricted (Houlton, 1951; Lelong *et al.*, 1952), but questions were raised about whether babies receiving high vs. low oxygen were otherwise similar.

IMPLICATING OXYGEN: EXPERIMENTAL EVIDENCE

One of many clinicians following these developments was Dr. Arnall Patz, then an ophthalmology resident at Gallinger Municipal Hospital in Washington, D.C. He, too, had become suspicious about a possible role for oxygen when he was called to see more and more babies with RLF after closed incubators were introduced. Although he had begun some animal studies, he reasoned that more direct and convincing evidence about whether oxygen supplementation was a cause of RLF in humans or simply an artifact would have to come from a study of human infants. Such a study would have to manipulate the level of oxygen delivery for premature babies, comparing outcomes in babies on high oxygen with outcomes among other babies on low oxygen. Patz and colleagues applied for, and eventually received, a $4,000 grant from the then-fledgling National Institutes of Health (NIH) to set up such a study.

Babies weighing under 3.5 pounds were assigned alternately to one of two groups. Group I was to receive 65–70% oxygen for 4–7 weeks. Group II was to receive oxygen only at 40% concentration or less, only in response to a clear clinical need, and only for 1–14 days. To help allay fears raised during review of their grant proposal about the possible risks of hypoxia, the investigators stipulated that all babies in both groups would be given enough oxygen to maintain a healthy pink color.

Nonetheless, it proved to be a difficult study to carry out: some nurses questioned the wisdom of curtailing oxygen for premature babies and turned up the oxygen concentration at night for some of them. Ultimately, 11 of 76 babies were excluded due to insufficiently constant oxygen levels or lack of follow-up data. Yet findings for the other 65 babies were striking: 17 of 28 (61%) in the high-oxygen group developed RLF, versus only 6 of 37 (16%) in the restricted-oxygen group. The researchers concluded that "…in view of the bizarre manner in which the incidence of the disease fluctuates, additional rigidly controlled observations are necessary…" (Patz *et al.*, 1952).

In view of the study's striking findings, that recommendation did not go unheeded. The National Institutes of Health soon convened a working group to plan a larger randomized experiment on oxygen supplementation. Ultimately, this study, one of the earliest randomized trials supported by NIH, was conducted in 18 hospitals that agreed to follow a common protocol. The study compared high vs. restricted oxygen regimens among babies with birth weights of 1500 grams or less who had survived at least 48 hours after birth. Because of the emerging concern about the safety of administering oxygen at high concentrations, for the first three months of the study, two babies were to be assigned to the restricted-oxygen regimen for every one assigned to the high-oxygen regimen. Thereafter, if no adverse effect of restricted oxygen on mortality appeared, all babies would receive the low-oxygen regimen. Babies in both groups were followed closely with standardized eye examinations to determine the incidence of RLF.

On September 19, 1954, results of the cooperative study were publicly announced, and they were published the following year (Kinsey, 1955). As shown in Table 1.3, the incidence of RLF was nearly threefold higher among babies in the high-oxygen group. Total mortality in both groups was similar. A smaller randomized trial of oxygen supplementation in Colorado was reported in the same year by Lanman *et al.* (1954), reaching similar conclusions.

DECLINING INCIDENCE

Early suspicions about possible adverse effects of oxygen had already begun to influence treatment in the early 1950s, but release of the National Cooperative Study findings hastened the trend toward restricting use of supplemental oxygen. The American Academy of Pediatrics and other influential

---

TABLE 1.3. THREE-MONTH RESULTS OF THE NATIONAL COOPERATIVE STUDY

Treatment group	Mortality		Incidence of RLF	
	Deaths/n	%	Cases/n	%
Routine high oxygen	15/68	22.0	12/53	22.6
Curtailed oxygen	36/144	25.0	8/104	7.7

(Based on data from Greenhouse [1990])

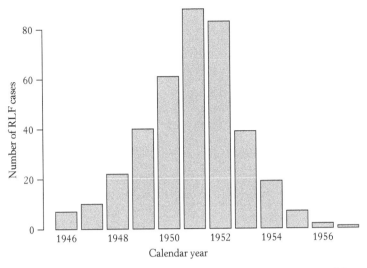

FIGURE 1.5 Number of retrolental fibroplasia (RLF) cases by calendar year in Southern California, 1946 to 1957. (Based on data from Silverman [1980])

professional organizations soon revised their recommendations to clinicians on care of premature babies, advocating more sparing use of oxygen and use of oxygen supplementation only when clinical circumstances necessitated it. Gratifyingly, the number of cases of RLF in the United States fell rapidly—Figure 1.5 shows the trend in Southern California. The RLF epidemic was over.

MECHANISM

A perplexing aspect of RLF was that implicating oxygen as a culprit seemed contrary to so much other biological knowledge. Oxygen was obviously essential for human life, and it was well known that premature babies often suffered from respiratory problems that led to low blood oxygen levels. Why was more of a good thing not better? Laboratory research on RLF was stymied for some time by lack of a good animal model for the disease. But in 1953, Ashton *et al.* reported research findings from studies on kittens. They found that the retina of a newborn kitten, like that of a prematurely born human baby, was incompletely vascularized. Development of retinal vessels was normally completed after birth, probably stimulated by mild hypoxia in areas of the retina that were not yet fully vascularized. Prolonged exposure to high oxygen levels after birth was found to produce constriction and ultimately obliteration of immature retinal vessels. When supplemental oxygen was then withdrawn, areas of the retina that had never become fully vascularized now became

severely oxygen-deprived. This led to inflammation and disordered vessel growth, followed in severe cases by scarring and destruction of the retina.

EPILOGUE

The rapid shift to more conservative use of oxygen supplementation in the 1950s is now generally credited as being the main reason for the rapid decline in RLF. But later evidence suggests that the change may not have occurred without cost. In 1960, Avery and Oppenheimer reported that deaths from hyaline membrane disease (subsequently termed *respiratory distress syndrome*) at Johns Hopkins Hospital had increased over the period from 1954–1958 after oxygen use was restricted. In the United States and in England and Wales, infant mortality on the first day of life, which had been declining steadily for more than 15 years, began to rise in the early 1950s and did not start falling again for another decade (James and Lanman, 1976). While many other changes in care were occurring during those years, it is thought that some clinicians may have been overzealous in their efforts to prevent RLF through sparing use of oxygen. None of the three experimental studies of oxygen described above had involved the number of participants that would be needed to detect small to moderate adverse effects of oxygen curtailment on mortality. In addition, the National Cooperative Study had only enrolled babies who had survived for at least 48 hours after birth. Its results thus did not directly address the possible consequences of oxygen restriction during the first two days of life, when many infant deaths occurred.

Retrolental fibroplasia has not disappeared. Its modern name is *retinopathy of prematurity*, a term that encompasses a wider spectrum of pathological features and that recasts prematurity from being a strong risk factor to being a required precondition. With further advances in neonatal care, survival of ever smaller premature babies has improved. Many such babies *must* have supplemental oxygen to survive. Fortunately, clinicians are now far better able to monitor and regulate oxygen levels in the tissues of premature infants undergoing treatment and can better steer a path between benefit and retinal toxicity.

CONCLUSIONS

As the first chapter in a book on epidemiologic methods, the foregoing story is intended not just to recount the history of one disease. Rather, the story illustrates the value of information gained from studying variations in disease frequency in human populations. Epidemiologic research turned out to occupy center stage in this episode of medical history, enabling relatively rapid recognition of an important cause of a disease that stemmed directly from the actions of well-meaning clinicians.

The history of RLF also suggests that some kinds of research should have greater impact than others on our beliefs and actions. One aim of this book is to highlight features of a research design that can make the results of one study more credible than those of another. For example, early enthusiasm for ACTH as treatment for RLF came from experience with a series of treated cases, but there was no comparable control group of cases treated without ACTH. When a control group was added in a subsequent study, conclusions about the effectiveness and safety of ACTH were completely reversed. Later, the sequence of research on oxygen and RLF evolved from observational studies to a small, non-randomized intervention trial, and eventually to a multi-center randomized trial. The broad conclusions of these studies proved to be similar, and the quality and consistency of evidence from better and better studies overcame skepticism and guided practice even before a mature biological theory of the pathogenesis of RLF had emerged.

From that viewpoint, some leading "characters" in the story of RLF are the study designs themselves.

Several of these designs will be explored in depth in chapters to come. To unmask some of these leading characters now:

- Owens and Owens conducted a *prospective cohort* study to confirm the role of prematurity. They first formed two groups of babies on the basis of birth weight, then monitored babies in both groups over time to measure and compare the incidence of RLF between groups.
- One of the studies carried out by Kinsey and Zacharias was a *case-control* study to investigate various perinatal risk factors. They first identified one group of babies with RLF and another group without RLF, then measured and compared the frequency of past exposure to various possible risk factors between those groups.
- In another part of the Kinsey and Zacharias study, and in the study by Campbell, an *ecological* research design was used to investigate possible hospital-level associations between treatment patterns and RLF incidence.
- Patz's study of oxygen supplementation was a *non-randomized intervention trial*. Whether a study baby received high- or low-dose supplemental oxygen was under the investigators' control. However, assignment of babies alternately between treatment regimens made the sequence of treatment-group assignments entirely predictable, not truly random.
- The National Cooperative Study was a true *randomized trial*. As in the Patz study, the investigators controlled which oxygen regimen each study baby received, but in this instance they used formal random assignment to do so.

The story of RLF also introduces several other key concepts in epidemiology to which we shall return in depth, including using counts and proportions as measures of disease frequency (Chapter 3), quantifying excess risk (Chapter 9), detecting and controlling confounding factors (Chapters 11 and 12), and determining whether associations are truly causal (Chapter 8).

Finally, it is worth noting that few of the investigators who conducted key studies on RLF considered themselves to be epidemiologists, even though they were using epidemiologic methods. At that time, most epidemiologists were busy working on infectious diseases, although the attention they paid to other kinds of health conditions had begun to grow. But epidemiologic concepts and methods are broadly applicable, and they are available to everyone. The overall goal of this book is to introduce many of the tools of epidemiology and to provide guidance about how to use them well.

Several detailed accounts of the history of RLF and its control have been published (James and Lanman, 1976; Reedy, 2004). Silverman (1980) includes personal anecdotes and reflections of several clinicians and researchers whose work is mentioned here. Jacobson and Feinstein (1992) reviewed a decade of clinical research on RLF and offered a detailed methodological critique. Duc (1999) reflected on lessons of the RLF story for practitioners seeking to apply evidence-based medicine.

REFERENCES

Ashton N, Ward B, Serpell G. Role of oxygen in the genesis of retrolental fibroplasia. A preliminary report. Br J Ophthalmol 1953; 37:513–520.

Avery ME, Oppenheimer EH. Recent increase in mortality from hyaline membrane disease. J Pediatr 1960; 57:553–559.

Blodi FC, Silverman WA, Day R, Reese AB. Experiences with corticotrophin (ACTH) in the acute stage of retrolental fibroplasia. Am J Dis Child 1951; 82:242–245.

Campbell K. Intensive oxygen therapy as a possible cause of retrolental fibroplasia: a clinical approach. Med J Australia 1951; 2:48–50.

Duc G. From observation to experimentation at the cotside: Lessons from the past. Pediatr Res 1999; 46:644–9.

Exline AL, Harrington MR. Retrolental fibroplasia: clinical statistics from the premature center of Charity Hospital of Louisiana at New Orleans. J Pediatr 1951; 38:1–7.

Greenhouse SW. Some historical and methodological developments in early clinical trials at the National Institutes of Health. Stat Med 1990; 9:893–901.

Houlton ACL. A study of cases of retrolental fibroplasia seen in Oxford. Tr Ophth Soc U 1951; 71:583–590.

Ingalls TH. Congenital encephalo-ophthalmic dysplasia. Pediatrics 1948; 1:315–325.

Jacobson RM, Feinstein AR. Oxygen as a cause of blindness in premature infants: "autopsy" of a decade of errors in clinical epidemiologic research. J Clin Epidemiol 1992; 45:1265–1287.

James LS, Lanman JT. History of oxygen therapy and retrolental fibroplasia. Pediatrics 1976; 52 (Suppl.):591–642.

Jefferson E. Retrolental fibroplasia. Arch Dis Child 1952; 27:329–336.

Kinsey VE. Etiology of retrolental fibroplasia and preliminary report of the Cooperative Study of Retrolental Fibroplasia. Tr Am Acad Ophth Otol 1955; 59:15–24.

Kinsey VE, Chisholm JF. Retrolental fibroplasia: evaluation of several changes in dietary supplements of premature infants with respect to the incidence of the disease. Am J Ophthalmol 1951; 34:1259–1268.

Kinsey VE, Zacharias L. Retrolental fibroplasia. Incidence in different localities in recent years and a correlation of the incidence with treatment given the infants. JAMA 1949; 139:572–578.

Lanman JT, Guy LP, Dancis J. Retrolental fibroplasia and oxygen therapy. JAMA 1954; 155:223–226.

Laupus WE. Comment on experiences with corticotrophin (ACTH) in the acute stage of retrolental fibroplasia. Am J Dis Child 1951; 82:243.

Lelong M, Rossier A, Fontaine M, LeMasson C, Michelin et Audibert J. Sur la retinopathie des prematures (fibroplasie retrolentale). Arch Fr Pediatr 1952; 9:897–914.

Owens WC, Owens EU. Retrolental fibroplasia in premature infants. Am J Ophthalmol 1949; 32:1–21.

Patz A, Hoeck LE, De La Cruz E. Studies on the effect of high oxygen administration in retrolental fibroplasia. Am J Ophthalmol 1952; 35:1248–1253.

Pratt EL. Comment on experiences with corticotrophin (ACTH) in the acute stage of retrolental fibroplasia. Am J Dis Child 1951; 82:243–244.

Reedy EA. The discovery of retrolental fibroplasia and the role of oxygen: a historical review, 1942–1956. Neonatal Netw 2004; 23:31–38.

Reese AB, Blodi FC, Locke JC, Silverman WA, Day RL. Results of use of corticotropin (ACTH) in treatment of retrolental fibroplasia. Arch Ophthalmol 1952; 47:551–555.

Silverman WA. Retrolental fibroplasia: a modern parable. New York: Grune and Stratton, 1980.

Terry TL. Extreme prematurity and fibroblastic overgrowth of persistent vascular sheath behind each crystalline lens. Am J Ophthalmol 1942; 25:203–204.

Terry TL. Retrolental fibroplasia in premature infants. V. Further studies on fibroplastic overgrowth of persistent tunica vasculosa lentis. Arch Ophthalmol 1945; 33:203–208.

2

Diseases and Populations

If public health is a branch of knowledge distinct from medicine, and the separation is believed well made, then public health must rest on some fundamental discipline which is characteristic of its activities and individual to it. Public health deals with groups of people, and epidemiology is the study of disease behavior as manifested by groups. For this reason epidemiology is stated to be the basic science of public health.

—JOHN GORDON

If you wish to converse with me, define your terms.

—FRANÇOIS VOLTAIRE

Epidemiology concerns describing and understanding patterns of disease occurrence in human populations, with the ultimate goal of preventing disease. It finds practical application every day in helping to lessen the burden of specific diseases in real populations, as illustrated by the retrolental fibroplasia example in the last chapter. But epidemiology is also based on a set of ideas that go beyond any one application. It has its own set of terms, its own body of theory, and its own methods. *Diseases* and *populations* are two of the most basic building blocks of that theory.

DISEASES

The scope of epidemiology is broad, and epidemiologic methods are widely applicable.[1] In that sense, *disease* can be defined very broadly to mean any departure from perfect health: any acute or chronic illness, congenital or acquired condition, medical diagnosis, psychiatric disorder, symptom, syndrome, injury, and so on. But for any particular epidemiologic study, a more explicit specification of the disease of interest is needed: a *case definition*.

Case Definition

An epidemiologic case definition is a set of rules for determining whether an individual does or does not

count as having the disease of interest for study purposes. A case definition can have major influence on the apparent frequency of a disease.

Example 2-1. During a severe heat wave in August, 2006, the chief medical examiner's office in New York City recorded 31 heat-related deaths. Noting that a previous heat wave in Chicago had resulted in hundreds of heat-related deaths, New York authorities attributed the difference to the success of "...efforts to find and save those at greatest risk." (*New York Times*, 2006)

On closer scrutiny by a careful journalist, however, the New York medical examiner's office was found to have classified deaths as heat-related only if heat stress was listed as the *immediate* cause of death on the death certificate. In contrast, during the earlier heat wave in Chicago, deaths had been classified as heat-related if heat stress was listed either as the immediate cause of death *or* as a significant contributing cause. Only about one-tenth of the deaths classified as heat-related in Chicago had heat stress listed as the immediate cause of death.

All case definitions are man-made, and they are developed for particular purposes and contexts.

Example 2-2. Consider the case definitions used in three different epidemiologic studies of diabetes mellitus:

- A study that sought to assess the frequency of diabetes, whether diagnosed or not, among United States adults used data from in-person interviews and examinations on a national sample. A case of diabetes was defined as an adult who either: (1) answered "yes" to the question "Have you ever been told by a doctor that you have diabetes or sugar diabetes?" or (2) underwent a fasting blood glucose test and had a result of ≥ 140 mg/dl (Wilder *et al.*, 2005).
- A study of time trends in the frequency of diabetes as a cause of death in the United States defined a case of diabetes as someone who had died and whose death certificate showed that the underlying cause of death had been assigned the code of 250 on the International Classification of Diseases, version 9 (Jemal *et al.*, 2005).
- A study of changes over time in the state-by-state frequency of diabetes among adult United States women involved adding standardized questions to a national telephone survey. A case of diabetes was defined as a woman who answered "yes" to the following question: "Have you ever been told by a doctor that you have diabetes?" (Ahluwalia *et al.*, 2005).

The case definitions of diabetes in these three studies were quite different. But note that no one of them would have been suitable for use in either of the other two studies of the same disease. A question about previously diagnosed diabetes in a telephone survey would be of little use for detecting undiagnosed diabetes, and it certainly would not yield much information if administered to a dead person. A test of fasting blood glucose could not be applied over the telephone or after death. A coded cause of death on a death certificate would not apply in a telephone survey or an in-person survey of living respondents.

Epidemiologic case definitions may thus justifiably differ from study to study. Nonetheless, a useful case definition should be: (1) based on objectively observable information, and (2) explicit about what features of the information qualify a person as meeting the case definition. In principle, a knowledgeable fellow researcher should be able to reproduce the results or apply the same case definition in another study with similar aims. A standardized case definition facilitates meaningful comparisons of disease frequency between studies that may involve different places, times, or population groups. A case definition that relies heavily on personal judgment or is only vaguely specified works against this goal.

Many epidemiologic case definitions rely heavily on clinical diagnoses. This is especially true when the research involves analysis of pre-existing data generated by clinicians, such as medical records or death certificates. Nonetheless, a clinical diagnosis and an epidemiologic case definition serve different purposes and may thus not be the same. A clinical diagnosis serves to guide treatment and provides a basis for forecasting likely outcomes. A clinical diagnosis thus focuses on events *after* illness is already established. In contrast, an epidemiologic case definition typically aims to group together people whose illnesses may have shared causes. Hence, its focus is on circumstances *before* illness developed. For example, an individual who seeks medical care after an arm injury might receive a clinical diagnosis of "Colle's fracture of the radius bone". That clinical diagnosis would be the same regardless of how the bone came to be broken. In an epidemiologic study of injuries, however, whether the same person qualifies as a case might instead depend heavily on the mechanism of injury. In a study of sports injuries, someone with a Colle's fracture after a fall in a soccer game might qualify as a case, along with players with injuries to other body parts. An otherwise identical Colle's fracture resulting from an automobile collision would not qualify as a case in such a study.

Moreover, epidemiologic case definitions must usually rely on information that is available or feasibly obtainable on a population scale. Use of invasive, costly, or exotic tests for this purpose is often impractical. Rarely, an epidemiologic study may involve costly tests on a carefully selected sample of individuals from a population of interest.

Where do epidemiologic case definitions come from? An epidemiologist rarely has to start from scratch. Often a case definition that was used in previous studies of the same disease remains suitable, saving time and effort and facilitating comparison of results; or it can at least be used as a starting point. For many infectious diseases, standard case definitions have been developed by the United States Centers for Disease Control and Prevention for use in its National Notifiable Diseases Surveillance System (2013).

When no precedent exists, as for a brand-new syndrome, epidemiologists can often collaborate with clinicians to develop a working case definition based on symptoms, examination findings, laboratory results, and the circumstances around illness onset.

Example 2-3. From November, 2002, to February, 2003, health officials in Guangdong Province, China, identified 305 cases of an acute respiratory illness of unknown etiology, including five deaths. The disease appeared to be readily transmitted to household contacts and health care workers. Travellers to the province later became ill when they arrived in Vietnam and Hong Kong, triggering new outbreaks. The condition became known as Severe Acute Respiratory Syndrome (SARS) (Centers for Disease Control and Prevention, 2003). To facilitate counting and investigating cases, a preliminary case definition was developed:

> Respiratory illness of unknown etiology with onset since February 1, 2003, meeting the following criteria:
>
> - Documented temperature > 38.0° C.
> - One or more symptoms of respiratory illness (e.g., cough, shortness of breath, difficulty breathing, or radiographic findings of pneumonia or acute respiratory distress syndrome)
> - Close contact[*] within 10 days of onset of symptoms with a person under investigation for or suspected of having SARS, or travel within 10 days of onset of symptoms to an area with documented transmission of SARS as defined by the World Health Organization (WHO)

The initial working case definition of SARS was very general: fever plus any of several fairly common respiratory symptoms. However, the additional epidemiologic criteria—occurring after February 1, 2003, and either travel to a SARS outbreak area or close contact with a known or suspected SARS case—limited who could qualify as a case of SARS. These features were based on a presumption that cases who shared those characteristics were more likely to have shared causes.

Later that year, a new strain of coronavirus was found to be the microbial agent responsible for

SARS, and antibody tests and cell-culture methods were developed to detect it. These developments led to formulation of two new case definitions to replace the original one. SARS-RUI (SARS report under investigation) continued to be defined based solely on clinical and epidemiologic features, while SARS-CoV (SARS due to coronavirus) additionally required laboratory evidence of infection with the new coronavirus.

Developing a case definition often involves striking a balance between competing aims. On one hand, a broad and inclusive case definition can be desirable in order not to miss cases that share similar causes. In a disease outbreak situation, it may be more efficient to set aside data on some cases later, rather than to backtrack and gather new data on cases who had been bypassed initially. This rationale favors an inclusive case definition and is further discussed in Chapter 20. On the other hand, an overly broad case definition can run the risk of mixing together heterogeneous illnesses with very different causes. If so, the study's ability to identify those causes can be weakened. Chapter 18 explores this issue further.

In part to cope with these competing aims, investigators can sometimes "hedge their bets" by collecting data in such a way that more than one case definition can be applied. In Example 2-1, researchers with access to Chicago death certificate data could apply either an inclusive or a restrictive case definition of heat-related deaths and evaluate the effect of this choice on the apparent frequency of that condition. In other situations, researchers may plan to compare their study results with those of previous studies that may have used different case definitions. Or a widely used case definition may have recently been revised because of new knowledge about the disease—for example, when a specific test for the coronavirus responsible for SARS became available.

Example 2-4. Several large epidemiologic studies of myocardial infarction (heart attack) have used a case definition based on: (1) cardiac chest pain; (2) certain abnormalities on the electrocardiogram; and (3) blood tests showing abnormally high levels of cardiac enzymes, which are released into the blood by dying heart muscle (White *et al.*, 1996; Tunstall-Pedoe *et al.*, 1994). Specific combinations of these features qualified a myocardial infarction case as meeting the study's case definition.

For many years, the third feature was assessed using the Creatine kinase MB isoenzyme (CK-MB)

---

[*]Defined as having cared for, having lived with, or having had direct contact with respiratory secretions and/or body fluids of a person suspected of having SARS.

test. But in 2000, a new test for a different cardiac enzyme, troponin, was substituted because it had been shown to detect smaller amounts of myocardial damage that were missed by the CK-MB test (Alpert et al., 2000).

An epidemiologic study in Olmsted County, Minnesota, identified cases of myocardial infarction over the 20-year period from 1987–2006 (Roger et al., 2010). Noting that changes in the case definition during the study period could affect time trends, the researchers collected data on both CK-MB and troponin test results for possible cases in 2000 and later. They found that 278 of the 1,127 cases occurring after the advent of the troponin test would not have qualified under the older case definition. By simply counting cases according to whichever case definition was current at the time, the frequency of myocardial infarction appeared to have been essentially constant over time. But when the same case definition was used throughout, the incidence of myocardial infarction was found to have decreased by about 20% from 1987 to 2006.

Sometimes the amount of available information about possible disease cases varies substantially from person to person, and it may not be feasible to gather additional data to fill the gaps. In such instances, it can be useful to categorize potential cases according to the level of available evidence. For example, in a study of variant Creutzfeld-Jakob disease, a rare and often fatal neurological condition, some cases were classified as *definite* if neuropathological confirmation was obtained at autopsy, while others were classified as *probable* if they had compatible clinical features but no neuropathological confirmation (Andrews *et al.*, 2000). Ultimately, the incidence of this disease was found to be increasing over time regardless of whether definite and probable cases were combined or if the analysis was restricted to definite cases, thus lending credence to conclusion that frequency of the disease was on the rise.

Disease Models

The approach to studying a disease epidemiologically must always take into account relevant aspects of disease biology—for example, who is biologically capable of developing the disease, how long episodes of disease can last, whether someone who has had the disease once can get it again, and so on. *State-transition* models provide a way to represent some of this information. They also lead naturally to other useful tools for visualizing how a disease is distributed in a population, and they underlie several common measures of disease frequency. Yet another attraction of state-transition models is that the mathematical theory of stochastic processes can be applied to them as an aid to understanding disease behavior in populations, as discussed in Chapter 4.

State-transition models involve specifying certain disease-related *states* that an individual can be in and the *transitions* that are possible between those states over time. Graphically, states are typically shown as boxes, and possible transitions are shown as arrows between the boxes. At any particular time, an individual is in one of the states. As time passes, he/she may remain in that state or may transition out of it along one of the arrows from the current state to another one.

Some of the most useful and widely applicable state-transition models are quite simple. Several such models will be considered here, some of them labelled with letters for later reference.

Model A

Probably the simplest model worth considering involves just two states—*non-diseased* and *diseased*—and a single transition between them:

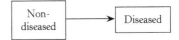

FIGURE 2.1

Under Model A, at any point in time, a person either has the disease of interest (according to some case definition) or does not have it. Over time, a person without the disease can get it, but no transition in the other direction is possible. Model A thus describes a disease that cannot be cured and from which no spontaneous recovery is possible. Examples include Alzheimer's disease, osteoarthritis, and atherosclerosis, none of which is presently reversible. Another example, using the term *disease* broadly, would be death from any cause.

The diseased state in Model A is sometimes called an *absorbing* state, because there are no arrows leading out of it. One implication of this model's structure is that the disease can occur at most once for an individual: i.e., it is non-recurrent.

Model B

For many other diseases, a more appropriate model involves the same two states, but with transitions possible in either direction:

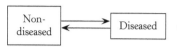

FIGURE 2.2

The arrow from diseased to non-diseased can represent spontaneous recovery or cure. Over time, a person can thus move back and forth between non-diseased and diseased states, implying that the disease can be recurrent. Examples include the common cold, depression, or urinary tract infection.

There is no inherent restriction in Model B as to how long a person who gets the disease remains in the diseased state. For some diseases, the duration of a disease episode may be very short, perhaps only an instant. Examples of this sort might include falls, cardiac arrhythmias, or epileptic seizures.

Non-susceptible States

For many diseases, certain classes of people are known *a priori* to be biologically incapable of developing the disease. For example, women cannot develop prostate cancer; men cannot develop cancer of the uterus. For such diseases, a non-diseased person can thus be in either of two states: susceptible or non-susceptible. By definition, no transition is possible from non-susceptible to diseased.

Besides disease biology, features of a case definition can also importantly affect susceptibility. For example, post-traumatic epilepsy can be defined as recurrent seizures following an episode of serious head trauma. People with no history of serious head trauma could not qualify as having post-traumatic epilepsy under this case definition, even if they were to develop an otherwise identical illness involving recurrent seizures.

For some diseases, a person may move directly from the susceptible state to the non-susceptible state, or vice versa. For example, a child who has never had mumps and hence is susceptible may be vaccinated against mumps and become non-susceptible. Someone who has never had surgery may then undergo a surgical procedure, thus becoming susceptible to a post-operative complication.

Several models can be constructed involving susceptible, non-susceptible, and diseased states,

depending on the transitions possible for a given disease. Appendicitis, for example, could be represented in the following three-state model:

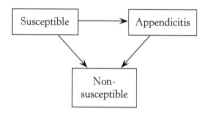

FIGURE 2.3

Anyone who has an appendix can develop appendicitis. Once appendicitis is diagnosed, standard treatment (at least in most of the developed world) is surgical removal of the appendix. Following appendectomy, the patient becomes permanently protected against ever having appendicitis again. Someone with an intact appendix who has never had appendicitis may also be rendered permanently non-susceptible by undergoing an "incidental" appendectomy—i.e., removal of a normal appendix as a preventive measure, usually during abdominal surgery performed for other reasons.

The term *at risk* is used in epidemiology as a synonym for *susceptible*—that is, capable of developing the disease. Someone who cannot become a case is *not at risk*. However, note also some fine points about this terminology:

- Being classified as *at risk* does not imply that a person will develop the disease with certainty in the future, or even that the risk of developing the disease is high. It just means that the risk is not zero. (Much epidemiologic research can be regarded as an attempt to discern *degrees* of risk among susceptibles.) In contrast, being classified as *not at risk* or *non-susceptible* implies zero risk of becoming a case under the case definition being used.
- Whether a person is or is not considered at risk may depend on how far into their future we look. For example, a woman who has just had a spontaneous abortion is not at risk for having another one the next day (assuming there is only one fetus). But over the longer term, she may become pregnant again and may have another spontaneous abortion. Hence, at the same moment, right after a spontaneous abortion, she could be considered both susceptible (over the long

term) and non-susceptible (over the short term). The *short-term* perspective is the one usually implied, unless stated otherwise. That is, a person is normally considered to be at risk at a certain time if, in the next instant, there is a non-zero probability that he/she could become a case.

- For most diseases, someone who already has the disease is considered not at risk. This is because someone who is already in a certain state cannot then transition into that state. (By analogy, you cannot *enter* a room if you are already inside it.)

The fullest possible model involving diseased, susceptible, and non-susceptible states is below:

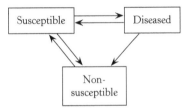

FIGURE 2.4

An example of this model might be occupational injury. The case definition for occupational injury would almost certainly require that an injury occur while on the job in order to qualify as 'occupational'. Accordingly, an individual would be susceptible to an occupational injury only while on the job, not while off duty. Employed individuals could thus move back and forth between susceptible and non-susceptible during the course of a typical day or week. If a minor injury occurred at work, the affected worker could remain on the job and thus be susceptible to another occupational injury. But if a more major injury occured, he/she would be likely to stop work in order to get treatment and/or to recover; during this period, the person would not be susceptible to an occupational injury.

Other State-Transition Models

State-transition models are often applied in infectious disease epidemiology: for example, some such models involve transitions among Susceptible, Infected, and Recovered states (Anderson and May, 1991; Cassels *et al.*, 2008).

More elaborate state-transition models can be constructed by adding states and possible transitions among them. For example, for some diseases, an intermediate state between non-diseased and diseased is thought to exist. A possible model for Alzheimer's disease is shown below:

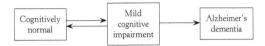

FIGURE 2.5

Under this model, individuals who are destined to develop dementia due to Alzheimer's disease first move from a cognitively normal state to a state of mild cognitive impairment. From that intermediate state, they may recover, or they may progress to full-blown Alzheimer's dementia. Once dementia occurs, it is irreversible. A further elaboration of this kind of model applies to disease screening (discussed in Chapter 19), which involves an ordered sequence of states between being disease-free and having disabling or fatal disease.

One reason to consider adding an intermediate state is that different factors may influence the probability of transition into and out of that state (Tyas *et al.*, 2007). Some of these factors may be modifiable and may identify opportunities for prevention at different stages on the way to disease. An ordered sequence of states can also be used to represent an increasing extent or severity of disease. For example, dental caries can be modeled as progressing from having no decayed teeth to having one decayed tooth, then two, and so on.

More than one state-transition model may be conceivable for a given disease. For example, two different models were described above for Alzheimer's disease, depending on whether mild cognitive impairment was included as an intermediate state. For falls in older adults, the simple two-state Model B above can be posited, recognizing that falls can recur. However, another possible model for fall occurrence in a person over time would be as shown below:

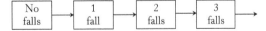

FIGURE 2.6

Here, each state represents the cumulative number of falls experienced so far by an older adult during a study period. Only someone who has not yet fallen is at risk for a first fall; only someone who has fallen exactly once is at risk for a second fall, and so on. One reason to consider such a model would be suspicion that the probability of transitioning from 0 falls to 1 fall may be quite different from that from 1 fall to 2 falls. And, in fact, much evidence suggests that having fallen once is a strong risk factor for falling again (Deandrea *et al.*, 2010).

These alternative models for the same disease are not contradictory; rather, they differ in their level of detail and purpose. Often an epidemiologic study focuses on a certain disease state and on certain transitions leading into or out of that state. A simple model may be adequate and most useful, as long as it captures the clinical and biological behavior of the disease as regards the states and transitions of interest while omitting other details.

Line Diagrams

Line diagrams are convenient tools for visualizing the disease-related experience of an individual over time. They build on the state-transition models considered above, adding information about the timing of changes from one state to another.

A person's history is shown as a horizontal line. Different states are denoted by differences in the appearance of the line, such as its thickness, shading, or color. Distance from left to right denotes elapsed time from a certain starting point. Any of several starting points can be used, depending on the context—for example, the time of birth, the time when the person first came under surveillance for possible disease occurrence, or a study-specific milestone such as assignment to a certain treatment group in a randomized trial.

To illustrate, suppose the disease of interest is wound infection at the site of a surgical incision. The line diagram below represents the experience of a hypothetical patient who develops a wound infection about 5.2 days after undergoing surgery. (Only the first week after surgery is shown.)

A transition into the diseased state is often referred to as a disease *event*. Conceptually, a disease event occurs at the point in time when the individual first meets the case definition. (Studies vary as to how precisely that time point can be ascertained.) How

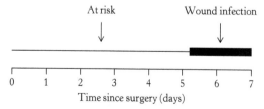

FIGURE 2.7

long the disease episode lasts does not affect the timing of the disease *event*: it occurs at time of *transition* into the diseased state.

If the amount of time spent in the diseased state is very short, a disease event may be shown on a line diagram as a vertical mark to make it visible. For example, the following line diagram could depict the occurrence of falls in an older adult during a certain year:

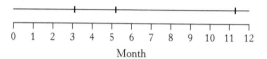

FIGURE 2.8

A more complex example might concern measles, involving three states: immune, susceptible, and ill with the measles. The line diagram below represents experience during the first year of life for a particular infant:

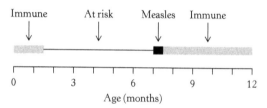

FIGURE 2.9

In this instance, while *in utero*, the baby received enough protective antibody across the placenta from his mother (who was herself immune) to render the baby immune to measles for several weeks after birth. After the maternally derived antibody dissipated, the infant was at risk for measles. He got sick with the measles for a few days at age 7 months, which stimulated antibody production that made him permanently immune thereafter.

Line diagrams will become especially useful when they are stacked vertically to represent disease experience in a population, as discussed later in this chapter.

POPULATIONS

Clinicians focus on each sick person as an individual. Clinical researchers often consider multiple cases of a certain disease—a case *series*—in order to describe their common features and differences. Epidemiologists view a set of disease cases in the context of the population from which they arose. This epidemiologic perspective allows several broader public health issues to be addressed. Among them, knowing the size of the source population from which cases arose lets us quantify how common or rare the disease is. Informally, the cases provide a *numerator*, while the population that generated them provides a *denominator*. In addition, comparing measures of disease frequency among population subgroups or across different populations can reveal factors associated with high (or low) frequency of disease, which in turn can provide clues about disease causation and possible opportunities for prevention.

Defined Populations

Before a population's size and composition can be known, the population must be defined. As with defining a case, defining a population involves specifying characteristics that all population members have in common and that set them apart from non-members. Characteristics often used for this purpose include *personal attributes*, such as age, gender, or membership in a predefined group, such as a factory work force or a health insurance plan; *geographic scope*, such as residence in a certain state or city; and the *time* or *time period* at which cases in the population can be identified and counted. Table 2.1 lists several examples of populations defined in terms of these characteristics.

Not every description of a group of people is sufficient to define it for epidemiologic purposes. For example, the characteristics of "a typical primary-care patient population" could vary greatly from one part of the world to another, or across historical time periods. A hypothetical group such as "people who would have been taken to Metropolitan General Hospital had they been injured in a motor-vehicle collision" may be possible to imagine, but in practice it would be almost impossible to ascertain the size

and characteristics of such a group. In short, like the rules for defining a case, the rules for defining a population must be specific enough to allow determining whether a certain person at a certain time would be included or not.

Defined Populations Observed over Time

Once the characteristics defining a population have been specified, it is straightforward in principle (if not always in practice) to determine its size and composition as of a single point in time. Everyone who meets the defining criteria at that time is a member, and counting them yields the population size.

But once we "start the clock" and monitor a population over a period of time, two possibilities need to be considered:

- The population's membership may remain stable throughout the time period of interest. No new members are added, and none of the original members are lost to follow-up. Such a population is termed *closed*.
- The population membership may change during the time period of interest. New members may be added, and members may be lost. Such a population is termed *open*.

The distinction between closed and open populations will be important when we choose an approach to measuring the incidence of new disease cases (Chapter 3), because it affects what kind of denominator is appropriate. But first, let us consider common situations that can involve closed or open populations, and some examples of each.

Closed Populations

A *closed population* is a defined set of individuals, all of them initially at risk, on whom we have complete data about how many of them become new disease cases during a certain fixed period of time. Specifically:

1. Every member is susceptible to the disease at the start of the observation period;
2. No new members are added during the observation period; and
3. Each of the original members can be classified at the end as having either (a) developed the disease, or (b) remained disease-free throughout the observation period.

TABLE 2.1. EXAMPLES OF DEFINED POPULATIONS

- The civilian, non-institutionalized population of the United States during 2010–2015
- All individuals inside the World Trade Center towers on September 11, 2001, when the first airplane struck
- All persons covered under the New York State Medicaid program as of April 1, 2010
- All babies born alive in Ghana during 2012
- Patients hospitalized in the surgical intensive care unit at Grady Memorial Hospital during August, 2013
- Residents of Dublin, Ireland, on June 16, 1904

In such a scenario, disease occurrence can be thought of in a statistical sense as the outcome of multiple Bernoulli trials, one for each population member. During the time period of interest, each person either becomes a case or does not. As will be discussed in Chapter 3, the proportion of persons initially at risk who become cases during the time period can be assessed directly in a closed population and is one natural measure of disease frequency. This proportion can also be interpreted as an estimate of the probability (or risk) of disease occurrence in an individual chosen at random from that population.

Some examples of closed populations are listed in Table 2.2. In each example, the time period of interest is essentially fixed and applies to all population members, and the population has a stable size and membership throughout that period, without gains or losses. One common situation that favors meeting these requirements is when the period of observation is short, as the first four examples illustrate. In the last example, however, the observation period is long—25 years. Deaths would be sure to occur in such a large population over such a long time. One might argue that people who die are lost from the population after death, and in this sense, the population membership could be viewed as changing over time. However, it is better to think of a closed population as the set of *original members*. Viewed in this way, the last example still satisfies our definition of a closed population because: (1) all members were alive at the beginning of follow-up and thus at risk for dying; (2) no new members could be added after the war ended, since they would have no opportunity to satisfy the population's eligibility criteria; and (3) the vital status of each original population member would be known at the end of the observation period.

Open Populations

Any defined population that does not qualify as *closed* under the above definition is considered *open*. Examples of open populations are shown in Table 2.3. In practice, open populations are more common than closed ones in epidemiologic research, chiefly because of the fairly stringent requirements for a closed population.

Many open populations in epidemiologic studies are defined by residence in a certain geopolitical area, such as a city, county, state, region,

TABLE 2.2. EXAMPLES OF CLOSED POPULATIONS

- Passengers on Air France Flight 447 while airborne
- Participants in a clinical trial in which all study procedures and observations are completed in a single encounter
- Motor-vehicle occupants involved in a police-investigated collision, considered from the moment of impact until police arrive
- Football players competing in a single play during a football game
- Soldiers who fought in and survived the Persian Gulf War, monitored for death from any cause for 25 years after the end of the war

TABLE 2.3. EXAMPLES OF OPEN POPULATIONS

- Residents of Chicago, Illinois, during 2009
- Factory workers employed at a certain automobile assembly plant at any time during a two-year study period
- High-school students in Miami public schools during a certain school year
- Washington State Medicaid program beneficiaries during 2010
- Enrollees in a certain Health Maintenance Organization (HMO) during a specified five-year calendar period

or nation. Population counts and health statistics are often routinely collected for such areas by government agencies. These populations gain new members over time through birth or in-migration; they lose members through death or out-migration.

Other open populations are defined administratively, not geographically. For example, being enrolled in a certain health insurance plan, or being a registered student in a certain school, may be one of the population's main defining characteristics. Often the link between person and organization can change, so that people gain or lose eligibility for membership over time.

Changes over time in eligibility for membership can also occur for other reasons. If the population is limited to persons in a certain age range, then people who were too young to qualify at the start of the study period may become old enough to join the population during the period. Likewise, members who originally met the age requirements may drop out during the study period once they pass the upper age limit.

State-Transition Models and Line Diagrams, Revisited

State-transition models were described earlier in terms of individual people, incorporating states that a person may occupy and changes from one state to another that a person can undergo over time. But state-transition models can also be used to represent disease occurrence in a population if we reinterpret the meaning of the boxes and arrows. Let a box now denote a *compartment* comprising all members of a population who are in a particular state at a certain time. Let an arrow represent the *flow* of people from one compartment to another over time. Right away, two measures of disease frequency in a population suggest themselves:

1. At a certain time, the number of people in the "diseased" compartment
2. Over a certain period of time, the number of people who move from the "susceptible" compartment into the "diseased" compartment

To anticipate Chapter 3, the first of these counts will be called the number of *prevalent* cases and is the numerator of a standard measure called *prevalence*. The second count will be called the number of *incident* cases, the numerator of *incidence*.

Line diagrams can be used to represent disease occurrence in a population by stacking them vertically and aligning them horizontally on a common time scale. Doing so can help clarify the distinction between closed and open populations. Figure 2.10 shows a closed population—perhaps people who ate at a picnic (shown as Time 0). Some developed gastrointestinal symptoms during the next four days. All ten members were at risk initially; nobody was added after Time 0; and all members were followed either until they became a case or until the end of the time period.

In contrast, Figure 2.11 shows an open population—perhaps patients in a certain intensive care unit (ICU), monitored for occurrence of intravascular catheter infection. Here, Time 0 is the start of a certain four-day calendar period, during which patients were admitted to, and discharged from, the ICU. The time line for a particular patient

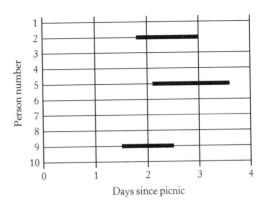

FIGURE 2.10

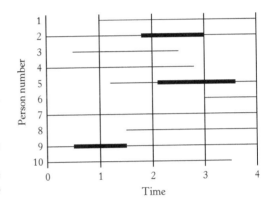

FIGURE 2.11

disappears during periods when he/she was not in that ICU.

In this example, ten different people were part of the ICU population for part or all of the time period of interest, but not all of them were there at Time 0. Some members (e.g., persons 3 and 4) also left the ICU before the end of the time period.

LINKING CASES WITH THE PROPER POPULATION BASE

Having now considered disease cases and populations separately, we should consider how the two fit together. Formal epidemiologic study of a problem typically begins, at least conceptually, by attempting to identify and count *all cases of disease in a defined population*. Often the population of interest is defined first, and then ways are sought to identify all disease cases within it. For example, one might be interested in determining the frequency of leukemia and lymphoma in the state of Iowa during 2010 for comparison with other states. The defined population of "Iowa residents during 2010" would be the starting point. Its size and composition could be estimated from census data. Iowa happens to have had a statewide cancer registry in 2010, which enumerated all new cancer cases in the state. This data source could be used to determine the total number of new leukemia and lymphoma cases among Iowa residents during 2010. For now, we will defer until Chapter 3 how an incidence rate would be calculated from these data.

Sometimes, however, the process is reversed: a set of cases comes to light first and triggers a search for the corresponding defined population.

Example 2-5.   In the mid-1990s, four cases of leukemia or lymphoma occurred among botanical researchers at the Rosenborg Laboratories of the Norwegian University of Science and Technology (Kristensen *et al.*, 2008). Over the next several years, four more such cases occurred among students in biology and chemistry departments that were housed in the same building. Concerns were raised that chemical exposures at the facility had caused these illnesses.

In order to determine whether eight cases of leukemia and lymphoma were more than would be expected, a denominator population was needed. To that end, the university's personnel and academic records were reviewed. A total of 7,189 individuals were identified who had been employees or students at Rosenborg Laboratories between 1976 and 2004. Those records were then matched up with the nationwide Cancer Registry of Norway to identify all leukemia or lymphoma cases among these employees and students during or after their time at Rosenborg. Twelve cases were identified—four more than the original eight. The investigators then calculated how many cases of leukemia and lymphoma would be expected among these Rosenborg Laboratories workers if they had experienced the same incidence rates as observed among all Norwegians of similar age, gender, and calendar year. The expected number was 11.3 cases. The investigation concluded that the overall frequency of leukemia and lymphoma was not much elevated among Rosenborg employees or students after all.

Identifying the proper base population after the fact can be tricky: a defined group of people that is conveniently available and that contains the cases may not necessarily qualify as the true population at risk for those cases. For proper correspondence

between a set of cases and a candidate population at risk, two conditions must hold:

1. If any person who became a case had *not* developed the disease, he or she would still have been included in the candidate population.
2. If any non-case in the candidate population had developed the disease, he or she would have been captured as a case.

Both requirements must be satisfied. They are based on *counterfactual* scenarios—"thought experiments" —in which a person's case/non-case status is hypothetically reversed. If requirement #1 is not met, then some of the cases at hand evidently arose from another, as-yet-unidentified group of people who are not part of the candidate population being considered. The candidate population is thus incomplete as the base for that set of cases. If requirement #2 is not met, then the mechanism for case ascertainment evidently misses some cases that arise in the candidate population. The case group may thus be incomplete.

To illustrate how these rules can be used in practice, consider the following example:

Example 2-6.   Suppose that a group of cardiologists has identified all cases of myocardial infarction who were admitted to a certain hospital during a certain year. You have been asked to help them use these cases as the starting point for an epidemiologic study of myocardial infarction. Your first task is to identify the corresponding population at risk.

First you might consider all patients who are admitted to the study hospital during the same year with any diagnosis. This group qualifies as a defined population—one could construct a list of them and thus specify exactly who is and who is not a member—and the group includes the heart attack cases. However, this population fails requirement #1: it is not necessarily true that each of the heart attack cases would have been admitted to the hospital with some *other* diagnosis during the year if he or she had not suffered a heart attack. Noting this leads you to realize that there are almost certainly other people "out there" who would have become cases at the study hospital if they had suffered a heart attack during the year. Thus, part of the real population at risk has not been captured by considering only hospitalized patients.

The population of all hospitalized patients may also fail requirement #2 if some patients who were hospitalized with other diagnoses would have gone elsewhere if they had had a heart attack. For example, if the hospital specializes in bone-marrow transplants, it may draw referrals from a wide region, even though many of those patients would have been hospitalized closer to home if they had had a heart attack.

You now realize that you must look outside the hospital for the population at risk. Accordingly, you might next consider trying to define a geographic "catchment area" from which the hospital is thought to draw its heart attack patients, then figure out the population of that catchment area. The distribution of hospitalized heart attack cases by place of residence might suggest such an area. To help meet requirement #1, you could exclude any heart attack cases who resided outside the catchment area. In most settings, however, this catchment area population would fail requirement #2. The study hospital may be just one of several local hospitals that treat heart attack patients, and there would be no guarantee that someone who resides in the catchment area would necessarily go to the study hospital if he or she suffered a heart attack. Thus, case ascertainment within the catchment area may be incomplete if only the study hospital's cases are included, and there may be no way to know how many other cases in it were missed unless data can be gathered from all other hospitals.

As this example shows, it is often not possible (unfortunately) to identify the true population at risk that generated the cases drawn from a particular clinical site. This limits the kinds of epidemiologic research that can be done with them. They are a clinical case series, but they do not necessarily represent all cases in a defined population at risk.

Fortunately, however, situations do exist in which a set of clinical cases *can* be linked to its corresponding population at risk. These situations are thus very favorable for epidemiologic research:

- There may be essentially only one source of care for a relatively isolated community. For example, the Mayo Clinic provides nearly all health care for residents of Rochester, Minnesota (Melton, 1996). The Marshfield Clinic does so for residents of Marshfield, Wisconsin (Nordstrom et al., 1994).
- There may be several sources of care, but all of them contribute to a single population-wide case registry. For example, the National Cancer Institute's Surveillance, Epidemiology,

and End Results program supports population-based cancer registries in several regions of the United States. (Hankey *et al.*, 1999).

- All health care for members of a single health insurance plan may be provided by, or billed to, that plan. In the United States, many Health Maintenance Organizations (HMOs) fit this description and have become important settings for epidemiologic research (Nordstrom *et al.*, 1994). Note that HMO enrollees constitute an administratively (not geographically) defined population.
- The research focuses only on the *outcome* of illness among patients at one or more clinical sites. These patients then become a defined population in their own right, and the research issue is complete ascertainment of disease outcomes among them. This kind of research has been called *clinical epidemiology* (Weiss, 2006).

NOTE

1. In fact, Miettinen (1985) has noted: "Given the applicability of the formal aspects of the epidemiologic discipline of research not only to nonmedical states and events in man but to nonhuman objects as well …it would be good to replace the term *epidemiology*—which refers to people—with something less specific, but an appealing suggestion has not yet been made."

REFERENCES

Ahluwalia IB, Mack KA, Mokdad A. Report from the CDC. Changes in selected chronic disease-related risks and health conditions for nonpregnant women 18–44 years old BRFSS. J Womens Health (Larchmt) 2005; 14:382–386.

Al-Abri SS, Beeching NJ, Nye FJ. Traveller's diarrhoea. Lancet Infect Dis 2005; 5:349–360.

Alpert JS, Thygesen K, Antman E, Bassand JP. Myocardial infarction redefined–a consensus document of The Joint European Society of Cardiology/American College of Cardiology Committee for the redefinition of myocardial infarction. J Am Coll Cardiol 2000; 36:959–969.

Anderson RM, May RM. Infectious diseases of humans: dynamics and control. New York: Oxford University Press, 1991.

Andrews NJ, Farrington CP, Cousens SN, Smith PG, Ward H, Knight RS, et al. Incidence of variant Creutzfeldt-Jakob disease in the UK. Lancet 2000; 356:481–482.

Cassels S, Clark SJ, Morris M. Mathematical models for HIV transmission dynamics: tools for social and behavioral science research. J Acquir Immune Defic Syndr 2008; 47 Suppl 1:S34–S39.

Centers for Disease Control and Prevention. Outbreak of Severe Acute Respiratory Syndrome—worldwide, 2003. MMWR Morb Mortal Wkly Rep 2003; 52:226–228.

Centers for Disease Control and Prevention. National Notifiable Diseases Surveillance System. http://wwwn.cdc.gov/nndss, 2013.

Deandrea S, Lucenteforte E, Bravi F, Foschi R, La Vecchia C, Negri E. Risk factors for falls in community-dwelling older people: a systematic review and meta-analysis. Epidemiology 2010; 21: 658–668.

Ellenberg JH, Nelson KB. Sample selection and the natural history of disease. Studies of febrile seizures. JAMA 1980; 243:1337–1340.

Hankey BF, Ries LA, Edward BK. The Surveillance, Epidemiology, and End Results program: a national resource. Cancer Epidemiol Biomarkers Prev 1999; 8:1117–1121.

Jemal A, Ward E, Hao Y, Thun M. Trends in the leading causes of death in the United States, 1970–2002. JAMA 2005; 294:1255–1259.

Kristensen P, Hilt B, Svendsen K, Grimsrud TK. Incidence of lymphohaematopoietic cancer at a university laboratory: a cluster investigation. Eur J Epidemiol 2008; 23:11–15.

Melton LJ. History of the Rochester Epidemiology Project. Mayo Clin Proc 1996; 71:266–274.

Miettinen OS. Theoretical epidemiology: principles of occurrence research in medicine. New York: Wiley, 1985.

New York Times. New York's Tally of Heat Deaths Draws Scrutiny (August 18, 2006). New York Times, P. 1, 2006.

Nordstrom DL, Remington PL, Layde PM. The utility of HMO data for the surveillance of chronic diseases. Am J Public Health 1994; 84: 995–997.

Roger VL, Weston SA, Gerber Y, Killian JM, Dunlay SM, Jaffe AS, et al. Trends in incidence, severity, and outcome of hospitalized myocardial infarction. Circulation 2010; 121:863–869.

Tunstall-Pedoe H, Kuulasmaa K, Amouyel P, Arveiler D, Rajakangas AM, Pajak A. Myocardial infarction and coronary deaths in the World Health Organization MONICA Project. Registration procedures, event rates, and case-fatality rates in 38 populations from 21 countries in four continents. Circulation 1994; 90:583–612.

Tyas SL, Salazar JC, Snowdon DA, Desrosiers MF, Riley KP, Mendiondo MS, et al. Transitions to mild cognitive impairments, dementia, and death: findings from the Nun Study. Am J Epidemiol 2007; 165:1231–1238.

Weiss NS. Clinical epidemiology. The study of the outcome of illness (3rd ed.). New York: Oxford University Press, 2006.

White AD, Folsom AR, Chambless LE, Sharret AR, Yang K, Conwill D, et al. Community surveillance of coronary heart disease in the Atherosclerosis Risk in Communities (ARIC) Study: methods and initial two years' experience. J Clin Epidemiol 1996; 49:223–233.

Wilder RP, Majumdar SR, Klarenbach SW, Jacobs P. Socio-economic status and undiagnosed diabetes. Diabetes Res Clin Pract 2005; 70:26–30.

Zitter JN, Mazonson PD, Miller DP, Hulley SB, Balmes JR. Aircraft cabin air recirculation and symptoms of the common cold. JAMA 2002; 288:483–486.

EXERCISES

1. A study sought to test the hypothesis that the risk of developing an upper respiratory infection (URI or "cold") following an airline flight is greater if the airliner recirculates cabin air rather than using fresh air from outside the plane to ventilate the cabin. The investigators recruited 1,501 passengers who were about to fly from an airport in the San Francisco area to Denver. Each person was classified according to whether his or her aircraft used fresh or recirculated air. Tracking information was also collected so that each person could be contacted again after 5–7 days to determine whether a new URI had developed.

   Which of the following would you consider to be suitable features of a practical case definition for such a study? Why?

   (a) Self-report of a cold
   (b) Self-report of a cold, but with certain specific symptoms required to be present (e.g., self-report of cold with at least symptoms A and B)
   (c) Any of several specific combinations of self-reported cold symptoms (e.g., symptoms A + B + C, or symptoms D + E, or symptoms A + F, etc.)
   (d) Visited a medical professional for symptoms that were diagnosed as a URI
   (e) Observed by a medical professional to have a reddened throat
   (f) Positive throat culture
   (g) Blood test positive for recent exposure to at least one common pathogen known to cause URIs

2. For each of the following diseases, would you consider the disease to be recurrent or non-recurrent? What is the population at risk?

   (a) Acute cholecystitis (inflammation of the gallbladder)

(b) Traveller's diarrhea

(c) Second primary breast cancer (new occurrence of breast cancer in the opposite breast in someone who previously had the disease)

(d) Gestational diabetes (diabetes that occurs during pregnancy)

(e) Workplace homicide

3. Sketch a state/transition diagram for each of the diseases named below. Ignore death for present purposes, except for part (a).

(a) Sudden cardiac death

(b) Headache

(c) Mumps

4. Febrile seizures occur at some time in about 2–4% of all children. While ill with a fever, the child loses consciousness and develops jerking movements, usually in all four limbs, sometimes lasting several minutes. Parents are often frightened to witness the seizure and are concerned about whether their child is likely to have recurrent seizures in later life.

At least 26 studies have followed up a group of such children to determine what proportion develop epilepsy, a chronic seizure disorder. On reviewing these studies, Ellenberg and Nelson (1980) noticed a pattern:

- 7 studies followed up all children who had experienced a febrile seizure in some defined population, such as a prepaid health plan or a geographic area. Estimates of the percentage of children who later developed epilepsy ranged across studies from 1.6% to 4.6%, with a median of 3.0%.

- 19 studies followed up all children with a febrile seizure who had been treated in a certain hospital clinic or by a particular specialist in seizure disorders. The results of these studies were much more variable but generally described a worse prognosis: the percentage of children who later developed epilepsy ranged across studies from 2.6% to 76.9%, with a median of 18.8%.

The definition of epilepsy and the duration and completeness of follow-up appeared to be generally similar across groups of studies. Why do you think the results differed so markedly between the groups of studies?

5. Classify each of the populations described below as *open*, *closed*, or *neither*.

(a) Boeing factory employees working on assembly of the 787 jetliner sometime during calendar 2010 and monitored for workplace injuries on that job.

(b) Your high school graduating class at the time the graduation photo of all of you was taken

(c) Your high school graduating class, tracked for death from any cause from graduation day to the present (assume for present purposes that all such deaths can be ascertained)

(d) All coronary artery bypass surgery patients at University Hospital during a certain three-year period, tracked for occurrence of a fatal or serious nonfatal intraoperative complication during the procedure.

(e) Members of a large prepaid health care plan who first took the drug rosiglitazone while a member during 2006 and who are monitored from then to now through plan's medical records to identify occurrences of heart attack (myocardial infarction)

6. The Department of Veterans Affairs (VA) operates a large network of hospitals and clinics that provide health care to people who have served in the United States military. Veterans have different levels of priority to receive VA care: priority is highest for veterans who were injured or became ill while in military service, for low-income veterans, and for certain other special target groups. Lower-priority veterans may receive VA care on a space-available basis. In 2008, there were an estimated 23.4 million United States veterans, of whom about 5.6 million received VA health care at least once during the year. Surveys have shown that about half of the veterans who receive VA care in a given year also receive health care outside the VA in that year.

Suppose you are interested in studying the degree to which veterans have an unusually high frequency of psychiatric hospitalization. Information on the incidence of psychiatric hospitalization among *non*-veterans is already available to you from other sources. You determine that, in 2008, about 102,000 veterans were hospitalized at least once for psychiatric illness at a VA facility. Can you identify the population at risk—i.e., the appropriate "denominator population"—that corresponds to those 102,000 psychiatric hospitalizations? Explain your answer briefly.

ANSWERS

1. Several features of the research problem influence how an epidemiologist would develop a suitable case definition in this instance:

- For many participants, Denver was the next stop on their journey but not their final destination. The study population was highly dispersed geographically after the study flight, so obtaining biological specimens or physical-examination data would be very difficult.

- URIs are caused by a wide variety of different bacteria and viruses, even though the symptoms and mechanisms of spread are generally similar.
- URIs are common, mild illnesses that are usually managed at home without involving a medical visit.

The investigators who conducted this study (Zitter *et al.*, 2002) hedged their bets by using three separate case definitions:

- Self-report of a cold
- Self-report of a cold with a runny nose
- A score of 14 or greater on a previously published checklist of eight URI symptoms (headache, sneezing, chilliness, sore throat, malaise, nasal discharge, nasal obstruction, cough), with each symptom rated on a 0-to-3 scale of severity.

These case definitions could all be applied to information obtained in a telephone interview with each person. Phone interviews were completed successfully for 73% of the original group. The results showed no significant association between aircraft air recirculation and later development of a URI according to any of the three case definitions.

The investigators probably chose not to use medical visits with a diagnosis of URI because most URIs would not trigger a medical visit by themselves and would thus be missed. Even if the investigators somehow managed to arrange a local medical visit for research purposes, presence of a reddened throat, as observed by a medical professional, would be hard to standardize in such a widely dispersed population. Likewise, throat cultures and blood tests could be logistically difficult to arrange. Moreover, although a positive throat culture could affect treatment, a URI related to the airplane ventilation system could nonetheless be present with or without a positive throat culture. Even if a blood sample could be obtained from everyone, doing blood tests for the many known microorganisms that produce URIs would be costly and would still run the risk of missing the particular agent involved in a certain person's illness.

2. (a) Cholecystitis is potentially recurrent. The population at risk would be anyone who does not currently have cholecystitis *and* who has a gallbladder. Anyone who has previously undergone a cholecystectomy is no longer susceptible.

(b) Traveller's diarrhea can definitely be recurrent. The case definition would probably require having a certain set of symptoms, such as the number and frequency of loose stools. But another feature of the case definition is built right into the name of the condition: a person must be a traveller to have traveller's diarrhea. For example, Al-Abri *et al.* (2005) used the following definition in their review:

> Traveller's diarrhoea is a common problem that may be defined as the passage of three or more unformed stools over 24 hours, with symptoms starting during or shortly after a period of foreign travel.

Hence the population at risk under such a definition would be confined to current or recent foreign travellers, however *those* terms are defined, who do not already have the disease. The same clinical symptoms could occur in a non-traveller and, in fact, could represent the same biological process, but the illness victim still would not meet one requirement of the case definition for traveller's diarrhea. As a consequence of this definition, someone who had not engaged recently in foreign travel would have to be considered not at risk.

(c) Second primary breast cancer is non-recurrent. (Even if some breast tissue were left in place after treatment of a second primary cancer, occurrence of yet another new breast cancer would have to be considered a *third* primary breast cancer, not a second.) The population at risk for second primary breast cancer would consist of people who have previously had one primary breast cancer and who still have some breast tissue. Note that not all such individuals are women.

(d) Gestational diabetes can recur in subsequent pregnancies. The population at risk would consist of pregnant women who do not already have diabetes, either pre-existing or gestational.

(e) Homicide clearly cannot recur in the same person. The population at risk would consist of workers while they are at work. A given individual can move in and out of the population at risk, even during the course of a single day. Hence the population at risk is clearly an open one whose membership can change over time.

3. (a) Clearly, sudden cardiac *death* is non-recurrent (although sudden cardiac *arrest* could recur).

Everyone would be at risk, so there is no third non-susceptible state to consider. A reasonable sketch would be:

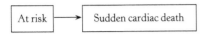

FIGURE 2.12

(b) Headaches can recur. Everyone is at risk except those who already have a headache. A reasonable sketch would therefore be:

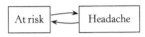

FIGURE 2.13

(c) Mumps can occur in anyone who has not previously had mumps and who has not been vaccinated. Recovery from mumps almost always confers lifelong immunity. People who have not had the mumps can be vaccinated and rendered non-susceptible. In addition, young infants can be non-susceptible by virtue of having antibodies inherited from an immune mother. A reasonable sketch would therefore be:

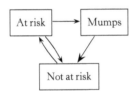

FIGURE 2.14

(Very rare cases of recurrent mumps are ignored here.)

4. A likely explanation is that the cases seen at hospital clinics or in the practices of seizure specialists may not be typical of all febrile seizure cases occurring in a defined population. Often these providers receive referrals of patients who have a relatively severe or difficult-to-manage form of the disease. Less complicated and less severe cases remain under the care of primary-care physicians and are seldom referred.

For example, the risk of epilepsy has been found to be greater in children who have had "atypical" febrile seizures — for example, "focal" seizures starting in one part of the body, or lasting an unusually long time, or occurring repeatedly within 24 hours. These are just the kinds of cases that a primary-care physician might be uncomfortable managing solo. Hence they tend to be over-represented in a clinic-based case series.

5. (a) This would be an open population. Although calendar year 2010 itself was of fixed duration, a worker could be hired or assigned to 787 assembly work any time during 2010 and could be fired or reassigned to another job any time

after starting that job. Thus, the worker population at risk changed members during the period of observation, with different workers on the job for different amounts of time at risk.

(b) The moment when the graduation photograph was taken was a single point in time, so the distinction between an open and a closed population would be irrelevant. The population's membership at a single moment in time is fixed and cannot change. The terms "open" and "closed" apply only to a population that is observed over a period of time.

(c) This would be a closed population. All members of the class were alive on graduation day and thus at risk. No new members can be added to the graduating class after graduation day. If all deaths are ascertained, then nobody is lost to follow-up. The time period from then to now is the same for all members.

(d) This could reasonably be regarded as a closed population. Care must first be taken to identify the appropriate time scale: it is *time since beginning of surgery*, not calendar time. Time 0 for each patient is when his/her surgery begins, and the patient's time at risk ends when his/her surgery finishes. Note that the number of calendar years over which cases were collected for study is irrelevant: each population member would be under observation for intraoperative complications only during the few hours in which he/she is in surgery, not continuously for several years. All patients are at risk at the beginning of surgery, and no population members are gained or lost during surgery.

It is true that surgery may last longer for some patients than for others. However, modest departure from the equal-time-periods assumption could probably be tolerated in this case. For practical purposes, what matters most is the proportion of such operations that involve serious intraoperative complications, regardless of how long the operation lasts.

(e) This would be an open population. Although no new population members could be added after 2006, some could be lost through disenrollment or death.

6. Unfortunately, the desired denominator population is quite elusive. One might initially be tempted to regard the 23.4 million United States veterans as a possible denominator population. But the statistics given indicate that only about 24% of veterans used any VA health care, either because many of the other veterans had low priority for VA care or because they chose to receive their care elsewhere. Hence there

were probably many veterans who were hospitalized for mental illness outside the VA. Because these cases were not captured in VA data, the overall veteran population does not really correspond to the 102,000 VA psychiatric hospitalizations.

One might also consider using the 5.6 million veterans who received some VA health care that year as the denominator population. Yet it is known that many of these veterans also received health care (possibly including psychiatric care) outside the VA, and any such non-VA psychiatric hospitalizations among them would not have been captured. Moreover, some of the veterans who *were* hospitalized for psychiatric illness during the year may have had no other reason for using VA care that year. Thus, they would not necessarily have been among the 5.6 million VA users if they had not had a VA psychiatric hospitalization.

In theory, the population at risk would consist of all veterans who would have been eligible for VA psychiatric hospitalization, and who would have chosen to use VA inpatient psychiatric care, if they developed mental illness requiring inpatient care during the year. Unfortunately, it is very difficult to identify those veterans and to estimate how many of them there are. Accordingly, most statistics about hospitalization frequency in the VA system use simple counts or express admissions for a particular cause as a proportion of all admissions.

3

Disease Frequency: Basic

In your otherwise beautiful poem, there is a verse which reads:

    Every moment dies a man

    Every moment one is born

It must be manifest that, were this true, the population of the world would be at a standstill. In truth the rate of birth is slightly in excess of that of death. I would suggest that in the next edition of your poem, you have it read:

    Every moment dies a man

    Every moment 1–1/16 is born

Strictly speaking this is not correct. The actual figure is a decimal so long that I cannot get it on the line, but I believe 1–1/16 will be sufficiently accurate for poetry. I am, etc.

—CHARLES BABBAGE, *inventor of the first programmable computer, in a letter to poet Alfred, Lord Tennyson*

Quantitative measures of disease frequency in a population are some of the most basic tools of epidemiology, and any epidemiologist needs to be skilled in their use. One aspect of skill is being able to choose the right tool for a job. This chapter provides an overview of the most commonly used measures of disease frequency, including what kind of question each measure answers, what kind of information it requires as input, and examples of its use. Finer details are omitted for now in an attempt to convey the "big picture."

Another aspect of skill is knowing your tools well. Chapter 4 discusses in more depth several of the measures introduced in this chapter, including some of their statistical properties and useful relationships among them.

ORIENTATION

In broad terms, most measures of disease frequency answer one of two kinds of questions. First, how common is a given disease *as of a certain time?* For example:

- Suppose that a newly published study shows that surgical bypass of atherosclerotic lesions in the carotid arteries is effective for preventing stroke. The medical director of a health insurance plan wants to know: How many of our enrollees currently have carotid atherosclerosis that would make them candidates for this surgery?

- Suppose that an international medical aid organization seeks to reduce chronic parasitic infection among children in villages in a less-developed country. They ask: What proportion of children are currently infected? In which villages is the proportion especially high?

These kinds of questions are answered by measures of disease *prevalence*, which quantifies the frequency of disease *as of a certain time*. Prevalence is a static measure: time is "frozen." Anyone who qualifies as being in the diseased state at the specified time is counted as a case. In the two examples above, the time point of interest is the present, but prevalence can also be applied to time on any of several time scales, including calendar time, age, or time after some salient event.

Second, how frequently do new cases of disease arise in a population as time passes? For example:

- Suppose that a health insurance plan has decided to fund a self-care program, designed to train people with newly diagnosed diabetes about how to monitor their glucose level and adjust their diet and insulin dosage. The plan's medical director asks: How many new cases of diabetes would be expected over the next year?
- Suppose that a few cases of connective-tissue disease have been reported in women with silicone breast implants. Affected women and their doctors may ask: Is connective-tissue disease any more likely to develop over time among women with such implants than among women without them?

These kinds of questions are best answered by measures of disease *incidence*, which concerns how often disease events occur *over a period of time*. Incidence is a dynamic measure, always involving the passage of time. The disease event of interest may be an instantaneous occurrence, such as death, or it may be the onset of a more persistent disease state, such as onset of diabetes. Sometimes only the frequency of fatal cases is of interest (or is the only information available). If so, measures of *mortality*—really a subtype of incidence that considers only fatal cases—are used.

In terms of the state/transition disease models considered in Chapter 2, prevalence concerns how a population of interest is distributed among the compartments (e.g., Figure 2.4) at some point in time: in particular, the number of people or the proportion of the population in the diseased state at that time. Incidence concerns the rate of flow along the arrow from the susceptible compartment to the diseased compartment. Each time someone changes from the susceptible state to the diseased state, a new disease event or *incident case* occurs.

Regardless of whether the need calls for prevalence or incidence, sometimes just counting the number of disease cases is sufficient. For example, the health plan medical director mentioned above simply needed to know the number of existing cases of carotid atherosclerosis, or the number of new cases of diabetes to expect over some time period.

But in many other situations, comparisons of disease frequency need to be made between populations of different sizes and/or that are observed over different periods of time. Case counts alone would not account for these differences. Instead, more valid comparisons require measures that relate the number of cases to the size of the population at risk and (for incidence) the amount of time over which they are observed. Most such measures take the form of a fraction: the numerator is the number of cases, and the denominator is the "base" for that number of cases. For prevalence, the denominator is simply the size of the population. For incidence, the denominator quantifies in some way the amount of at-risk experience that generated those cases. Depending on the type of incidence measure, the denominator can be either the number of people initially at risk, or the total amount of person-time at risk experienced by population members during the time period of interest.

Sometimes information needed for the desired denominator—such as the size of the true population at risk—is unobtainable. Instead, a proxy denominator may be available that is better than no denominator at all, particularly if it is safe to assume that the proxy denominator will be approximately proportional to the true one.

All of the measures described below can be applied either to a full population or to each of several subpopulations within it—e.g., to each of several age groups, or to males and females separately. Doing so permits comparisons of disease frequency among those subpopulations, even if they have different sizes. Whenever a subpopulation-specific measure is computed, both its numerator and its denominator (if there is one) are restricted to members of that subpopulation. In other words, each subpopulation is treated as a mini-population in its own right.

PREVALENCE

The *count of prevalent cases* of a disease is the number of people who are in the diseased state at a specified time. *Prevalence* is a proportion, obtained by dividing the count of prevalent cases by the population size at that time:

$$\text{Prevalence} = \frac{\text{Number of prevalent cases}}{\text{Size of population}}$$

Prevalence can be visualized in terms of line diagrams. On an appropriate time scale, the point in time at which prevalence is assessed determines the horizontal position of a vertical line that cuts across the time lines for all population members. In Figure 3.1, two of five people are in the diseased state at that time, so the prevalence would be $2/5 = 40\%$.

Example 3-1. Concerned about infections acquired in health care settings, the Veterans Health Administration commissioned a study of the prevalence of nursing home–acquired infections in its 133 nursing homes (Tsan *et al.*, 2008). On November 9, 2005, personnel at all such VA facilities reviewed the medical records of all 11,475 residents on that day to determine each resident's infection status, according to a standardized case definition. A total of 591 residents qualified as having at least one nursing home–acquired infection on that day, for an overall prevalence of 591/11,475 = 5.2%. The three most common types of infection were symptomatic urinary tract infection (181 cases, 1.6%), asymptomatic bacteriuria (79 cases, 0.7%), and pneumonia (60 cases, 0.5%). All of these prevalence estimates pertained to a single calendar day: November 9, 2005—in effect, a point in calendar time.

Prevalence involves "stopping the clock" and assessing disease frequency at a point in time. However, the point in time need not necessarily be a point in calendar time. It can can refer instead to a point on another relevant time scale, as illustrated in the following example:

Example 3-2. In 1944, the cities of Newburgh and Kingston, New York, took part in a study of the effects of water fluoridation for prevention of tooth decay in children (Ast and Schlesinger, 1956). Initially, the water in both cities had low fluoride concentration. In 1945, Newburgh began adding fluoride to its water to increase the fluoride concentration tenfold, while Kingston left its water supply unchanged. At baseline, the frequency of dental caries among children in both cities appeared to be similar. To assess the effect of water fluoridation, a dental health survey was conducted among all schoolchildren in certain grades in both cities during the 1954–1955 school year. One measure of dental decay in children aged 6–9 years was whether at least

one of a child's deciduous cuspids or first or second deciduous molars was missing or had clinical or X-ray evidence of caries. Of the 216 first-graders examined in Kingston, 192 had decay by this definition, compared with 116 of the 184 first-graders examined in Newburgh.

Overall, there were 192 *prevalent cases* of dental decay among first-graders in Kingston at the time of the study and 116 in Newburgh. These counts themselves could be useful to local health officials for estimating the number of dental personnel and other resources needed to provide restorative dental care for children in each city. However, a fair comparison of the frequency of dental decay in the two cities would need to account for differences in the number of children examined. Prevalence serves this purpose. The *prevalence* of dental decay was 192/216 = 89% in Kingston and 116/184 = 63% in Newburgh.

Figure 3.2 diagrams the data collection process in, say, Newburgh for the dental-decay example. A total of 184 first-graders were examined, each corresponding to a row in the figure, arranged here in chronological order by examination date. The dental-decay status of each child was known only at his or her survey examination, shown as a small "window" through which we glimpse a tiny portion of the child's dental-disease time line. As in Chapter 2, that line is thick if the child was a case at the time, and thin if not. Given the brevity of the examination in relation to the pace at which dental decay develops, in effect each child's disease status was assessed at a point in time. The rest of his or her time line was unobserved, as implied by dots to the left and right of the window.

The figure shows that these examinations were not all done simultaneously—which would have required 184 examination teams—or even on the same day. Instead, they were distributed over several months during the school year as the examiners worked their way through different schools and grades. The point in time to which the prevalence refers is thus not a point in calendar time. Nor is it a point on the age time scale: the first-graders were examined at various ages, albeit within a fairly narrow range. Rather, the point in time is the *time of examination* for each child. The key feature is the fact that each child's disease status was observed only as of one point in that child's lifetime, not monitored over a period of time. The calendar time period and age range over which the examinations

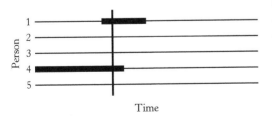

Time

FIGURE 3.1

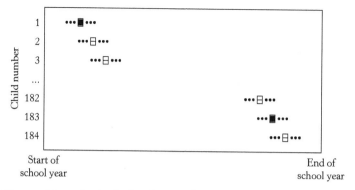

FIGURE 3.2 Diagram of data collection for dental survey of Newburgh, NY, first-graders.

were done are relevant as descriptors, along with place and other population-defining characteristics, to put the prevalence estimate in its proper context. Prevalence can be compared across time periods or age groups, just as can other disease frequency measures.

The format in which prevalence is expressed can be chosen for convenience to avoid an awkward number of leading or trailing zeros, or for ease of comparison with other published estimates. For example, the prevalence of dental decay among Newburgh first-graders could be expressed as 63%, as 0.63, as 630 per 1000, as 6,300 per 10,000, etc.

INCIDENCE

Incidence concerns how frequently people who are at risk for disease become disease cases during a defined period of observation. Incidence is based on disease events, each representing a transition from being at risk to being diseased.

An *incident case* occurs when an individual changes from being susceptible to being diseased, by the study's case definition. The *count of incident cases* is the number of such events that occur in a defined population during a specified time period. Recurrent disease events in the same person may or may not qualify as incident cases, depending on the study's purpose and case definition.

A simple count of incident cases can sometimes be sufficient to quantify the extent of a problem or to guide health planning. For example, knowing the number of lower-extremity amputations per year in a certain health plan could be used to project the number of limb prostheses likely to be needed. Comparing the counts of incident cases across different diseases can also reflect patterns of relative incidence

if the diseases in question share essentially the same population at risk.

Example 3-3. In 2010, 1,307,893 new cases of genital *Chlamydia trachomatis* infection were reported to the United States Centers for Disease Control and Prevention, compared with 309,341 new cases of gonorrhea (Centers for Disease Control and Prevention, 2011). Assuming similar completeness of reporting for both diseases, these counts by themselves would support a conclusion that the incidence of genital *C. trachomatis* infection was about 4.2 times as high as the incidence of gonorrhea. This is because the sizes of the populations at risk for each disease would be the same (or nearly so, after subtracting prevalent cases).

Counts may also be adequate for comparing incidence among populations that can safely be assumed to be of similar size.

Example 3-4. Over a two-year period, Gruska *et al.* (2005) identified all episodes of out-of-hospital cardiac arrest in greater Vienna, Austria, through the Municipal Ambulance Service, which handles almost all calls for emergency medical assistance in the city. The 1,498 arrest episodes were distributed among the days of the week as shown in Figure 3.3. Significantly more cardiac arrests occurred on a Monday than on any other day of the week.

Although no attempt was made to quantify the size of the Viennese population at risk that generated these cases, it is probably safe to assume that the size of population at risk was approximately constant among days of the week. Thus, even without

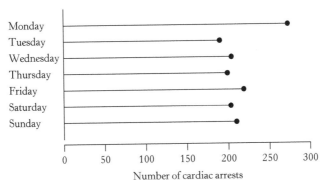

FIGURE 3.3 Occurrence of out-of-hospital cardiac arrests by day of the week: Vienna, Austria, 1995–1996. (Based on data from Gruska *et al.,* 2005)

a denominator, it is very likely that the day-to-day variation in case counts alone reflects true variation in incidence, highest on Mondays.

Very often, however, one needs to compare the frequency of new disease occurrence between populations of different sizes, or over time periods of different durations. Then a simple count of incident cases is inadequate; a denominator is needed. Two main approaches to quantifying incidence are used in such situations: *cumulative incidence* and *incidence rate*. The approach used is driven chiefly by whether the defined population is closed or open.

Cumulative Incidence

Cumulative incidence is the proportion of initially susceptible individuals in a closed population who become incident cases during a specified time period.

$$\text{Cumulative incidence} = \frac{\text{Number of incident cases}}{\substack{\text{Number of persons} \\ \text{initially at risk}}}$$

Cumulative incidence is also sometimes called *incidence proportion* or *attack rate*. It is the simplest measure of incidence that accounts explicitly for the size of the population at risk.

Example 3-5. A jumbo jet full of tourists bound from Tokyo to Copenhagen stopped at Anchorage, Alaska, for refueling and reprovisioning. Upon reaching cruising altitude again, the crew served breakfast. Somewhere over the polar ice cap, an illness characterized by cramps, vomiting, and diarrhea swept through the plane, and by the time they reached Copenhagen, 196/344 = 57% of passengers had become ill. Epidemiologists who investigated the outbreak used interview data and food service records to calculate the cumulative incidence of illness among those who did and those who did not eat various food items. Eating ham proved to be strongly associated with becoming ill. Among those who ate ham that had been prepared by a particular cook, 86% got sick, compared with none of those who ate ham prepared by a different cook. Microbiological tests found heavy staphylococcal contamination of the suspected ham, which was eventually found to have resulted from improper food handling by one of the cooks (Eisenberg *et al.,* 1975).

Figure 2.10 in Chapter 2 illustrates how cumulative incidence relates to line diagrams. It shows the occurrence of gastrointestinal illness in a closed population of picnic attendees. Cumulative incidence can be calculated at any of various time points after the picnic (time 0). Initially, ten people were at risk, which determines the denominator. The one-, two-, three-, and four-day cumulative incidences would be 0/10, 2/10, 3/10, and 3/10, respectively.

Two key features of cumulative incidence are related to the fact that it is a *proportion*. First, cumulative incidence can be measured directly only in a closed population: the population cannot gain or lose members during the period of follow-up, except for losses that occur after the person has already become a case. Otherwise, the case count in the numerator would not correspond to the defined population at risk in the denominator. For example, if a new member were to join the population partway through follow-up and then become a case, he or she would be added to the numerator, even though he or she had not been counted as a member of the denominator population at risk. (Chapter 4 describes how

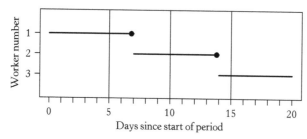

FIGURE 3.4 Two injuries among three workers.

cumulative incidence can sometimes be estimated indirectly, under certain assumptions, when some of the original population members are lost to follow-up during the study period.)

Second, each person who becomes a case is counted only once in the numerator, even if he/she has more than one disease episode during the period of interest. Without this rule, at the extreme, the numerator could conceivably exceed the denominator, yielding a ratio that would clearly not be interpretable as a proportion.

Ideally, the time period to which cumulative incidence refers should be constant for all members of the study population. For example, the proportion of patients undergoing a surgical procedure who develop deep venous thrombosis during the two weeks after surgery could be termed the "two-week cumulative incidence" of that complication. Nonetheless, cumulative incidence is sometimes calculated when the time period is not strictly constant among individuals. For example, the cumulative incidence of death before discharge among hospitalized patients is sometimes used as a measure of disease severity or outcome. Because of differences in length of hospital stay, the amount of time at risk for death actually varies somewhat among patients.

Incidence Rate

The need for a another kind of incidence measure is motivated by the following hypothetical example.

Example 3-6. Suppose that a sawmill recently installed a fast new saw that greatly improves the rate at which logs can be turned into finished lumber. Unfortunately, from time to time, the blade catches on a flaw in a log and expels wood back toward the operator, sometimes causing injury.

During the first 20 days of machine use, three workers operate the machine. Worker #1 runs it for 7 days until injured on Day 7. Worker #2 runs it for

the next 7 days until injured on Day 14. Worker #3 runs it without injury through Day 20. Figure 3.4 shows this information graphically.

In response to workers' concern, the sly sawmill owner makes no changes to the machine but alters employee assignments. For the next 20 workdays, a different worker operates the new saw each day. Injuries occur on days 7 and 14, as shown in Figure 3.5. But at the end of this period, the sawmill owner claims a big reduction in the incidence of injury, from $2/3 = 67\%$ to $2/20 = 10\%$.

The sawmill owner's comparison is clearly not a fair one, because the amount of *time at risk* for injury per worker is much less during the second period than during the first. Another measure of incidence—the *incidence rate*—can account for this difference.

The *incidence rate* is the count of incident cases divided by the aggregate amount of at-risk experience from which they arose. Its denominator is usually measured in units of *person-time at risk*.

$$\text{Incidence rate} = \frac{\text{Number of incident cases}}{\text{Amount of at-risk experience}}$$

Recurrent disease events in the same person may or may not be counted in the numerator, depending on the study's purpose and case definition, as discussed in Chapter 2.

The incidence rate also goes by several other names, including *incidence density*, *person-time incidence rate*, or sometimes simply *incidence*. The idea behind it is straightforward. Other things being equal, the number of new cases of disease in a population should be proportional to (1) the size of the population at risk and (2) the amount of time over which susceptible individuals are observed for occurrence of new cases. The denominator of the incidence rate combines these two factors. The number of cases in

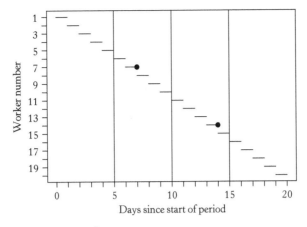

FIGURE 3.5 Two injuries among 20 workers.

the numerator is a unitless count, while the denominator is expressed in time units. Hence the incidence rate has units of $(\text{time unit})^{-1}$, such as years^{-1} or days^{-1}.

Example 3-7. Gardner *et al.* (1999) studied on-the-job back sprains and strains among 31,076 material handlers employed by a large retail merchandise chain. Payroll data for the 21-month study period were linked with job injury claims, which provided data on the timing of each injury, body part injured, and mechanism of injury. A total of 767 qualifying back injuries occurred during 54,845,247 work hours, yielding an incidence rate of 1.40 back injuries per 100,000 worker-hours. Higher incidence was found among males and among employees whose work was more physically demanding.

The work force in this example was an open population. Thousands of workers joined or left the company during the study period. Only on-the-job back injuries were of interest, so each worker's at-risk experience consisted of many discontinuous time periods at work, separated by periods away from work. These features of the situation made an incidence-rate approach to measuring disease frequency attractive and a good match to the available data.

Incidence rates can be used in a wide range of epidemiologic research situations. They can be applied to both closed and open populations, with or without detailed information on time at risk for each individual population member, and for both recurrent or non-recurrent disease events—circumstances in

which cumulative incidence may be impossible to apply.

Estimating the Incidence Rate with Detailed Data on Individual Times at Risk

In some research situations, detailed information can be obtained on the amount of time at risk for each individual population member and the timing of each disease event. In the back-injury example above, payroll records provided each worker's time on the job right down to the hour, and injury claims provided the number and timing of back injuries. The numerator was the total number of qualifying back injuries, and the denominator was the sum of hours worked across all workers.

As noted earlier, recurrent disease events in the same person may or may not qualify for inclusion, depending on the study's purpose. Whether recurrent cases count or not clearly can affect the numerator. Less obviously, it also can also affect the denominator. Consider the line diagram on the left side of Figure 3.6. In this example, horizontal lines indicate the timespan over which each of five population members is observed, and black dots indicate when cases occur. The table at right in the figure shows the contribution of each person to the numerator and denominator of the incidence rate, depending on whether recurrent cases in the same individual do or do not qualify for inclusion.

Contributions to the numerator differ only for person #5, whose second disease event would count under one case definition but not the other. But also note that if only initial cases count, then any person-time after the occurrence of a person's first disease event is not added to the denominator. This

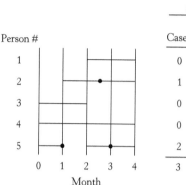

| | | If recurrences do count | | If recurrences do not count | |
Person #		Cases	Person-months	Cases	Person-months
1		0	2	0	2
2		1	3	1	1.5
3		0	2	0	2
4		0	4	0	4
5		2	3	1	1
		3	14	2	10.5

FIGURE 3.6 Calculation of number of cases and person-time, depending on whether recurrent cases do or do not count.

is because any recurrent disease event during that time would not be counted as a case, and therefore that person-time is not time at risk for a qualifying disease event. This rule affects the person-time contribution of any person who has an initial disease event. If the disease is rare, such that only a very small proportion of individuals have disease events, the effect of the difference on total person-time may be small. But for more common diseases, it can be too large to ignore.

Estimating the Incidence Rate Without Detailed Data on Individual Times at Risk

Often detailed information about each population member's time at risk is unknown and not feasibly obtainable. This problem often arises, for example, when the defined population of interest consists of residents of a geographic area over some time period. The number of incident cases may be readily available, but the larger challenge is to estimate the total amount of person-time at risk from which those cases arose.

Two approaches to estimating total person-time at risk can be explained and justified algebraically. Again, a line-diagram example helps in visualizing how they work. Consider a simple example in which detailed information about each person's time at risk actually *is* available. Figure 3.7 shows a small open population of eight people who are at risk over different time intervals during a certain ten-day period. To simplify the arithmetic, we require that on any given day, each person is at risk for the entire day or for none of it, so the number of days at risk for a person can take on only integer values. (In principle,

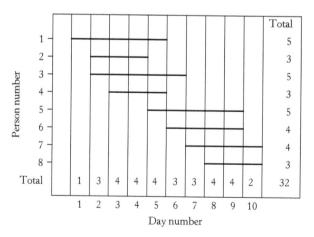

FIGURE 3.7 Line diagram showing two approaches to calculating total person-time.

time could be divided into arbitrarily small intervals to sidestep this restriction without changing the method.)

Total person-time at risk—here, 32 person-days—can be calculated either of two ways. First, each individual's contribution of time at risk can be determined, then these values can be summed across all individuals. This method corresponds to the column of numbers at the right. Second, the number of individuals at risk on each day can be determined, then these values can be summed across all days. This method corresponds to the row of numbers at the bottom.

More formally, let $x_{ij} = 1$ if person i is at risk on day j, or 0 otherwise. Let N be the total number of individuals who contribute any person-time (here, $N = 8$); let D be the duration of the study time period (here, $D = 10$ days); and let T be total person-time at risk (here, $T = 32$ person-days). Then:

$$T = \sum_i \sum_j (x_{ij}) = \sum_j \sum_i (x_{ij})$$

which are the two approaches just described for calculating T.

Now define:

$\bar{d}$ = average time at risk per person

  $= T/N$

$\bar{n}$ = average number of people at risk per day

  $= T/D$

In the example, $\bar{d} = 32/8 = 4$ days at risk per person, and $\bar{n} = 32/10 = 3.2$ persons at risk per day. These definitions can be rearranged to give two expressions for T:

$$T = N \cdot \bar{d} \qquad (3.1)$$

$$T = D \cdot \bar{n} \qquad (3.2)$$

Equations (3.1) and (3.2) lead to two strategies for estimating T without detailed information on each person:

1. N may be known exactly and $\bar{d}$ approximately. For example, a published paper may report that 120 people were monitored for deep vein thrombosis for an average of 2.8 years, and that 6 cases were detected. Even without knowing exactly how long each study participant was followed, the incidence

rate of deep vein thrombosis can be estimated as $\frac{6}{120 \times 2.8 \text{ years}} = 0.018 = 1.8$ cases per 100 person-years.

2. D may be known exactly and $\bar{n}$ approximately. For example, suppose that 12 new cases of West Nile virus infection are identified during a given year in a certain state, and that the state's population at mid-year is known from census data to be about 2.4 million people. Technically, 2.4 million may not be the exact average of the state's population during that year, but it is probably a pretty good approximation. The incidence rate of West Nile virus infection can then be estimated as $\frac{12}{2,400,000 \times 1 \text{ year}} = 5$ cases per million person-years.

Sometimes more than a single mid-period estimate of the size of the population at risk may be available, permitting a more refined estimate of total person-time based on method 2. For example, suppose that estimates of the size of the population at risk are available for the beginning and end of a period, but not at any intermediate time points, as shown graphically in Figure 3.8. Total person-time corresponds to the area of the shaded trapezoid, which would be $\frac{1000 + 800}{2} \times 2$ person-years. The first factor can be seen to be the average population at risk during the time period, assuming a linear decline over time.

This method of approximation can be extended to make use of multiple population-size estimates over time, possibly at irregular time intervals. In Figure 3.9, total person-time at risk would be approximated as the summed area of the five trapezoids:

$$T = \left[\frac{N_0 + N_1}{2} \times (t_1 - t_0) \right]$$
$$+ \left[\frac{N_1 + N_2}{2} \times (t_2 - t_1) \right] + \cdots$$
$$+ \left[\frac{N_4 + N_5}{2} \times (t_5 - t_4) \right]$$

For some diseases, the prevalence of disease may be high enough, or a separate not-at-risk state common enough, that the discrepancy between total population size and size of the true population at risk is too large to ignore. Corrections may then need to be based on the estimated prevalence of disease or the estimated proportion of the population that is not at risk. For example, the estimated incidence of dementia in the elderly has been found to increase considerably when prevalent cases of dementia are subtracted from the denominator

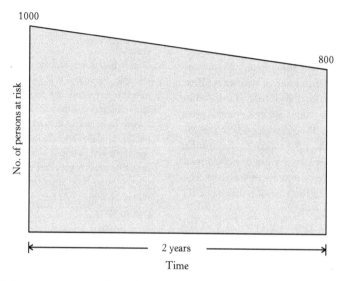

FIGURE 3.8 Estimating person-time when only start-of-period and end-of-period estimates of population at risk are available.

(Rocca *et al.*, 1998). For uterine cancer, higher and almost certainly more accurate incidence estimates have been obtained when the estimated number of women who no longer have a uterus (due to prior hysterectomy) were subtracted from the denominator (Marrett, 1980).

Denominators Other Than Person-Time

In some areas of epidemiologic research, including study of injuries, denominators other than person-time are often used to quantify the amount of at-risk experience from which a set of incident cases arose.

For example, the incidence of motor-vehicle collision injuries can be expressed as injuries per 100,000 person-years, as injuries per 100,000 licensed-driver-years, or as injuries per million vehicle-miles traveled. The extent to which older adults are a high-risk group for motor-vehicle collision injuries has been shown to depend on which denominator is used (Massie *et al.*, 1995). At the time of the study, a smaller percentage of older adults than of younger adults had a valid driver's license. Moreover, population surveys showed that even those older adults who did have a driver's licence drove fewer miles per year than did

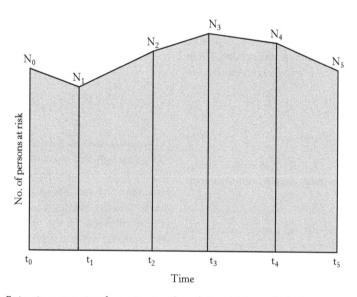

FIGURE 3.9 Estimating person-time from estimates of population at risk at multiple time points.

TABLE 3.1. COMPARISON OF CUMULATIVE INCIDENCE AND INCIDENCE RATE

Characteristic	Cumulative incidence	Incidence rate
Units	None	$(\text{Time unit})^{-1}$
Range	0–1	0–infinity
Directly calculable by:	Observing a closed population over time	Observing a closed or open population over time with detailed data on individual times at risk
Indirectly calculable by:	Survival-analysis methods in presence of censoring[a]	Estimating total person-time as (average size of population at risk) × (duration of observation period)
Individual-level counterpart	Risk (probability)	Hazard rate[a]

[a] Discussed in Chapter 4

younger drivers. Hence the increase in incidence by age was more marked when the denominator was vehicle-miles traveled.

Comparison of Cumulative Incidence and Incidence Rate

The differences between cumulative incidence and the incidence rate are both conceptual and statistical. These distinctions were appreciated by early epidemiologists and health statisticians (Vandenbroucke, 1985). Table 3.1 summarizes and contrasts several properties of these two measures of incidence. Despite the differences, the generic term *incidence* is widely applied to both cumulative incidence and incidence rate throughout the medical literature. The specific kind of incidence being discussed must often be inferred from the context.

Chapter 4 describes how confidence limits for incidence rates can be obtained; how cumulative incidence and the incidence rate are related mathematically; how, under certain assumptions, one can be computed from the other; and how incidence rates in a population have a counterpart (the hazard rate) at the individual level.

Variants of Incidence

Incidence can actually be regarded as a family of disease-frequency measures. Some members of this family traditionally go by names of their own, but on closer examination they can be seen to be just special types of incidence.

Mortality

Mortality is the incidence of fatal cases of a disease in the population at risk for dying of the disease. The denominator includes both prevalent cases of the disease as well as persons who are at risk for developing the disease. Subtypes are *cumulative mortality* and *mortality rate*. *Death rate* and *mortality density* are essentially synonyms for the mortality rate.

Example 3-8. Over the 5-year period from 2002–2006, some 258,205 deaths due to traumatic brain injury were recorded in the United States (Faul *et al.*, 2010). Essentially the entire United States population was considered to be at non-zero risk for dying of traumatic brain injury, although the level of risk clearly varied greatly from person to person. Hence the denominator for the mortality rate was (estimated average size of the United States population during 2002–2006) × (length of observation period) = 293,235,577 × 5 years. The mortality rate for traumatic brain injury during that period was thus $258,205/(293,235,577 \times 5 \text{ person-years}) = 17.6$ deaths per 100,000 person-years.

Case Fatality

Case fatality refers to the incidence of death from a disease *among persons who develop the disease.* Case fatality reflects the prognosis of the disease among cases, while mortality reflects the burden of deaths from the disease in the population as a whole.

In principle, *cumulative fatality* and *fatality rate* could be defined as special types of cumulative incidence and incidence rate, respectively, with appropriate restrictions on who counts toward the numerator and denominator. In practice, these terms are rarely used, although the underlying theory would still apply. Instead, *case fatality* is most commonly used:

$$\text{Case fatality} = \frac{\text{Number of fatal cases}}{\text{Total number of cases}}$$

Case fatality can be viewed as the cumulative incidence of death due to the disease among those who develop it. A fixed time period after disease onset may or may not be explicitly specified and must often be inferred from the context. As a variant of cumulative incidence, case fatality is most readily applied for diseases of relatively short duration, in which there are few losses to follow-up or deaths from other causes.

Example 3-9.   The National Highway Traffic Safety Administration (2010) reported that 4,092 deaths occurred in the United States during 2009 when a pedestrian was struck and killed by a motor vehicle. They estimate that 59,000 pedestrians were injured in pedestrian/motor-vehicle collisions during that year. Based on these data, the case fatality of pedestrian/motor-vehicle collision injury in 2009 was 4,092/59,000 = 6.9%.

Proxy Measures of Incidence

Sometimes good denominator data for the desired measure of incidence cannot feasibly be obtained. Yet case counts alone are likely to be inadequate for comparing incidence between populations that differ in size or other key characteristics. Under those circumstances, a proxy denominator may be better than none at all.

Proportional Mortality

The *proportional mortality* for a disease is:

$$\text{Proportional mortality} = \frac{\text{Deaths from the disease}}{\text{Deaths from all causes}}$$

As its name implies, it is simply the proportion of all deaths that are due to a particular cause in a specified population and time period of interest. This proportion can provide useful descriptive information in its own right: for example, the statement that heart disease accounted for 25% of all deaths among Americans in 2007 refers to proportional mortality (National Center for Health Statistics, 2011).

For purposes of comparing disease frequency between populations, the main advantage of proportional mortality is that its denominator—total number of deaths—can usually be ascertained from the same source that furnishes its numerator. The count

of all deaths serves as a proxy for person-time at risk under the assumption that, other things being equal, one would expect total deaths to vary in proportion to population size and duration of the monitoring period.

A potential limitation of comparing proportional mortality between populations or subpopulations can be illustrated by an example:

Example 3-10.   Berkel and de Waard (1983) studied mortality among Seventh-Day Adventists (SDA) in the Netherlands over a ten-year period. Members of that church are prohibited from using tobacco or alcoholic beverages and are encouraged to follow a vegetarian diet. Hence the investigators expected a reduced death rate among SDA from cancer (particularly lung cancer, which is strongly related to smoking) and heart disease.

The results are summarized in Table 3.2. Among deaths in SDA for which a cause of death could be ascertained, 2.5% were due to lung cancer and 47.1% to cardiovascular disease. Those percentages were found to be quite similar to the corresponding proportional-mortality percentages for the Netherlands population of similar age and gender, suggesting little or no health benefit for SDA.

But in this instance, the investigators also had detailed year-by-year data on the size of the SDA population, from which they could determine person-time at risk contributed by SDA during the study period by age and gender. They obtained the age- and gender-specific mortality rates for the Netherlands as a whole from published sources. By applying these published mortality rates to the SDA person-time data, they estimated how many deaths would have been expected among SDA if this group had experienced the mortality rates observed among all Netherlands residents of similar age and gender. The rightmost two columns of Table 3.2 shows these results, which lead to quite a different conclusion. The observed numbers of lung cancer and cardiovascular disease deaths in SDA were in fact sharply lower than the number of such deaths expected based on mortality rates for the general population. But deaths from *other* causes were also substantially lower than expected among SDA. Hence the *proportions* of SDA deaths from lung cancer and heart disease differed very little from those in the Netherlands as a whole. Results from the proportional-mortality analysis alone would have been misleading in this instance because total number of deaths was a poor proxy for person-time at risk.

TABLE 3.2. PROPORTIONAL MORTALITY AND MORTALITY RATE ANALYSES OF DEATHS AMONG DUTCH SEVENTH-DAY ADVENTISTS (SDA)

| | Proportional mortality[a] | | Number of deaths in SDA | |
Cause of death	SDA	Netherlands	Observed	Expected from Netherlands mortality rates
Lung cancer	2.5%	2.5%	12	26.7
Other cancer	21.4%	18.9%	103	203.9
Cardiovascular disease	47.1%	50.8%	227	547.4
Other known cause	29.0%	27.7%	140	298.6
Unknown	–	–	40	–
All causes	100.0%	100.0%	522	1,076.6

[a] As percent of deaths with known cause
(Based on data from Berkel and de Waard [1983])

Proportional Incidence

Proportional incidence is based on the same basic idea, but ignoring whether cases are fatal or not. For example, hospital admissions for diabetes may be expressed as a proportion of all hospital admissions if no good data are available on the size of the true population at risk for hospitalization. Similarly, incident cases of colon cancer may be expressed as a proportion of all incident cancer cases. Note that the denominator of proportional incidence may be less obvious than for proportional mortality. But in general, the *proportional incidence* of disease X, say, can be defined as:

$$\text{Proportional incidence of X} = \frac{\text{Incident cases of X}}{\text{Incident cases in a larger disease category that contains X}}$$

The same potential pitfall applies. The comparisons mentioned above could be misleading if the overall hospitalization rate or the overall cancer incidence rate were to differ between populations being compared. Contrasts based on proxy measures must therefore be cautiously interpreted.

Fetal Death Ratio

In perinatal epidemiology, the frequency of fetal death in a certain population over a specified time period is often expressed as:

$$\text{Fetal death ratio} = \frac{\text{Number of fetal deaths}}{\text{Number of live births}}$$

The denominator for a cumulative-incidence measure of fetal death would be the total number of pregnancies. But some pregnant women may undergo spontaneous or elective abortions that can be difficult to ascertain and to count. Hence the number of live births is used as a proxy for the total number of pregnancies.

In contrast to proportional mortality, the fetal death ratio and other analogues that do not include the numerator as part of the denominator are not proportions and thus require different data analysis methods.

PERIOD PREVALENCE

Earlier, prevalence was described as reflecting the frequency of the diseased state at a specified point in time. Hence the term *point prevalence* is sometimes used to emphasize this feature (Porta, 2008). In contrast, *period prevalence* is really a hybrid of prevalence and cumulative incidence. Like cumulative incidence, it refers to a period of time rather than a point in time. However, cases counted in its numerator include both (1) prevalent cases that already exist at the beginning of the observation period, and (2) new cases that occur during the period. Referring to Figure 3.10, persons #1, #3, #4, and #5 would

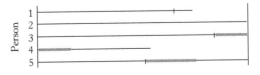

FIGURE 3.10 Diagram of period prevalence.

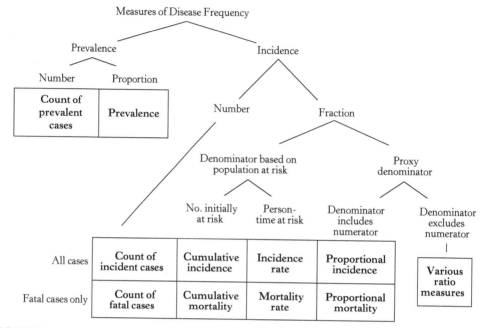

FIGURE 3.11 Overview of measures of disease frequency.

all count as cases. The denominator includes both (1) persons at risk when the period starts, as well as (2) extant cases when the period starts. For Figure 3.10, the period prevalence would thus be 4/5 = 0.8.

Period prevalence is essentially uninterpretable except in a closed population, for the same reasons that apply to cumulative incidence. For a closed population, if P = point prevalence when the observation period starts and CI = cumulative incidence among individuals at risk at that time, then period prevalence can be seen to be:

$$\text{Period prevalence} = P + (1 - P) \cdot CI \qquad (3.3)$$

For Figure 3.10, this would be $1/5 + (1 - 1/5) \times 3/4 = 0.8$.

The main limitation of period prevalence is that point prevalence and cumulative incidence convey very different kinds of information about disease frequency. The distinction is lost when they are combined in this way, which limits the usefulness of period prevalence as a summary measure. When possible, point prevalence and cumulative incidence are generally better kept separate as two more interpretable components.

Nonetheless, sometimes this separation cannot be made from the data available, and "period prevalence" may be an accurate descriptive term for a

frequency measure that *can* be calculated. For example, the United States Centers for Disease Control (1998) reported that 25.3 per 1,000 United States women who delivered a liveborn infant during 1993–1995 had diabetes during the pregnancy, according to data on the baby's birth certificate. Some of these mothers had diabetes before becoming pregnant, while others developed diabetes during pregnancy. In any event, all reportedly had diabetes sometime during the period of pregnancy, so 25.3/1,000 is probably best regarded as a period prevalence. A subsequent revision of the birth certificate in most states allowed distinguishing between pre-existing diabetes and diabetes with onset during pregnancy (gestational diabetes) (Osterman *et al.*, 2009).

RECAP

Figure 3.11 shows a classification scheme for most of the measures covered in this chapter and some of the key distinctions among them.

REFERENCES

Ast DB, Schlesinger ER. The conclusion of a ten-year study of water fluoridation. Am J Public Health 1956; 46:265–271.

Babbage C. Letter to Alfred, Lord Tennyson. Quoted in: Newman JR (ed.). The world of mathematics. Volume 3, p. 1487. New York: Simon and Schuster, 1956.

Berkel J, de Waard F. Mortality pattern and life expectancy of Seventh-Day Adventists in the Netherlands. Int J Epidemiol 1983; 12: 455–459.

Centers for Disease Control and Prevention. Diabetes during pregnancy—United States, 1993–1995. MMWR 1998; 47:408–414.

Centers for Disease Control and Prevention. Sexually Transmitted Disease Surveillance 2010. Atlanta, GA: U.S. Department of Health and Human Services, 2011.

Eisenberg MS, Gaarslev K, Brown W, Horwitz M, Hill D. Staphylococcal food poisoning aboard a commercial aircraft. Lancet 1975; 2:595–599.

Faul M, Xu L, Wald MM, Coronado VG. Traumatic brain injury in the United States: emergency department visits, hospitalizations and deaths 2002–2006. Atlanta, GA: Centers for Disease Control and Prevention, National Center for Injury Prevention and Control, 2010.

Gardner LI, Landsittel DP, Nelson NA. Risk factors for back injury in 31,076 retail merchandise store workers. Am J Epidemiol 1999; 150: 825–833.

Gruska M, Gaul GB, Winkler M, Levnaic S, Reiter C, Voracek M, et al. Increased occurrence of out-of-hospital cardiac arrest on Mondays in a community-based study. Chronobiol Int 2005; 22:107–120.

Guskiewicz KM, McCrea M, Marshall SW, Cantu RC, Randolph C, Barr W, et al. Cumulative effects associated with recurrent concussion in collegiate football players: the NCAA Concussion Study. JAMA 2003; 290:2549–2555.

Landon MB, Spong CY, Thom E, Hauth JC, Bloom SL, Varner MW, et al. Risk of uterine rupture with a trial of labor in women with multiple and single prior cesarean delivery. Obstet Gynecol 2006; 108:12–20.

Lavados PM, Sacks C, Prina L, Escobar A, Tossi C, Araya F, et al. Incidence, 30-day case-fatality rate, and prognosis of stroke in Iquique, Chile: a 2-year community-based prospective study (PISCIS project). Lancet 2005; 365:2206–2215.

Marrett LD. Estimates of the true population at risk of uterine disease and an application to incidence data for cancer of the uterine corpus in Connecticut. Am J Epidemiol 1980; 111:373–378.

Massie DL, Campbell KL, Williams AF. Traffic accident involvement rates by driver age and gender. Accid Anal Prev 1995; 27:73–87.

National Center for Health Statistics. Health, United States, 2010 with special feature on death and dying. Hyattsville, MD: National Center for Health Statistics, 2011.

National Highway Traffic Safety Administration. Traffic Safety Facts: 2009 data. Washington, D.C.: U.S. Department of Transportation, 2010.

Osterman MJK, Martin JA, Menacker F. Expanded health data from the new birth certificate, 2006. National Vital Statistics Reports, Vol. 58, No. 5. Hyattsville, MD: National Center for Health Statistics, 2009.

Porta M (ed.) A dictionary of epidemiology (5th edition). New York: Oxford, 2008.

Rocca WA, Cha RH, Waring SC, Kokmen E. Incidence of dementia and Alzheimer's disease. A reanalysis of data from Rochester, Minnesota, 1975–1984. Am J Epidemiol 1998; 148:51–62.

Sloan JH, Kellermann AL, Reay DT, Ferris JA, Koepsell T, Rivara FP, et al. Handgun regulations, crime, assaults, and homicide. A tale of two cities. N Engl J Med 1988; 319:1256–1262.

Tsan L, Davis C, Langberg R, Hojlo C, Pierce J, Miller M, et al. Prevalence of nursing home-associated infections in the Department of Veterans Affairs nursing home care units. Am J Infect Control 2008; 36:173–179.

Vandenbroucke JP. On the rediscovery of a distinction. Am J Epidemiol 1985; 121:627–628.

Van Landingham MJ. Murder rates in New Orleans, LA, 2004–2006. Am J Public Health 2007; 97:1614–1616.

EXERCISES

1. A study of time trends in the frequency of HIV infection is being planned in a small African country. Due to the high cost of testing a truly random sample of the population, the study will involve testing sentinel groups that can be accessed at low cost. Inmates in federal prisons have been chosen as a captive population.

   Over the last few years, the incarcerated population has averaged 1,200 persons. The study team plans to obtain a serum sample from each incoming prisoner over a 2-year period. It is estimated that 800 new prisoners will be incarcerated during the study period. Suppose that 40 of the serum samples test positive for HIV, and that all 800 incoming prisoners are different individuals (i.e., none are repeat offenders). Which of the following will the investigators be able to calculate from the study data? For each that can be calculated, do so using the hypothetical results, and name the defined population to which it applies.

   (a) Incidence rate of HIV infection

(b) Cumulative incidence of HIV infection
(c) Prevalence of HIV infection

2. A large study by Landon *et al.* (2006) sought to determine the risk of uterine rupture during labor among women attempting to deliver a baby vaginally, in relation to the number of previous deliveries each had had by Cesarean section (C-section). Among 16,915 women with a single prior C-section, 115 experienced uterine rupture during the attempt to deliver vaginally. By comparison, 9 uterine ruptures occurred among 975 women who had had two or more C-sections before trying to deliver vaginally.

(a) What kind of disease-frequency measure would be appropriate here to express the frequency of uterine rupture in each group of mothers?
(b) Was the risk of uterine rupture higher or lower among women who had had multiple prior C-sections, compared to women with one prior C-section?

3. If a hen and a half lay an egg and a half in a day and a half, how many eggs would one hen lay in three days?

4. Iquique, Chile, is a coastal city of about 200,000 people with a predominantly Hispanic-Mestizo population. An epidemiologic study (Lavados *et al.*, 2005) sought to estimate the incidence of first strokes in Iquique for comparison with rates observed in other settings.

During a 2-year period from July 1, 2000, to June 30, 2002, all patients who were admitted with their first-ever stroke at any hospital in the city were identified and counted.

(a) The breakdown of these first-ever stroke cases by age was:

TABLE 3.3.

Age group	No. of patients	Percent
0–24	8	2.7
25–34	4	1.4
35–44	14	4.8
45–54	43	14.7
55–64	73	25.0
65–74	64	21.9
75–84	66	22.6
85+	20	6.8
Total	292	100.0

Do these results indicate that the risk of experiencing a first stroke in that setting was greatest among persons 55–64 years of age? Explain briefly.

(b) A published report from the project states:

> In 2000, the population of [Iquique] was 181,984 according to the projections of the 1992 national census, and in 2002, it was 214,526 according to the 2002 national census. … We calculated incidence rates using the sum of the two populations as the denominator—i.e., the projected population in Iquique in 2000, according to the 1992 national census projections, plus the actual population of 2002, according to the 2002 national census.

The two population estimates were summed for each age group, yielding the following totals:

TABLE 3.4.

Age group	2000 + 2002 population
0–24	179,054
25–34	66,462
35–44	62,300
45–54	43,174
55–64	23,682
65–74	13,838
75–84	6,366
85+	1,836
Total	396,712

We will ignore the slight discrepancy between this total and the sum 181,984 + 214,526 = 396,510 from the previous paragraph. Note, however, that either number is roughly twice the population size of Iquique.

The investigators described these totals as the "number at risk" in each age group. They then calculated the incidence of first stroke in each age group by dividing the number of cases in that age group (from the first table) by the corresponding "number at risk" (from the second table).

In principle, a better approach to quantifying incidence in this open population would be to calculate an incidence rate for each age group as (no. of cases)/(person-years at risk). Assume for present purposes that essentially the entire population was at risk for a first stroke. From the data given, can you calculate the appropriate age-specific incidence rates? If so, do so; if not, why not?

(c) The investigators reported that the overall incidence of first-ever strokes was 292/396,712 = 73.6 per 100,000. In the same study, the investigators also identified 68 persons with recurrent strokes and reported that the incidence of recurrent stroke was 68/396,712 = 17.1 per 100,000.

   i. Does this imply that, in this setting, once a person had a first stroke, the risk of having another one was actually lower than the risk of having the initial one? Why or why not?

   ii. Suppose that a community survey in Iquique showed that 5% of its population had a past history of stroke. How could this information be used to obtain better estimates of the overall incidence of first strokes and of recurrent strokes? (Hint: what is the population at risk for each type of event?)

5. During 2004, there were 264 recorded murders in New Orleans, Louisiana, for a homicide rate of 57.1 per 100,000 person-years—about four times the national rate. The number of murders in New Orleans fell to 210 during 2005. However, Hurricane Katrina struck on August 29, 2005, and the city was virtually depopulated for several weeks before some former residents began to return.

   The best available estimates of the city's population during 2005 come from Census Bureau estimates before Katrina hit and from the New Orleans Emergency Operations Center and the Louisiana Recovery Authority afterward. An approximate summary is:

   (a) From January 1–August 28, the city's population size was fairly stable at an estimated 462,269 persons (the 2004 mid-year population estimate).

   (b) From August 29–September 30, New Orleans had been almost completely evacuated.

   (c) During October, people returned steadily, and by the end of the month, about 71,000 residents had come back.

   (d) During November and December, the influx of returnees was more gradual. By the end of 2005, the estimated population of the city was 91,000.

   Estimate the homicide rate for New Orleans during 2005, and compare it to the homicide rate for the previous year.

6. Vancouver, British Columbia and Seattle are geographically near each other and are quite similar with regard to population size and several measures of socioeconomic status. For the period 1980–1986, the following data were obtained from the respective police departments concerning homicides, according to weapon used.

TABLE 3.5. PERCENTAGE OF HOMICIDES COMMITTED USING EACH WEAPON TYPE

Type of weapon	Seattle	Vancouver
Firearm	42.5%	14.3%
Knife	27.4%	50.0%
Other	30.1%	35.7%
	100.0%	100.0%

A newspaper reporter is sitting beside you when these data are shown at a press conference. He voices his conclusion that a Seattle resident may be more likely than a Vancouver resident to be shot to death by someone else, but that Seattleites can at least take comfort in knowing that they are less likely to be stabbed to death or killed by other weapons than are Vancouver residents. Do you agree? Why or why not?

7. CDC estimates that about 300,000 sports-related concussions occur each year in the United States. A study of concussion among collegiate football players involved surveillance for concussion among 4,251 player-seasons (Guskiewicz *et al.*, 2003). (A single player monitored for a full football season contributed one player-season.) Overall, 184 players experienced at least one concussion, and 12 players experienced a repeat concussion within the same season.

   Assume for present purposes that all of the study data were collected during a single playing season. From these results, can you determine whether the incidence of repeat concussion is greater than the incidence of a first concussion? Explain your answer briefly.

8. Atrial fibrillation (AF) is a heart rhythm abnormality that can be either chronic or "paroxysmal" (occurring in repeated episodes). AF increases the risk of stroke, but the excess risk can be significantly reduced by taking anticoagulants.

   To estimate the prevalence of AF among older adults in a certain region of England, 4,843 persons were sampled at random from a list of all persons aged 65 years or older who were registered with a National Health Service primary care physician. Of the 3,678 who participated and had an electrocardiogram, 207 were found to have AF.

   To check for participation bias, medical records were also reviewed for a sample of participants and for a sample of nonparticipants. A diagnosis of AF was found somewhere in the medical record for 139/1,413 in the participant sample and for 40/382 in nonparticipants.

(a) Based on these results, what is your best estimate of the prevalence of AF among older adults in the region?

(b) Do the results from medical records review for a subsample of participants and nonparticipants suggest that persons with AF were any more or less likely to be surveyed?

(c) Why do you think the percentage of patients with AF in the medical records substudy was so much higher than the percentage found to have AF in the survey?

ANSWERS

1. Only (c) can be calculated, and it is 40/800 = 5%. It is the prevalence of HIV infection among incoming prisoners at the time of entry into prison.

   The length of the study period and the size of the total prison population are not really relevant here. The prevalence figure given above tells us nothing about HIV infection among inmates who were already in prison, since none were tested. Although the tests are to be performed over a 2-year period, each incoming inmate being tested is observed only once, not over a period of time after being determined to be at risk, as would be required for any measure of incidence. Hence the appropriate time scale is not calendar time, but time since prison entry, and we observe all study subjects at time 0 on this scale.

2. (a) Cumulative incidence would be a natural choice. The issue is how frequently women experience a change in state from having an intact uterus to having a ruptured uterus during the time period of labor. The study population was a closed one—no women would join the study in mid-labor, and few if any would be lost to follow-up for such a short-term outcome. The duration of labor may differ among women, but what matters most clinically is whether the uterus ruptures during childbirth, not the rupture rate per minute or the timing of rupture. Cumulative incidence has the nice feature of being readily interpretable as an estimate of the probability of rupture for a randomly chosen woman from the group on which cumulative incidence was calculated.

   (b) The cumulative incidence of uterine rupture was higher among those with two or more previous C-sections: $9/975 = .0092 = 9.2$ per 1,000 women at risk, versus $115/16,915 = .0068 = 6.8$ per 1,000 women. Incidentally, however, the observed difference could easily have occurred by chance in the absence of any true difference: $p = 0.49$ by chi-square test (with continuity correction).

3. This familiar riddle is actually an incidence rate problem. The number of eggs laid should be proportional to the number of hens and to the amount of time spent waiting for eggs. The "incidence rate" of egg-laying is 1.5 eggs/(1.5 hens $\times$ 1.5 days) = 2/3 eggs/hen-day. One hen on the job for three days amounts to 3 hen-days, so we would expect $3 \times 2/3 = 2$ eggs.

4. (a) No, these are just case counts ("numerator data") and do not take into account the size of the population at risk in each age group. The small number of cases among adults age 85+ years, for example, might simply result from there being relatively few people that old in Iquique.

   (b) Although the investigators described the 2000 + 2002 population totals as "numbers at risk" and described them as numbers of *people*, in this case these numbers can more properly be interpreted as *person-years* at risk. To see this, consider the following diagram for a single age group:

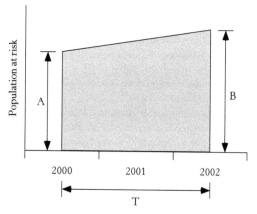

FIGURE 3.12

   The investigators calculated their denominator as $A + B$. The desired denominator, in person-years, would be the area of the shaded trapezoid, which is $\frac{(A+B)}{2} \times T$. But in this case, T = 2 years, the duration of the study. Hence $\frac{(A+B)}{2} \times 2 = A + B$, so the two approaches yield the same numerical values, albeit with different units and interpretations.

   We now have the necessary numerator and denominator data and can divide them to obtain the desired age-specific incidence rates (Table 3.6).

   Note that the incidence of first strokes actually increased steadily with age, in contrast to the percentages in the first table, which were based simply on case counts.

   (c) i. No. The problem is that the total population of Iquique was used as the denominator for both incidence rates. This treated everyone

TABLE 3.6.

Age (years)	No. of cases	Person-years at risk	Incidence rate[a]
0–24	8	179,054	4.5
25–34	4	66,462	6.0
35–44	14	62,300	22.5
45–54	43	43,174	99.6
55–64	73	23,682	308.3
65–74	64	13,838	462.5
75–84	66	6,366	1,036.8
85+	20	1,836	1,089.3

[a] Cases per 100,000 person-years

in the city as being at risk both for a first stroke and for a recurrent stroke. In fact, only persons who had no history of a previous stroke would be at risk for a *first* stroke, and only those who previously had at least one stroke would be at risk for a *recurrent* stroke.

The discrepancy between the total population and the true population at risk may not have been very great for first strokes—a large majority of Iquique residents probably had never had a stroke and thus were indeed at risk for a first one. But the discrepancy would have been much larger for recurrent strokes. This problem makes the reported incidence of recurrent stroke largely uninterpretable in terms of risk.

ii. The population at risk for a *first* stroke is people who have never had a stroke. The survey indicates that 95% of the city's population falls into that category. A corrected estimate of the incidence of first strokes would then be $292/(0.95 \times 396,712) = 77.5$ cases per 100,000 person-years.

The population at risk for a *recurrent* stroke is people who have previously had a stroke. The survey indicates that 5% of the city's population falls into that category. A corrected estimate of the incidence of recurrent strokes would then be $68/(0.05 \times 396,712) = 342.8$ per 100,000 person-years. Although the survey results are hypothetical, these calculations show that it is quite possible, given the data presented, for the risk of having another stroke to be sharply elevated among those who have already had at least one.

5. Figure 3.13 shows the changing size of the New Orleans population during 2005:
The total number of person-years at risk corresponds graphically to the combined areas of the rectangle, triangle, and trapezoid in the figure. This quantity can be calculated as shown in Table 3.7.

The homicide rate for 2005 was thus $210/320,290 = 65.6$ homicides per 100,000 person-years—about 15% higher than the rate in 2004, despite the smaller number of murders in 2005.

This problem was based on a paper by Van Landingham (2007), which used a slightly different method to estimate person-years at risk during the last three months of 2005 but reached a similar conclusion.

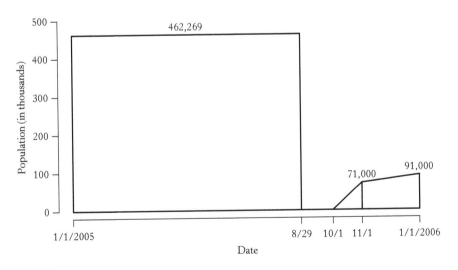

FIGURE 3.13

TABLE 3.7.

Period	Duration (years) (A)	Average population (B)	Person-years (A × B)
Jan 1 – Aug 28	240/365.25	462,269	303,750
Aug 29 – Sep 30	33/365.25	0	0
Oct 1 – Oct 31	31/365.25	$\frac{0+71,000}{2} = 35,500$	3,013
Nov 1 – Dec 31	61/365.25	$\frac{71,000+91,000}{2} = 81,000$	13,528
TOTAL	365/365.25		320,290

6. The table concerns only proportional-mortality data on the distribution of homicides by weapon type. It does not show whether the actual incidence (mortality) of homicides, overall or of any type, is higher in one city than in the other.

Here are the actual homicide incidence rates from the two cities during those years:

TABLE 3.8.

Type of weapon	Homicide rate[a] Seattle	Vancouver
Firearm	4.8	1.0
Knife	3.1	3.5
Other	3.4	2.5
All types	11.3	7.0

[a] Homicides per 100,000 person-years
(Based on data from Sloan et al. (1988))

The overall incidence of homicide was higher in Seattle, and the difference in rates for firearms accounted for most of the excess. The incidence of homicide carried out with knives was slightly higher in Vancouver, but the incidence of murder involving other weapons was actually higher in Seattle than in Vancouver (Sloan et al., 1988).

7. We wish to compare two incidence rates, one for *first* concussions and the other for *repeat* concussions during the same season. Identifying the two numerators is straightforward: there were 184 players with a first concussion, and 12 with a repeat concussion.

Obtaining denominators for these rates is more challenging. The only players at risk for a first concussion are those who have had no concussions so far during the season. The only players at risk for a repeat concussion are those who have already had a concussion during the season. Those are the only two possibilities, so all player-time must accrue toward one

denominator or the other. In other words, the denominators of the two rates of interest must add up to 4,251 player-seasons. Say that the number of player-seasons at risk for repeat concussion is x; then the number of player-seasons at risk for first concussion must be $4,251 - x$.

Calculating x would be easy in principle if we had detailed data about how much playing time each athlete with a first concussion accrued during the rest of that season. However, even without such detailed information, we can set bounds on x. As noted above, the only athletes who contributed any player-time toward x were the 184 with a first concussion. At one extreme, if all 184 athletes had their first concussion at the very beginning of the season, and all continued to play for the rest of the season, they would accrue a maximum of 184 player-seasons at risk for a repeat concussion. At the other extreme, if all 184 athletes had their first concussion very near the end of the season, they would accrue very little time at risk for a repeat concussion. The lower bound for x is 0.

Now suppose that $x = 184$ player-seasons, its maximum possible value. Then the incidence rate of first concussions would be $184/(4,251 - 184) = 4.5$ first concussions per 100 player-seasons at risk. The incidence rate of repeat concussions would be $12/184 = 6.5$ repeat concussions per 100 player-seasons at risk. At any smaller value of x, the first rate would decrease while the second would increase. Thus we can safely conclude that the incidence of repeat concussions must have exceeded the incidence of first concussions.

8. (a) Prevalence = $207/3,678 = 0.056$
   (b) AF was found for $139/1,413 = 9.8\%$ of participants and $40/382 = 10.5\%$ of nonparticipants, suggesting little participation bias.
   (c) The kind of prevalence measured in the community survey was *point prevalence* as of the

time the electrocardiogram was taken for each participant. The kind of prevalence measured in the medical record review is better considered *period prevalence*. It referred not to the proportion of patients who had AF at a particular point in time, but over the period of time during which patients had received care from the clinic whose medical record was reviewed.

4

Disease Frequency: Advanced

Chapter 3 introduced several widely used measures of disease frequency in populations. This chapter takes a closer look at several of these measures, focusing on their interpretation and statistical properties and relationships among them.

People enter the study of epidemiology with varying amounts of prior statistical training. This chapter assumes knowledge of algebra and introductory biostatistics, including statistical notation and a few probability distributions (binomial, Poisson, normal, χ^2, and F). Readers without that background may find parts of this chapter challenging but are encouraged to try to follow the basic reasoning and conclusions without getting bogged down in mathematical details. Readers with more statistical experience should find connections between new terminology and familiar concepts.

POPULATION DISEASE FREQUENCY AND INDIVIDUAL DISEASE RISK

Many common measures of disease frequency can be viewed in two ways: (1) as a measure of disease burden in a population, and (2) as an estimate of disease probability or risk for an individual. Epidemiologists are used to moving freely between these two perspectives. The same quantity may be referred to sometimes as the *cumulative incidence* of disease and sometimes as the *risk* of developing the disease.

Example 4-1. Gestational diabetes mellitus (GDM) is a form of carbohydrate intolerance involving abnormally high blood glucose levels that develops anew during pregnancy. Women with GDM are more likely to have complications in late pregnancy and delivery, and metabolic abnormalities are more common in their newborns.

From March 2004, through December 2007, some 635,785 women in Florida without pre-existing diabetes gave birth to a singleton baby (i.e., not twins, triplets, etc.). Among these mothers, 30,419 (4.78%) developed GDM during the pregnancy, by a standard case definition (Kim *et al.*, 2012).[1]

The number 4.78% in this example can be interpreted in two ways. First, it can be viewed as the frequency[2] of GDM in a certain population at a certain place during a certain time period. It quantifies an aspect of the health burden of GDM in a defined population of Florida women. Public health workers can compare it with the frequency of GDM in other states, track changes over time to determine if the problem in Florida is getting better or worse (possibly in response to prevention efforts), compare the frequency of GDM with that of other pregnancy complications in Florida women, and so on. All of these public health issues focus on the frequency of GDM in the population as a whole.

Second, the number 4.78% can be interpreted as the *probability* or *risk* that a woman in this study population would develop GDM during her pregnancy. From this perspective, the population is viewed as a collection of individuals with certain characteristics in common—in other words, as a set of replicate observations. This view provides a basis for inductive inference: predictions about the likely fate of one person can be based on the observed experience of others. Estimates of individual risk can be important for clinical care, for personal decisions about health behavior, and for insurance, among other purposes.

Estimating disease risk in an individual from disease frequency in a population involves dealing with some special challenges, however, both theoretical and practical. The train of logic involved is described here, using the GDM study as context.

To begin, if the aim is to estimate disease risk for an individual, whom do we have in mind? Strictly speaking, the probabilistic interpretation mentioned above applies most directly to an individual selected at random *from the population actually studied.* But an estimate of disease risk is not usually needed for those specific people, whose disease status is already known. Far more often, an estimate of disease risk is needed instead for a target individual, real or hypothetical, from *outside* the study population.

In order to extrapolate results from a study population to a target individual outside it, we need to think of both the study population and the target individual as samples from a larger *superpopulation*. Figure 4.1 shows a conceptual diagram. The superpopulation must necessarily have broader criteria for membership than the study population, because the superpopulation includes the target individual as well. It will hence be larger in size than the study population, possibly much larger. Its exact size and composition may be unknown, and disease frequency in the full superpopulation is not directly observed.

The concept of a larger universe from which a study sample has been drawn is a familiar idea in statistics and is the basis for confidence limits and statistical significance testing. Here, disease frequency in the study population serves to provide an estimate of disease frequency in a larger superpopulation. However, the study population is rarely a truly random sample of the superpopulation, which raises the possibility of a biased estimate. Confidence limits around the estimate do not account for any such bias, but they can nonetheless be useful as a guide to the

amount of random error due to sampling that affects the estimate, which in turn depends on the size of the sample. Methods for obtaining confidence limits for a measure of disease frequency are covered later in this chapter.

Example 4-2. It is June of 2012. A clinician in Tampa, Florida, has just begun caring for a 34-year-old pregnant Asian woman, a married college graduate. She has two previous children and no personal or family history of diabetes. She is overweight, with a pre-pregnancy weight of 215 pounds and height of 5 feet 6 inches, corresponding to a body mass index (BMI) of 35.8 kg/m^2. Ultrasonography indicates a single fetus. The baby is expected to be born in December of 2012. The clinician would like to estimate this woman's risk of GDM, in order to help decide how closely to monitor her metabolic status and to provide cautionary advice or reassurance.

An estimate of the woman's risk of GDM can come from results of the Florida GDM study mentioned earlier, under certain assumptions. The woman in question meets most of the study's eligibility criteria. However, the Florida GDM study ended in 2007, and the clinician's patient is expected to have her baby in 2012. Hence a superpopulation that includes both must cover a longer time period. A reasonable choice would be all Florida mothers at risk for GDM and delivering a singleton baby from March 2004 through December 2012. If GDM frequency during the study years can be assumed to remain stable through 2012, then the Florida study findings should provide a valid estimate of GDM frequency in the superpopulation. Among study women, the cumulative incidence of GDM was 4.78%, which is a point estimate of GDM frequency in the superpopulation. Because the estimate was based on over 635,000 mothers, 95% confidence limits for true GDM frequency in the superpopulation are very narrow, from 4.73% to 4.84%, indicating a high level of precision.

Second, if we are willing to assume that this particular woman was, in effect, selected at random from the superpopulation, then her estimated risk of GDM would be the estimated proportion of women in the superpopulation who developed GDM, or 4.78%.

The two assumptions mentioned in this example merit further comment. Each corresponds to an arrow in Figure 4.1. First, an assumption was required that the Florida GDM study population was

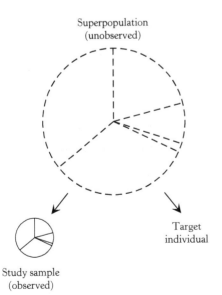

FIGURE 4.1 Study population and target individual as samples from a hypothetical superpopulation.

representative of the superpopulation from which our target woman's risk estimate would be derived. How well this assumption holds depends on how similar the criteria for membership are between the study population and the superpopulation to which results are being extrapolated. In this case, the clinician's patient already met most criteria for membership in the Florida GDM study population, so only a modest expansion of the criteria for membership was needed to form a superpopulation that would include her. A key issue is whether the frequency of GDM in pregnancies from 2004–2007 would still apply in 2012. No direct evidence was available, but other indirect evidence might enable an informed judgment. In principle, within the Florida study data, GDM frequency could be tracked year by year to see if it was rising, falling, or stable during the study years. Rising or falling GDM frequency would call into question whether the study results could be extrapolated to 2012. (No such information was provided in the published study.) In addition, information about GDM frequency from 2004 through 2012 might also be available from other settings, such as other nearby states or the United States as a whole. Seeing no important time trends elsewhere could favor an assumption that GDM frequency was stable over time in Florida as well.

The second assumption in Example 4-2 was that the clinician's patient had, in effect, been selected at random from the superpopulation. If nothing else were known about her beyond meeting criteria for the superpopulation, or if none of the known information about her were related to GDM frequency, then 4.78% would indeed be the best available estimate of her risk of GDM.

But of course more *is* known about her. Moreover, evidence from the Florida GDM study showed that the study population was heterogeneous and that GDM was not equally common among different subgroups. As suggested by the "pie slices" in Figure 4.1, each subgroup in the Florida GDM study population has a corresponding subgroup in the superpopulation. By our earlier logic, GDM frequency in a subgroup of the Florida GDM study population provides an estimate of GDM frequency in the corresponding subgroup of the superpopulation. Rather than using estimated GDM frequency in the entire superpopulation as an estimate of the target woman's GDM risk, a more individualized estimate could come from using GDM frequency in a subgroup that matches her particular characteristics.

How do we identify such a subgroup? Ideally, it would consist of a large number of people who resemble the target woman in every respect. Unfortunately, that goal is unattainable, as it is impossible to match on everything. Epidemiologic analysis can take us partway, however, by helping to identify characteristics that matter and providing an estimate of risk for a combination of a few such characteristics that match our target individual.

In the case of GDM, besides reporting on the frequency of GDM overall, the Florida study examined it in relation to several characteristics of mothers as recorded on Florida birth certificates. Two of the most important ones proved to be the race/ethnicity of the mother and her pre-pregnancy body-mass index (BMI). Figure 4.2 shows how GDM frequency varied among race/ethnicity groups and, for Asian/Pacific Islander mothers, how it varied by mother's BMI.

Among all study mothers, the cumulative incidence of GDM was 4.78%. The 95% confidence interval for this estimate, and for others in the figure, are shown at right in the figure. They specify a numerical range within which GDM frequency would be likely to fall in the superpopulation if the study population were a random sample of it. For all women, the 95% confidence interval is from 4.73% to 4.84%—so narrow that the vertical lines marking the two ends of the interval fall nearly on top of each other. Among Asian/Pacific Islander mothers, GDM frequency was 9.98%, roughly twice as high as for all other mothers. Among Asian/Pacific Islander mothers with pre-pregnancy BMI between 35.0 and 39.9, GDM frequency was 20.1% (95% confidence interval: 14.2% – 27.2%). Clearly, the clinician's patient is at well-above-average risk for GDM. But note how the width of the confidence interval around this risk estimate is fairly wide, because it is based on a much smaller group of study mothers.

As discussed later in this book, other statistical approaches are available for estimating individual risk as a function of multiple risk factors besides the recursive-partitioning approach used above. To some extent, they help circumvent the limitation of small subgroup size as more individual characteristics are taken into account, but at the price of requiring stronger assumptions about how multiple factors jointly affect risk.

Sometimes results from more than one epidemiologic study are available to serve as the source for individual risk estimates. Because of the uncertainties involved in extrapolating from a study

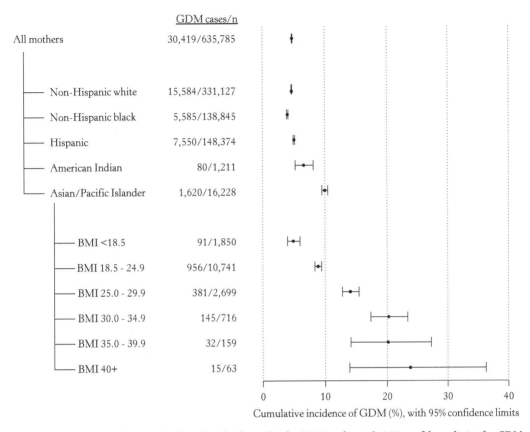

GDM cases/n

	GDM cases/n
All mothers	30,419/635,785
Non-Hispanic white	15,584/331,127
Non-Hispanic black	5,585/138,845
Hispanic	7,550/148,374
American Indian	80/1,211
Asian/Pacific Islander	1,620/16,228
BMI <18.5	91/1,850
BMI 18.5 - 24.9	956/10,741
BMI 25.0 - 29.9	381/2,699
BMI 30.0 - 34.9	145/716
BMI 35.0 - 39.9	32/159
BMI 40+	15/63

Cumulative incidence of GDM (%), with 95% confidence limits

FIGURE 4.2 Tree diagram of selected results from Florida GDM study, with 95% confidence limits for GDM frequency in each group.

population to an individual outside it, the estimates may disagree, as in the following example.

Example 4-3. The American Heart Association has recommended that anyone with a 10% or greater chance of developing coronary heart disease (CHD) in the next ten years should consider taking low-dose aspirin for prevention (Pearson *et al.*, 2002). As an advocate of evidence-based medicine, a 48-year-old male physician in New England sought to estimate his own 10-year risk of developing CHD. He found that the 10-year cumulative incidence of CHD had been measured in two seemingly relevant populations: (1) 2,489 adult men in the nearby community of Framingham, Massachusetts; and (2) 10,724 adult male physicians from throughout the United States. No CHD incidence data were available from either source on a subgroup of men exactly like himself with regard to age, blood pressure, cholesterol level, smoking status, and other factors thought to influence CHD risk. However, data from each

population had been used to develop a multivariable statistical model designed to predict 10-year CHD risk as a function of several personal characteristics, including those just mentioned.

After doing the necessary calculations, the physician found that, according to the Framingham data, his 10-year risk of developing CHD was 7%. According to the physician data, his 10-year risk was 3%. Fortunately, both estimates led to the same conclusion as to whether he should take aspirin for CHD prevention. But he noted wryly that one way to reduce his risk of CHD by more than half was simply to self-identify with his occupational peer group rather than with his neighbors! (Kent and Shah, 2012)

To summarize, the task of estimating disease risk in an individual from disease frequency in a population almost always involves extrapolation to an individual outside the original study population. Formally, that extrapolation involves generalizing study results to a "superpopulation" that would be broad enough to include the target individual. Confidence limits for disease frequency in the study population (or a subgroup thereof) can help quantify the amount of uncertainty in risk estimation due to sampling error. However, those confidence limits do not account for qualitative differences between the study population and a broader superpopulation that would encompass the target individual. Judging the likely effect of those differences must be guided by subject-matter knowledge and by indirect evidence from other sources. Despite these limitations, epidemiologic studies can provide valuable guidance for estimating disease risk in an individual by: (1) helping to identify personal attributes or other factors that are importantly associated with risk, and (2) quantifying disease frequency in a group of people who share at least some relevant characteristics with the target individual.

Confidence Limits

When all cases of a disease have been identified and counted in a defined population, and interest focuses on that population alone, it can be argued that the resulting measure of disease frequency is not subject to sampling error. For example, it is a statement of historical fact that 4.78% of Florida mothers who bore a singleton infant between March 2004 and December 2007 developed GDM during their pregnancy. No random error is involved.

Often, however, a population in which disease frequency has been measured is viewed as providing information about disease frequency in some larger, unobserved domain. For example:

1. It may not be feasible to ascertain disease status on everyone in a large population, but it may be possible to do so on a sample. For example, the United States National Health and Nutrition Examination Survey (NHANES) conducts in-person measurements of health-related characteristics on a carefully selected sample of about 5,000 United States residents each year. The prevalence of, say, hypertension among adults in the NHANES sample in a given year can be used to obtain an estimate of the prevalence of hypertension among all United States adults in that year.

2. Sometimes disease occurrence in a study population is regarded as providing information about an ongoing *disease-generating process* that is assumed to operate before, during, and after the study period in that setting. The study population is regarded as a sample

in time, rather like a sample of water drawn from a flowing river.

3. As illustrated earlier, sometimes a study population is regarded as a sample drawn from a larger *superpopulation*, not necessarily confined to the study setting.

In each situation, disease frequency in the study population is used to estimate the unobserved true disease frequency in a larger domain from which the study population has been sampled. One implication of this view is that if the study were repeated, possibly many times, new samples would be selected and could yield a different result each time. Confidence limits provide a numerical range within which the unobserved true frequency of disease in the larger domain is likely to fall.

The amount of sampling error in an estimate depends on several factors. These include the statistical nature of the quantity being estimated (e.g., whether a rate or a proportion), the sampling design, and the sample size. In situation #1 above, choosing a study sample from a larger defined population of interest may involve using a different sampling approach for different population strata (e.g., urban vs. rural), sampling pre-existing clusters of people (e.g., neighborhoods) rather than sampling people individually, and/or giving certain kinds of people (e.g., minorities) a higher probability of being included in the sample. The size of the larger source population may also be finite and known, making it possible to obtain narrower confidence limits by applying a *finite population correction*.

In this book, methods for obtaining confidence limits are described only for situations in which the study population can be regarded as a simple random sample of independent observations from an infinite source population. Situations #2 and #3 above can approximate these conditions, and situation #1 may as well, if the study population is a simple random sample from a much larger source population. Fuller statistical treatment of confidence limits for other kinds of parameters and sampling plans can be found in, e.g., Levy and Lemeshow (2009); Korn and Graubard (1999); Cochran (1977); Lumley (2011).

Most commonly used disease-frequency measures can be classified statistically as either a rate or a proportion. Appendix 4A provides computational details on confidence limits for rates and proportions. A few other measures described in Chapter 3 are raw counts without a denominator, but confidence limits for a count itself are rarely required as an end result in practice.

A CLOSER LOOK AT SEVERAL SPECIFIC MEASURES OF DISEASE FREQUENCY

Prevalence

Prevalence and Length-Biased Sampling
Not all cases of a disease necessarily have an equal chance of being included in a set of prevalent cases. The reason is that the time course of many diseases is quite variable from person to person, and an individual's chance of being a case at the time of a prevalence survey often depends on how much time he or she spends in the diseased state.

Coronary heart disease, for example, can take several forms, including cardiac chest pain (angina pectoris), acute myocardial infarction, or sudden cardiac death. Figure 4.3 shows the time course of coronary heart disease for three hypothetical cases in a workforce population of middle-aged men during a one-year period. At mid-year, case #1 develops chronic angina pectoris, which lasts through the end of the year and beyond. Case #2 experiences a myocardial infarction early in the year and dies a week later. Case #3 remains disease-free until late in the year, when he suddenly collapses with ventricular fibrillation and dies almost immediately of sudden cardiac death.

Now suppose that an employee health survey seeks to measure the prevalence of coronary heart disease by enumerating all prevalent cases in the workforce. For simplicity, say that a questionnaire is sent to all employees simultaneously and that all eligible cases among survey recipients are correctly identified. This protocol is tantamount to drawing a vertical line somewhere in Figure 4-3 at a horizontal position reflecting the date of the survey and counting all active cases crossed by that line. If a survey date is chosen at random, case #1 has about a 50% chance of being active on the survey date chosen and thus of being included as a prevalent case. Case #2 has about a 1/52 of being included, because only a

few potential survey dates would fall within the week when he is an active case. Case #3 has an infinitesimal chance of being included—the survey would have to reach him between the onset of ventricular fibrillation and when he dies minutes later.

Other things being equal, a person's probability of being captured as a prevalent case is proportional to the duration of his or her disease. Unlike a set of incident cases, a set of prevalent cases thus tends to be skewed toward cases with more chronic forms of the disease. This principle has important implications for the design of some kinds of epidemiologic research, particularly case-control studies, to be discussed in Chapter 15. For example, a set of prevalent cases may not be ideal for use in a case-control study of etiologic risk factors, because any risk factor that is also associated with chronicity of the disease may be unusually common among such cases (Wang *et al.*, 1999). The same principle arises in evaluating the effects of disease screening programs. Screening for disease is like a prevalence survey, and cases detected by screening tend to be skewed toward more slowly progressive forms of pre-symptomatic disease, as discussed in Chapter 19.

Confidence Limits for Prevalence
Statistically, prevalence is a proportion. Confidence limits for a proportion can be obtained by methods described in Appendix 4A.

Cumulative Incidence

Estimating Cumulative Incidence in the Presence of Censoring
Sometimes we want to estimate cumulative incidence but cannot do so directly because some members of the study population at the start of an observation period drop out during the period, even though they had not become a case before dropping out. Disease occurrence information among dropouts who were still at risk for the disease of interest when they dropped out is termed *censored*. Censoring can occur for many reasons, including voluntary withdrawal, leaving a disease-surveillance system's coverage area, or the scheduled end of study data collection.

When censoring is present, the study population is no longer strictly closed; on the other hand, no new members may be added, as could happen in a completely open population. (The term "semi-closed" has been sometimes been used.) *Survival analysis* is a family of statistical methods that can

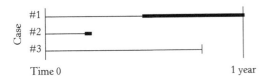

FIGURE 4.3 Three hypothetical cases of coronary heart disease.

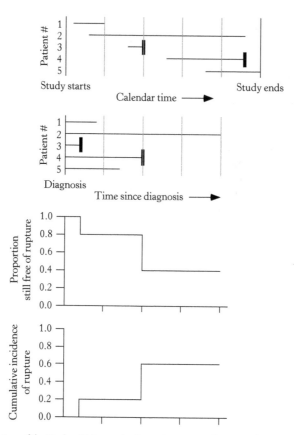

FIGURE 4.4 Application of the Kaplan-Meier method to estimate cumulative incidence for five hypothetical subjects.

allow estimation of cumulative incidence in the presence of censoring, under certain assumptions (Clark et al., 2003; Kalbfleisch and Prentice, 2002; Hosmer and Lemeshow, 2008; Selvin, 2008). A simple and widely used method that requires relatively few assumptions is described here: the *Kaplan-Meier* or *product-limit* method (Kaplan and Meier, 1958).

To see how the method works, a specific context will be helpful. An abdominal aortic aneurysm is a balloon-like expansion of the abdominal aorta caused by weakening of the aortic wall. Biomechanical theory posits that as an aneurysm grows, its wall becomes thinner and weaker, thus increasing the chance of still further expansion and potentially catastrophic rupture. However, surgical repair of an unruptured aneurysm involves significant risk, pain, and cost. To help decide between early surgery and watchful waiting, doctors and patients need to know the risk of rupture and how it varies over time.

As a "thought experiment," we can imagine monitoring a group of newly diagnosed aneurysm patients over time, without censoring. The cumulative incidence of rupture would rise over time. How high

and how quickly the risk rises would help determine the urgency of elective surgery.

In practice, however, aneurysm patients would be diagnosed on widely varying calendar dates, and it would be almost impossible to follow them all until rupture occurred. Censoring could happen due to elective surgical repair, patient leaving the study area, or the scheduled end of data collection. Patients could also die of other causes before rupture occurred.

Example 4-4. A study by Nevitt and colleagues (1989) involved tracking the experience of 176 residents of Rochester, Minnesota, who were first diagnosed with an unruptured abdominal aortic aneurysm between 1951 and 1984. Among them, 11 ruptures were identified within eight years after diagnosis. However, even by five years after diagnosis, only 76 of the original patients were actually still at risk for rupture and being followed. Had all 176 patients been tracked for a full eight years without censoring, the cumulative incidence of rupture no doubt would have exceeded 11/176, possibly by a large amount.

Figure 4.4 portrays five hypothetical patients who are diagnosed with an aneurysm on various calendar dates during a five-year study period. In the top panel, each patient's experience is shown as a horizontal line that begins at date of diagnosis and terminates either with rupture (a bold vertical bar) or with censoring (a vanishing line).

In the second panel, the time scale is changed to time *since diagnosis*, which bears more directly on the research question at hand. To make this time-scale conversion, each person's line is moved leftward to align its start with the vertical axis, keeping its length and manner of termination unchanged.

The third panel is the Kaplan-Meier survival curve derived from these data. (Such "curves" normally have a stair-step shape like this one.) Although we are mainly interested in cumulative incidence, it is mathematically more convenient to focus first on "survival"—here, the probability of *not* having had a rupture. To construct the curve, we proceed from left to right. By definition, all patients with a newly discovered unruptured aneurysm are free of rupture at diagnosis (time 0), so the survival curve begins at height 1.0. Here, no ruptures occurred until halfway through the first year. Of the five patients then under surveillance, four remained rupture-free immediately after patient #3's rupture. Hence the curve drops at that point to $1.0 \times (4/5) = 0.8$. Before the next rupture occurred, patients #1 and #5 dropped out due to censoring. Those losses have no effect on the height of the survival curve at the times they occur. However, they increase the amount by which it drops whenever any subsequent ruptures occur. The next rupture (patient #4) occurred two years after diagnosis. At that time, one of the two patients still at risk and under surveillance remained rupture-free after patient #4's rupture. Hence the curve drops to $0.8 \times (1/2) = 0.4$ at that time. This relatively large drop is because patient #4 represented a larger *proportion* of the study population then remaining at risk. After that rupture, no further ruptures occurred through year 4, when the last person under surveillance dropped out.

The bottom panel of Figure 4-4 shows the desired plot of cumulative incidence over time, obtained by calculating cumulative incidence = 1− (proportion still free of rupture) at each follow-up time. In effect, it is the third panel turned upside-down. Note that the estimated cumulative incidence

of rupture at 4 years is 0.6, not $2/5 = 0.4$, as might have been guessed naïvely without accounting for censoring.

When there is no censoring, the Kaplan-Meier method yields the same cumulative incidence estimate as the simpler direct method described in Chapter 3. When censoring is present, the method uses the experience of those remaining at risk and under follow-up to estimate the shape of the curve. The validity of the resulting curve and cumulative incidence estimates depends on an assumption that censoring is unrelated to risk. In other words, it is assumed that, had they been observed to completion, the survival curve for persons with censored data would look the same as the curve for everyone else, aside from sampling variability. This assumption is usually not empirically testable, but a judgment about its plausibility can often be informed by considering the reasons for censoring. In the aneurysm example, censoring due to the arbitrary end of the study period might well be unrelated to risk and create no bias. However, censoring due to surgical repair might be triggered by onset of symptoms or by evidence of rapid aneurysm growth, so that the surgeon's hand may have been forced by impending rupture. To the extent that censoring for that reason is common, we might suspect that the cumulative incidence of rupture without surgical intervention would be underestimated by the Kaplan-Meier method.

Sometimes study subjects can also have their follow-up cut short by *competing risks*—i.e., other kinds of events whose occurrence makes it biologically impossible for a subject to experience the outcome event of main interest thereafter. For example, a patient who dies of some other cause cannot subsequently experience a ruptured aneurysm. Under those conditions, the Kaplan-Meier estimate of cumulative incidence is interpretable as cumulative incidence among subjects who do not have a competing risk event (Satagopan *et al.*, 2004).

The Kaplan-Meier method is described more formally in Appendix 4B. Survival analysis also includes several other conceptually similar but computationally more complex methods for estimating cumulative incidence when adjustment must be made for subject characteristics that may differ across comparison groups. More details can be found in survival analysis references (Kaplan and Meier, 1958; Kalbfleisch and Prentice, 2002; Selvin, 2008).

Confidence Limits for Cumulative Incidence

Statistically, cumulative incidence is a proportion. When no censoring is involved and cumulative incidence is estimated as described in Chapter 3, confidence limits can be obtained as detailed in Appendix 4A. When the data are subject to censoring and cumulative incidence must be estimated indirectly by the Kaplan-Meier method or a related method, a more complicated statistical approach is required to set confidence limits—see, e.g., Rosner (2006, p. 747).

Incidence Rate

Incidence Rate and Hazard Rate

Earlier in this chapter we noted that cumulative incidence in a population can also be interpreted as disease probability or risk in an individual chosen at random from that population. One might wonder: does the incidence rate, which is usually measured as disease events per quantity of person-time, also have an interpretation at the individual-person level?

It does, in terms of a quantity called the *hazard rate*. Imagine a person who is at risk for a given disease at some time t and who is observed for the next small increment of time—from t to $t + \Delta t$, say. The hazard rate can be defined as:

$$\lim_{\Delta t \to 0} \left[\frac{\Pr(\text{disease event in interval} \ (t, t + \Delta t) \mid \text{susceptible at } t)}{\Delta t} \right]$$

The hazard rate is a kind of "instantaneous" incidence rate: it is the probability of experiencing a disease event, per unit of person-time, at a particular moment in the life of a person at risk. Computed as the ratio of a unitless probability to an amount of time, the hazard rate has units of (time unit)$^{-1}$, just as does the incidence rate. The hazard rate is important in many forms of survival analysis, including proportional-hazards regression (discussed in Chapter 12).

For some diseases, the hazard rate no doubt varies greatly over time within a person. For example, the hazard rate for being struck by a motor vehicle is surely much greater while crossing the street than while asleep at home in bed. It can also vary from person to person: at any given time, the hazard rate of injury due to gun violence is no doubt greater for an urban gang member than for a suburban church minister. For other conditions, such as dementia or arthritis, the hazard rate may be much less variable within and among population members.

Regardless of how the hazard rate varies over time and among people, the incidence rate in a population can be shown to be a grand average of the hazard rate over the aggregate of person-time in its denominator (Koepsell and Weiss, 2003). The overall incidence rate can also be viewed as an average of person-specific incidence rate contributions from individual population members, each of which is in turn an average hazard rate for that individual. But note that the overall incidence rate is a *weighted* average: the weight for each person's contribution is the fraction of total person-time that he/she contributes to the total. In an open population, members can contribute different amounts of person-time and thus are weighted unequally.

One example of the consequences of this differential weighting is the so-called "healthy worker survivor effect" (Arrighi and Hertz-Picciotto, 1994). Active employees of a company monitored over several years make up an open population: members can come and go as they join or leave the work force. Longer-term employees must, among other things, be healthy enough to keep working, and hence they contribute more person-time at risk. Less-healthy workers who die or become disabled stop working earlier and contribute less person-time. The overall incidence rate of illness or injury among the company's active employees thus tends to be skewed toward the experience of relatively healthy workers, usually toward a lower overall rate.

Confidence Limits

The conventional method for obtaining confidence limits for an incidence rate is to treat the denominator as a fixed quantity and to base confidence limits for the rate on confidence limits for the numerator alone, treating it as a Poisson-distributed count. Appendix 4A provides computational details and an example.

In many contexts, the conventional Poisson-based method may give at best only approximate confidence limits, however, because it is based on an implicit assumption of a constant hazard rate. When the hazard rate is indeed constant across individuals and over time, all person-time within the observation period is freely interchangeable. An analogy from physics is decay of a radioactive element: the hazard rate of fissioning in a certain atom at a certain moment is thought to be constant across all atoms of the same isotope and over time. In the human health arena, there are probably not many exact counterparts—perhaps the hazard of being struck by a giant meteor from outer space. Nonetheless, some situations come closer than others. Three situations are described here in which a constant-hazard assumption would be plausible or not-so-plausible. When it is seriously violated, conventional confidence limits based on the Poisson distribution can be too narrow (Glynn and Buring, 1996; Clayton, 1994).

Homogeneous population

The constant-hazard assumption is more likely to be met for a relatively homogeneous population observed over a relatively short time period. "Relatively homogeneous" and "relatively short" must be interpreted in the context of the disease in question. In occupational epidemiology, for example, cases and person-time at risk are routinely accumulated in multiple categories defined by job title, age range, gender, and calendar year, with the incidence rate being estimated separately for each of the resulting categories (Checkoway *et al.*, 2004). Within categories, the at-risk population is thought to be relatively homogeneous, favoring a constant-hazard assumption.

Hazard varying randomly among individuals

In some situations, theory and/or available data suggest that the hazard rate varies among individuals, even after accounting for measured differences in exposure to risk factors and other personal characteristics. This variation could arise, for example, from differences in genetic susceptibility, differences in exposure to unmeasured risk factors, or just biological variation. In the biostatistical literature, random inter-individual differences in hazard rates are called differences in *frailty* (Aalen, 1994; Clayton, 1994).

This situation often applies to studies of recurrent illness (Glynn *et al.*, 1993; Glynn and Buring, 1996; Cumming *et al.*, 1990). Under the constant-hazard assumption, someone who has had one disease event is no more or less likely than anyone else to have another event in the future. But for many diseases, evidence suggests that future risk is often elevated among persons who have already experienced an initial event. For example, victims of assault have been found to be at greatly increased risk of being assaulted again (Dowd *et al.*, 1996). Children treated for an unintentional injury are more likely than are other children to experience a future unintentional injury (Johnston *et al.*, 2000). Postmenopausal women who experience a vertebral fracture are at high risk of having an additional fracture

within the next year (Lindsay *et al.*, 2001). Possible mechanisms include continued exposure to a hazardous environment, existence of a chronic underlying health condition that predisposes to recurrent complications, or effects of the initial illness event itself, as might occur if an assault victim confronted his or her attacker. Whatever the reason, an initial event may serve as a marker for a subpopulation with a higher hazard rate.

Several statistical approaches have been proposed to deal with this problem (Glynn and Buring, 1996; Clayton, 1994; Sturmer *et al.*, 2000). One involves computing an individual event rate for each population member based on his or her observed number of events and person-time at risk, and basing confidence limits for the overall incidence rate on the observed variance in those event rates across persons (Glynn and Buring, 1996; Stukel *et al.*, 1994). More complex multivariable methods include logistic regression using generalized estimating equations, Poisson regression with correction for overdispersion, negative-binomial regression, or adaptations of proportional-hazards survival analysis (Thomsen and Parner, 2006; Sturmer *et al.*, 2000).

Hazard varying over time

The constant-hazard-rate model can be expected to hold best over relatively short observation periods. As time passes, changes in such factors as exposure to environmental causes, diagnostic methods, and disease classification can occur and affect the hazard rate. Closed populations also age. To reduce variation in hazard over time in the face of these factors, a long period of observation can be subdivided into shorter sub-periods or "time bands" for analysis. Other analytic strategies include modeling the effects of time itself on incidence—for example, by including time as a predictor in the kinds of multivariable models to be described later (Chapter 12).

Often, however, changes in hazard rates over time are not of main interest and are instead just a potential source of bias when making comparisons among subgroups or populations. This viewpoint has helped make the proportional-hazards model popular in epidemiology (Cox, 1972; Kalbfleisch and Prentice, 2002; Selvin, 2008). Briefly, under this model, the "baseline" hazard may change over time in an arbitrary way, and these changes are assumed to apply to all individuals (or those within a defined stratum). But at any given moment, an individual's hazard relative to that of other individuals then at risk is assumed to depend on his or her measured personal characteristics, at least one of which is exposure to a potential risk factor of main interest. The quantity estimated is then the *hazard ratio* for the exposed condition compared to the unexposed condition.

Incidence Rate and Mean Time to Disease Onset

An incidence rate whose denominator is measured in person-time has units of $(\text{time unit})^{-1}$—for example, years^{-1} or days^{-1}. Under certain idealized conditions, the *reciprocal* of incidence can be interpreted as the mean time to disease onset. Although this odd fact is perhaps of more theoretical than practical importance, its basis is explained here. It will soon play a role in linking different measures of disease frequency.

As an aid to intuition, consider a hypothetical closed population of N susceptible individuals who are followed indefinitely for development of a non-recurrent disease. Say that the incidence rate remains constant at some value IR throughout the follow-up period. If there are no competing risks, and if the population is followed long enough, then everyone in it must eventually develop the disease. Before becoming a case, person i contributes a certain amount of person-time at risk, T_i. Total person-time, $T = \sum_i T_i$, stops increasing when the last case occurs. At that time, N cases would have occurred in T person-time. By definition, the incidence rate was constant throughout follow-up, so $IR = N/T$.

Now suppose we are interested in how much time goes by, on average, until a susceptible person becomes a case. This would be $(\sum_i T_i)/N = T/N = 1/IR$. In other words, the reciprocal of the incidence rate estimates the mean time to disease onset under the circumstances described.

Example 4-5. Say that upper respiratory infections occur at the (very high) incidence rate of 3 per person-year. The average time to the next upper respiratory infection for a person at risk would be $1/(3 \text{ year}^{-1})$, or 4 months.

For low-incidence diseases, the required assumption of no competing risks will rarely be satisfied, in which case the resulting numerical estimate of

mean time to disease onset may not be very meaningful. However, the algebraic relation itself will prove useful below.

Odds

The *odds* of disease can be defined as $\frac{\text{No. of cases}}{\text{No. of non-cases}}$. If the numerator counts all new cases in a closed population during a specified time period, and the denominator counts those who do not become cases during that period, then their ratio represents the odds of *developing* disease during the period (*incidence odds*). If instead the numerator and denominator count cases and non-cases, respectively, in a defined population at a point in time, then their ratio represents the odds of having disease at that point in time (*prevalence odds*).

Cumulative incidence and prevalence, as proportions, tend to be more readily interpretable measures of disease frequency than incidence odds and prevalence odds. For that reason alone, cumulative incidence and prevalence are usually preferred for purposes of description and comparison. However, some epidemiologic study designs (particularly the case-control design) and some multivariable analysis methods (particularly logistic regression) that will be discussed in later chapters produce results that are most directly interpretable in terms of disease odds. The importance of odds as a disease-frequency measure stems mainly from the usefulness of those designs and analytic techniques.

A convenient feature of odds is that, in many situations, the proportion of persons with disease (e.g., cumulative incidence or prevalence) is low enough that disease odds closely approximate that proportion. Say that a is the number of cases and b the number of non-cases. Cumulative incidence or prevalence, as proportions, can be written as $\frac{a}{a+b}$. If the disease is rare, then b is much larger than a, and $\frac{a}{a+b} \approx \frac{a}{b} = \text{odds}$. The rarer the disease, the closer the approximation.

RELATIONSHIPS AMONG MEASURES OF DISEASE FREQUENCY

Populations and Their Subpopulations

Many measures of disease frequency take the form of a fraction, C/D. The numerator, C, is typically the number of cases, while the denominator, D, is typically the population size or a total amount of person-time at risk. Prevalence, cumulative incidence, person-time incidence rate, mortality rate, case fatality, and various other measures all fit this description.

Suppose that a population of interest can be divided up into two or more mutually exclusive and collectively exhaustive subpopulations. This partitioning could, for example, be by gender (male or female), by age (all 10-year age groups, perhaps), by presence or absence of some genetic marker, by smoking status (never, current, or past smoker), or by any other exposure or trait on which information is available. Subpopulations could also be defined by unique combinations of such factors—e.g., young male smokers—as long as all such combinations are included. Say that there are J subpopulations in all, let C_j be the number of cases in subpopulation j, and let D_j be the corresponding denominator. Then:

$$\frac{C}{D} = \frac{C_1 + C_2 + \cdots + C_J}{D}$$

$$= \frac{C_1}{D} + \frac{C_2}{D} + \cdots + \frac{C_J}{D}$$

$$= \frac{D_1}{D} \cdot \frac{C_1}{D_1} + \frac{D_2}{D} \cdot \frac{C_2}{D_2} + \cdots + \frac{D_J}{D} \cdot \frac{C_J}{D_J}$$

$$= \sum_j \frac{D_j}{D} \cdot \frac{C_j}{D_j}$$

In words, disease frequency in a full population is a *weighted average* of disease frequency in its subpopulations. Each subpopulation's disease frequency (C_j/D_j) is weighted by the fraction of the full-population denominator that comes from that subpopulation (D_j/D).

Example 4-6. In a population of 700 women and 300 men, there are 35 prevalent cases of diabetes among women and 30 cases among men. The overall prevalence of diabetes is thus $(35+30)/(700+300)$ $= 65/1{,}000 = 6.5\%$, while the gender-specific prevalences are $35/700 = 5\%$ in women and $30/300 = 10\%$ in men.

The overall prevalence, 6.5%, is a weighted average of 5% and 10%. The weight for 5% is 0.7, because women compose 700/1,000 of the overall study population; the weight for 10% is 0.3 because men compose 300/1,000 of the overall study population. Thus $6.5\% = (0.7)(5\%) + (0.3)(10\%)$.

Figure 4.2, discussed earlier, is another illustration. The overall frequency of GDM in all study women was a weighted average of GDM frequency in the five race/ethnicity groups. The frequency of GDM among Asian/Pacific Islander mothers was, in turn, a weighted average of GDM frequency among subgroups of Asian/Pacific Islander mothers formed according to pre-pregnancy BMI.

The weighted-average rule, while simple, is very important. Among other applications, it underlies several measures of excess risk, as well as the techniques of direct and indirect rate adjustment, which will be covered in later chapters.

A few special cases are worth noting. Suppose that the measure of interest is a proportion, such as prevalence or cumulative incidence. If disaggregation of the population is carried to the extreme, such that each subpopulation consists of a single individual, then $C_j/D_j = 1/1$ for each case and $0/1$ for each non-case. Thus, $C/D = \sum_j \frac{1}{D} \cdot \frac{C_j}{1}$, each population member's contribution being weighted equally by $1/D$.

Suppose instead that the disease frequency measure is a *rate* with a person-time denominator. Let C/T be the full-population rate, where T is total person-time at risk. Similar algebra shows that $C/T = \sum_j \frac{T_j}{T} \cdot \frac{C_j}{T_j}$ where T_j is the person-time contributed from subpopulation j. Each weight T_j/T is now the proportion *of total person-time* that comes from subpopulation j. As before, the weights sum to 1. As noted earlier in this chapter, if the population is disaggregated into individual people, different people may get different weights: each person's weight depends on how much person-time he/she contributes to the total, and those contributions may be unequal.

Finally, if all of the subpopulations have the same disease frequency, that shared constant value will also equal the full-population value.

Cumulative Incidence and Incidence Rate

A useful relationship between the two main measures of incidence can be developed for non-recurrent diseases. One application is to enable a fair comparison between an incidence rate from one source and a cumulative incidence from another source.

Consider a closed population at risk that is observed over a specified time period for occurrence of a non-recurrent disease. (This is Model A from

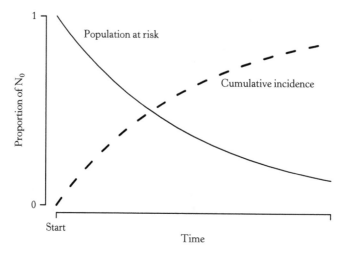

FIGURE 4.5 Increasing cumulative incidence and decreasing proportion of original population remaining at risk over time when incidence rate is constant.

Chapter 2.) Cumulative incidence can be measured directly in this situation. But suppose that new disease occurs in this population at a constant incidence *rate*. Let N_0 be the number of persons initially at risk. At first, during each increment of time Δt, the population experiences $N_0 \cdot \Delta t$ person-time at risk. But once the first case occurs, the population at risk decreases by one. Hence the amount of person-time contributed in the next Δt time increment is $(N_0 - 1) \cdot \Delta t$—slightly less than before. Given a constant incidence rate, this decrease in person-time at risk translates to a slightly lower expected number of cases during a time interval of duration Δt. And as each new case occurs, the population at risk shrinks further, leading to fewer and fewer expected cases in each time increment Δt.

It can be shown with calculus that the population at risk would decline *exponentially* over time—a process analogous to the exponential decay of a radioactive element. Let N_t be the number remaining at risk at time t, and let IR be the incidence rate (here, a constant). Then:

$$N_t = N_0 \cdot e^{-IR \cdot t}$$

where e is the base of natural logarithms, approximately 2.71828. The expression e^x is also sometimes written $\exp(x)$.

Because of the steadily declining population at risk, a smaller and smaller number of new cases occur per unit of time. Meanwhile, the denominator of cumulative incidence, N_0, remains constant. Hence cumulative incidence continues to rise, but

with decreasing slope. Specifically, the cumulative incidence expected at time t is:

$$CI_t = \frac{N_0 - N_t}{N_0}$$

$$= \frac{N_0 - N_0 \cdot \exp(-IR \cdot t)}{N_0}$$

$$= 1 - \exp(-IR \cdot t) \qquad (4.1)$$

Figure 4.5 illustrates this relationship graphically.

Equation (4.1) can be handy when comparing results from two or more studies that used different incidence measures. As we have seen, the incidence rate applies to a broader range of populations and disease types, while cumulative incidence is more easily interpretable in terms of disease probability or risk. Equation (4.1) provides a way to use incidence rate data to address questions involving cumulative incidence.

Example 4-7. Clinicians caring for elderly patients who are hospitalized after major trauma, such as a motor vehicle crash or a serious fall, have observed that even if these patients survive the hospitalization, many do poorly and never fully recover. To help clarify the prognosis after hospitalization for major trauma in older adults, Davidson *et al.* (2011) linked Washington State hospital discharge records for trauma patients with death certificate data over an 8-year period. Among 8,100 trauma patients age 85+ years who were discharged alive, 32% were found to have died within a year thereafter. But given the advanced age of these patients, the question arose: what percentage of them would be expected to die within a year under normal circumstances?

This question can be addressed by using mortality data from Washington State. During the same 8-year period, the estimated average population age 85+ years in Washington State was 93,094, and there were 106,964 deaths among Washington residents in that age group during the period.

The trauma group was a closed population of 8,100 persons observed over a one-year period, namely the year after hospital discharge. The comparison group was an open population of elderly Washington residents. In this open population, the number at risk did not decline steadily as cases occurred; rather, it was replenished by younger people who graduated into the 85+ age group during the study period and/or by net in-migration from outside the state. Note that 93,094 was the *average* number of people in this age group. During the 8-year study period, people aged 85+ years contributed $93,094 \times 8 = 744,752$ person-years, for a mortality rate of $106,964/744,752 = 0.1436$ deaths per person-year. The expected one-year cumulative mortality for a population subjected to that mortality rate would be $1 - \exp(-0.1436 \cdot 1) = 0.134 = 13.4\%$. The observed cumulative mortality of 32% among elderly hospitalized trauma patients thus represented a large excess.

In many situations, the outcome event is rare enough and/or the observation period short enough that very little reduction in the size of the population at risk takes place during the period of interest. It can be shown mathematically that when cumulative incidence is near zero, $CI = 1 - \exp(-IR \cdot t) \approx IR \cdot t$. For example, an incidence rate of 10 cases per 1,000 person-years over a one-year period would produce $CI = 1 - \exp(-10/1,000 \cdot 1) = 0.00995$, very close to $10/1,000 \cdot 1 = 0.010$. The relation $CI \approx IR \cdot t$ can be a convenient "back-of-the-envelope" approximation when cumulative incidence is low and no calculator is available. But equation (4.1) applies regardless of outcome frequency and is only slightly more complicated.

Prevalence, Incidence, and Duration

We now consider a different situation in which prevalence, incidence, and disease duration can be shown to be related. Imagine a closed population in which a recurrent disease state occurs, such as urinary tract infection, the common cold, or depression. (This is Model B from Chapter 2.) Assume that all individuals who do not have the disease are susceptible— that is, there is no third "not-at-risk" state. Say also that the incidence rate is constant at some value I among all susceptibles and over time. Under this simple two-state model, people move back and forth between the diseased and susceptible states over time, as shown in Figure 4.6.

The flow along the disease-onset path, expressed as the number of new cases per unit of time, depends on (1) the size of the susceptible pool and (2) the incidence rate I. Because the disease can be recurrent, there is also a counter-flow of individuals from diseased back to susceptible, which we may call *recovery*. The number of recoveries per unit of time depends on (1) the size of the diseased pool, and (2) what can be called a *recovery rate*, which is just like the incidence rate but operates in the opposite direction. Let us further assume that this recovery rate is constant over time and is the same for all diseased individuals at some value R.

As noted earlier in this chapter, $1/I$ can be interpreted as the mean time to disease onset among susceptibles. By similar logic, $1/R$ can be interpreted as mean time to recovery among diseased individuals. In other words, $1/R$ is the *mean duration* of disease, which it will be convenient to call $\bar{d}$.

Now suppose that all individuals start out in the susceptible state, and imagine what happens over time. People begin to develop the disease at a rate determined by I. In the process, they start emptying the susceptible compartment and start filling the diseased compartment. As the diseased compartment accumulates prevalent cases, recoveries begin to occur. The more prevalent cases accumulate, the more recoveries occur, which tends to empty the diseased compartment and to refill the susceptible compartment. As long as the two opposing flows are unequal, one compartment will grow and the other shrink, which in turn will act to equalize the two flows. Eventually an equilibrium is reached, in which the flow of incident cases is exactly balanced by the flow of recoveries. Because the flows into and out

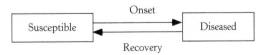

FIGURE 4.6 Two-state model to illustrate relationship among prevalence, incidence, and duration of disease.

of each compartment are equal at that point, both compartments maintain a stable size.

More formally, suppose that the flows and compartment sizes at equilibrium are labelled as follows:

S = number of susceptible persons

D = number of diseased persons (prevalent cases)

i = number of incident cases per time unit Δt

r = number of recoveries per time unit Δt

At equilibrium,

$$i = r$$
$$S \cdot I \cdot \Delta t = D \cdot R \cdot \Delta t$$
$$\frac{D}{S} = I \cdot \frac{1}{R}$$
$$= I \cdot \bar{d} \qquad (4.2)$$

Relation (4.2) says that, under the specified conditions and at equilibrium, D/S is the product of the incidence rate and mean duration of disease. D/S is not quite the prevalence of disease, however, which would be $D/(S + D)$. Rather, D/S is the *prevalence odds*. But as was noted earlier in discussion of odds, when the prevalence of disease is low, S is much larger than D, and thus $D/(S + D) \approx D/S$. In many realistic situations, disease prevalence is indeed known or can be assumed to be low, so the approximation (prevalence) $\approx$ (prevalence odds) would hold. The final result is then:

Prevalence $\approx$ (Incidence rate)

$\times$ (Mean disease duration)   (4.3)

Relation (4.3) links two key measures of disease frequency, prevalence and incidence. It is a time-honored rule of thumb in epidemiology. Nonetheless, it is probably best regarded as a conceptual aid rather than as a relation that can be expected to hold true consistently in real data. The main reason is that the assumptions behind our hypothetical model are often only approximately met under real-world conditions. For example, the incidence rate and recovery rate may not remain constant over time long enough for an equilibrium to be achieved, because of changes in environmental or behavioral exposures, disease-control activities, diagnostic technologies, treatments, and so on. Also, the population of interest may not be closed, so that in- and out-migration of prevalent cases may occur. Nonetheless, relation (4.3) remains quite useful as a reminder of

the two main determinants of disease prevalence. It can also be used to help predict how prevalence may change as a result of changes in incidence or disease duration.

Example 4-8. Imagine a population of married women aged 15–45 years in whom the incidence and prevalence of pregnancy are studied. Table 4.1 shows three scenarios. In the "base case," the incidence rate of pregnancy is 8 per 100 woman-years. Full-term pregnancies last 9 months, or 0.75 years. If all pregnancies go to term, and if incidence has been stable long enough for equilibrium to be reached, then a prevalence survey would be expected to find about $8/100 \times 0.75 = 6/100 = 6\%$ of women pregnant on a random survey date.

Now suppose that highly effective oral contraceptives become available for the first time, and a random 50% of women choose to use them. No other changes in reproductive practices occur. Use of the "pill" should reduce the incidence of pregnancy by half, to 4 per 100 woman-years, but it should not affect the duration of pregnancies that do occur. Once a new equilibrium is achieved, we would expect another prevalence survey to find about 3/100 women pregnant on a random date.

Starting over from the "base case" without oral contraceptives, suppose instead that elective abortions become available. A random 50% of women who become pregnant decide to terminate the pregnancy at three months, while the rest carry the child to term. Elective abortions would not affect the rate at which women become pregnant, so the incidence

---

TABLE 4.1. INCIDENCE, DURATION, AND PREVALENCE OF PREGNANCY IN A HYPOTHETICAL POPULATION OF WOMEN OF REPRODUCTIVE AGE

| Birth control use | Pregnancy | | |
	Incidence rate[a]	Duration (years)	Predicted prevalence (approx.)
None	8	0.75	6%
50% use "pill"	4	0.75	3%
50% have abortion at 3 months	8	0.50	4%

[a] Pregnancies per 100 woman-years

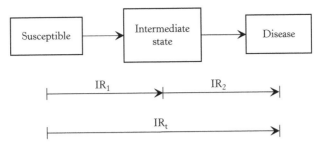

FIGURE 4.7 Disease model with an intermediate state.

of pregnancy would remain at 8 per 100 woman-years. But abortions would reduce the average duration of a pregnancy from 9 months to $(0.5)(3) + (0.5)(9) = 6$ months. Hence we would expect fewer women—about $4/100$—to be in the pregnant state on a random survey date.

Additivity of Rates

Often two or more diseases of interest can occur in the same population. If the diseases are mutually exclusive and share the same population at risk, then their incidence rates can be added to give an overall incidence rate of developing any of the diseases. This rule applies naturally to mortality rates for different causes of death, mortality rates being just a special type of incidence rate. For example, if in a certain population the mortality rate from cardiovascular disease is 200 deaths per 100,000 person-years, and the mortality rate from non-cardiovascular causes is 600 deaths per 100,000 person-years, then the population's overall mortality rate must be 800 deaths per 100,000 person-years.

Additivity of Sojourn Times

In some situations, development of a certain disease is thought to involve progression through one or more intermediate states. For example, women who develop cervical cancer are thought to pass through a state of having atypical, but not frankly cancerous, cervical cells that can be detected on a Pap smear. Not all people in the intermediate state need necessarily progress to the final disease state, just as not all people at risk necessarily develop the intermediate state.

Figure 4.7 illustrates this kind of model and three incidence rates: IR_1 is the incidence rate of developing the intermediate state, IR_2 the incidence rate from the intermediate state to the final disease state, and IR_t the overall incidence rate from susceptible to final disease.

IR_1 and IR_2 cannot simply be added or multiplied to obtain IR_t. However, use can again be made of the fact that $1/IR$ is interpretable as the mean time spent in one state before transitioning to another. Here, the reciprocal of each incidence rate is termed a *sojourn time*—that is, the mean time spent in one state before progressing to the next state.

$$1/IR_1 = s_1 = \text{mean time from susceptible to intermediate state}$$

$$1/IR_2 = s_2 = \text{mean time from intermediate state to final disease state}$$

$$1/IR_t = s_t = \text{mean time from susceptible state to final disease state}$$

Sojourn times can be added: $s_t = s_1 + s_2$. In words, the expected (i.e., mean) time required to go from susceptible to final disease is the mean time from susceptible to intermediate plus the mean time from intermediate to final disease (Morrison, 1979). Hence the three incidence rates can be related as follows:

$$s_t = s_1 + s_2$$

$$= 1/IR_1 + 1/IR_2$$

$$IR_t = \frac{1}{1/IR_1 + 1/IR_2}$$

Sojourn times are important in the theory of screening. The duration of an asymptomatic, preclinical stage that could be detected by a test bears on the feasibility of screening and on how frequently the screening test would need to be applied (Zheng and Rutter, 2012; Brenner *et al.*, 2011; Fenton and Weiss, 2004).

Mortality, Incidence, and Case Fatality

The following relations follow directly from the definitions of mortality, incidence, and case fatality:

$$\text{Mortality rate} \approx \text{incidence rate} \times \text{case fatality}$$

$$\text{Cumulative mortality} \approx \text{cumulative incidence} \\ \times \text{case fatality}$$

Intuitively, we can think of the risk of dying of a disease as (the risk of getting the disease) × (the risk of dying of it if you get it). These relations are shown as approximations because (1) the denominators of mortality and incidence differ slightly with regard to inclusion of prevalent cases; and (2) some time must pass between disease onset and death from the disease. The incidence rate that is current when disease-related deaths occur may differ from the rate in effect when those cases arose.

For the pedestrian/motor-vehicle collision injury example described in Chapter 3, neither of these caveats would be of serious concern. In 2009, an estimated 58,000 pedestrians were injured when struck by a motor vehicle, and 4,092 deaths resulted. The United States population in 2009 was about 306,800,000. Hence:

$$\text{Mortality rate} \approx \frac{4{,}092 \text{ deaths}}{306{,}800{,}000 \text{ person-years}}$$

$$\approx \frac{59{,}000 \text{ cases}}{306{,}800{,}000 \text{ person-years}}$$

$$\times \frac{4{,}092 \text{ deaths}}{59{,}000 \text{ cases}}$$

$$\approx (\text{incidence rate}) \times (\text{case fatality})$$

OTHER COMPOSITE MEASURES OF POPULATION DISEASE BURDEN

The disease frequency measures described in Chapter 3 are widely used and will probably continue to be so. Nonetheless, measures based on counting cases or deaths, with or without a denominator, have been criticized as providing only limited information about the impact of disease on the overall health of affected individuals or communities (McKenna et al., 2005; Murray, 1994). Several other measures of population disease burden have been suggested to address this shortcoming (Molla et al., 2003; Murray

et al., 2000; U.S. Burden of Disease Collaborators, 2013). Two examples will be described briefly here.

Years of Potential Life Lost (YPLL) is based on the idea that "premature" deaths—those occurring at younger ages—may have greater social and economic impact than do deaths in old age. If so, then age at death should be considered when quantifying the population impact of fatal disease (Gardner and Sanborn, 1990; Centers for Disease Control and Prevention, 1986). A version of YPLL that has been used in reporting of national health statistics for the United States is:

$$\text{YPLL} = \sum_{a=1}^{X} d_a (X - a)$$

where a denotes age at death (in years), d_a denotes number of deaths at age a, and X denotes a particular cutoff age, often age 65, 70, or 75 years. YPLL weights each death by the number of years before age X at which the death occurs. Deaths of young children thus get large weights; deaths at or after age X years get zero weight. YPLL can be expressed per 1,000 population (say), but this is not really necessary if all comparisons are made within the same population. When ranked by YPLL rather than mortality rates, diseases that cause death at younger ages, such as injuries or congenital anomalies, move higher in the ranking (National Center for Health Statistics, 2012, p. 116).

Criticisms of YPLL include the fact that the choice of a cutoff age X is somewhat arbitrary. YPLL can also vary depending on the age distribution of the population at risk, which affects comparability of YPLL between populations with different age structures. YPLL also involves an implicit assumption that persons who died of a certain disease before age X would otherwise have lived to age X or beyond (Gardner and Sanborn, 1990; Lai and Hardy, 1999).

Disability-Adjusted Life Years (DALYs) is a more complex composite measure of population disease burden (Murray, 1994; Murray and Acharya, 1997; U.S. Burden of Disease Collaborators, 2013). DALYs add together: (1) person-years of life lost due to premature death from a disease, relative to life expectancy without the disease; and (2) person-years of *healthy* life lost due to disability. The latter involves weighting each person-year of life lived with disease-related disability by a value ranging from 0 (perfect health) to 1 (death), reflecting the degree of adverse impact of the disability on function and quality of life. The weights have been estimated using survey techniques in a sample from the population of interest or, if necessary, from external sources.

Incidence, prevalence, and mortality data all provide input to calculation of DALYs through a complex formula presented and explained by Murray *et al.* (1994; 1997). The measure was designed as a tool for priority-setting among diseases and for evaluating disease control efforts, among other purposes. Estimates of DALYs associated with different diseases have been presented for different regions of the world (Murray and Lopez, 1997) and for the United States (McKenna *et al.*, 2005). As with YPLL, diseases that cause death at younger ages tend to appear higher on lists of diseases ranked by DALYs than on lists ranked by mortality rates. Also, diseases that often cause long-term disability, such as alcohol abuse, depression, and arthritis, tend to rank relatively high on DALYs.

Criticisms of DALYs have included concerns about the availability and quality of the data needed to implement them, especially in less-developed countries; representativeness of the samples and validity of the survey methods used in ascribing weights to disability levels; and implicit devaluation of person-years lived by people with disabilities (Almeida *et al.*, 2001).

APPENDIX 4A: CONFIDENCE LIMITS FOR RATES AND PROPORTIONS

The methods described here assume that the study population is a simple random sample from an infinite source population and that individuals have been sampled independently. Confidence limits for measures derived from multi-stage samples, such as those used in several United States national health surveys, require more complex statistical methods that account properly for stratification, clustering, and/or varying sampling probabilities among individuals (Levy and Lemeshow, 2009; Korn and Graubard, 1999; Lumley, 2011).

Methods for obtaining exact confidence limits are given priority. These formulas require as input critical values of either the χ^2 distribution (for rates) or the F distribution (for proportions). Those critical values can be obtained easily nowadays by using built-in functions in standard statistical packages or spreadsheet programs, or from published statistical tables. Because powerful, fast, free statistical software is so widely available, there is rarely a need to consider alternatives to exact methods. However,

methods based on normal-distribution approximations are also described. These approximations are useful for rough calculations when a computer or statistical tables are unavailable, or for very large sample sizes.

Rates

Rates take the form c/T, where c is the number of disease events and T is the amount of at-risk experience underlying c, usually measured in units of person-time. Confidence limits for the rate are developed by treating T as fixed and estimating confidence limits for c, which is commonly treated as following a Poisson distribution (Fleiss *et al.*, 2003, p. 342).

Exact $(1 - \alpha) \times 100\%$ lower (R_L) and upper (R_U) confidence limits for the unobserved true rate are:

$$R_L = \frac{\chi^2_{2c;\,\alpha/2}}{2T}$$

$$R_U = \frac{\chi^2_{2c+2;\,(1-\alpha/2)}}{2T}$$

In the formula for the lower limit, $\chi^2_{2c;\,\alpha/2}$ is the critical value of the χ^2 distribution with $2c$ degrees of freedom that puts $\alpha/2$ probability in the lower tail. For the upper limit, $\chi^2_{2c+2;\,(1-\alpha/2)}$ is the critical value of the χ^2 distribution with $2c+2$ degrees of freedom that puts $1 - \alpha/2$ probability in the lower tail (or, equivalently, $\alpha/2$ in the upper tail).

As an example, suppose that 9 cases are observed in 60 person-years, for a point estimate of 15 cases per 100 person-years. For exact 95% confidence limits, $\chi^2_{2c;\,\alpha/2} = \chi^2_{18;\,0.025} = 8.23$, and $\chi^2_{2c+2;\,(1-\alpha/2)} = \chi^2_{20;\,0.975} = 34.17$. Thus, $R_L = 8.23/(2 \cdot 60) = 0.069 = 6.9$ cases per 100 person-years, and $R_U = 34.17/(2 \cdot 60) = 0.285 = 28.5$ cases per 100 person-years.[3]

Observing zero disease events poses a special problem. The true rate cannot be negative, so R_L must be zero. All of the uncertainty is in the upper limit. The exact method still works for R_U, but now $R_U = \frac{\chi^2_{2;\,1-\alpha}}{2T}$ for a *one-sided* confidence interval. The upper 95% confidence limit when $c = 0$ is about $2.996/T$. This fact is the basis of the so-called "rule of three": if no events are observed, one can be 95% confident that the unobserved true rate is less than about $3/T$ (Hanley and Hand-Lippman, 1983).

For rates based on large numbers of events (say, $c > 100$), a method based on the normal approximation to the Poisson distribution is reasonably accurate (Armitage and Berry, 1994, p. 142):

$$R_L \approx \frac{c - Z\sqrt{c}}{T}$$

$$R_U \approx \frac{c + Z\sqrt{c}}{T}$$

where Z is the critical value of the normal distribution that puts $1 - \alpha/2$ probability in the lower tail. For 95% confidence limits, $Z \approx 1.96$.

Proportions

Several measures of disease frequency are *proportions*, including prevalence, cumulative incidence, and proportional mortality. Let c be the number of cases in the numerator and n the number of persons in the denominator. Exact $(1 - \alpha) \cdot 100\%$ lower (P_L) and upper (P_U) confidence limits for the unobserved true proportion can be obtained as follows (Fleiss et al., 2003, pp. 25–26):

$$P_L = \frac{c}{c + (n - c + 1) \cdot F_{2(n-c+1),\, 2c;\, 1-\alpha/2}}$$

$$P_U = \frac{(c+1) \cdot F_{2(c+1),\, 2(n-c);\, 1-\alpha/2}}{n - c + (c+1) \cdot F_{2(c+1),\, 2(n-c);\, 1-\alpha/2}}$$

In the formula for the lower limit, $F_{2(n-c+1),\, 2c;\, 1-\alpha/2}$ is the critical value of the F distribution with $2(n - c + 1)$ and $2c$ degrees of freedom that puts $1 - \alpha/2$ probability in the lower tail (or, equivalently, $\alpha/2$ in the upper tail). For the upper limit, $F_{2(c+1),\, 2(n-c);\, 1-\alpha/2}$ is the critical value of the F distribution with $2(c + 1)$ and $2(n - c)$ degrees of freedom that puts $1 - \alpha/2$ probability in the lower tail.

As an example, suppose that 8 cases are observed in a denominator population of 160, for a point estimate of $8/160 = 0.05$. Then, for exact 95% confidence limits,

$$F_{2(n-c+1),\, 2c;\, 1-\alpha/2} = F_{306,\, 16;\, 0.975} = 2.343,$$

and

$$F_{2(c+1),\, 2(n-c);\, 1-\alpha/2} = F_{18,\, 304;\, 0.975} = 1.796.$$

Thus,

$$P_L = \frac{8}{8 + 153 \times 2.343} = 0.0218,$$

and

$$P_U = \frac{9 \times 1.796}{160 - 8 + 9 \times 1.796} = 0.0961.$$

A special problem arises when $c = 0$ or $c = n$. The true proportion being estimated cannot be less than 0 or greater than 1. Hence, if $c = 0$, then P_L must be 0; if $c = n$, then P_U must be 1. One confidence limit is thus already known, and all of the uncertainty is in the other limit. The exact method still works for the remaining confidence limit, but $\alpha/2$ is replaced by α in its expression, giving a one-sided confidence interval. In these situations, reference to the F-distribution is not really necessary, however: exactly the same result can be obtained by taking $P_U = \alpha^{1/n}$ if $c = 0$, or by taking $P_L = 1 - \alpha^{1/n}$ if $c = n$.

If $c \geq 10$ and $n - c \geq 10$, the normal approximation to the binomial distribution gives reasonably accurate confidence limits (Armitage and Berry, 1994, p. 122). Let $\hat{p} = c/n$. Then:

$$P_L \approx \hat{p} - Z\sqrt{\frac{\hat{p}(1 - \hat{p})}{n}}$$

$$P_U \approx \hat{p} + Z\sqrt{\frac{\hat{p}(1 - \hat{p})}{n}}$$

where Z is the critical value of the normal distribution that puts $1 - \alpha/2$ probability in the lower tail. For 95% confidence limits, $Z \approx 1.96$.

APPENDIX 4B: ALGORITHM FOR THE KAPLAN-MEIER METHOD

The following notation is used:

t_i = Time point at which a case or censoring event occurs, indexed from earliest to latest

$N(t_i)$ = Number at risk at t_i

$C(t_i)$ = Number of cases occurring at t_i

$L(t_i)$ = Number of persons censored at t_i

$S(t_i)$ = Proportion still disease-free just after t_i

$CI(t_i)$ = Cumulative incidence just after t_i

Set starting values as follows:

$N(t_0)$ = Initial number of persons at risk

$S(t_0) = 1$

At each time point t_i, working from earliest to latest, set:

$$N(t_i) = N(t_{i-1}) - C(t_{i-1}) - L(t_{i-1})$$

$$S(t_i) = S(t_{i-1}) \times \frac{N(t_i) - C(t_i)}{N(t_i)}$$

$$CI(t_i) = 1 - S(t_i)$$

Once N drops to 0, S and CI become undefined.

NOTES

1. For present purposes, a small number of women from "other" races or with missing GDM status have been excluded, so numerical results appearing here differ slightly from those in the published paper.
2. Specifically, the *cumulative incidence* of GDM over the time interval of pregnancy. Some authors have called the same quantity *prevalence*, evidently referring to period prevalence during pregnancy. Equation (3.3) in Chapter 3 shows that as long as no women have pre-existing GDM at the start of pregnancy, as is required by the case definition, then period prevalence and cumulative incidence would be equivalent.
3. In the public-domain *R* statistical language (R Development Core Team, 2012), for instance, the statement R.L <- qchisq(0.025, 2 * 9) / (2 * 60) immediately gives the lower 95% confidence limit.

REFERENCES

Aalen OO. Effects of frailty in survival analysis. Stat Methods Med Res 1994; 3:227–243.

Almeida C, Braveman P, Gold MR, Szwarcwald CL, Ribeiro JM, Miglionico A, et al. Methodological concerns and recommendations on policy consequences of the World Health Report 2000. Lancet 2001; 357:1692–1697.

Armitage P, Berry G. Statistical methods in medical research (3rd ed.). London: Blackwell, 1994.

Arrighi HM, Hertz-Picciotto I. The evolving concept of the healthy worker survivor effect. Epidemiology 1994; 5:189–196.

Barrow SM, Herman DB, Córdova P, Struening EL. Mortality among homeless shelter residents in New York City. Am J Public Health 1999; 89:529–534.

Beral V, Bull D, Green J, Reeves G, Million Women Study Collaborators. Ovarian cancer and hormone replacement therapy in the Million Women Study. Lancet 2007; 369:1703–1710.

Brenner H, Altenhofen L, Katalinic A, Lansdorp-Vogelaar I, Hoffmeister M. Sojourn time of preclinical colorectal cancer by sex and age: estimates from the German national screening colonoscopy database. Am J Epidemiol 2011; 174:1140–1146.

Center JR, Bliuc D, Nguyen TV, Eisman JA. Risk of subsequent fracture after low-trauma fracture in men and women. JAMA 2007; 297:387–394.

Centers for Disease Control and Prevention. Premature mortality in the United States: public health issues in the use of years of potential life lost. MMWR 1986; 35:1S–11S.

Checkoway H, Pearce NE, Kriebel D. Research methods in occupational epidemiology (2nd ed.). New York: Oxford, 2004.

Clark TG, Bradburn MJ, Love SB, Altman DG. Survival analysis part I: basic concepts and first analyses. Br J Cancer 2003; 89:232–238.

Clayton D. Some approaches to the analysis of recurrent event data. Stat Methods Med Res 1994; 3:244–262.

Cochran WG. Sampling techniques (3rd ed.). New York: Wiley and Sons, 1977.

Cox DR. Regression models and life tables (with discussion). J R Stat Soc B 1972; 34:187–220.

Cumming RG, Kelsey JL, Nevitt MC. Methodologic issues in the study of frequent and recurrent health problems. Falls in the elderly. Ann Epidemiol 1990; 1:49–56.

Davidson GH, Hamlat CA, Rivara FP, Koepsell TD, Jurkovich GJ, Arbabi S. Long-term survival of adult trauma patients. JAMA 2011; 305:1001–1007.

Dowd MD, Langley J, Koepsell T, Soderberg R, Rivara FP. Hospitalizations for injury in New Zealand: prior injury as a risk factor for assaultive injury. Am J Public Health 1996; 86:929–934.

Fenton JJ, Weiss NS. Screening computed tomography: will it result in overdiagnosis of renal carcinoma? Cancer 2004; 100:986–990.

Fleiss JL, Levin B, Paik MC. Statistical methods for rates and proportions (3rd ed.). New York: Wiley and Sons, 2003.

Gardner JW, Sanborn JS. Years of potential life lost (YPLL)–what does it measure? Epidemiology 1990; 1:322–329.

Glynn RJ, Buring JE. Ways of measuring rates of recurrent events. BMJ 1996; 312:364–367.

Glynn RJ, Stukel TA, Sharp SM, Bubolz TA, Freeman JL, Fisher ES. Estimating the variance of standardized rates of recurrent events, with application to hospitalizations among the elderly in New England. Am J Epidemiol 1993; 137:776–786.

Hanley JA, Hand-Lippman A. If nothing goes wrong, is everything all right? Interpreting zero numerators. JAMA 1983; 249:1743–1745.

Hosmer DW, Lemeshow S. Applied survival analysis: regression modeling of time-to-event data (2nd ed.). Hoboken, NJ: Wiley Interscience, 2008.

Johnston BD, Grossman DC, Connell FA, Koepsell TD. High-risk periods for childhood injury among siblings. Pediatrics 2000; 105:562–568.

Kalbfleisch JD, Prentice RL. The statistical analysis of failure time data (2nd ed.). Hoboken, NJ: Wiley and Sons, 2002.

Kaplan EL, Meier P. Nonparametric estimation from incomplete observations. J Am Stat Assoc 1958; 53:457–481.

Kent DM, Shah ND. Risk models and patient-centered evidence: should physicians expect one right answer? JAMA 2012; 307:1585–1586.

Kim SY, England L, Sappenfield W, Wilson HG, Bish CL, Salihu HM, et al. Racial/ethnic differences in the percentage of gestational diabetes mellitus cases attributable to overweight and obesity, Florida, 2004–2007. Prev Chronic Dis 2012; 9:E88.

Koepsell TD, Weiss NS. Epidemiologic methods: studying the occurrence of illness (1st ed.). New York: Oxford University Press, 2003.

Korn EL, Graubard BI. Analysis of health surveys. New York: Wiley, 1999.

Lai D, Hardy RJ. Potential gains in life expectancy or years of potential life lost: impact of competing risks of death. Int J Epidemiol 1999; 28:894–898.

Levy PS, Lemeshow S. Sampling of populations: methods and applications (4th ed.). New York: Wiley, 2009.

Lindsay R, Silverman SL, Cooper C, Hanley DA, Barton I, Broy SB, et al. Risk of new vertebral fracture in the year following a fracture. JAMA 2001; 285:320–323.

Lumley T. Complex surveys: A guide to analysis using R. New York: Wiley and Sons, 2011.

McKenna MT, Michaud CM, Murray CJL, Marks JS. Assessing the burden of disease in the United States using disability-adjusted life years. Am J Prev Med 2005; 28:415–423.

Molla MT, Madans JH, Wagener DK, Crimmins EM. Summary measures of population health: report of findings on methodologic and data issues. Hyattsville, MD: National Center for Health Statistics, 2003.

Morrison AS. Sequential pathogenic components of rates. Am J Epidemiol 1979; 109:709–718.

Murray CJ. Quantifying the burden of disease: the technical basis for disability-adjusted life years. Bull World Health Organ 1994; 72:429–445.

Murray CJ, Acharya AK. Understanding DALYs (disability-adjusted life years). J Health Econ 1997; 16:703–730.

Murray CJ, Lopez AD. Global mortality, disability, and the contribution of risk factors: Global Burden of Disease Study. Lancet 1997; 349:1436–1442.

Murray CJ, Salomon JA, Mathers C. A critical examination of summary measures of population health. Bull World Health Organ 2000; 78:981–994.

National Center for Health Statistics. United States, 2011: with special feature on socioeconomic status and health. Hyattsville, MD: National Center for Health Statistics, 2012.

Nevitt MP, Ballard DJ, Hallett, Jr JW. Prognosis of abdominal aortic aneurysms: a population-based study. N Engl J Med 1989; 321:1009–1014.

Pearson TA, Blair SN, Daniels SR, Eckel RH, Fair JM, Fortmann SP, et al. AHA guidelines for primary prevention of cardiovascular disease and stroke: 2002 update: consensus panel guide to comprehensive risk reduction for adult patients without coronary or other atherosclerotic vascular diseases. American Heart Association Science Advisory and Coordinating Committee. Circulation 2002; 106:388–391.

R Development Core Team. R: a language and environment for statistical computing. R Foundation for Statistical Computing, Vienna, Austria 2012. URL: http://www.R-project.org. ISBN 3-900051-07-0.

Rosner B. Fundamentals of biostatistics (6th ed.). New York: Duxbury Press, 2006.

Satagopan JM, Ben-Porat L, Berwick M, Robson M, Kutler D, Auerbach AD. A note on competing risks in survival data analysis. Br J Cancer 2004; 91:1229–1235.

Selvin S. Survival analysis for epidemiologic and medical research: a practical guide. New York: Cambridge University Press, 2008.

Stukel TA, Glynn RJ, Fisher ES, Sharp SM, Lu-Yao G, Wennberg JE. Standardized rates of recurrent outcomes. Stat Med 1994; 13:1781–1791.

Sturmer T, Glynn RJ, Kliebsch U, Brenner H. Analytic strategies for recurrent events in epidemiologic studies: background and application to hospitalization risk in the elderly. J Clin Epidemiol 2000; 53:57–64.

Thomsen JL, Parner ET. Methods for analysing recurrent events in health care data. Examples from admissions in Ebeltoft Health Promotion Project. Fam Pract 2006; 23:407–413.

US Burden of Disease Collaborators. The state of U.S. health, 1990–2010. Burden of diseases, injuries, and risk factors. JAMA 2013; 310:591–608.

Wang HX, Fratiglioni L, Frisoni GB, Viitanen M, Winblad B. Smoking and the occurrence of Alzheimer's disease: cross-sectional and longitudinal data in a population-based study. Am J Epidemiol 1999; 149:640–644.

Zheng W, Rutter CM. Estimated mean sojourn time associated with hemoccult SENSA for detection of proximal and distal colorectal cancer. Cancer Epidemiol Biomarkers Prev 2012; 21: 1722–1730.

TABLE 4.2.

Patient no.	Date of admission	Date of first fall	Date of discharge	Comment
1	1/6	1/18	–	
2	1/14	–	–	
3	1/26	3/1	3/26	Discharged home
4	2/2	–	2/28	Admitted to hospital on 2/28
5	2/12	2/14	–	
6	2/15	–	3/22	Transferred to other facility
7	2/20	–	–	
8	2/28	3/15	–	
9	3/1	–	3/28	Discharged home
10	3/10	–	–	
11	3/12	–	3/26	Admitted to hospital on 3/26
12	3/20	3/29	–	

EXERCISES

1. Falls are a common problem among nursing home residents. In preparation for implementation of a new fall-prevention program, the staff of a particular nursing home unit that cares for patients with Alzheimer's disease have assembled baseline data about the incidence of falls among patients on the unit. The occurrence of first falls was monitored among all patients who were admitted to the unit during the 3-month period from January through March. The data have been summarized as shown in Table 4.2.

    Residents for whom no date of first fall was listed did not fall while on the unit. Those for whom no discharge date was listed were still on the unit as of April 1.

    You have been asked to assist with quantifying the baseline incidence of falls. They are particularly interested in the cumulative incidence of falls during the first 30 days after admission, for comparison with such statistics from other facilities. Recognizing that the sample size is small, what is your best estimate of the 30-day cumulative incidence of falls after admission to the unit?

2. The local health department where you work has received funding to set up one new prenatal clinic in some needy area of the county. You and your colleagues decide that the birth prevalence of low birth weight will be used as the primary indicator of need. You are helping the department decide whether to put the clinic in Allenville or Bakertown. Allenville's population is predominantly black, while Bakertown's population is predominantly white; neither community contains any significant number of residents other than blacks or whites.

    At your request, a data technician has compiled some statistics from birth certificate data for babies born in each town over the last two years. Unfortunately, in his haste, he forgot to write down which town was which. Here are the results he shows you:

TABLE 4.3.

Race	% of babies weighing < 2,500 grams at birth	
	Town 1	Town 2
Black	12%	18%
White	6%	9%
All babies	8%	15%

He apologizes and is about to set off to re-do his analysis and identify the towns. Instead, you ponder the data carefully, then thank him for giving you all the information you need to determine that the needier community is Allenville. How did you reach that conclusion?

3. A study of mortality among homeless men in New York City identified 332 middle-aged men in homeless shelters on a particular night in 1987 (Barrow et al., 1999). Through linkage to the National Death Index, it was determined that 43 (13.1%) of these men died during the following 7 years.

    Vital statistics for New York City showed that the mortality rate for comparably aged males at that time was about 9.1 deaths per 1,000 person-years. If this mortality rate had applied to the 332 homeless men in the sample, how many deaths would have been expected during the 7-year period?

4. Bone fractures that occur with low-level trauma can indicate underlying osteoporosis. A study of older women was conducted in Australia to assess the risk of

TABLE 4.4.

Age (years)	First fracture		Second fracture	
	Fractures	Person-years at risk	Fractures	Person-years at risk
60–69	147	6,833	43	1,209
70–79	378	14,154	111	1,758
80+	380	7,674	99	1,109

TABLE 4.5.

	HRT use		
	Never	Past only	Current
Number of:			
Participating women	474,682	186,751	287,143
Ovarian cancer cases	1,142	391	740
Ovarian cancer deaths	819	275	497
Average length of follow-up (years) for:			
Cancer occurrence	5.30	5.05	5.34
Death	6.92	6.72	6.89

another (second) fracture in women who experienced an initial low-trauma fracture (Center *et al.*, 2007). A total of 2,245 women age 60 years or older were monitored for fracture occurrence over a 16-year study period. A summary of the results appears in Table 4.4.

Suppose that an Australian woman suffers a low-trauma fracture of the wrist on her 65th birthday. What is the probability that she will experience another fracture by the time she reaches age 80? Assume that the incidence rates above apply to her and that she does not die before her 80th birthday.

5. Genital infection with human papillomavirus (HPV) is strongly associated with increased risk of cervical cancer in later life, even though HPV infection itself may be asymptomatic. Women become infected with HPV mainly through sexual contact, and acquiring HPV infection is common among younger, sexually active women.

Say that the incidence rate of HPV infection among sexually active women in college is 25 per 100 woman-years and stays constant through the college years. Out of 100 sexually active women who are HPV-negative when they enter college, how many would be expected to have been infected with HPV by the time they graduate four years later?

6. The Million Women Study (Beral *et al.*, 2007) sought to investigate possible links between use of hormone replacement therapy (HRT) and development of ovarian cancer. Some 948,576 postmenopausal British women with no previous cancer and who had not already undergone surgical removal of both ovaries entered the study when screened for breast cancer during 1996–2001. Each woman completed a questionnaire that asked about current or past use of HRT and other topics. A second similar mailed questionnaire about 3 years later was completed by 64% of the women. Identifying information on participants was then linked with population-based cancer registry data and with death records maintained by the British National Health Service. Cancer registry data were available through the end of 1999, 2003, or 2004, depending on area of residence; death records were available through the end of 2005 nationwide.

A summary of results appears in Table 4.5.

Changes in hormone-use status during the study were rare and can be ignored for present purposes.

(a) Calculate and compare the incidence of ovarian cancer in HRT never-users, past-only users, and current users.

(b) Estimate the case fatality of ovarian cancer among all participating women. What key assumption(s) must be true for your estimate to be valid?

7. The following sentence appeared in a recent issue of a prominent medical journal: "Despite the effectiveness of several forms of treatment for heart failure, the

prevalence of heart failure continues to rise." If the "effectiveness" to which the statement refers included a reduced risk of death, would you be surprised to see an increased prevalence of heart failure in relation to more widespread use of these forms of treatment? Explain.

8. The "cause of death" field on the death certificate in most states provides four lines for the certifying official to complete. They appear approximately as follows:

      Immediate cause: A ————————

Due to or as a consequence of: B ————————

Due to or as a consequence of: C ————————

Due to or as a consequence of: D ————————

The last-listed condition is regarded as the *underlying* cause of death. In most tabulations of cause-specific mortality statistics, deaths are assigned to this underlying cause.

However, it has been found that the total contribution to mortality of many conditions, such as diabetes, may be underestimated if deaths are linked to that condition only when it is listed as the underlying cause of death. To circumvent this limitation, the National Center for Health Statistics makes available Multiple Cause of Death data files, which contain the number of deaths for which each medical condition is listed on *any* line, A–D, of the death certificate. In the case of diabetes, for example, nearly four times as many deaths are counted as diabetes-related if it is allowed to appear on *any* line, as opposed to being listed as the underlying cause of death.

For a certain year, you are trying to estimate the overall mortality rate for lung disease-related deaths in the United States. To avoid understating the importance of lung diseases, you have located a table based on the Multiple Cause of Death data files. A key part reads as follows:

TABLE 4.6.

Lung condition	Mortality rate[a]
Acute bronchitis and bronchiolitis	1.3
Influenza and pneumonia	84.0
Influenza	2.6
Pneumonia	81.4
Bronchitis, emphysema, and asthma	24.5
Chronic or unspecified bronchitis	4.7
Emphysema	19.1
Asthma	2.8

[a] Deaths per 100,000 person-years

You decide to accept, for present purposes, the union of all conditions listed in Table 4.6 as a reasonable working definition of lung disease. Would it be fair to add the mortality rates from the three major categories listed—that is, 1.3 for acute bronchitis and bronchiolitis; plus 84.0 for influenza and pneumonia; plus 24.5 for bronchitis, emphysema, and asthma— to get the total mortality rate for lung-disease–related death? Why or why not?

ANSWERS

1. A few residents on the unit were under surveillance for falls throughout the first 30 days and beyond, but it is also possible and desirable to use information about several other residents who did not spend at least 30 days on the unit. The Kaplan-Meier method would be useful here. Discharge home, transfer to another facility, admission to the hospital, and ending of the surveillance period on April 1 can all be treated as forms of *censoring*, or loss to follow-up.

The relevant time scale is really time since admission, not calendar date. The calculations are thus simplified if the data for each resident are recast in terms of the number of days from admission (their "start" date) to (a) their first fall, or (b) their censoring date, whichever came first (their "end" date). The results are as follows:

TABLE 4.7.

Patient no.	Start date	End date	Follow-up time	Fell?
1	1/6	1/18	12	Yes
2	1/14	4/1	77	No
3	1/26	3/1	34	Yes
4	2/2	2/28	26	No
5	2/12	2/14	2	Yes
6	2/15	3/22	35	No
7	2/20	4/1	40	No
8	2/28	3/15	15	Yes
9	3/1	3/28	27	No
10	3/10	4/1	22	No
11	3/12	3/26	14	No
12	3/20	3/29	9	Yes

Only the last two columns are needed to carry out the calculations for the Kaplan-Meier method. It is convenient to sort the rows according to duration of follow-up, so that the timing of falls and censoring events is ordered from earliest to latest (Table 4.8).

The proportion *not* falling ("surviving") can then be calculated by the Kaplan-Meier method, as shown in Table 4.9. The rightmost column shows the final

TABLE 4.8.

Patient no.	Follow-up time	Fell?
5	2	Yes
12	9	Yes
1	12	Yes
11	14	No
8	15	Yes
10	22	No
4	26	No
9	27	No
3	34	Yes
6	35	No
7	40	No
2	77	No

estimates of cumulative incidence, calculated as (1 − proportion surviving). In this table, all the data were used, although follow-up times beyond 30 days are not needed to estimate 30-day cumulative incidence.

The cumulative incidence of falls over time can be summarized graphically as shown in Figure 4.8.

The estimated 30-day cumulative incidence of falls would be 0.344, or 34.4%.

2. You knew that the overall rate (here, the overall prevalence of weighing under 2,500 grams at birth) in a population is always a weighted average of subgroup-specific rates within that population, and that the weights are the proportion of the population in each subgroup. Because most of Allenville's pregnant mothers would be black, the prevalence for "All babies" in Allenville must lie closer to the prevalence for black mothers than to the prevalence for white mothers. For Town #1, the overall prevalence of 8% is closer to the 6% for whites than it is to the 12% for blacks, so Town #1 cannot be Allenville; it must be Bakertown. For Town #2, the overall prevalence of 15% is closer to the 18% prevalence for blacks than to the 9% prevalence in whites, which makes sense if it is, in fact, Allenville.

Having identified which town is which, it is easy to decide which is needier. The race-specific and overall prevalences of low birth weight are all higher in Allenville, so it gets the clinic.

3. The cumulative mortality (CM) in a closed population that is subject to a mortality rate (MR) of 9.1 deaths per 1,000 person-years for 7 years would be:

$$CM = 1 - \exp(-MR \times t)$$
$$= 1 - \exp(-9.1/1,000 \times 7)$$
$$= 0.0617$$

No. of deaths expected $= 332 \times 0.0617$
$$= 20.5$$

One might initially be tempted to think that 332 men followed for 7 years would experience 332×7 person-years at risk. Applying the rate of 9.1 per 1,000 person-years would then yield an estimate of $332 \times 7 \times .0091 = 21.1$ deaths. This answer would be not too far off, but it is an overestimate. The problem is that not all 332 men in this closed population would remain alive for all 7 years. Those who die would stop

TABLE 4.9.

Days since admission	No. at risk	No. of falls	No. of censorings	Proportion "surviving"	Cumulative incidence
0	12	0	0	1.000	0.000
2	12	1	0	$1.000 \times 11/12 = 0.917$	0.083
9	11	1	0	$0.917 \times 10/11 = 0.833$	0.167
12	10	1	0	$0.833 \times 9/10 = 0.750$	0.250
14	9	0	1	0.750	0.250
15	8	1	0	$0.750 \times 7/8 = 0.656$	0.344
22	7	0	1	0.656	0.344
26	6	0	1	0.656	0.344
27	5	0	1	0.656	0.344
34	4	1	0	$0.656 \times 3/4 = 0.492$	0.508
35	3	0	1	0.492	0.508
40	2	0	1	0.492	0.508
77	1	0	1	0.492	0.508

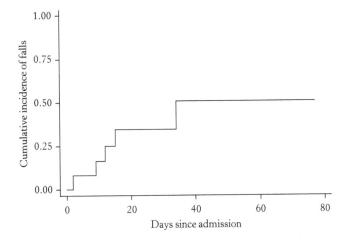

FIGURE 4.8

contributing person-years as soon as they died. The population at risk for dying would thus decline over time and would not experience a total of $332 \times 7 = 2{,}324$ person-years. (They would instead contribute about 2,251.5 person-years. Can you figure out how to get this number?) Assuming a constant mortality rate during the 7-year follow-up period, the first method automatically accounts for the declining population at risk over time.

4. The desired probability can be estimated as the cumulative incidence of second fracture in a hypothetical cohort of, say, 1,000 such women over the 15-year period from age 65 to age 80 years. For the first 5 years (ages 65 to 70), the cohort would be subject to an incidence rate of $43/1{,}209$ second fractures per woman-year at risk. For the next 10 years (ages 70 to 80), the rate would increase to $111/1{,}758$. Thus:

$$N(0) = \text{No. at risk for a second fracture}$$
$$\text{at time 0 } (= \text{age 65})$$

$$= 1{,}000$$

$$N(5) = \text{No. still at risk for a second fracture}$$
$$\text{at year 5 } (= \text{age 70})$$

$$= N(0) \cdot e^{(-IR \times t)}$$

$$= 1{,}000 \cdot e^{(-43/1{,}209 \times 5)}$$

$$= 837.1$$

$$N(15) = \text{No. still at risk for a second}$$
$$\text{fracture at year 15 } (= \text{age 80})$$

$$= 837.1 \cdot e^{(-111/1{,}758 \times 10)}$$

$$= 445$$

The results are shown graphically in Figure 4.9.

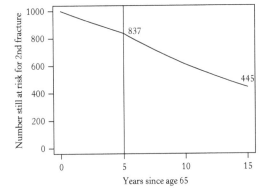

FIGURE 4.9

The desired 15-year cumulative incidence would be $(1{,}000 - 445)/1{,}000 = 0.555$, or 55.5%.

5. One might naïvely think that 100 women initially at risk and observed for four years would experience 400 woman-years at risk, yielding $400 \times 25/100 = 100$ HPV infections—in other words, that all 100 women would become infected. The fallacy of this method becomes obvious if the observation period is extended to five years, yielding 125 newly HPV-infected women out of 100 women for a cumulative incidence of 125%—clearly an impossibility.

Instead, the number of women remaining at risk for HPV infection would decline steadily during the four-year college period. As soon as a woman becomes HPV-infected, she is no longer "at risk" for HPV infection and stops contributing person-time at risk. Fortunately, decline in the population at risk is accounted for in the formula $CI = 1 - \exp(-IR \cdot t)$. In this case, the expected four-year cumulative incidence of HPV infection would be $1 - \exp(-25/100 \cdot 4) \approx 0.63$. In other words, we expect

TABLE 4.10.

	HRT use			
	Never	Past only	Current	Total
Cases	1,142	391	740	2,273
No. of women	474,682	186,751	287,143	
Average no. of years at risk	5.30	5.05	5.34	
Total woman-years at risk	2,515,815	943,093	1,533,344	4,992,278
Incidence rate[a]	45.4	41.5	48.3	45.5

[a] Cases per 100,000 woman-years at risk

TABLE 4.11.

	HRT use			
	Never	Past only	Current	Total
Deaths	819	275	497	1,591
No. of women	474,682	186,751	287,143	
Average no. of years at risk	6.92	6.72	6.89	
Total woman-years at risk	3,284,799	1,254,967	1,978,415	6,518,181
Mortality rate[a]				24.4

[a] Deaths per 100,000 woman-years at risk

that 63 of the 100 women would become HPV-infected.

6. (a) Although no new women were added after recruitment was complete, women were followed during the study for widely varying lengths of time. A woman's time at risk depended on her year of entry into the study, on the last year for which cancer registry data were available in her area, and on whether she died during the study. Hence a person-time approach to quantifying incidence is more suitable than a cumulative-incidence approach.

Total person-time at risk for each exposure group can be estimated as (number of women) × (average time at risk). (A Total column has been included in Table 4.10 for later use in part (b).)

Compared to never-users of HRT, the incidence of ovarian cancer was slightly higher in current users and slightly lower in past users.

(b) Time under surveillance for death averaged nearly 7 years, while time under surveillance for incident cancer averaged a little over 5 years. Because they were ascertained over time periods of different length, it would not be valid simply to divide the total number of deaths by the total number of cancer cases. However, if it is assumed that incidence and mortality rates were stable over time, we can use the relation (mortality) ≈ (incidence) × (case fatality). It can be re-expressed as (case fatality) ≈ (mortality) / (incidence).

The overall incidence rate can be calculated as (total cases) / (total woman-years), as shown in Table 4.10, giving 45.5 cases/100,000 woman-years. The overall mortality rate can be similarly calculated as shown in Table 4.11.

The estimated case fatality would thus be 24.4/45.5 = 0.54 = 54%.

7. No. The prevalence of heart failure depends on two things: the incidence of heart failure and the average duration of the condition among those who get it. There is no reason to expect that the new forms of treatment would affect the incidence of heart failure in any way, because these treatments would be applied only to those who had heart failure, not to susceptibles. However, if the new treatments prolonged survival of heart failure patients (without curing the condition), then the average heart failure patient would have the disease for a longer period of time. This longer average duration would be expected to lead, in turn, to an *increased* population prevalence of heart failure.

8. No, because the different lung condition categories being added together are not mutually exclusive. A death from acute bronchitis or pneumonia could

occur in a person who had chronic bronchitis, emphysema, or asthma as an underlying contributing condition. Hence the same death could be counted twice: once for the acute bronchitis or pneumonia, and again for the underlying chronic lung condition. Note, for example, that the three subcategories under bronchitis, emphysema, and asthma add to more than the category total, probably because the same death certificate could list more than one of the subcategory conditions.

To be additive, incidence or mortality rates must be based on *non-overlapping* case definitions—a requirement not met in this example.

5

Overview of Study Designs

We're all of us guinea pigs in the laboratory of God.

—TENNESSEE WILLIAMS

An epidemiologic study generally begins with a question. Once the research question has been specified, the next step in trying to answer it is to choose a study design.

A study design is a plan for selecting study subjects and for obtaining data on them. Study subjects in epidemiology are typically individual people, but at times they can be other kinds of "observation units", such as social groups, places, time periods, even published studies. Information on study subjects can come from pre-existing sources or can be gathered anew by various methods, including direct observation, interviews, questionnaires, physical examinations, or physiological measurements.

In principle, the number of possible study designs is infinite. But in practice, a few standard designs account for most epidemiologic research. Collectively, these standard designs are flexible enough and efficient enough to address a wide range of research questions. Knowledge of their pros and cons can usually guide the investigator to a study design that is well matched to a particular research question. This chapter aims to provide a broad overview by introducing several standard study designs and terms that are commonly used to describe them and distinguish them from each other. Later chapters cover several specific designs in more depth.

Design Tree

Just as there are many possible study designs, there are many possible ways to classify them, depending on which features are highlighted. Figure 5.1 is a tree diagram that organizes designs according to important distinguishing features. Major branches of this tree include:

- *Descriptive* studies are often among the earliest studies done on a new disease, in order to characterize it, quantify its frequency, and/or determine how its frequency varies in relation to demographic characteristics, place, and time. Their distinguishing characteristic is that they are undertaken without a specific hypothesis about causes or patterns of association.
- *Analytic* studies are undertaken to test one or more specific hypotheses, usually about whether a certain exposure influences the risk of a disease. Analytic studies, in turn, can be divided into two main kinds:

  - In *randomized* studies, random chance is used to assign subjects to different exposure groups.
  - In *non-randomized* studies, no formal chance mechanism governs which subjects are exposed and which are not. Sometimes the investigator has the ability to assign subjects to different exposure conditions and elects to do so non-randomly. But more often the investigator is merely a passive observer, with no control at all over subjects' exposure to the factor of interest. Several of the most commonly used non-randomized analytic study designs are described in this chapter, with brief mention of a few others.

Another feature that distinguishes study designs is the unit of study itself. In most epidemiologic research, the study subjects are individual people, each of whom can be determined to have been exposed or not and diseased or not. In *ecological*

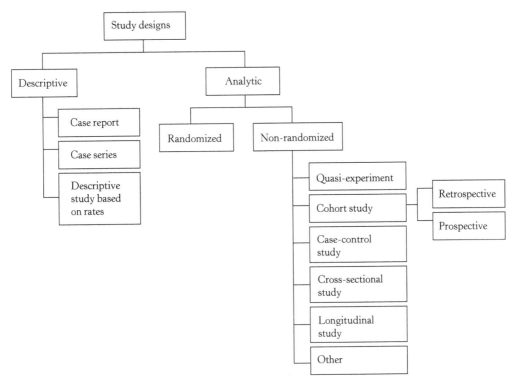

FIGURE 5.1 Major epidemiologic study designs.

studies, the units of study are entire groups of people, as for example when mortality rates by state are examined in relation to each state's per-capita income. As discussed in Chapter 16, ecological studies can themselves be categorized in much the same way as can studies of individuals. The unit of study can thus be regarded as a separate dimension or "layer" on which studies can be classified, beyond those shown in Figure 5.1.

DESCRIPTIVE STUDIES
The hallmark of a descriptive study is that it is undertaken without a specific hypothesis.

Case Reports
A *case report* describes some notable clinical occurrence, such as an unusual combination of signs and symptoms, experience with a novel treatment, or a sequence of events that may suggest a previously unsuspected causal relationship. German physician Alois Alzheimer introduced the medical world to the disease that came to bear his name through a case report describing the clinical and neuropathological features he observed in just one afflicted woman (Alzheimer, 1906). A case report can alert others to

be on the lookout for similar occurrences, lead to more formal attempts to quantify the magnitude of the problem, or suggest a possible association for follow-up in other studies. It is generally reported simply as a clinical narrative.

Example 5-1. Roselle *et al.* (2008) reported on a 62-year-old woman who sought care for an illness of several weeks' duration, characterized by nausea, vomiting, fever, diarrhea, and flu-like symptoms. During clinical evaluation, she reported having taken red yeast rice capsules as a nutritional supplement twice daily for several months. Blood tests showed a sharply elevated levels of aspartate aminotransferase (which suggests abnormal liver function), and abdominal ultrasonography showed an enlarged liver. A liver biopsy showed changes consistent with drug-induced hepatitis. Investigating further, her physicians found that red yeast supplements contain lovastatin, a lipid-lowering agent, which can cause hepatitis as a side effect. Her symptoms cleared up over several weeks after being advised to stop taking red yeast supplements. Her physicians published a brief description of her clinical story as an alert to other medical professionals about a possibly unappreciated side effect of a commonly used herbal supplement.

Strictly speaking, a case report may not fully qualify as a "study design." It often results from serendipity, rather than as a planned strategy for answering a research question that was specified in advance. Nonetheless, a case report can often provide the first suggestion of a possible new problem or association, which is then explored further with other study designs.

Case Series

A case report shows that something can happen once; a *case series* shows that it can happen repeatedly. A case series also provides an opportunity to identify common features among multiple cases and to describe patterns of variability among them.

Example 5-2. Between June 2005 and February 2008, more cases of avian influenza A (H5N1) ("avian flu") were identified in Indonesia than in any other country (Kandun *et al.*, 2008). This disease, which can be transmitted from birds to humans, is of special concern because it is clinically more severe than illness due to other strains of the influenza virus. Mutation of the virus could potentially allow it to spread from human to human and cause many deaths in an influenza pandemic.

Indonesian investigators described the clinical features of 127 avian flu cases who met a case definition set by the World Health Organization. Almost all (93%) had fever within the first two days of illness, but only 35% had a cough, 17% had rhinorrhea, and 1% had muscle aches, all of which are considered typical flu symptoms. Many patients did develop respiratory symptoms as their illness progressed. Case fatality was very high: 103/127 = 81%. Factors associated with a fatal outcome included delayed initiation of antiviral treatment and not being part of a cluster of cases who shared exposure to the same source. The researchers stressed the need for rapid, specific laboratory tests for avian flu in view of the non-specific clinical picture, as such a test could facilitate earlier treatment initiation and disease control efforts.

As noted in Chapter 2, a case series that includes *all* cases in a defined population can be of special value because it avoids the selection bias that can accompany referral of certain kinds of patients to a particular clinical center. Extrapolating results from one setting to another must always be done with caution, but one can at least be more confident that the cases in a population-based case series are representative of cases in the setting where they arose.

Descriptive Studies Based on Rates

A *descriptive study based on rates* combines data on a population-based set of cases with denominator data. It quantifies the population burden of disease, using incidence, prevalence, mortality, or other measures of disease frequency, as discussed in earlier chapters. Often such studies use data from existing sources, such as birth and death certificates, ongoing disease registries or surveillance systems, or periodic health surveys. New data collection may be undertaken if the problem is important enough and there are no satisfactory pre-existing data.

A descriptive epidemiologic study based on rates often involves exploratory comparisons of disease frequency in relation to personal characteristics, place, and time. Ordinarily these comparisons are made without advance hypotheses about what they might show, so the term *descriptive* still fits. These studies can be a rich source of hypotheses that lead to later analytic studies.

Example 5-3. Methicillin-resistant *Staphylococcus aureus* (MRSA) is a bacterial pathogen that can infect various body sites, causing serious and sometimes fatal illness. Many cases arise in health care settings, where the bacteria can enter normally sterile body cavities via catheters, surgery, or other invasive procedures. MRSA infection can be difficult to treat because of the organism's resistance to antibiotics that historically were effective against *S. aureus*.

Community-wide surveillance for invasive MRSA infection has been coordinated by the U.S. Centers for Disease Control and Prevention. In one investigation (Kallen *et al.*, 2010), qualifying cases were identified and reported by clinical laboratories in nine U.S. metropolitan areas with a collective population of about 15 million people. During a four-year study period, 21,503 invasive MRSA cases were identified, about 72% of them apparently hospital-acquired and the rest community-acquired. Overall incidence declined during the four-year study period from 3.21 to 2.63 cases per 10,000 person-years. Incidence rates varied nearly 100-fold by age, being highest in infants and older adults, and lowest in children beyond infancy. Invasive MRSA incidence was greater in males than females and higher in African-Americans than in other racial groups.

The researchers noted that the encouraging downward trend in the incidence of invasive MRSA over time might have been due in part to aggressive programs to prevent MRSA transmission within health care settings.

ANALYTIC STUDIES

The hallmark of an analytic study is that it is undertaken to test a hypothesis. In epidemiology, a typical hypothesis concerns whether a certain *exposure* causes a certain *outcome*, such as whether cigarette smoking causes lung cancer. Diagrammatically:

$$\text{Exposure} \xrightarrow{\;?\;} \text{Outcome}$$

FIGURE 5.2

The term *exposure* is used very generally in epidemiology to refer to any trait, behavior, environmental factor, or other characteristic being investigated as a possible cause. Closely related terms include *potential risk factor, putative cause, independent variable,* or *predictor.*

The *outcome* in epidemiologic studies of disease etiology is occurrence of disease. However, the same research designs that can be used to study disease etiology can also be used to study disease consequences. For example, a randomized trial can be used to determine whether receiving a new vaccine reduces the risk of developing a disease, and a randomized trial can also be used to study whether one treatment is better than another at prolonging survival among patients who develop the disease. The broader term *outcome* thus has the advantage of applying to both etiologic and clinical studies. Essentially synonymous terms include *end-point, response,* or *dependent variable.*

Why is presence or absence of a hypothesis so important? Specifying a primary exposure and a primary outcome quickly narrows the field of suitable design choices and guides the final selection among them. Characteristics of the primary exposure and outcome largely dictate which study designs would be feasible and, among the feasible designs, which ones have the potential to yield the most valid results and greatest efficiency. Important characteristics of the exposure include whether it is potentially modifiable, whether it is potentially modifiable *by the investigator,* how common it is in a potential study population, and where data on the exposure status of study subjects would come from. Important characteristics of the outcome include its frequency in a potential

study population and how a study subject's outcome status would be determined. The frequency of the exposure and outcome are also key determinants of how large a study would need to be.

The directional arrow from exposure to outcome in Figure 5.2 is worth noting. It indicates that the hypothesis motivating an analytic study nearly always concerns whether the exposure actually *causes* the outcome, not merely whether the two are associated. Chapter 8 discusses the kinds of evidence that support an inference of causality. One firm requirement is that the exposure must *precede* the outcome in time. Some analytic study designs provide stronger evidence than others about whether this condition is met.

Closely related to the goal of evaluating the effect of an exposure on an outcome is the idea of *counterfactuals* or *potential outcomes.* As a thought experiment, an ideal way to determine whether a certain exposure causes a certain outcome for a certain individual would be to:

1. Arrange for the individual to be exposed to the factor of interest, and examine his/her outcome after a suitable time interval; then...
2. "Turn back the clock," and arrange for the same individual to be *un*exposed to the factor of interest under identical circumstances, and examine his/her outcome after the same time interval.

Given the outcomes under both conditions, it would be self-evident whether the exposure is or is not a cause of the outcome for that person. If both outcomes are the same, then it made no difference whether the person was exposed or not, and exposure cannot be said to be a cause. But if the two outcomes differ, then the exposure did affect the outcome. If the outcome under condition #1 was better than that under condition #2, then the exposure was beneficial; otherwise, it was harmful.

Needless to say, this study design is not among the designs described later in this chapter, mainly because it cannot actually be carried out. It is not possible to compare outcomes for the same person under both exposed and nonexposed conditions at the same time under the same circumstances. In the real world, only one of the two exposure conditions prevails: a given study subject is either exposed or not exposed, and he/she experiences a certain outcome. The other exposure condition is *counterfactual*—an imaginary condition that did not actually occur. Viewed from another angle, the outcome under whichever exposure condition actually occurred is the outcome observed, while the outcome that would have occurred under the other exposure condition is a *potential* outcome that is not observed.

Even though such a thought experiment cannot actually be carried out, different real-world study designs can be viewed as producing different kinds of evidence about what would have occurred under counterfactual conditions. In a randomized trial, for example, observed outcomes in the control group provide an estimate of what would have happened in the intervention group if they had not been intervened upon. In a simple before–after study, a subject's pre-exposure status is assumed to provide an estimate of what his/her post-exposure status would have been in the absence of exposure; any before–after difference is ascribed (rightly or wrongly) to the exposure.

Another distinction between the idealized thought experiment and real-world epidemiologic studies is that most epidemiologic studies do not actually produce estimates of causal effects *for individual study subjects*. Rather, most designs produce evidence about the effect of the exposure on the outcome *on average*. With a few exceptions, the key comparisons in most epidemiologic study designs are between groups, not within individuals. This is not necessarily a limitation if, as in most research situations, the eventual goal is to gauge the likely effects of an exposure in other people besides the individuals who actually take part in a study. Average effects can serve this purpose.

Randomized Trials

Randomized trials occupy a special place among epidemiologic research designs. Other things being equal, results from randomized trials can offer a firmer basis for an inference of causality than results obtained from any other study design. The design's key feature is that a formal chance mechanism is used to assign participants either to receive an intervention (exposure) of interest or to serve as a control. Subjects are then followed over time to measure one or more outcomes, such as occurrence of a disease. Chapter 13 covers randomized trials in some depth, including several design variations.

A generic two-arm, parallel-groups randomized trial is diagrammed in Figure 5.3. From some source of potential study subjects, such as patients receiving care from a given source, potential candidates

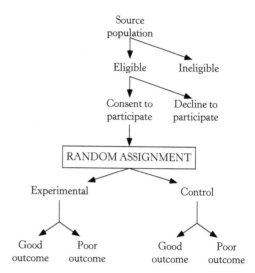

FIGURE 5.3 Two-arm parallel-groups randomized trial.

are screened for eligibility. Those found to be eligible are then asked to give their informed consent to participate in the trial. Consenting subjects are then randomized by a formal chance mechanism to one of two groups or *arms* of the trial, here called *experimental* and *control*. Subjects in the experimental arm receive a study intervention to be evaluated; those in the control arm do not receive that intervention and instead receive no intervention, a placebo, a specific alternative treatment, or "usual care". Both groups are then followed over time, and the incidence of one or more outcomes is compared between groups.

Example 5-4. Older adults who experience a fall are known to be at high risk for falling again, which can result in injury and impaired mobility. Researchers in central England sought to evaluate a program that was intended to reduce recurrent falls (Logan *et al.*, 2010). Emergency medical personnel in four primary-care districts screened adults age 60 years or older who had fallen and for whom an ambulance was called, but who did not require transport to a hospital. Of 252 such fallers, 230 were found to meet study eligibility criteria (i.e., were well enough to participate and were not already enrolled in a fall-prevention program), and 204 of them consented to participate in the trial. They were randomly assigned to two equal-sized groups, experimental and control. Nearly all of those assigned to the experimental group received a multifaceted program that included supervised balance and strength training exercises, home environmental modification to remove trip hazards and install grab bars in the bathtub or shower, medical review by a nurse to avoid overmedication and maintain good blood pressure control, and group seminars on fall prevention. Those assigned to the control group received a letter advising them to continue using social and medical services as usual. All participants kept a diary in which they recorded any falls they experienced, mailing in a summary monthly. Telephone follow-up calls were made as needed each month to obtain complete outcome data.

During the year following enrollment, the incidence rate of falls was 3.46 falls per person-year in the experimental group—still high, but less than half the incidence rate of 7.68 falls per person-year in the control group. The incidence of fall-related ambulance calls was also 40% lower in the experimental group, and several measures of physical health also showed improvement. The researchers concluded that the fall-prevention program had been beneficial and suggested that it be implemented and evaluated in other settings.

Randomization generally provides excellent control over *confounding* (discussed below), even by factors that may be hard to measure or that may be unknown to the investigator. A difference in outcomes between the groups formed by randomization that exceeds the limits of chance can be ascribed with high confidence to the difference in exposure status that the study was designed to investigate. As this example shows, randomized trials also provide information on the actual incidence of outcome events, because they involve monitoring two or more groups over time. Finally, they can be used to compare multiple outcomes between treatment arms without having to alter the basic study design.

For all their virtues, randomized trials have not been the source of data for most inferences regarding disease causation. Some exposures, such as genetic markers or family history, are not readily modifiable. For many other exposures of concern, such as cigarette smoking or water pollution, it is not feasible or ethical to allow chance to dictate which persons are to incur them. Randomized trials can also be too expensive or impractical if the primary outcome of interest is very rare, or if long periods of follow-up would be required before intervention effects would appear.

Non-randomized Studies

In non-randomized studies, regardless of the nature of the exposure—a genetic trait, a lifestyle choice, a feature of the physical or social environment, or whatever—the researcher must assume that it is not distributed at random in the population. Inevitably there are various other differences between exposed and non-exposed persons, and some of the characteristics on which they differ may also affect disease risk in their own right. Hence a key methodological issue in all non-randomized studies is *confounding*: distortion of an exposure–outcome association due to their mutual association with another factor or factors. Confounding is discussed in depth in Chapters 11 and 12.

Most non-randomized studies are termed *observational* studies, because the investigator plays the more passive role of observer rather than experimenter. (An exception would be *quasi-experiments*, discussed below, which involve an intervention.)

Non-randomized Intervention Studies ("Quasi-experiments")

In a *non-randomized intervention trial* or *quasi-experiment*, the investigator actually controls the assignment of study subjects to either an experimental or a control condition, but elects to do so by a process other than randomization. The term *quasi-experiment*, borrowed from the social sciences (Campbell and Stanley, 1966), distinguishes these studies from randomized trials, which have been called "true" experiments. A non-randomized intervention trial design is most useful when the investigator has some control over which study subjects are exposed to which condition, but when cost, logistics, or political considerations preclude using randomization to make those assignments. A design diagram for a quasi-experiment would look just like Figure 5.3, except that "random assignment" would be replaced by "non-random allocation."

Example 5-5. The Living 4 Life study sought to test the effectiveness of a school-based, youth-driven program to decrease obesity among adolescents in New Zealand (Utter *et al.*, 2011). Six schools in southern Auckland were studied: four intervention schools in the Mangere region and two schools with similar ethnic and socioeconomic composition that were far enough from the intervention schools to minimize possible spillover of the intervention. The intervention was developed in consultation with community leaders and student health councils.

Components included lunch and breakfast activities (some involving exercise), dances, "health weeks," changes to the eating environment in schools, and attempts to reduce television viewing time and to improve the quality of foods available at school. Over the three-year intervention period, the prevalence of obesity actually increased from 32% to 35% at intervention schools and from 29% to 30% at control schools. The investigators concluded that the intervention lacked sufficient potency to cause meaningful changes in eating and exercise behavior, and that obesity prevention efforts may need to start earlier than adolescence to be effective.

In this example, the exposure status of each student was determined by which school he/she attended, each school being assigned non-randomly to intervention or control conditions. Having all four experimental schools be located near one another facilitated involving community leaders in developing the intervention, and having two control schools in a separate region was intended to prevent their "contamination" by intervention activities at experimental-group schools.

An important potential problem with non-randomized trials is that the non-random process of exposure assignment can cause the comparison groups to differ systematically on factors that influence study outcomes. This places a greater burden on the researcher to deal with such potential confounding, and it can be a challenge to identify, measure, and control for all relevant confounding factors. Because confounding is also a key methodological issue in observational studies, non-randomized trials are often regarded as more closely akin to cohort studies (discussed below) than to randomized trials.

Cohort Studies

A *cohort study* involves comparing disease incidence over time between groups that differ on their exposure to a factor of interest. The cohort study design is discussed in depth in Chapter 14.

Example 5-6. Oral contraceptives were first approved for public use in the early 1960s. Although clinical testing had shown them to be highly effective for preventing pregnancy, there was concern that because they contain biologically active doses of female sex hormones, they might also affect the risk of cancer of the female reproductive organs and

breast. Detecting effects on the risk of rare but serious cancers would require studying large numbers of women.

During a 14-month period beginning in May 1968, about 47,000 women of reproductive age were identified from among the patients of 1,400 British physicians who were members of the Royal College of General Practitioners (Hannaford *et al.*, 2007; Beral *et al.*, 1988). By design, about half of these women were using oral contraceptives at the time of their recruitment, and the other half were never-users. All were either married or living as married.

For the next 28 years, participating physicians provided updated data twice per year on all study women who remained under their care, including month-by-month data on oral contraceptive use and on the occurrence of various fatal or non-fatal illnesses. Women who were initially in the never-user group but who later began using oral contraceptives were switched to the ever-user group at that time. After 1996, active follow-up through physicians was discontinued, but most participants had agreed to allow passive follow-up thereafter for cancer occurrence through British population-based cancer registries.

Results of the study were published regularly over many years as evidence accumulated. Through 2004, about 744,000 woman-years at risk had accrued in ever-users of oral contraceptives and 339,000 woman-years among never-users. Table 5.1 summarizes the number of cases and incidence rates for selected cancers. The incidence rates shown were adjusted for several potential confounding factors, using techniques to be covered in Chapter 11, to make the comparisons between groups more valid. The ratio of rates in ever-users to that in never-users is also shown as a measure of strength of the exposure–outcome association, with 95% confidence limits to convey the precision of that estimated ratio. Overall, ever-use of oral contraceptives was associated with lower risk of cancers of the uterine body and ovary. A small elevation was seen in the incidence of invasive cervical cancer, and a slight reduction in that of breast cancer, but both of these observed associations were within the bounds of chance given no true association.

The Royal College of General Practitioners Oral Contraception Study illustrates several features of a cohort study. The first step was to identify two groups of women, exposed and non-exposed— here, oral contraceptive users and non-users. As is

TABLE 5.1. INCIDENCE OF CANCER OF REPRODUCTIVE ORGANS AND BREAST IN RELATION TO ORAL CONTRACEPTIVE USE AMONG WOMEN IN THE ROYAL COLLEGE OF GENERAL PRACTITIONERS ORAL CONTRACEPTION STUDY

Cancer type	No. of cases		Incidence rate[a]		Relative incidence (A ÷ B)	
	Ever-users	Never-users	Ever-users (A)	Never-users (B)	Est.	(95% CI)
Uterus						
Invasive cervix	118	36	14.9	11.2	1.33	(0.92–1.94)
Uterine body	81	75	11.3	19.5	0.58	(0.42–0.79)
Ovary	96	93	13.2	24.7	0.54	(0.40–0.71)
Breast	891	448	121.5	124.2	0.98	(0.87–1.10)

[a] Cases per 100,000 woman-years, adjusted for age, parity, smoking, and social class
(Based on data from Hannaford *et al.* [2007])

common in cohort studies, the relative sizes of these two groups did not necessarily reflect the prevailing frequency of exposure in the study setting. Rather, two equal-sized groups of about 23,000 women each were chosen for scientific reasons—namely, to enhance the power of the study to find exposure–outcome associations if they existed. Forming two equal-sized exposure groups at the outset thus involved selecting oral contraceptive users and non-users with different sampling probabilities from the clientele of participating physicians. In this case, a woman's exposure status could change over time. A never-user who began using oral contraceptives during the study switched to the ever-user group thereafter. Hence the relative sizes of the groups shifted over time. Because each exposure group was an open population, person-time incidence rates were used to quantify the frequency of cancer.

Two major subtypes of cohort studies can be distinguished: *prospective* and *retrospective*. Figures 5.4 and 5.5 diagram the two subtypes. The key difference concerns when the outcomes of interest occur relative to when the study is begun in calendar time. As Figure 5.4 shows, in a prospective cohort study, the study is initiated before any of the outcomes that will eventually be counted and analyzed have occurred. The Royal College of General Practitioners Oral Contraception Study was a prospective cohort study: subject recruitment began in 1968, and all of the cancer cases of interest occurred in subsequent years as the research proceeded.

In contrast, Figure 5.5 shows a retrospective cohort study. The key difference is that the outcomes of interest *have already occurred* by the time the study is mounted. Essentially, a retrospective cohort study involves reconstructing a cohort study that has already taken place. Yet the basic architecture of the study design is the same: first, exposed and non-exposed groups of subjects are formed; and second, the two groups are monitored over time to assess the incidence of outcomes of interest.

Example 5-7. Hydroxymethylglutaryl coenzyme A reductase inhibitors, commonly called *statins*, are among the most widely prescribed medications in the United States. They are mainly used to reduce blood cholesterol levels and thus to prevent heart disease, but studies in experimental animals have suggested that statins could also reduce age-related loss of bone density. If this effect of statins carried over to humans, reduced risk of a fracture could be a beneficial side effect of taking statins.

In 2000, Ray *et al.* initiated a retrospective cohort study of statin use in relation to incidence of hip fractures. The study used automated databases from the Tennessee Medicaid program, which paid for prescription medications and hospitalization costs for low-income state residents. The researchers identified 12,506 Medicaid enrollees who had begun using statins at some time during the ten-year period from 1989–1998. For comparison, they identified 4,798 enrollees who had begun using a non-statin cholesterol-lowering drug during the same period, and 17,280 demographically similar persons selected

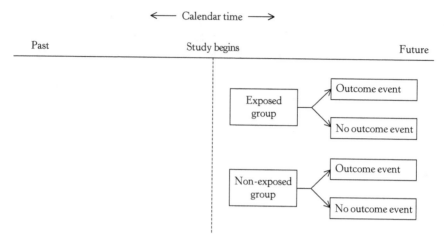

FIGURE 5.4 Prospective cohort study.

at random from among the many Medicaid enrollees who had not used either type of drug. Hip fracture incidence was then ascertained for these three exposure groups from computerized hospital discharge billing records through 1998.

Among statin users, 49 hip fractures occurred in 24,512 person-years, for an incidence rate of 2.00 hip fractures per 1,000 person-years. The corresponding rate in users of non-statin cholesterol-lowering drugs was 17/8,990 = 1.89 fractures per 1,000 person-years, and that in non-users was 120/33,189 = 3.62 fractures per 1,000 person-years. The investigators concluded that statins may indeed reduce the risk of hip fracture and that the other cholesterol-lowering drugs studied may have a similar effect. Alternatively, the underlying condition for which a cholesterol-lowering drug is prescribed may itself

be causally or non-causally associated with lower hip fracture risk, regardless of how the condition is treated (Ray *et al.*, 2002).

Two features of retrospective cohort studies are illustrated by this example. First, even though the study involved up to 10 years of follow-up for hip fracture occurrence in study subjects, completing the study took much less time—essentially, the time needed to perform the analysis on computerized databases that already existed. Second, the study depended heavily on having suitable pre-existing data that had been collected for other purposes. Unlike the prospective cohort study in Example 5-6, investigators on the retrospective cohort study did not have the option of collecting additional data from study subjects at baseline or during follow-up to meet

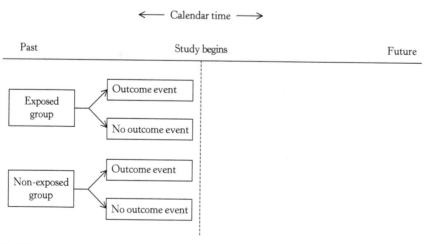

FIGURE 5.5 Retrospective cohort study.

the needs of their research. In this case, little information was available in Medicaid databases on other potential confounding factors such as smoking and obesity status—an acknowledged limitation of the study.

The terms *prospective* and *retrospective* have historically been troublesome because of ambiguity about the time scale to which they refer. In times past, *cohort study* and *prospective study* were sometimes treated as synonyms. And if the time scale is the life history of a study subject, then all cohort studies do indeed involve "looking forward" from the time of exposure toward possible occurrence of an outcome event later in life. But if the time scale is calendar time relative to when the study is begun, then some cohort studies involve looking backward at past outcome events, while others involve looking forward toward future outcome events. The inconsistency in meaning led to confusing, apparently self-contradictory study design labels such as "retrospective prospective study." Fortunately, the earlier ambiguous meaning is now deprecated (Porta, 2008) and largely abandoned. Most epidemiologists use the terms as they are used in this book.

Cohort studies have several generic strengths:

- Because they involve monitoring people over time for disease occurrence, cohort studies provide estimates of the actual incidence of disease in exposed and non-exposed persons. For example, Table 5.1 suggested that the incidence of invasive cervical cancer may have been about 1/3 higher among women who had used oral contraceptives than among never-users, but the study also showed that this form of cancer was still quite rare in both groups. This information could be helpful to women (and their physicians) who are weighing risks and benefits when deciding whether to begin oral contraceptive use.
- By design, exposure status is determined and recorded before any outcome events of interest have been identified in study subjects. In most instances, this feature provides unambiguous evidence that exposure preceded outcome, as required for causal inference.
- Like intervention trials, cohort studies also facilitate studying multiple outcomes in relation to the same exposure. As Table 5.1 shows, the Royal College of General

Practitioners Oral Contraception Study compared the incidence of several different forms of cancer between the same two exposure groups. In other analyses, the investigators also compared the incidence of cardiovascular, rheumatic, and other diseases as new hypotheses about possible effects of oral contraceptives came to light.
- Cohort studies are well suited to studying rare exposures. This is because the relative number of exposed and non-exposed persons in the study need not reflect true exposure prevalence in the population at large. This advantage was exploited in Example 5-7. Statin use was much less common in the 1990s than later. The investigators included all statin users but needed to study only a small fraction of the many non-statin users to provide an adequate comparison group.

Like intervention trials, prospective cohort studies are an inefficient way to study rare outcomes and/or outcomes that appear only long after exposure. Nonetheless, these problems can be overcome with very large study populations and/or by monitoring disease occurrence in them for a prolonged period. The oral-contraception study example shows that this strategy is possible, given sufficient resources and time.

Case-Control Studies

A *case-control study* involves comparing the frequency of past exposure between *cases* who develop the disease (or other outcome of interest) and *controls* who do not. The controls serve to estimate of the frequency of exposure in the population at risk that generated the cases. In terms of counterfactuals, the controls provide an estimate of the expected frequency of past exposure among cases if the cases had not developed the outcome. Figure 5.6 shows

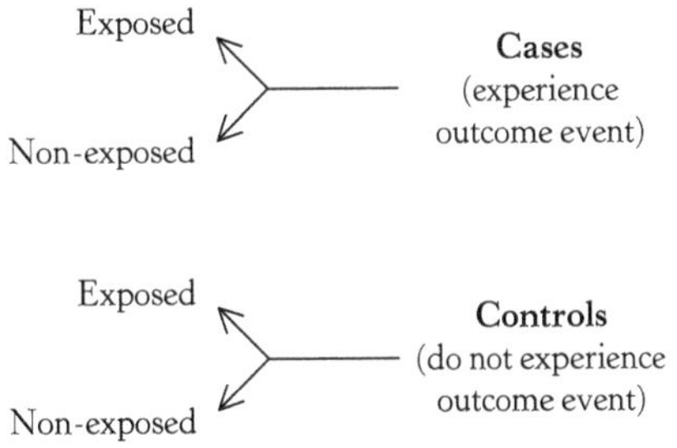

FIGURE 5.6 Case-control study.

a diagram of the case-control design, which is discussed more fully in Chapter 15.

Example 5-8.   An earlier study of statins and hip fracture, which had provided a stimulus for the retrospective cohort study in Example 5-7, employed a different study design (Wang *et al.*, 2000). It used data from three government-funded health care programs in New Jersey, which together paid for medications and hospitalizations for elderly indigent state residents. Over a 4.5-year period, 1,222 program enrollees had been hospitalized for a hip fracture, and they were termed the *cases*. The date of hospitalization for hip fracture became each case's *index date*. For comparison, 4,888 program enrollees were then selected who had not had a hip fracture, and they were termed the *controls*. The controls were sampled from the large number of enrollees without hip fracture in such a way that the control group would resemble the case group with regard to age and gender. Each control was assigned an index date, which was chosen at random from the distribution of index dates among cases. The researchers then determined past use of a statin or a non-statin cholesterol-lowering drug prior to each subject's index date, using computerized prescription records.

The results showed that 27 (2.2%) of the cases had used a statin drug in the 180 days before their index date, compared to 213 (4.4%) of the controls. A non-statin cholesterol-lowering drug had been used by 17 (1.4%) cases and by 81 (1.7%) controls during the same time period.

At first, a case-control study may appear to be attacking the problem backwards by proceeding from effect to cause. The paradox can be resolved, however, by noting that two different time sequences are at play. One is the causal chain of events leading to the disease or other outcome. As always, to qualify as a cause, the exposure must precede the outcome in a subject's lifetime. In the above example, the investigators examined only medication use prior to the occurrence of hip fracture in cases, or prior to a comparable index date in controls.

The other time sequence is the order in which information is gathered on exposure and disease in the process of carrying out the study. In a case-control study, the first step is to ascertain a subject's status on the outcome in order to determine whether he or she she qualifies as a case or control. Often cases are scarce while potential controls are plentiful, so all eligible cases may be included but only a fraction of all potential controls. The second step is then to gather information about past exposure for each case and control.

Estimating relative incidence from case-control data

The case-control study by Wang *et al.*, showed that previous use of a statin was less common among hip fracture cases (2.2%) than among controls (4.4%). The retrospective cohort study by Ray *et al.* showed that hip fracture incidence was lower among statin users (2.00 per 1,000 person-years) than among non-users (3.62 per 1,000 person-years). Thus, the two studies broadly agreed in finding a negative association between statin use and hip fracture, consistent with the hypothesis that statin use might be protective.

Perhaps surprisingly, however, it is possible to quantify the exposure–outcome association in a case-control study in such a way that it can be compared directly with results from a cohort study. The key measure of association that permits such a comparison is *relative incidence*, defined as $\frac{\text{Incidence in exposed persons}}{\text{Incidence in non-exposed persons}}$. This measure will be discussed in depth in Chapter 9 and is also known as the *relative risk*; or, when incidence is expressed as a rate, as the *rate ratio*. It is a very commonly used measure of strength of association. Calculating relative incidence from results of a cohort study is straightforward, because both the numerator and denominator are measured directly. In the retrospective cohort study by Ray *et al.*, the relative incidence was (2.00 hip fractures per 1,000 person-years) ÷ (3.62 hip fractures per 1,000 person-years) = 0.55. In words, hip fracture incidence in statin users was 0.55 times the incidence in non-users. It can also be interpreted as implying $(1 - 0.55) \times 100\% = 45\%$ lower incidence in users compared to non-users.

Estimating relative incidence from results of a case-control study is not so straightforward, because incidence is not directly measured in a case-control study. Consider the following exposure–outcome results from the Wang *et al.* case-control study:

TABLE 5.2.

Statin use?	Hip fracture?	
	Yes	No
Yes	27	213
No	1,195	4,675

(Based on data from Wang *et al.* [2000])

Any initial temptation to view $27/(27 + 213) = 0.1125$ as the "incidence" of hip fracture among statin users must be resisted, because it does not meet the definition of incidence. The population at risk underlying those 27 hip fracture cases in statin users was not just the $27 + 213 = 240$ statin users who made their way into the study; rather, the population at risk for those cases was *all statin users in the source population from which cases and controls were drawn*—a much larger denominator population, whose size cannot be determined from the data shown.

Even though neither the incidence in exposed nor the incidence in non-exposed groups can be obtained from case-control data alone, the *odds ratio* usually provides a good estimate of relative incidence from case-control data. Appendix 5A demonstrates why this is so. For the above table, the odds ratio is $\frac{27 \times 4,675}{213 \times 1,195} = 0.50$. It can be interpreted as meaning that the incidence of hip fracture in statin users was 0.5 times that in non-users. This result agrees well with the relative incidence of 0.55 from the retrospective cohort study by Ray *et al.* In both studies, additional analysis using techniques to be covered later yielded an *adjusted* relative incidence or odds ratio, and confidence limits for it. These results also agreed well between the two studies.

Case-control studies have several generic strengths:

- They are well suited to studying rare diseases. This is because a study's ability to detect an association between exposure and the risk of a rare disease is usually limited mainly by the small number of cases available. Under a case-control design, the investigator can start by casting a wide net for cases, perhaps through surveillance in a large population at risk or over a long time period. All qualifying cases that are found can then be included. But gathering exposure data on *all* non-cases in a large source population is seldom necessary and would, in fact, be a waste of resources, as will be illustrated later in this chapter.
- Case-control studies are also well suited to studying multiple exposures in relation to the same outcome. Once the case and control groups have been formed, studying an additional exposure may require little more than adding another question to an interview or another item to a data collection form.

- Case-control studies can often yield an answer relatively quickly, even when exposure affects outcome only after a long time period—an advantage they share with retrospective cohort studies. The reason is that case-control studies begin by ascertaining the outcome, and by that time, any long delay between exposure and outcome has already occurred.

Among their limitations, case-control studies do not directly yield information about the absolute incidence of disease in exposed and non-exposed persons. As discussed in Chapter 15, however, sometimes additional information about the sampling method and sampling fraction for controls, or about total disease incidence in the source population, can be combined with the results from a case-control study to estimate incidence in exposed and non-exposed individuals.

In contrast to the example on statin use and hip fracture, some case-control studies involve interviews with cases and controls to ascertain past exposure status. By the time the cases are interviewed, they are usually well aware that they have developed the disease, and this knowledge can influence their recall and/or reporting of past exposures. Cases may "ruminate" about the past in search of an explanation for their health misfortune and report an exposure that would have been overlooked or dismissed by a control. Alternatively, cases may purposefully deny a socially undesirable past exposure, such as a history of risky sexual behavior, if seeking to avoid blame. In either situation, differences in reporting of the same exposure by cases and controls are known as *recall bias*. This and other potential sources of error in measuring exposure status in case-control studies will be discussed further in Chapter 15.

Later in this chapter, we return to show how cohort study and case-control study designs employ different sampling strategies to investigate exposure–outcome associations. This difference is a major determinant of the number of study subjects required under each design, which often guides a choice between them.

Cross-Sectional Studies

All of the analytic study designs described thus far consider only exposures that precede the outcome in time. Intervention trials and cohort studies establish the exposure status of all subjects before any outcomes have occurred, while case-control studies limit themselves to exposures that occur prior to becoming a case.

In contrast, the distinguishing feature of a *cross-sectional study* is that exposure and outcome are ascertained as of the same point or period in time:

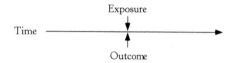

FIGURE 5.7

Example 5-9. Peart *et al.* (2011) studied 2,368 children aged 12–19 years who had participated in the National Health and Nutrition Examination Survey, in order to assess the relationship between television watching and body-mass index, a measure of fatness. At a single examination session, each child was asked standardized questions about their usual amount of television viewing. Height, weight, and other anthropometric measurements were also taken. Adolescents who reported watching two or more hours of television per day were significantly more likely to be overweight or obese than those who reported watching fewer than two hours of television per day.

This study found an association between obesity and watching more television, but it was not designed to determine which came first. Causality could work in either direction: prolonged physical inactivity from watching television could lead to obesity, or obesity could make a teenager less inclined to engage in vigorous exercise and more inclined to watch television.

Potential ambiguity about the direction of causality is a common limitation of cross-sectional studies. However, sometimes the causal arrow could plausibly point in only one direction—for example, if a cross-sectional study found an association between a genetic marker and disease, it would not be plausible that disease occurrence caused the genetic marker to appear or disappear.

Cross-sectional studies also characterize the exposure and disease status of study subjects as of a certain point in time or during the same short time interval. The cases are *prevalent* cases, not incident cases. As noted in Chapter 4, under this sampling scheme, the sample of cases tends to be skewed toward cases of longer duration. Hence an association found between exposure and disease in a cross-sectional study may actually represent an association with the chronicity of disease rather than with its incidence.

Unfortunately, as in many other fields of science, terms are not always used consistently in epidemiology. Sometimes "cross-sectional" has been used to refer to how subjects are sampled, rather than to the temporal relationship between exposure and outcome. In particular, some authors have used "cross-sectional" to mean that subjects are selected from a source population without regard to either exposure or outcome—a "cross-sectional sample" (Fleiss *et al.*, 2003). One must sometimes infer from the context which meaning was intended.

Longitudinal Studies

A longitudinal study involves measuring an outcome repeatedly over time on study subjects.

Example 5-10. New York City firefighters and emergency medical services personnel who responded to the World Trade Center attacks on September 11, 2001, were exposed to dense clouds of particulate matter from disintegrating building materials and chemicals from combustion. Aldrich *et al.* (2010) studied pulmonary function over time in 12,781 of those responders. All had had at least one lung-function examination (spirometry) before the disaster date, and repeat spirometry was scheduled every 12–18 months thereafter for the next six years. Average forced expiratory volume in one second (FEV_1), a measure of airway obstruction, was found to decline substantially in the year following the disaster, and it continued to decrease more gradually thereafter.

In this example, breathing contaminated air during the World Trade Center disaster was the exposure. The outcome, FEV_1, was measured before and repeatedly after the exposure. There was no separate control group; rather, any effects of exposure were inferred from the time path of FEV_1.

A pitfall with many longitudinal studies is that factors other than the exposure of interest may be partly or even fully responsible for any observed differences in outcomes. This problem can be considered a form of confounding. Variants of longitudinal designs can involve tracking aggregate measures of disease frequency over time in a population. As discussed in Chapter 21, these designs can be used as tools for evaluating the health effects of environmental changes or of policies—contexts in which it may be difficult or impossible to identify a concurrent non-exposed comparison group.

Other Study Designs

The study designs described above probably account for a large majority of epidemiologic research. However, various other designs have been developed for specialized purposes. A few among many are mentioned here.

The *case-crossover* design can be used to study effects of transient exposures on risk of acute conditions, such as injury, stroke, or myocardial infarction (Maclure, 1991; Maclure and Mittleman, 2000). The exposure status of cases at the time disease occurs is compared with their exposure status at one or more past reference times—e.g., the same day of the week and time of the day, but one week earlier. No disease-free control group is studied. For example, the case-crossover design has been used to study an association between a driver's use of a cellular telephone and the risk of a motor-vehicle crash (Redelmeier and Tibshirani, 1997). Case-crossover studies are discussed further in Chapter 18. A related design has been called the *self-controlled case series* design, which compares incidence rates between exposed and non-exposed periods within the same persons. It has been used to study a possible association between use of antipsychotic drugs and the risk of stroke (Douglas and Smeeth, 2008).

The *case-cohort* design involves comparing the exposure status of cases with that of a random sample of people (the "subcohort") selected from the full population that generated the cases (Prentice, 1986). Unlike the case-control design, cases may also be members of the subcohort. This design permits comparison of several case groups to the same subcohort. Among other applications, it can be an efficient alternative to a retrospective cohort study design when additional data collection is needed to obtain data on potential confounding factors.

The *case-only* design can be useful for studying gene–environment interactions (Khoury and Flanders, 1996). Using data from cases only, the investigator examines the association between presence of a genetic marker and presence of an environmental exposure. If these two characteristics can be assumed to occur independently in the population at large, then their co-occurrence among cases (more than would be predicted from the frequency of each one alone among the cases) can be interpreted as evidence of gene–environment interaction. Other applications of the case-only design are described in Chapter 15.

A *two-stage* study design can be useful for investigating a possible association between a rare exposure and a rare outcome (White, 1982). Even when exposure and outcome data are available or can be obtained inexpensively on a large population, additional data collection may still be required on additional variables, such as potential confounding factors. Different sampling fractions are used for subjects in each cell of a 2 × 2 table cross-classifying exposure and outcome, giving subjects in the less-populated cells a higher probability of being sampled for additional data collection.

Cohort and Case-Control Study Designs as Different Sampling Plans

Two of the main "workhorses" in observational epidemiologic research are the cohort and case-control study designs. Many research problems can be studied with either design, as illustrated by the statins and hip fracture examples described earlier, so an investigator is often faced with a choice.

The key distinction between the designs concerns how subjects are sampled to form the comparison groups. The two sampling strategies have different implications as to the number of study subjects required, which is one important factor in choosing a design. Contrasting the designs in terms of sampling plans also clarifies how a case-control study differs from a retrospective cohort study, both of which investigate exposure–outcome associations involving events that occurred in the past.

Consider a hypothetical research situation in which the aim is to determine whether a certain exposure is associated with occurrence of a certain disease. Say that all members of a closed population of 10,000 people were initially at risk three years ago, at which time some unknown fraction had the exposure. Between three years ago and the present time, an unknown number of disease cases have occurred.

Determining the association between exposure and disease can be framed in terms of the standard 2 × 2 table:

TABLE 5.3.

Exposed?	Diseased? Yes	No	Total
Yes			
No			
Total			10,000

A "brute force" option would be to gather exposure, disease, and any other necessary data on all 10,000 population members. But such a large undertaking may be needlessly costly and inefficient if the research question could be answered satisfactorily by gathering data on a much smaller subset of the full population. It is also possible that collecting data on all 10,000 people could be a wasted effort if it turns out that even 10,000 people are too few to provide a conclusive answer.

To choose an efficient study design, and to gauge whether it is likely to answer the research question, the investigator must first: (1) estimate the likely frequency of exposure in the study population; (2) estimate the likely frequency of disease; and (3) specify the size of the exposure–outcome association that the study should be able to detect. Estimates (1) and (2) can sometimes be based on pilot data, on previous research in the same or similar settings, or, in the absence of data, on opinions of people with subject-matter expertise and knowledge of the setting. Specifying (3) involves deciding how large an effect would matter for theory or practice. That target may be larger or smaller than observed associations in any previous studies or pilot investigations.

In this example, suppose that after exploring those sources, the investigator's best estimates are that: (1) about 25% of the population would have the exposure, and (2) the three-year cumulative incidence among non-exposed individuals would be about 1 per 100. The researcher also judges that if the relative incidence is 2.0 or greater, the study needs to be able to detect it. Under these assumptions and hypothesis, a possible retrospective cohort study and a possible case-control study can be sketched out and compared.

Cohort Study Approach

A cohort study would involve: (1) forming two groups of exposed and non-exposed persons as of three years ago, and then (2) ascertaining whether each member of each group subsequently developed disease. (Other data on potential confounding factors might also be needed on them.)

How many subjects would be required? Appendix 5B describes statistical methods for answering that question. It is not necessary for present purposes to understand all the details, only to know that such methods exist, what they require as inputs, and how the results can guide the choice of a study design. Reasonable inputs for sample-size calculations in this instance would be:

TABLE 5.4.

Input	Value	Description
α	0.05	Threshold for statistical significance; $\alpha = 0.05$ maps to $Z_\alpha \approx 1.96$ for two-tailed hypothesis tests
β	0.2	Specifies that study should have at least a $(1 - 0.2) = 0.8$ probability of yielding a statistically significant result if the true relative incidence is 2.0 or greater; $\beta = 0.2$ maps to $Z_\beta = 0.84$
p_0	1/100	Projected cumulative incidence in non-exposed group
p_1	2/100	Projected cumulative incidence in exposed group
k	1	Planned ratio of group sizes (non-exposed:exposed); $k = 1$ specifies equal-sized groups

Results of the calculations show that 2,319 exposed and 2,319 non-exposed subjects would be needed, for a total of 4,638 subjects. It is reassuring that, if the estimated frequency of exposure of 25% is close to the truth, there should be about 2,500 exposed and 7,500 non-exposed individuals in the full population. Thus, enough potential subjects appear to be available to populate both study groups.

Given that non-exposed persons are thought to outnumber exposed persons by 3:1 in the full population, why not mimic this ratio in the sizes of the two study groups? With this change (now $k = 3$), the sample-size calculations show that 1,435 exposed and 4,305 non-exposed subjects would be needed, for a total of 5,740 subjects. Using unequal-sized groups is less efficient: it requires collecting data on $5,740 - 4,638 = 1,102$ more study subjects than with equal-sized groups to achieve the same statistical power. More generally, Figure 5.8 shows that the fewest total study subjects are required when the groups are about equal in size.

Case-Control Study Approach

A case-control study would involve: (1) forming a case group of people who developed the disease within the previous three years and a control group of those who did not, and then (2) determining whether each case and control had previously been exposed. (Other data on potential confounding factors might also be needed on them.)

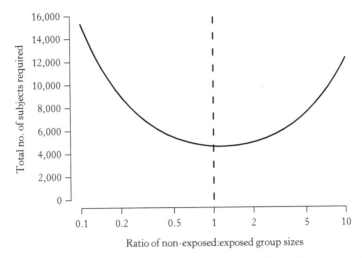

FIGURE 5.8 Total number of subjects needed for a hypothetical cohort study, in relation to ratio of study group sizes.

How many cases and controls would be required? The same statistical approach that was used for a cohort-study design can be used again, but with different inputs:

TABLE 5.5.

Input	Value	Description
α	0.05	Same as before
β	0.2	Same as before
p_0	0.25	Projected frequency of exposure among controls
p_1	0.4^a	Projected frequency of exposure among cases
k	1	Specifies equal-sized case and control groups (for now)

[a] This value results from use of the *odds ratio* to estimate relative incidence in a case-control study. When $p_1 = 0.4$ and $p_0 = 0.25$, odds ratio = 2.0. See Appendix 5B for a general formula.

The results are that 152 cases and 152 controls would be needed, for a total of 304 subjects. That is far fewer than the number of subjects needed for even the most efficient cohort-study design, and it illustrates why case-control studies can be very attractive for study of rare diseases. In this example, disease is relatively rare, while exposure is common.

But there is a problem. Using the best available estimates of exposure and disease frequency (mentioned above) and a hypothesized relative incidence

of 2.0, the projected 2×2 table for the entire source population would be:

TABLE 5.6.

	Diseased?		
Exposed?	Yes	No	Total
Yes	50	2,450	2,500
No	75	7,425	7,500
Total	125	9,875	10,000

Only 125 cases are projected to be available, while 152 cases are needed to achieve the desired study power under the case-control design being considered.

Fortunately, a scarcity of cases can be offset to some extent by an abundance of potential controls. In this example, if the control group is allowed to be twice the size of the case group (now $k = 2$), sample-size calculations show that 112 cases and 224 controls would give the same statistical power as 152 cases and 152 controls. The total number of subjects increases from 304 to 336, which may increase data collection costs, but 112 is a more achievable and defensible target number of cases. And 336 total subjects under the case-control design remains far fewer than the 4,638 subjects required under the most efficient cohort design.

There are limits on the extent to which more controls can compensate for a scarcity of cases, however. Figure 5.9 shows how study power varies in relation to the control: case ratio when the number

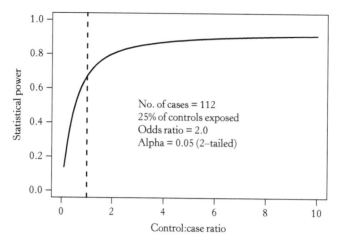

FIGURE 5.9 Study power in relation to control:case ratio for a hypothetical case-control study.

of cases is fixed at 112 and other design assumptions remain the same. Having more controls per case always increases power, but with decreasing incremental gains. Beyond about 3–4 controls per case, gains in power are small. The scarcity of cases imposes a ceiling on study power. Sometimes it may simply not be possible to break through that ceiling, even with an infinite number of controls; there may be no alternative but to find ways to increase the number of cases.

In any event, sample-size calculations show that either design is a viable possibility in this example. Despite a clear advantage in efficiency for the case-control design, it may not necessarily win the competition. As noted earlier in this chapter, cohort studies have certain advantages, including the ability to obtain direct estimates of the absolute incidence of disease among exposed and non-exposed persons and the ability to extend the design easily to study other outcomes of the same exposure. These features may be important enough to offset the difference in efficiency. Also, sometimes a pre-existing data source is rich enough in content to support study needs without new data collection. If so, including 5,000 or even 10,000 subjects in the study may be no more costly than studying 336 subjects. On the other hand, case-control studies also have advantages, including making it easy to study possible effects of other exposures besides the one of primary interest, without altering the basic study design.

Both Designs Applied

In this hypothetical scenario, it is instructive to imagine how *both* designs might play out, even though in practice an investigator would choose one design or the other. Say that the topmost table in Figure 5.10 shows the actual (but unobserved) distribution of exposure and disease status in all 10,000 people. In actuality, 30% of the population was exposed (not 25%, as assumed in study planning), the three-year cumulative incidence of disease was 1.5 per 100 (not 1 per 100) among the non-exposed, and the true relative incidence was 1.8. The two alternative designs involve sampling from this topmost table in different ways, even though the investigator never observes the entire table.

The left branch of Figure 5.10 follows the cohort design. As planned, 2,319 exposed and 2,319 non-exposed persons are drawn at random from their respective source populations. To do this, the investigator may first need to ascertain exposure status for all 10,000 people in the source population, perhaps from a data source that contains exposure (but not necessarily outcome) information. The 2,319 subjects in the exposed study group would then be a random sample from all 3,000 exposed persons, and the 2,319 subjects in the non-exposed study group would be a random sample from all 7,000 non-exposed persons.[1] The second step would then be to ascertain subsequent disease status (and possibly other data on confounding factors) on all individuals in the exposed and non-exposed study groups. The lower left table in Figure 5.10 shows the expected number of persons in all four cells, rounding to the nearest whole number. The actual cell counts would vary at random around these expected values. If the exposed study group is representative of all exposed persons in the source population, then the number of disease cases should be $81/3000 \times 2,319 \approx 63$, and likewise for the non-exposed group.

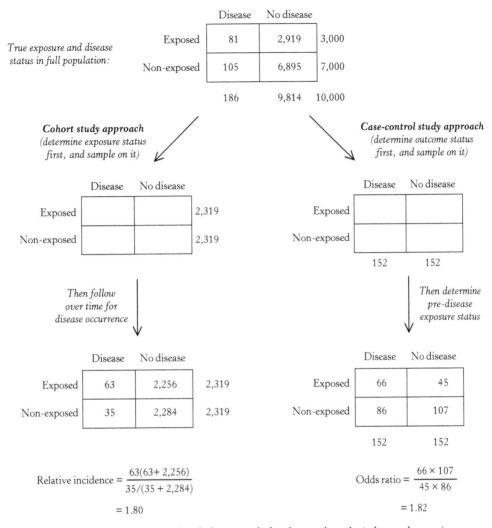

FIGURE 5.10 Cohort and case-control study designs applied to the same hypothetical research scenario.

The right branch of Figure 5.10 follows the case-control design. The first step is to form the case and control groups. To do this, the investigator would initially need to ascertain whether each of the 10,000 people in the source population did or did not develop disease during the three-year study period, perhaps from an existing data source that contains outcome (but not necessarily exposure) information. In this instance, that step would show that 186 total cases had occurred. That number is greater than the 125 cases projected during study planning. In view of the larger-than-expected number of cases, the investigator might revisit the control:case ratio and revert to equal-sized case and control groups of 152 persons each to save on data collection costs. The 152 cases studied would then be a random sample from all 186

cases in the source population, and the 152 controls group would be a random sample from all 9,814 non-diseased persons. The next step would then be to ascertain prior exposure status (and possibly other data on confounding factors) on all individuals in the case and control groups. The lower right table shows the expected number of persons in all four cells, rounding to the nearest whole number. If the case group is representative of all diseased persons in the source population, then the number of exposed cases should be $81/186 \times 152 \approx 66$, and likewise for the control group. Under the case-control design, the odds ratio would be used to estimate relative incidence. In this example, the expected odds ratio is slightly greater than, but still close to, the true relative incidence in the full source population.

To summarize, this comparison of cohort and case-control designs for a hypothetical research situation illustrates several points. The relative efficiency of the two designs depends on the frequency of disease and exposure: case-control studies are efficient for rare diseases, and (by symmetry, although not shown explicitly in this example) cohort studies are efficient for rare exposures. Under either design, when plenty of potential subjects are projected to be available for both comparison groups, forming equal-sized groups tends to maximize efficiency—that is, it requires the fewest total subjects to achieve a target level of study power. If instead the size of one comparison group is limited by a scarcity of subjects, increasing the size of the other comparison group can help to compensate, but little additional power is gained by making one group more than about 3–4 times as large as the other. Finally, while sample-size and power calculations can help guide the choice of an efficient study design, other pros and cons of competing designs also come into play and may trump sample-size considerations when the final selection is made.

KEY FACTORS IN CHOOSING A STUDY DESIGN

Every study design has strengths and weaknesses. Choosing the most suitable design for a given research problem nearly always involves weighing pros and cons on several dimensions, and no simple algorithm can provide an optimal answer for every situation. Still, it may be useful to review a few key questions that an investigator should usually think about when seeking to match a research aim to a study design. Answers to them can greatly narrow the field of design choices to a few good alternatives:

- What kind of research question is being asked? If the main goal is simply to "get the lay of the land," exploring a disease or other outcome about which hardly anything is known, then a descriptive study may be a logical starting point. It can provide basic information about frequency and patterns of variation according to person, place, and time, which will serve as a foundation for later studies solving into possible causes. Alternatively, if the main goal focuses on a specific factor as a possible cause of a specific outcome, an analytic study design is likely to offer a more appropriate research framework and greater efficiency.

- Can the investigator manipulate the exposure? If so, then a randomized trial design is worth considering, even if it should ultimately prove infeasible. Other things being equal, randomized trials offer superior protection against confounding factors and can answer the research question most definitively. Barring that option, a quasi-experiment may be the next best alternative, albeit more vulnerable to confounding. If the exposure cannot be manipulated, then the choice is among observational analytic study designs.

- Where would the data come from? The costs, in time and money, of conducting a study usually depend on the nature and extent of new data collection required. Sometimes good fortune makes available pre-existing data whose content, size, and quality are sufficient to address the main research question without additional data collection. If so, then a retrospective cohort study or a case-control study are strong possibilities. If insufficient pre-existing data are available, then a prospective cohort study or a case-control study requiring primary data collection may be needed.

- How common is the outcome? If it is rare, then a case-control study design can offer major advantages in efficiency. However, the relative disadvantage of a cohort-study approach may be overcome by the availability of extensive pre-existing data or by the overriding importance of obtaining incidence estimates.

- How common is the exposure? If it is rare, then a cohort study can offer major advantages in efficiency.

Beyond these general principles, it is helpful to be aware of the many "niche" designs that have been developed for specialized purposes so that their strengths can be exploited should an opportunity to use them arise.

CONCLUDING REMARKS

We finish this overview of epidemiologic study designs with two general remarks, both of which acknowledge that life is complicated. First, what constitutes a "study" is not always obvious. For instance, the Framingham Heart Study began in 1948 by interviewing and examining a sample of adult residents of Framingham, Massachusetts, and tracking them over time for onset of cardiovascular disease. By 2011, that "study" had burgeoned to involve six different cohorts being followed on different time scales under different protocols addressing a multitude of research aims. In the interim, it had generated over 2,300 scientific publications, addressing dozens of different exposures and outcomes, many of which had never been envisioned by the originators (Framingham Heart Study, 2012).

For the purposes of classifying and understanding epidemiologic study designs, it is better think of a study more narrowly: as a formal attempt to answer a focused research question in a particular population and setting at a certain time. That focused question often concerns whether a certain exposure causes a certain outcome. From that viewpoint, the Framingham Heart Study is best considered a multifaceted research program that encompasses many studies, each with a design of its own.

Second, some of the features that are commonly used to distinguish research designs are not necessarily mutually exclusive. A cohort study may involve exposed and non-exposed groups that are re-examined repeatedly over time on some outcome, thus making the study both a cohort study and a longitudinal study. A cohort study can involve exposed and non-exposed groups that were formed in the distant past, have been followed for outcome occurrence from the distant past through the recent past (a retrospective cohort study), and then continue to be followed on into the future (a prospective cohort study). Results of a randomized trial may be analyzed two different ways, once by comparing the groups formed by random assignment (a true randomized trial) and again by comparing groups formed according to the intervention actually received (a quasi-experiment). A case-control study may have been motivated by the need to evaluate a hypothesized effect of a certain primary exposure (an analytic study), but it may also have gathered data opportunistically on many other characteristics in an exploratory way without any additional hypotheses (technically, a descriptive study).

As noted at the beginning of this chapter, the number of possible research designs is limitless. Examples in this chapter were chosen to be relatively "pure" illustrations of each study design as an aid to learning. And many epidemiologic studies do indeed fit quite neatly into one of the standard design types described here. But sometimes an unusual study design mixes features in such a way that no standard design label can convey adequately how the study

groups were formed and the protocol under which data were collected on them. Ultimately, a key motivation for classifying and naming study designs is to promote efficient communication and comprehension. Each standard design has certain well-known strengths and vulnerabilities. Using a familiar design label can quickly guide a fellow scientist toward issues commonly involved in conducting and interpreting that kind of study. But if a standard label fits poorly and could be misleading, it may be better simply to describe what was done, allowing brevity to give way to clarity.

APPENDIX 5A: WHY THE ODDS RATIO PROVIDES AN ESTIMATE OF RELATIVE INCIDENCE IN A CASE-CONTROL STUDY

Imagine that full information is available on a large, closed population at risk with regard to new disease occurrence among persons with and without a given exposure. At the end of a fixed time interval, the data could be organized as follows:

TABLE 5.7.

	Disease	No disease	Total
Exposed	a	b	$a+b$
Not exposed	c	d	$c+d$

where a, b, c, and d are the number of persons in each cell. The cumulative incidence of disease among exposed persons is $\frac{a}{a+b}$, and the cumulative incidence of disease in non-exposed persons is $\frac{c}{c+d}$. The *relative incidence* is their ratio, $\frac{a/(a+b)}{c/(c+d)}$.

Now further assume that the disease is rare—that is, the number of cases in each exposure group is small in comparison to the number of non-cases. Under this assumption, $\frac{a}{a+b} \approx \frac{a}{b}$, and $\frac{c}{c+d} \approx \frac{c}{d}$, so $\frac{a/(a+b)}{c/(c+d)} \approx \frac{a/b}{c/d}$. The quantity $\frac{a/b}{c/d}$ is known as the *odds ratio* because it is the ratio of the odds of disease among exposed persons (a/b) to the odds of disease in non-exposed persons (c/d). When the disease is rare in both exposure groups, the odds ratio thus approximates the relative incidence. This fact is not especially important when full information on the entire population is available, or in a cohort study, because the desired relative incidence can be calculated directly.

However, note that $\frac{a/b}{c/d} = \frac{ad}{bc} = \frac{ad}{cb} = \frac{a/c}{b/d}$. That is, the odds ratio can written as a ratio of two quantities: a/c, which represents the odds of *exposure* among diseased persons, and b/d, which represents the odds of *exposure* among non-diseased persons.

Now suppose that a case-control study is done within this same study population by including all of the cases and a 1% random sample of the many non-cases as controls. If the controls are representative of all non-cases, then the expected odds of exposure among the controls should be $\frac{0.01 \cdot b}{0.01 \cdot d} = \frac{b}{d}$. The sampling fraction for controls (here, 1%) cancels out. The net result is that one can estimate from case-control data two quantities, a/c and b/d, whose quotient is the odds ratio. This relationship holds even if the sampling fractions for cases and non-cases differ.

Here is a hypothetical example:

TABLE 5.8.

	Disease	No disease	Total
Exposed	150	99,900	100,000
Not exposed	100	199,900	200,000

With full information, relative incidence could be calculated directly as $\frac{150/100,000}{100/200,000} = 3.000$.

If all cases and a 1% random sample of non-cases are studied in a case-control study, the expected results would be:

TABLE 5.9.

	Cases	Controls
Exposed	150	999
Not exposed	100	1,999

The odds ratio would be $\frac{150 \times 1,999}{999 \times 100} = 3.0015$, very close to the true relative incidence of 3.000 in the full source population.

Note that the rare-disease assumption refers to disease frequency *in the source population* from which cases and controls are drawn, not among subjects in the case-control study itself. This assumption is not empirically testable from case-control data

alone. The apparent (often high) frequency of disease among case-control study subjects is usually just a consequence of having used a much larger sampling fraction for cases than for non-cases.

The scenario described above concerned closed populations of exposed and non-exposed persons, in which cumulative incidence would be the natural measure of incidence. In exposed and non-exposed open populations, incidence *rates* with a person-time denominator would be used instead. The basic data layout is:

TABLE 5.10.

	Cases	Person-time
Exposed	a	T_1
Not exposed	c	T_0

Relative incidence would be $\frac{a/T_1}{c/T_0}$, which can be written as $\frac{a/c}{T_1/T_0}$. The numerator, a/c, is the odds of exposure among all disease cases, which can be estimated from a representative sample of cases. The denominator, T_1/T_0, is the odds of exposure in the base of person-time from which the cases arose. If controls in a case-control study are chosen in such a way as to sample in an unbiased way the frequency of exposure in this base of person-time, then the odds of exposure among controls provides a valid estimate of T_1/T_0. Under these conditions, the odds ratio provides an unbiased estimate of relative incidence without requiring a rare-disease assumption (Rodrigues and Kirkwood, 1990).

APPENDIX 5B: ESTIMATING THE REQUIRED SIZE OF COHORT AND CASE-CONTROL STUDIES

This appendix assumes basic familiarity with principles of statistical hypothesis testing, including null (H_0) and alternative (H_A) hypotheses, Type I and Type II errors, α, β, and power.

Case-Control Studies and Cohort Studies in Closed Populations

Case-control studies involve comparing the proportion of subjects exposed between cases and controls. Cohort studies in closed populations typically involve comparing cumulative incidence between exposed and non-exposed groups. Both designs thus compare a certain proportion between two groups that may be of different sizes, and the basic statistical approach to sample-size estimation is the same. The method described here assumes two independent unmatched samples with binary exposure and outcome variables. The possible need to control for confounding factors by stratification or other means during data analysis is ignored for present purposes. Methods for cohort or case-control designs that involve matching or stratification, and for other designs, are described in, e.g., Rosner (2006) and Fleiss *et al.* (2003).

The following inputs are always required:

TABLE 5.11.

Z_α = Critical value that puts probability $\alpha/(\text{no. of tails in hypothesis test})$ in the upper tail of the normal distribution, where α is the maximum tolerable probability of a Type I error. For a two-tailed test at $\alpha = 0.05$, $Z_\alpha \approx 1.96$.

Z_β = Critical value of the normal distribution that puts probability β in the upper tail, where β is the maximum tolerable probability of a Type II error. Power is defined as $1 - \beta$. For $\beta = 0.2$, $Z_\beta \approx 0.84$.

Three additional inputs shown in Table 5.12 are required. The meaning of each depends on the type of study design.

Then let:

$$\bar{p} = \frac{p_1 + kp_0}{1 + k}$$

$$n_1 = \frac{\left[\begin{array}{c} \sqrt{\bar{p}(1-\bar{p})(1+1/k)} \cdot Z_\alpha \\ + \sqrt{p_1(1-p_1) + p_0(1-p_0)/k} \cdot Z_\beta \end{array} \right]^2}{(p_1 - p_0)^2}$$

$$(5.1)$$

For a cohort study, n_1 is the required number of exposed subjects, and kn_1 is the required number of non-exposed subjects. For a case-control study, n_1 is the required number of cases, and kn_1 is the required number of controls.

Cohort Studies in Open Populations

Cohort studies in open populations typically compare incidence rates between exposed and non-exposed groups. The method described here estimates the total amount of person-time at risk required (T), which may be divided unequally between exposed and non-exposed groups. The method assumes independent, unmatched samples and at most one outcome event per person. A key quantity is the proportion exposed among cases (p), which has a different expected value under H_0 and H_A.

Required inputs for the method are Z_α and Z_β, as defined above, and those shown in Table 5.13.

TABLE 5.12.

Input	Interpretation under:	
	Cohort design	Case-control design
p_0	Expected cumulative incidence in non-exposed group	Expected proportion exposed among controls
p_1	Expected cumulative incidence in exposed group under H_A. Set $p_1 = p_0 \cdot RR$, where RR = relative risk under H_A.	Expected proportion exposed among cases under H_A. Set $p_1 = \dfrac{p_0 \cdot OR}{1 + p_0 \cdot (OR - 1)}$, where OR = odds ratio under H_A.
k	Ratio of group sizes (non-exposed / exposed)	Ratio of group sizes (controls / cases)

TABLE 5.13.

f = proportion (fraction) of total person-time T
    contributed by exposed group
IR_0 = projected incidence rate in non-exposed group
RR = rate ratio under H_A

Total required person-time T is estimated in three steps:

1. Calculate p^*, the expected value of p under H_A:

$$p^* = \frac{(\text{No. exposed cases})}{(\text{No. exposed cases}) + (\text{No. non-exposed cases})}$$

$$= \frac{(T \cdot f \cdot IR_0 \cdot RR)}{(T \cdot f \cdot IR_0 \cdot RR) + [T \cdot (1-f) \cdot IR_0]}$$

$$= \frac{f \cdot RR}{1 + f \cdot (RR - 1)}$$

(Under H_0, $p = f$, paralleling the distribution of person-time.)

2. Calculate c, the required number of cases needed to test $H_0 : p = f$ against $H_A : p = p^*$ at the specified α and β, using a one-sample binomial test (Rosner, 2006, p. 761; Fleiss *et al.*, 2003, p. 32):

$$c = \left[\frac{\sqrt{f \cdot (1-f)} \cdot Z_\alpha + \sqrt{p^* \cdot (1-p^*)} \cdot Z_\beta}{p^* - f} \right]^2$$

3. Calculate the total amount of person-time T needed to generate c cases under H_A. As in step 1, the number of cases expected in T person-time is (no. of exposed cases) + (no. of unexposed cases) = $(T \cdot f \cdot IR_0 \cdot RR) + [T \cdot (1-f) \cdot IR_0]$. Solving for the value of T that would generate c cases gives:

$$T = \frac{c}{IR_0 \cdot [1 + f \cdot (RR - 1)]}$$

Required person-time at risk is then $T \cdot f$ in the exposed group and $T \cdot (1 - f)$ in the non-exposed group. Person-time in either group depends on the mean number of people at risk and the length of time over which they are followed for outcome events, both of which may be modifiable by the investigator.

NOTE

1. If there is a cost per subject to determining exposure status, a more efficient method may be to put the list of 10,000 people into random order and determine exposure status one by one, working down this list until both study groups are filled.

REFERENCES

Aldrich TK, Gustave J, Hall CB, Cohen HW, Webber MP, Zeig-Owens R, et al. Lung function in rescue workers at the World Trade Center after 7 years. N Engl J Med 2010; 362:1263–1272.

Alzheimer A. Über einen eigenartigen schweren Erkrankungsprozeßder Hirnrinde. [On an unusual illness of the cerebral cortex.] Neurologisches Centralblatt 1906; 23:1129–1136.

Beral V, Hannaford P, Kay C. Oral contraceptive use and malignancies of the genital tract. Results from the Royal College of General Practitioners' Oral Contraception Study. Lancet 1988; 2: 1331–1335.

Campbell DT, Stanley JC. Experimental and quasi-experimental designs for research. New York: Rand McNally, 1966.

Cruz MA, Katz DJ, Suarez JA. An assessment of the ability of routine restaurant inspections to predict food-borne outbreaks in Miami-Dade County, Florida. Am J Public Health 2001; 91:821–823.

Douglas IJ, Smeeth L. Exposure to antipsychotics and risk of stroke: self controlled case series study. BMJ 2008; 337:a1227.

Fleiss JL, Levin B, Paik MC. Statistical methods for rates and proportions (3rd ed.). New York: Wiley and Sons, 2003.

Framingham Heart Study. http://www.framingham-heartstudy.org/, 2012.

Hannaford PC, Selvaraj S, Elliott AM, Angus V, Iversen L, Lee AJ. Cancer risk among users of oral contraceptives: cohort data from the Royal College of General Practitioner's oral contraception study. BMJ 2007; 335:651.

Jenab M, Bueno-de Mesquita HB, Ferrari P, van Duijnhoven FJB, Norat T, Pischon T, et al. Association between pre-diagnostic circulating vitamin D concentration and risk of colorectal cancer in European populations: a nested case-control study. BMJ 2010; 340:b5500.

Kallen AJ, Mu Y, Bulens S, Reingold A, Petit S, Gershman K, et al. Health care-associated invasive MRSA infections, 2005–2008. JAMA 2010; 304:641–648.

Kandun IN, Tresnaningsih E, Purba WH, Lee V, Samaan G, Harun S, et al. Factors associated with case fatality of human H5N1 virus infections in Indonesia: a case series. Lancet 2008; 372: 744–749.

Khoury MJ, Flanders WD. Nontraditional epidemiologic approaches in the analysis of gene-environment interaction: case-control studies with no controls! Am J Epidemiol 1996; 144:207–213.

Logan PA, Coupland CAC, Gladman JRF, Sahota O, Stoner-Hobbs V, Robertson K, et al. Community falls prevention for people who call an emergency ambulance after a fall: randomised controlled trial. BMJ 2010; 340:c2102.

Maclure M. The case-crossover design: a method for studying transient effects on the risk of acute events. Am J Epidemiol 1991; 133:144–153.

Maclure M, Mittleman MA. Should we use a case-crossover design? Annu Rev Public Health 2000; 21:193–221.

Peart T, Velasco Mondragon HE, Rohm-Young D, Bronner Y, Hossain MB. Weight status in US youth: the role of activity, diet, and sedentary behaviors. Am J Health Behav 2011; 35: 756–764.

Porta M (ed.) A dictionary of epidemiology (5th edition). New York: Oxford University Press, 2008.

Prentice RL. A case-cohort design for epidemiologic cohort studies and disease prevention trials. Biometrika 1986; 73:1–11.

Ray WA, Daugherty JR, Griffin MR. Lipid-lowering agents and the risk of hip fracture in a Medicaid population. Inj Prev 2002; 8:276–279.

Redelmeier DA, Tibshirani RJ. Association between cellular-telephone calls and motor vehicle collisions. N Engl J Med 1997; 336:453–458.

Rodrigues L, Kirkwood BR. Case-control designs in the study of common diseases: updates on the demise of the rare disease assumption and the choice of sampling scheme for controls. Int J Epidemiol 1990; 19:205–213.

Roselle H, Ekatan A, Tzeng J, Sapienza M, Kocher J. Symptomatic hepatitis associated with the use of herbal red yeast rice. Ann Intern Med 2008; 149:516–517.

Rosner B. Fundamentals of biostatistics (6th edition). New York: Duxbury Press, 2006.

Sidney S, Petitti DB, Soff GA, Cundiff DL, Tolan KK, Quesenberry CP Jr. Venous thromboembolic disease in users of low-estrogen combined estrogen-progestin oral contraceptives. Contraception 2004; 70:3–10.

Strömberg B, Dahlquist G, Ericson A, Finnström O, Köster M, Stjernqvist K. Neurological sequelae in children born after in-vitro fertilisation: a population-based study. Lancet 2002; 359:461–465.

Utter J, Scragg R, Robinson E, Warbrick J, Faeamani G, Foroughian S, et al. Evaluation of the Living 4 Life project: a youth-led, school-based obesity prevention study. Obes Rev 2011; 12 Suppl 2: 51–60.

Wang PS, Solomon DH, Mogun H, Avorn J. HMG-CoA reductase inhibitors and the risk of hip fractures in elderly patients. JAMA 2000; 283:3211–3216.

White JE. A two-stage design for the study of the relationship between a rare exposure and a rare disease. Am J Epidemiol 1982; 115: 119–128.

Williams T. Camino Real (block twelve). Norfolk, CT: New Directions, 1953.

EXERCISES

1. Individuals stricken with a spinal cord injury can be left with permanent paralysis of the legs, arms, or both. Bones in the paralyzed limbs become osteoporotic and highly susceptible to fracture, with even minor trauma.

   Investigators at U.S. Department of Veterans Affairs hospitals have planned a study involving veterans with spinal cord injury who experience a fracture in a paralyzed limb. These veterans will be compared with other paralyzed veterans without a fracture in a paralyzed limb. The study's main aim is to ascertain possible differences between the groups on subsequent use of medical care and risk of other complications or death. Fracture patients will be recruited as fractures occur and will then be matched with otherwise-similar non-fracture patients. Information about both groups will be drawn from computerized medical records.

   How would you classify the study design?

2. In venous thromboembolism (VTE), blood clots form in large veins, then break free and are carried in the bloodstream to lodge in the lungs. Although relatively rare, VTE is nonetheless the most common vascular disease among women of childbearing age. Years ago, epidemiologic studies indicated increased risk of VTE among users of early oral contraceptives (OCs), which contained relatively high doses of estrogen. OCs in use today contain much lower estrogen doses or none at all.

   Sidney et al. (2004) sought to determine the degree to which the risk of VTE is elevated among current users of modern OCs. Over about two years, all recognized VTE cases among women aged 18–44 years were identified in a large California prepaid health plan. They were compared to a sample of female enrollees of similar age without VTE. Both groups were interviewed about OC use at the time of VTE (or at a comparable index time for controls) and about other risk factors. An excerpt of the results is shown in Table 5.14.

   Consider each of the following quantities. If it can be calculated from the data shown, do so. If not, so state and briefly explain why not.

   (a) Incidence of VTE among current OC users

TABLE 5.14.

Current OC user?	No. of VTE cases	No. of non-cases
Yes	69	64
No	84	247

(Based on data from Sidney *et al.* [2004])

(b) Incidence of VTE among women who were not currently using OCs

(c) $$\frac{\text{Incidence of VTE among current OC users}}{\text{Incidence of VTE among women who were not currently using OCs}}$$

3. Advances in in-vitro fertilization (IVF, or "test-tube" conception) have led to growing use of the technique worldwide. In Sweden, about 2% of babies born in recent years were conceived through IVF. A group of Swedish investigators sought to determine the extent to which IVF may increase the risk of several adverse postnatal and early childhood outcomes, especially low birth weight, cerebral palsy, congenital malformation, mental retardation, and chromosomal abnormality. Data sources available to them included:

• The Swedish Medical Birth Registry, which included birth certificate data on all children born in Sweden
• Records of the National Board of Health and Welfare, which received reports from all 14 IVF clinics in Sweden about which mothers underwent IVF and when they had the procedure
• Reasonably accurate diagnosis data on patients treated at all 26 childhood disability centers in Sweden, which provided care to children with the various congenital and developmental abnormalities of interest under a national health care system

All of these data sources had been maintained for at least 20 years and were expected to continue. Sweden also assigned a unique personal identification number to each citizen, including mothers and newborns, that could be used to link data across data sources.

If you were a member of the investigative team, what type of epidemiologic study design would you suggest as best suited to the research aims and data resources available? Briefly justify your choice.

4. Vitamin D has a well-known role in calcium regulation and bone metabolism. Significant sources of vitamin D include foods, endogenous vitamin D made by skin cells after sunlight exposure, and vitamin supplements. Recent laboratory studies suggest that vitamin D may also be involved in modulating cell growth and blood-vessel formation, both of which are important in the genesis of cancer.

1992–1998, a multinational collaborative study in Europe recruited about 520,000 cancer-free adults from the general population or through screening programs (Jenab *et al.*, 2010). At recruitment, all participants donated a blood sample and completed a standardized dietary questionnaire. Occurrence of cancer was then monitored through population-based cancer registries and death certificates in each country. By 2003, 1,248 participants had developed colorectal cancer. Each of them was matched to a study participant of the same age, gender, and area of residence who was known to be alive and had not developed colorectal cancer. Stored blood samples and questionnaire data were then analyzed to compare the two groups. The results showed lower blood vitamin D levels among those who developed colorectal cancer than among those who did not. However, essentially no differences were found with regard to dietary intake of foods high in vitamin D.

(a) Classify the study design.
(b) The results for blood levels of vitamin D differed from the results for self-reported dietary intake of vitamin D. Could this difference be due to recall bias in the self-reported dietary data? Explain briefly.
(c) The study results were considered encouraging by cancer-control experts, because blood level of vitamin D may be a potentially modifiable risk factor for colorectal cancer. What type of study design might best establish whether raising a person's blood level of vitamin D reduces his or her risk of colorectal cancer?

5. Cruz *et al.* (2001) sought to evaluate the effectiveness of routine restaurant inspections for preventing foodborne illness outbreaks in greater Miami. Each of the approximately 8,000 restaurants in the area was scheduled for four inspections each year. Each inspection assessed 12 critical items, such as storing food at proper temperatures, absence of vermin, and excluding sick employees from food handling.

During a one-year period, 60 confirmed foodborne outbreaks that were traced to a restaurant occurred in the Miami area. The investigators reviewed past inspection reports for the 60 affected restaurants, as well as for 120 other area restaurants chosen at random from among those that had been inspected in the same calendar months. Among the 60 restaurants where a foodborne illness outbreak had occurred, 54.9% had had at least one violation on a critical item at their most recent inspection before the outbreak. Among the 120 other restaurants, 44.7% had had at least one critical violation at the time of their corresponding inspection.

(a) How would you classify the overall study design?
(b) From the information given, can you estimate the following quantity?

$$\frac{\text{Incidence of outbreaks in restaurants with 1+ critical violations}}{\text{Incidence of outbreaks in restaurants with no critical violations}}$$

If so, estimate it. If not, explain why not.

6. Anxiolytic drugs, also called "minor tranquilizers," are prescribed for anxiety and related symptoms. They can also produce sedation, drowsiness, and inattentiveness. Suppose that a study is being planned to investigate whether current use of an anxiolytic drug increases the risk of being injured in a motor-vehicle crash. A large Health Maintenance Organization (HMO) that provides prescription drugs at low cost to enrollees has implemented a computerized pharmacy system that makes it possible to determine which enrollees fill drug prescriptions at what times. It also appears feasible, with suitable confidentiality protections, to link HMO enrollment records with a state police database that captures all police-reported motor vehicle crashes in the state, with or without injury.

The HMO has 120,000 members aged 16 years or older (i.e., who are old enough to drive), and enrollment is expected to remain about the same over the next few years. Preliminary analysis of the computerized pharmacy data has shown that about 2% of HMO enrollees in that age group are receiving an anxiolytic at any given time. Federal traffic safety agencies report that the motor-vehicle crash injury rate among licensed drivers was about 1,060 per 100,000 person-years in recent years. If a prospective cohort study is begun this year, how long would it take to accumulate enough data to test whether the crash injury rate among licensed drivers in the HMO is at least 50% higher in those receiving anxiolytics than in those who are not? Assume that:

- 90% of HMO members aged 16 years or older are licensed drivers
- Use of anxiolytics is equally common among comparably aged enrollees with and without a driver's license
- Non-exposed drivers would experience injuries at the national rate

- Repeat injury episodes in the same person within the study period would be rare enough to ignore
- The study should have 80% power to detect the hypothesized association
- The threshold for statistical significance will be 0.05, using two-tailed hypothesis tests

ANSWERS

1. The study will be a prospective cohort study. The groups being compared will be paralyzed veterans with or without a fracture in a paralyzed limb. Note that experiencing a fracture is the *exposure*, not the outcome. The outcomes are medical care use, incidence of complications, and death. The study is prospective because none of the fractures or outcomes to be studied will have occurred before data collection begins.

2. (a) This quantity cannot be calculated from the data shown. Neither cumulative incidence nor incidence rates can be estimated directly from case-control data, because the frequency of disease within the study population is chiefly determined by different sampling fractions for cases and non-cases.
   (b) This quantity also cannot be calculated from the data shown, for the same reason.
   (c) This quantity, *relative* incidence (or relative risk, RR), *can* be estimated from case-control study data using the odds ratio. Here,
   $$RR \approx OR = (69 \times 247)/(64 \times 84) = 3.17.$$

3. Strömberg *et al.* (2002) chose a retrospective cohort study design, probably because:

- The exposure was relatively rare (2% of births). All of the IVF-conceived babies born in the past two decades could be used and compared with a comparably sized sample of the many non-IVF babies born during the same years. In the actual study, two matched non-IVF babies were compared with each IVF baby.
- There was a single exposure (IVF) of main interest, but several outcomes: low birth weight, cerebral palsy, congenital malformation, mental retardation, and chromosomal abnormality. This features lends itself to a cohort-study approach.
- They could directly measure the birth prevalence, or subsequent incidence, of each outcome event. That feature provided useful information about absolute risk, not just *relative* risk.
- Doing the study retrospectively was possible and desirable because of the excellent data resources available in Sweden for this purpose. Although IVF

was rare, they could use all IVF babies over a 20-year period to bolster sample size.

A randomized trial of this exposure is unlikely ever to be done due to infeasibility and low power.

A case-control design would be possible, but it would be complicated by the need for several case groups—one for each outcome of interest. Moreover, each case group would probably require a different control group. A single control group that had *none* of the abnormalities listed would not be ideal for any particular abnormality. For example, excluding all low birth weight babies from the control group would omit some babies who were actually at risk for cerebral palsy but who did not develop it and who thus should have been included in a control group for cerebral palsy. Moreover, the case-control design would not lead directly to estimates of the absolute risk of any of the abnormalities of interest.

A prospective cohort study is also possible, but, given the rarity of IVF, it could take a long time to accumulate enough IVF babies to permit detection of the rarer adverse outcomes with reasonable statistical power. Given the availability of suitable data going back two decades, a retrospective cohort design would offer large numbers and could be completed much sooner than a prospective cohort study.

In this instance, all of the necessary data had already been collected and were available from existing sources. Had that not been so, a *case-cohort* design might have been another appealing option. A single "subcohort" representative of all births (including both IVF and non-IVF) would be sampled and compared with each of several several case groups.

4. (a) This was a case-control study. Colorectal cancer cases and cancer-free controls were chosen from a previously formed cohort of study subjects. (When cases and controls are drawn from a pre-existing cohort, the design is sometimes called a *nested* case-control study.) For efficiency, only the exposure information (blood vitamin D levels and dietary vitamin D intake levels) on 1,248 cases and 1,248 controls was analyzed, not on everyone in the full cohort of 520,000 people.

(b) No. Like the blood sample, the dietary information had been obtained at the time of recruitment into the study cohort, before colorectal cancer had occurred in any cohort members. *Recall bias* refers to differences in the reporting of past exposure by cases vs. non-cases due to awareness of their disease status at the time they answer questions about exposure.

Differentially biased recall could not have occurred in this study, because at the time they provided the dietary data, none of the subjects knew whether or not they would later develop colorectal cancer.

(c) A randomized trial would offer the most definitive evidence. Willing volunteers could be randomly assigned to take either vitamin D supplements or a placebo. The dose of vitamin D would be chosen as high enough to achieve a blood level that should put most study subjects into a presumably low-risk exposure category, but low enough to minimize side effects. Cancer incidence would then be monitored in the supplement and placebo groups. Because the incidence of colorectal cancer is fairly low, the study would need to be quite large and/or extend over several years. The researchers who conducted the case-control study did, in fact, suggest such a randomized trial as a logical next step.

5. (a) This was a case-control study—a somewhat unusual one in that restaurants, not people, were the units of study. Sixty "case" restaurants where an outbreak had occurred were compared with 120 "control" restaurants with no outbreak. The exposure was whether a violation on a critical item had been found at the time of the most recent inspection prior to the outbreak.

(b) This quantity is *relative incidence*, or *relative risk*. It cannot be calculated directly from case-control data alone, because the high frequency of adverse outcomes within the study sample is simply a result of sampling cases with a much higher sampling fraction than controls.

However, although neither the numerator nor the denominator of relative risk can be estimated directly, their quotient *can* be estimated using the odds ratio from case-control data. In this instance, because there were only 60 outbreaks among the 8,000 or so Miami-area restaurants under surveillance, the rare-disease assumption is easily satisfied.

From the data given, the following 2 × 2 table summarizes the results of the case-control study:

TABLE 5.15.

No. of violations	Cases	Controls
One or more	33	54
None	27	66
Total	60	120

The odds ratio would be $OR = \frac{33 \times 66}{54 \times 27} = 1.49$, which should be a good estimate of the relative risk.

(Incidentally, the OR can also be calculated directly from the exposure frequencies among cases and controls as $\frac{0.549 \times (1 - 0.447)}{0.447 \times (1 - 0.549)}$, giving the same result apart from rounding error. This shortcut avoids the extra step of actually constructing the 2×2 table of counts.)

In this instance, we also know from the background information that there were approximately 8,000 restaurants in the Miami area. We can use this added information to illustrate that the odds ratio is a good estimate of relative risk. Suppose that there were, in fact, exactly 8,000 restaurants. Of these, 60 were case restaurants, and all of the other 7,940 were non-cases (i.e., potential controls). If the 120 controls actually studied were representative of all 7,940 potential controls, then the frequency of violations observed among these 120 controls (44.7%) should be a good estimate of violation frequency in all potential controls. If full information were available on all 8,000 restaurants, they should be distributed approximately as follows:

TABLE 5.16.

No. of violations	Cases	Non-cases
One or more	33	3,549
None	27	4,391
Total	60	7,940

In this table, $33/(33 + 3,549)$ *would* be a valid estimate of the (cumulative) incidence of outbreaks among restaurants with one or more violations, and $27/(27 + 4,391)$ would be the incidence of outbreaks among restaurants with no violations. Their ratio would be 1.51, very close to the 1.49 obtained by using the odds-ratio approximation. Normally we do not bother to construct this last table because: (1) a good estimate of the total number of non-cases in the source population may not be available; (2) the numbers in the non-cases column are projections, not directly observed values, and cannot be treated the same way statistically for purposes of hypothesis testing; and (3) if the outcome of interest can safely be assumed to be rare in both exposure groups, we know that we can rely on the $OR \approx RR$ approximation without further ado.

6. The method in Appendix 5B for cohort studies in open populations can be used. Based on the background information provided and the assumptions allowed, inputs to the method are as follows:

TABLE 5.17.

Input	Value	Comment
α	0.05	Maps to $Z_\alpha \approx 1.96$ for two-tailed hypothesis tests
β	0.2	Power $= 1 - \beta = 0.8$; $\beta = 0.2$ maps to $Z_\beta \approx 0.84$
f	0.02	Fraction of population (and hence person-time) exposed
IR_0	$\frac{1,060}{100,000}$	Assumed incidence rate in non-exposed group
RR	1.5	Hypothesized relative incidence among exposed

Under the null hypothesis, 2% of cases would be using anxiolytics at the time of the crash—the same percentage as in controls. But if $RR = 1.5$, the expected proportion of cases exposed would be:

$$p^* = \frac{f \cdot RR}{1 + f \cdot (RR - 1)}$$

$$= \frac{0.02 \cdot 1.5}{1 + 0.02 \cdot (1.5 - 1)}$$

$$\approx 0.0297$$

The number of cases required to test the null hypothesis (true proportion of cases exposed $= 0.02 = f$) against the alternative hypothesis (true proportion of cases exposed $= 0.0297 = p^*$) would be:

$$c = \left[\frac{\sqrt{f \cdot (1 - f)} \cdot Z_\alpha + \sqrt{p^* \cdot (1 - p^*)} \cdot Z_\beta}{p^* - f} \right]^2$$

$$\approx \left\{ \left[\frac{\sqrt{0.02 \cdot (1 - 0.02)} \cdot 1.96 + \sqrt{0.0297 \cdot (1 - 0.0297)} \cdot 0.84}{0.0297 - 0.02} \right] \right\}^2$$

$$= 1,848$$

The total number of person-years required to generate 1,848 cases would be:

$$T = \frac{c}{IR_0 \cdot [1 + f \cdot (RR - 1)]}$$

$$= \frac{1,848}{1,060/100,000 \cdot [1 + 0.02 \cdot (1.5 - 1)]}$$

$$\approx 172,614 \text{ person-years}$$

If 90% of the 120,000 HMO members are licensed drivers, they would contribute $120,000 \times 0.9 = 108,000$ person-years each study year, so it would take $172,614/108,000 \approx 1.6$ study years to accumulate enough crash injury cases.

6

Sources of Data on Disease Occurrence

Knowledge is of two kinds. We know a subject ourselves, or we know where we can find information upon it.

—SAMUEL JOHNSON

Epidemiologists are often data scavengers. Using pre-existing data can allow a study to be done more cheaply, more quickly, and often on a larger scale than if new data collection were required.

As we have seen, most epidemiologic studies quantify disease frequency in terms of rates or proportions. All such measures have a numerator and a denominator, which may come from different sources. Figure 6.1 provides an overview of several common sources through which disease cases can be identified. In other words, it shows sources of numerator data. The most suitable data source for a particular study depends partly on the nature of the disease: whether it is commonly fatal; whether it tends to occur only near the time of birth or later in life; whether it typically prompts victims to seek medical care, and if so, what kind of care is usually provided. The kinds of pre-existing data available also vary greatly in different parts of the world and from one research setting to another.

Denominator data generally come from fewer sources. Sometimes the denominator can come from the same source that provides the numerator: for example, birth certificates can be used both to identify cases of some perinatal diseases as well as to enumerate and characterize the population at risk. Otherwise, for geographically defined populations, such as residents of an American city or state, census data or intercensal estimates are often available from the U.S. Census Bureau or from state or local government agencies. For administratively defined populations, such as enrollees of a health insurance plan or employees of a company, membership lists are often available through the organization in question.

Unfortunately, pre-existing information was not necessarily collected with the researcher's needs in mind. Hence, dealing with data limitations is often an important part of conducting and interpreting epidemiologic research. This chapter considers strengths and weaknesses of several commonly used kinds of pre-existing data, as well as some techniques for assessing and dealing with data limitations. It focuses mainly on data resources available in the United States.

Use of pre-existing data in epidemiology has been revolutionized in recent years by technological advances and the growth of information technology. Information once found only in musty reference libraries and obscure government publications has become instantly available over the Internet from almost anywhere in the world. The World Wide Web is often the first place to look for many kinds of health statistics, with traditional paper sources serving only as a backup. However, the location, organization, and content of information on the Web change often. Appendix 6A provides URLs for a few key websites that are likely to remain stable and that can be used as starting points for data searching. The U.S. Centers for Disease Control and Prevention (CDC) maintains an on-line data archive called WONDER that includes a variety of population health-related data sets (Centers for Disease Control and Prevention, 2012; Friede *et al.*, 1993).

NUMERATOR DATA

Death Records

Death and epidemiologic research have long gone hand-in-hand. John Graunt began analyzing parish "bills of mortality" in 17th-century London, calling

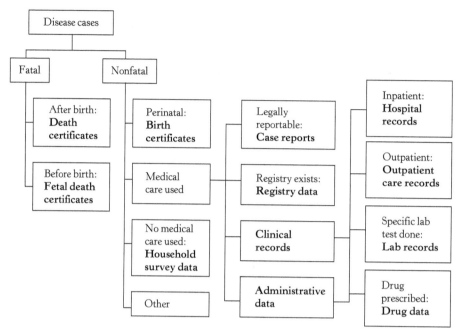

FIGURE 6.1 Common data sources for identification of disease cases.

attention to what could be learned by tracking the number of deaths due to plague and other causes from year to year. Two centuries later, William Farr, medical statistician for England and Wales, began compiling and disseminating cause-specific mortality statistics. Farr's system for organizing causes of death became the basis for the International Classification of Diseases (ICD).

In modern times, a great deal of epidemiologic research continues to be based on mortality statistics. Some conditions, such as homicide and suicide, are fatal by definition. For some other diseases, case fatality is very high—pancreatic cancer and amyotrophic lateral sclerosis (ALS), for example—so that mortality is a good approximation to incidence. Even for diseases that may or may not cause death, the fatal cases may arguably be those of greatest public health impact and those that we most want to prevent. As Farr put it, "Stone cold hath no fellow" (Fredrickson, 1968).

Registration of all deaths has been required by law in most developed countries for many years. A death certificate is also needed by survivors to claim life insurance, Social Security payments to next of kin, and other benefits. Accordingly, records of death certificates maintained at government vital records offices in the developed world are believed to capture almost all deaths that occur within their jurisdictions, and the data can span many decades.

In the United States, registration of births and deaths is a state function. The original copies of birth and death certificates are filed in state vital statistics offices. Although states have ultimate responsibility and authority, the National Center for Health Statistics (NCHS) provides a model death certificate that has historically been used with minor modifications by all states and local death registration areas in the United States. Its content and format are revised periodically. The 2003 revision is shown in Appendix 6B. Personal information about the decedent (items 1–23 and 51–55) is gathered and recorded by whoever is responsible for disposition of the body, usually the funeral director. Information about the time, cause, manner, and circumstances of death (items 24–50) normally comes from the physician in attendance at the time of death. If there is any suspicion of foul play or suicide, if death occurred accidentally, or if no physician was in attendance, legally the case must be referred to a medical examiner (a physician, often a forensic pathologist) or coroner (a public official, not necessarily a physician). The medical examiner or coroner decides whether an autopsy is necessary.

Cause-of-death information is recorded on the death certificate in a hierarchy that works backwards from immediate cause to underlying cause. For example, this section might show *myocardial rupture*; due to or as a consequence of *acute myocardial infarction*; due to or as a consequence of *coronary artery thrombosis*; due to or as a consequence of *atherosclerotic coronary artery disease*. The last-listed cause in the sequence—here, atherosclerotic coronary artery disease—is considered the *underlying* cause of death and used in most compilations of mortality statistics. Public-use data are also available that retain all causes listed in the hierarchy, which lessens the chance that a disease of interest will be missed due to inconsistencies in how death certificates are completed or coded. Space is also provided on the death certificate for recording other significant medical conditions that the certifier judges to have contributed to death.

The training and motivation of physicians in assigning cause of death is uneven (Smith Sehdev and Hutchins, 2001), and the certifying physician may not have complete medical knowledge of the case. Autopsies in non-criminal cases are rarely performed nowadays (Hoyert *et al.*, 2007), and even when they are, the cause of death listed on the death certificate may not necessarily be updated to reflect autopsy results (Kircher *et al.*, 1985). Unfortunately, no widely used routine mechanism is in place to check the listed cause of death against other clinical information. For these reasons, cause-of-death data must be assumed to be subject to misclassification, the extent of which can vary by disease, reporting jurisdiction, or other factors (Gittelsohn and Royston, 1982). Validation substudies, discussed below, are one way to gauge the extent of misclassification. Despite these limitations, much useful knowledge has been gleaned from imperfect death certificate data, so that errors in cause of death need not necessarily be a fatal flaw.

Coding and grouping of causes of death follows the International Classification of Diseases (ICD), discussed in Chapter 10. The ICD is revised about every 10–15 years by the World Health Organization (World Health Organization, 2011).

In the United States, death certificates are first filed with city and county health departments, who check them for completeness and consistency and retain copies for local use. They are then forwarded to state vital statistics offices, where they are checked again and archived. States transmit death certificate data electronically to the National Center for Health Statistics. National mortality data are available to epidemiologists from NCHS in electronic media containing counts of deaths by year, state and county

of residence, age group, gender, race/ethnicity, and underlying cause of death (ICD code). Custom tables of U.S. mortality statistics by combinations of these variables can be obtained over the Internet from CDC's WONDER system. Mortality data are also available from state and local health departments.

NCHS initiated the National Death Index in 1979. Researchers can use it to determine who within a set of study subjects has died anywhere in the United States. The user sends identifying information about subjects, such as name, date of birth, gender, and/or Social Security number, to NCHS, then receives information about probable and possible matches to the National Death Index, including date of death, state of death, and (at extra cost) cause of death. Ascertainment of deaths by this method has been found to be nearly complete (Cowper *et al.*, 2002; Boyle and Decoufle, 1990). Other sources of vital status data are also available for selected populations, such as U.S. veterans (Boyko *et al.*, 2000) and Social Security recipients (Cowper *et al.*, 2002).

Example 6-1. Speizer *et al.* (1968) examined deaths due to asthma in England and Wales for the years 1952–1966. In contrast to trends in other countries, where asthma mortality had been stable or declining, rates in England and Wales had increased steadily after about 1960. Figure 6.2 shows that the rise had been especially marked among children aged 10–14 years. The researchers also noted the following:

- Asthma in younger children can often be hard to distinguish from bronchiolitis, and asthma in adults can be confused with chronic obstructive pulmonary disease, but asthma among 10–14 year olds would be less likely to be misclassified as another disease.
- The increase in deaths from asthma was not accompanied by a decrease in deaths from bronchitis, chronic respiratory disease, or pneumonia, as might be expected if shifts in diagnosis assignment or coding were the only explanation.
- There had been no concurrent increase in visits to physicians for asthma, suggesting that the rise in mortality was more likely to have been due to increased case fatality than to increased incidence.
- The increase corresponded in time to rapid increases in sales of high-potency sympathomimetic aerosols as treatment for asthma.

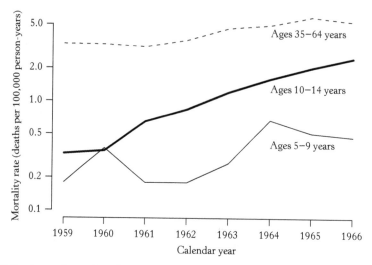

FIGURE 6.2 Death rates from asthma, by age: England and Wales, 1959–1969.

Later research raised further concerns about the side effects of high-potency inhalers and led to greater caution in their therapeutic use. But even at its peak, asthma mortality in the highest-risk age group was only about 2.5 deaths per 100,000 person-years, making it extremely unlikely that an individual physician would see enough asthma deaths to notice the increase. Tracking deaths on a large-population scale made it possible to detect the epidemic.

Birth Records

Registration of births is also legally required in most developed countries. NCHS provides a model birth certificate that is used, with minor modifications, by all U.S. states. The 2003 model birth certificate is shown in Appendix 6C. States vary as to when they actually change from older to revised birth certificates.

The upper *public* part of the model birth certificate (items 1–13) contains identifying and demographic information about the baby and parents. The lower *confidential* part is retained by vital statistics offices, which publish statistics and make the data available for approved research. The lower part contains many items of interest to epidemiologists, including parents' race, education, and marital status; mother's pregnancy history; baby's birth weight, gestational age, and birth order; medical and behavioral factors for the current pregnancy; labor and delivery complications; obstetrical procedures; complications affecting the newborn; and the presence of congenital anomalies.

Demographic information and mother's pregnancy history are recorded by the physician or midwife or by hospital personnel in consultation with the mother. These data are generally quite complete, except for items about the father if the mother is unmarried (Ventura *et al.*, 2000). The physician or midwife records medical information in the confidential part, mostly by marking checkboxes. Validation studies have found considerable underreporting on these items (Lydon-Rochelle *et al.*, 2005; DiGiuseppe *et al.*, 2002). Nonetheless, birth certificate data have proven to be a fertile information resource for epidemiologic research on maternal and infant health.

Example 6-2. The proportion of pregnant American mothers whose child is delivered by Cesarean section began rising steadily in the mid-1990s. One hypothesis was that a larger percentage of pregnant women were gaining too much weight during pregnancy, leading to an increased frequency of unusually large babies (fetal macrosomia) who may not fit through the birth canal and must be delivered by Cesarean section. Using national birth certificate data files on babies born from 1990–2000, Rhodes *et al.* (2003) investigated trends over time in the frequency of high maternal weight gain, fetal macrosomia, and Cesarean delivery among first full-term singleton deliveries. They found that the proportion of mothers who gained at least 40 pounds while pregnant had increased steadily during that decade. However, within each weight-gain category, the prevalence of fetal macrosomia had actually declined, while the frequency of Cesarean section had increased. These findings suggested that fetal macrosomia was a relatively unimportant contributing cause to the rise in Cesarean sections.

Fetal Death Records

Most states require registration of fetal deaths if the fetus had reached a gestational age of at least 20 weeks. (Some states mandate reporting of all fetal deaths regardless of gestational age.) NCHS issues a model fetal death certificate, which captures demographic and medical data as on the model birth certificate and cause-of-death data as on the model death certificate. Fetal death records are also compiled nationally and available for research (Martin and Hoyert, 2002). However, registration of fetal deaths has been found to be much less complete than registration of live births or of deaths that occur after birth, especially for fetal deaths that occur at earlier gestational ages (Harter *et al.*, 1986; Greb *et al.*, 1987). Moreover, cause-of-death information is often non-specific or incomplete and has been found to correspond poorly with autopsy reports (Lammer *et al.*, 1989). Accordingly, fetal death certificates have so far been less used for epidemiologic research than have other vital records.

Disease Reports

Under state and local laws, certain diseases must be reported to health authorities by any health care provider who encounters a new case (Centers for Disease Control and Prevention, 2012; Roush *et al.*, 1999). The list of reportable diseases varies somewhat among jurisdictions, but it generally includes infectious diseases for which timely information on case occurrence is needed for disease prevention and control. Some conditions, such as polio, syphilis, and tuberculosis, are transmissible from person to person. Reporting of individual cases can trigger public health efforts aimed at the protection of other individuals who may already have been in contact with the reported case, or those who might have future contact with it. Other diseases, such as botulism or paralytic shellfish poisoning, occur after an environmental exposure such as contaminated food, and reporting can trigger a public health response to prevent others from being exposed.

State and local laws typically require more rapid notification of authorities for diseases that pose an immediate threat to others of potentially fatal or disabling illness. For example, in Washington State, a new case of rabies must be reported immediately, while three working days are allowed for reporting a new case of AIDS, and a month is allowed for reporting a new case of chronic hepatitis B infection.

Passive reporting of this kind is thought to be fairly complete for rare, clinically severe diseases of clear public health importance, such as botulism or plague. But for many other legally reportable diseases, under-ascertainment of cases is a serious problem (Doyle *et al.*, 2002; Marier, 1977). Some conditions, such as hepatitis A or salmonellosis, can be clinically mild and may never result in a medical care encounter. If care is sought but the illness is non-specific, the necessary diagnostic tests may not be done, and the diagnosis may be missed. For example, a study of passive reporting for shigellosis in the United States estimated that of every 100 cases, 76 were symptomatic, 28 consulted a physician, 9 had a stool culture, and 7 had a positive stool culture (Rosenberg *et al.*, 1977).

Even when a reportable disease is diagnosed, physicians often fail to submit a case report (Doyle *et al.*, 2002). One survey found that non-reporting physicians were unaware that they had this responsibility or that the particular disease was legally reportable, or were unfamiliar with reporting forms or procedures, or were concerned about patient confidentiality, or were unmoved by the incentives or sanctions in place (Konowitz *et al.*, 1984). For all of these reasons, the reported cases of many notifiable infectious diseases probably represent only a fraction of all truly occurring cases.

Approaches that have been used to enhance reporting include the following:

- *Sentinel physicians* agree in advance to report all patient encounters for a target disease for a certain time period. For example, about 3,000 health care providers report outpatient visits for influenza-like illness weekly as part of ILINet, a network for influenza surveillance in the United States (Centers for Disease Control and Prevention, 2010). This approach to case identification sacrifices comprehensive population coverage for more complete ascertainment among patients of relatively motivated care providers.
- *Laboratory-based reporting* is mandated for some diseases and jurisdictions when a specific test is routinely done to diagnose a

disease. For example, clinical laboratories in Washington State are legally required to report immediately to their local health department any positive culture for *Corynebacterium diphtheriae*, which causes diphtheria. Because there are many fewer clinical laboratories than individual health care providers, compliance with reporting requirements is easier to monitor and promote.

- *Active surveillance* involves outreach to providers and sometimes directly to the public to identify cases who would be missed by passive reporting. Active surveillance was an important part of the successful program to eradicate smallpox—a disease spread only person-to-person and for which an effective vaccine has long been available (Foege *et al.*, 1971). In the late 1960s, smallpox persisted in eight West and Central African nations where full vaccination of the population was practically impossible to achieve. Fortunately, full vaccination also proved unnecessary. The smallpox eradication team instead focused on early detection and aggressive control of local outbreaks. Their active-surveillance approach used newspapers, radio, teachers, mail carriers, village and area chiefs, and regular contacts with health care providers and volunteer agencies to identify cases not captured by the passive smallpox reporting system. As incidence declined, a larger and larger proportion of cases were identified only through active surveillance. The final smallpox-eradication push was timed to coincide with the seasonal dip in incidence. By mid-1969, the disease was completely wiped out from the region. Because of the added cost and effort, active surveillance is most often used only temporarily and locally as part of special programs for disease control or research.

Disease Registries

Registries collect standardized data, often from multiple sources, on individual cases of disease. Use of more than one data source enhances completeness of case ascertainment, and linkage across sources prevents duplicate counting of the same cases. Here are some examples of diseases for which well-developed registries exist:

- *Cancer.* The National Cancer Institute funds population-based cancer registries in many areas of the United States as part of the Surveillance, Epidemiology, and End Results (SEER) program, begun in 1973. Collectively, SEER registries cover about 28% of the U.S. population and identify about 450,000 new cancer cases each year. Cases are identified from review of records of hospital discharges and pathology laboratories. Pathology reports are also used to classify tumors by histological type, and medical records are abstracted to obtain demographic and clinical information, including stage at diagnosis and type of treatment. Survivorship is tracked through state vital records and the National Death Index. Cancer cases identified through SEER are regularly used in case-control studies of cancer etiology. SEER registries identify nearly all cancer cases in their geographically defined populations, which become sampling frames for selection of controls.
- *Birth defects.* Federally funded population-based birth defects registries exist in 14 U.S. states and territories, covering about 1.3 million live births each year. A particularly well-developed registry is the Metropolitan Atlanta Congenital Defects Program, begun in 1967, which seeks to identify all birth defects among the approximately 50,000 infants born annually in five counties composing greater Atlanta (Correa-Villaseñor *et al.*, 2003). Case finding uses birth and death certificates, hospital and physician records, and genetic laboratory test results, which collectively are thought to ascertain about 87% of cases (Honein and Paulozzi, 1999).
- *Selected bacterial infections.* Population-based laboratory surveillance covers ten areas of the United States to identify cases of infection due to six bacteria of clinical and public health importance (group A or B *Streptococcus*, *Streptococcus pneumoniae*, *Haemophilus influenzae*, *Neisseria meningitidis* and methicillin-resistant *Staphylococcus aureus*). The system exploits the growing use of computerized laboratory records, supplemented by regular calls to designated contacts at other laboratories in the coverage area.

Because of the expense of ongoing data collection, linkage, quality control, and database maintenance, registries exist for only a few diseases, and most are limited in geographic scope. Moreover, not all disease registries are population-based: some hospital- or clinic-based registries are set up mainly to create a list of potential participants for clinical research and are thus of more limited use to epidemiologists for lack of a denominator.

Health Care Utilization Data

For illnesses that prompt the use of health care, information generated in the process of providing that care can be valuable for epidemiologic purposes.

- *Clinical records* are a rich source of patient-specific data from clinical examinations, laboratory tests, drug prescriptions, and procedures. The growth of electronic medical record systems has greatly increased the volume and scope of the data potentially available for research and lowered data-gathering costs (Klompas *et al.*, 2012). But in many settings, medical records remain largely paper-based, and extracting the information for epidemiologic research involves coping with several challenges: accessing the records, which may not be archived indefinitely; and dealing with the uneven organization, completeness, and legibility of the records themselves. Sometimes a patient may also receive care from more than one source, and each source may keep its records in a different format.
- *Administrative data* that are generated as a byproduct of clinical care are sometimes easier than clinical records to access and to use for research (Jutte *et al.*, 2011). The data are typically computerized and in a standardized format. When care is provided on a fee-for-service basis, each service typically appears on a billing claim containing a patient identifier and the date, provider, and nature of the service. The patient's disease may be implicit in the service itself, as with coronary artery bypass grafting; claims also usually include one or more diagnosis codes to justify delivery of the service.

    In some care settings, no bill is generated because the care is not paid for on a fee-for-service basis. Examples include Health Maintenance Organizations (HMOs),

veteran's hospitals, and military hospitals. Nonetheless, these organizations often track utilization for their own administrative purposes. An internal record may thus document each delivery of a service, containing much the same data as might otherwise have appeared on a billing claim.

Epidemiologists must keep in mind that administrative data do not exist primarily to support epidemiologic research and may be prone to both random and systematic errors (Ray, 2011; Weiss, 2011). The data systems themselves and the meaning of information in them can also change over time. For example, Helms (1987) described a "pseudo-epidemic" of septicemia among Medicare patients in Iowa hospitals, which, strangely, did not appear to be localized to any particular hospital or due to any specific organism. The time course of the increase in cases coincided, however, with introduction of a new reimbursement system for Medicare patients based on Diagnosis-Related Groups (Cohen *et al.*, 1987). The new payment system created financial incentives for hospitals to increase reporting of septicemia on billing claims, which may have occurred either through more complete reporting or by shifts in how diagnoses were coded.

Inpatient Care

Some diseases, such as appendicitis, hip fracture, or meningitis, almost always involve treatment in a hospital. For these conditions, hospital discharge data can be a valuable resource for identifying cases. Discharge abstract data typically include at least demographic information, date and length of hospitalization, diagnoses, surgical procedures, and vital status on discharge.

The usefulness of such data for epidemiologic purposes is further enhanced if the hospitals generating the data provide essentially all inpatient care for a defined population, allowing calculation of incidence rates. This situation is fully or nearly satisfied in several American states, in which all hospitals contribute records of discharges to a statewide database (Steiner *et al.*, 2002). Nationally, NCHS has gathered data on inpatient discharges since 1965, based on a probability sample of about 500 non-federal, short-stay U.S. hospitals with about 300,000 discharges annually (National Center for Health Statistics, 2012). After 2010, data-gathering at the sampled hospitals was expanded to include both inpatient and outpatient care, ambulatory surgery, and emergency care, composing what is now called the National Hospital Care Survey.

Population-based hospital discharge data are also available for several kinds of administratively defined populations. Inpatient care for an estimated 95% of the U.S. population over age 65 years is covered by Medicare (Lauderdale et al., 1993; Hennessy et al., 2007), albeit with some variation in coverage by age and race (Fisher et al., 1990). Medicare data have been used, for example, to study the incidence and case fatality of hip fracture among New England Medicare beneficiaries (Fisher et al., 1991).

The Department of Veterans Affairs (VA) operates about 172 hospitals that provide care for U.S. veterans (Boyko et al., 2000). It has gathered computerized discharge data on all hospitalizations since 1970 and uses electronic medical records systemwide. Use of the Social Security number as the primary patient identifier is a special advantage, facilitating linkage across hospitalizations, across facilities, or with other VA data. The population base for these data is less clear, however, because many veterans receive part or all of their health care outside the VA system. Linkage of VA and Medicare data may strengthen the epidemiologic research potential of both by enhancing completeness of case ascertainment for veterans age 65 years or older (Fleming et al., 1992; Hynes et al., 2007). Several large HMOs also maintain extensive computerized databases on health care use by their members, including hospitalizations (Fishman and Wagner, 1998; Selby, 1997; Psaty et al., 1991).

Outpatient Care

Many diseases routinely lead to use of health care but seldom require hospitalization—for example, rheumatoid arthritis, migraine headache, and urinary tract infection. Medically treated cases of these illnesses must therefore be sought using ambulatory-care medical records and/or administrative data that pertain to outpatient care.

For geographically defined populations, few settings have an ongoing mechanism in place to identify all cases of diseases treated on an outpatient basis. The Rochester Epidemiology Project in Rochester, Minnesota, is one such place, where medical records at the Mayo Clinic and at offices of a few independent care providers are regularly reviewed to gather diagnostic information community-wide (St. Sauver et al., 2011; Melton, 1996). For example, this

resource has been used to study the incidence and descriptive epidemiology of autism (Barbaresi et al., 2005) and of epilepsy (Hauser et al., 1993), both of which are treated mainly outside the hospital.

Increasing use of electronic health records has made possible *syndromic surveillance* in some settings. Data abstracted from emergency department visits are transmitted electronically to local public health authorities soon after the clinical encounters, allowing rapid detection of unusual increases in the frequency of certain chief complaints, syndromes, or diagnoses of possible public health importance. This approach has been used for surveillance of influenza (Bellazzini and Minor, 2011) and of illness related to West Nile virus (Chung et al., 2013).

Nationally, NCHS conducts two main ongoing surveys of ambulatory care (National Center for Health Statistics, 2012). The National Ambulatory Medical Care Survey involves a probability sample of approximately 180,000 outpatient visits each year to over 15,000 U.S. physicians in office-based practice, capturing data on patient demographics, diagnoses, and treatments. A complementary activity, the National Hospital Ambulatory Medical Care Survey, captures similar data on about 100,000 outpatient visits annually to about 480 hospital-associated clinics or emergency departments nationwide. These systems yield reasonably precise national and regional estimates but generally include too few observations from any one state or community to yield stable state or local estimates. Ability to link repeated encounters by the same person over time is also limited.

Pharmacy Records

Besides providing a source of data on exposure to prescription drugs, computerized pharmacy data can also be used to identify cases of a disease linked to a particular drug. For example, records of prescriptions for insulin can be used to identify people with diabetes. Medicaid data have also been especially useful for pharmacoepidemiologic research, because exposure to a prescription drug can be ascertained from billing claims in settings where the Medicaid program covers them (Ray and Griffin, 1989).

Population Health Surveys

Some nonfatal illnesses rarely result in a medical care encounter—for example, minor injuries, headaches, upper respiratory infections, and chronic fatigue. Although they may be medically less severe, many such diseases are very common and, in the aggregate, can constitute a significant public health burden. Yet the data sources listed above, which rely on the health care system, may not be adequate for case identification. Obtaining more complete population-based data on their occurrence often requires a health survey: that is, sampling persons from the target population and gathering data about them by mail, telephone, face-to-face contact, or other means not dependent on their use of medical care. Three large ongoing national surveys that use different methods of data collection exemplify this approach:

- The *National Health Interview Survey* (NHIS), conducted by NCHS, is a continuous survey of the civilian, non-institutionalized U.S. population. It currently involves about 40,000 households comprising about 100,000 individuals each year. Households are selected using multistage probability sampling, with oversampling of blacks, Hispanics, and Asians. Data are collected by in-person interview with an adult household member about household and family characteristics. In addition, one adult and one child (if applicable) are randomly sampled in each study household to gather more information on personal health characteristics. Core questions cover sociodemographics, family structure, income, occupation, acute and chronic conditions, injuries, overall health status, activity limitations, health behavior, immunizations, insurance status, perceived access to care, and health care use. This core set of questions is supplemented by others on special topics that change from year to year, such as use of cancer screening, or children's mental health.

  > **Example 6-3.**   Respiratory infections are common among schoolchildren and are easily spread among them. Tak *et al.* (2011) studied whether teachers, whose work brings them into regular close contact with children, are at increased risk for developing head or chest colds. Combining seven years of NHIS data, they found that the proportion of subjects responding yes to the question "Did you have a head cold or chest cold that started during the last 2 weeks?" was indeed higher among teachers than among other workers (odds ratio = 1.28,

  > 95% confidence interval 1.17 – 1.41), after accounting for demographic factors, smoking status, and the number of children in the respondent's household. The higher two-week cumulative incidence among teachers was greatest when the interview had been conducted during the school year; during the summer months, no excess incidence among teachers was observed.

- The *National Health and Nutrition Examination Survey* (NHANES), conducted by NCHS, uses mobile examination vans to carry out standardized in-person interviews, physical examinations, nutritional assessments, and diagnostic tests on a sample of about 5,000 people annually throughout the United States in randomly selected communities. Blacks, Hispanics, Asians, and persons over age 60 years are oversampled. This survey produces estimates of the prevalence of undiagnosed, often asymptomatic conditions, such as diabetes, hypertension, osteoporosis, and iron-deficiency anemia.

  > **Example 6-4.**   Impaired hearing in youth can interfere with their social development and education. Adolescents are of special concern because of the growing popularity of personal audio devices with earphones capable of playing music at volume levels loud enough to damage their hearing. Shargorodsky *et al.* (2010) used audiometric data from the National Health and Nutrition Examination Survey to track trends in the prevalence of hearing impairment among U.S. adolescents aged 12–19 years. They found that from 1988–1994 to 2005–2006, the prevalence of measurable hearing loss in that age group increased from 14.9% to 19.5%, with higher-frequency audio acuity being especially affected.

- The *Behavioral Risk Factor Surveillance System* (BRFSS), conducted by the CDC, involves telephone interviews with a probability sample of over 500,000 U.S. adults aged 18 years or older who are reachable by telephone in all 50 states. It is the largest ongoing telephone survey in the world. As its name suggests, BRFSS focuses on health-related behaviors, such as smoking, alcohol use, immunizations, and use of screening tests. But it also obtains information about selected health conditions reported by respondents, including hypertension, diabetes, asthma, dental disease, obesity, and HIV/AIDS. Core questions are asked of everyone in the sample, and states may add questions of their own or include optional "modules" that cover other health topics. In recent years, BRFSS has faced several challenges common to telephone surveys, including widespread use of answering machines or voice mail to filter calls, saturation of the public by telemarketing, and the growing percentage of the population with only cellular telephones. Response proportions have suffered, raising concerns about the representativeness of the respondent sample. Within-sample comparisons among subgroups may be less jeopardized. The BRFSS sampling frame has been expanded in recent years to include cellular telephone numbers as well as land-line telephone numbers in an attempt to reduce bias.

Example 6-5. Diez-Roux et al. (2000) used BRFSS data to investigate whether the extent of inequality in the distribution of income within U.S. states was associated with hypertension. Self-reported data on each respondent's hypertension status, family income, and other personal characteristics were drawn from the survey, while data on the income distribution in each state were drawn from the U.S. Census. Multilevel statistical modeling was then used to account simultaneously for the effects of both individual-level and state-level factors. Even after adjustment for individual income, hypertension was found to be more common among respondents living in states with more unequal income distributions—an association felt to represent a possible contextual effect of income inequality on health. Such a study would have been difficult or impossible without survey data on a large number of participants in each state.

Information about these surveys and other, more specialized health surveys can be obtained from the World Wide Web sites of the respective agencies (Appendix 6A), including copies of survey instruments, data collection protocols, sampling details, and guidance on proper data analysis. All three surveys yield fairly precise estimates for the entire United States and for large, multistate geographic regions. Samples sizes in BRFSS are generally large enough to yield fairly precise state-specific estimates as well. All three surveys involve complex sampling schemes that require the use of specialized analytic methods to obtain valid confidence limits and significance tests (Korn and Graubard, 1991, 1999; Levy and Lemeshow, 2009; Lumley, 2011).

DENOMINATOR DATA

Denominator data for geographically defined populations in the United States are usually based directly or indirectly on the decennial census. Counts from the most recent census are available online by age, gender, race/ethnicity, and sociodemographic characteristics at various levels of aggregation. Several of the most commonly used area types are summarized in Table 6.1 (U.S. Census Bureau, 2010). Note that ZIP code areas are defined, used, and sometimes changed by the U.S. Postal Service, not the Census Bureau, and are therefore not on this list. The Census Bureau does define ZIP Code Tabulation Areas that approximate ZIP code areas as of the most recent decennial census by aggregating census blocks (Grubesic and Matisziw, 2006).

The Census Bureau also prepares population estimates for calendar years between decennial censuses by age, gender, and race for counties and larger areas, and total population counts for certain areas smaller than a county. These intercensal estimates use information from births, deaths, number of federal tax returns and Medicare enrollees, and immigration statistics. Many state and local governments supplement Census Bureau statistics with their own intercensal estimates.

Census data can be purchased on computer media from the Census Bureau, downloaded from the Census Bureau's own extensive World Wide Web site, or obtained from CDC WONDER.

Although other sources of error may be greater in many epidemiologic applications, raw census counts

TABLE 6.1. SELECTED COMMONLY USED TYPES OF CENSUS AREAS

Area type, in order of decreasing size	Description	No. in 2010
Nation	–	1
Region	Combination of states	4
Division	Combination of states	9
State, plus D.C.	–	51
County	–	3,143
Census tract	Small area within a county, usually with about 2,500–8,000 residents and boundaries that follow visible features	73,057
Block group	Area with about 250–550 housing units, averaging 1/4 of a census tract	217,740
Block	Small area bounded by streets, streams, or other natural or legal boundaries	11,078,297

have been found to underestimate population size. The extent of undercounting varies among population subgroups. The Census Bureau's own estimates of degree of undercounting in the 2010 census, based on independent post-enumeration surveys, showed that the proportion undercounted tended to be greater among minorities and younger adult males, but was less than 5% in all of these groups (U.S. Census Bureau, 2012).

For administratively defined populations, a list of enrollees or population members almost always exists and may be continuously updated. For populations such as employee work forces, insurance plan enrollees, and school students, detailed data may also be available on member characteristics and each person's membership history, often in computerized form. These records can be used to obtain accurate estimates of the number of people or amount of person-time at risk.

USES OF MULTIPLE DATA SOURCES

When information on disease occurrence is obtainable from two or more sources for the same population, it can be possible to exploit them to obtain more accurate estimates of disease frequency. One data source can be used to evaluate, and sometimes to circumvent, limitations of another.

Validation Studies

A common problem is the possibility of "false positives"—that is, persons who are identified as cases in a data source but who do not actually qualify

under the study's case definition. This problem can occur in various ways, including diagnostic errors, coding mistakes, or having insufficient data to judge eligibility. Sometimes it can be addressed by a validation substudy that uses a second data source with more detailed or accurate information. Even if it is not feasible to check the second data source for all cases initially identified, it may be feasible and worthwhile to do so for a sample. Because medical records contain relatively detailed clinical information, they are often used as a secondary source for validation.

Example 6-6. Jiang *et al.* (1995) sought to measure the incidence of Guillain-Barré syndrome (GBS), a rare form of ascending paralysis, in southwest Stockholm, Sweden, using a population-based registry that relied chiefly on hospital discharge records. They expected that patients with GBS diagnosis codes—those labelled as "Guillain-Barré polyradiculitis" or "acute inflammatory polyneuropathy (Guillain-Barré syndrome)"—should qualify. But they were also concerned that some qualifying cases might be coded as "non-specific polyneuropathy," even though this catch-all category could also include patients with a variety of other neurological conditions. Accordingly, they conducted a validation study. A neurologist reviewed the medical records for 83 of the 103 patients discharged with a diagnosis code indicating GBS during an 18-year period, and for 40 patients discharged with non-specific polyneuropathy, using published criteria for GBS developed by the U.S. National Institutes of Health. They found that 83% of patients discharged with a GBS diagnosis code indeed met the diagnostic criteria for GBS, while no patients with non-specific polyneuropathy met them. As a result, the investigators reported a lower incidence estimate for GBS than the registry data alone suggested. They were also able to report that very few cases were missed through miscoding as non-specific polyneuropathy.

Estimating the Number of Missed Cases

The opposite problem can be thought of as "false negatives"—persons who meet the case definition but who are missed by a data source. Population-based registries often try to minimize under-ascertainment by seeking cases through two or more data sources, recognizing that no one source captures them all.

Perhaps surprisingly, having multiple data sources available for case identification can make it possible not only to estimate the number of cases missed by each source but also to estimate indirectly the number of cases missed by all sources combined, under certain assumptions. The statistical methods for doing so are based on *capture-recapture sampling* (Hook and Regal, 1995). The basic idea can be illustrated by considering just two data sources, which are assumed to cover the same base population over the same time period. Cases may be captured by both sources, by source #1 only, by source #2 only, or by neither source, as summarized in Table 6.2. The counts a, b, and c are thus known, while d is unknown. However, d can be estimated if the probability of capturing a case in source #1 can be assumed to be independent of the probability of capture in source #2. This independence assumption would imply that $a/(a+c) = b/(b+d)$. Solving this equation for the one unknown quantity, $d = bc/a$ is an estimate of the number of cases missed by both sources.

Example 6-7. *Chlamydia trachomatis* infection is the most commonly reported sexually transmitted disease in the United States, even though many medically recognized cases go unreported. The diagnosis is established when a medical laboratory finds a positive culture for the organism on a urethral or cervical swab specimen submitted by a physician or other clinician. In Massachusetts, both laboratories and clinicians are legally required to report every new case of *C. trachomatis* infection within 24 hours. Over a six-month period, a total of 5,259 cases were reported to the Massachusetts Department of Public

TABLE 6.2. SAMPLE DATA LAYOUT WHEN CASES CAN BE IDENTIFIED FROM TWO SOURCES

| | | Captured by source #2? | |
		Yes	No
Captured by source #1?	Yes	a	b
	No	c	d

Health. Some of these cases were reported by clinicians, some by laboratories, and some by both, as follows:

TABLE 6.3.

| Reported by clinicians | Reported by laboratories | | |
	Yes	No	Total
Yes	1,730	2,036	3,766
No	1,493	x	
Total	3,223		

It is evident from this table that neither clinicians nor laboratories reported all of the cases that had been medically recognized, despite the legal requirement to do so. Among the 3,223 cases reported by laboratories, only 1,730 (53.7%) of them had been reported by physicians. Among the 3,766 cases reported by physicians, only 1,730 (45.9%) had been reported by laboratories. The capture-recapture method is based on an assumption that if physician reporting was 53.7% complete among laboratory-reported cases, then it was also 53.7% complete among cases *not* reported by laboratories. If so, then $2,036 = 0.537 \cdot (2,036 + x)$, so that $x = 1,757$. The same result is obtained if the roles of the two data sources are reversed. Computationally, the easiest formula is $x = 2,036 \times 1,493/1,730 = 1,757$. Adding the estimated 1,757 doubly missed cases to the 5,259 reported cases yields an estimated total of 7,016 medically attended cases (Centers for Disease Control and Prevention, 2005).

Independence of case ascertainment between data sources is a fairly strong assumption and one not easily checked. Still, assuming instead that $x = 0$ flies in the face of evidence within the table that each data source is incomplete. In this example, assuming that $x = 0$ would be tantamount to saying that among laboratory-reported cases, physicians reported only 53.7% of them, but among cases *not* reported by laboratories, physicians reported 100.0% of them. Extensions of the capture-recapture method allow the independence assumption to be relaxed if there are three or more data sources (Hook and Regal, 1995; Ton *et al.*, 2010; Dunbar *et al.*, 2011).

Expanding Opportunities for Research Through Data Linkage

Beyond the ability to cross-check data sources, a wide range of substantive research questions can be addressed by linking data on disease occurrence from one data source with exposure data drawn from another source.

Example 6-8. Daling *et al.* (1982) investigated whether characteristics related to homosexual behavior were associated with the incidence of anal cancer in men. Taking care to protect confidentiality, names of men identified in western Washington State's population-based cancer registry as having anal cancer were linked to names in the state syphilis registry, which is based on disease reports from clinicians and medical laboratories. Eight of 47 men with anal cancer were found to have had a positive syphilis test result. Based on the proportion of men with cancer of other body sites who also had a positive test result in the syphilis registry, only 0.40 syphilis-positive anal cancer cases would have been expected.

The investigators also used data from ten U.S. population-based cancer registries to determine that 24.4% of male anal cancer cases had never been married, compared with 7.8% of men with colorectal cancer. Because both syphilis and being single were known to be associated with male homosexuality, the researchers suggested that anal intercourse could be a risk factor for anal cancer. This hypothesis was later supported by case-control studies that measured this exposure directly through personal interviews.

CONCLUSION

Besides the broadly useful data sources described in this overview, a variety of other specialized or localized resources can also be used for epidemiologic studies. Examples include armed forces intake examinations, screening programs, school or workplace absenteeism records, employer or union data, law enforcement and regulatory agency records, among others. More information about them can be found in references on public health surveillance (Lee *et al.*, 2010; Teutsch and Churchill, 2000) and administrative data sources (Virnig and McBean, 2001; Jutte *et al.*, 2011). The National Center for Health Statistics also publishes an annual volume entitled *Health, United States*, which includes a detailed appendix describing many sources of health data.

APPENDIX 6A: SELECTED WORLD WIDE WEB SITES

TABLE 6.4.

Organization	URL
Centers for Disease Control and Prevention	www.cdc.gov
CDC WONDER data retrieval system	wonder.cdc.gov
National Center for Health Statistics	www.cdc.gov/nchs
U.S. Census Bureau	www.census.gov
World Health Organization	www.who.int

APPENDIX 6B: MODEL DEATH CERTIFICATE

U.S. STANDARD CERTIFICATE OF DEATH

LOCAL FILE NO.   STATE FILE NO.

1. DECEDENT'S LEGAL NAME (Include AKA's if any) (First, Middle, Last) | 2. SEX | 3. SOCIAL SECURITY NUMBER

4a. AGE-Last Birthday (Years) | 4b. UNDER 1 YEAR (Months / Days) | 4c. UNDER 1 DAY (Hours / Minutes) | 5. DATE OF BIRTH (Mo/Day/Yr) | 6. BIRTHPLACE (City and State or Foreign Country)

7a. RESIDENCE-STATE | 7b. COUNTY | 7c. CITY OR TOWN

7d. STREET AND NUMBER | 7e. APT. NO. | 7f. ZIP CODE | 7g. INSIDE CITY LIMITS? □ Yes □ No

8. EVER IN US ARMED FORCES? □ Yes □ No | 9. MARITAL STATUS AT TIME OF DEATH □ Married □ Married, but separated □ Widowed □ Divorced □ Never Married □ Unknown | 10. SURVIVING SPOUSE'S NAME (If wife, give name prior to first marriage)

11. FATHER'S NAME (First, Middle, Last) | 12. MOTHER'S NAME PRIOR TO FIRST MARRIAGE (First, Middle, Last)

13a. INFORMANT'S NAME | 13b. RELATIONSHIP TO DECEDENT | 13c. MAILING ADDRESS (Street and Number, City, State, Zip Code)

14. PLACE OF DEATH (Check only one: see instructions)

IF DEATH OCCURRED IN A HOSPITAL: □ Inpatient □ Emergency Room/Outpatient □ Dead on Arrival | IF DEATH OCCURRED SOMEWHERE OTHER THAN A HOSPITAL: □ Hospice facility □ Nursing home/Long term care facility □ Decedent's home □ Other (Specify):

15. FACILITY NAME (If not institution, give street & number) | 16. CITY OR TOWN, STATE, AND ZIP CODE | 17. COUNTY OF DEATH

18. METHOD OF DISPOSITION: □ Burial □ Cremation □ Donation □ Entombment □ Removal from State □ Other (Specify): | 19. PLACE OF DISPOSITION (Name of cemetery, crematory, other place)

20. LOCATION-CITY, TOWN, AND STATE | 21. NAME AND COMPLETE ADDRESS OF FUNERAL FACILITY

22. SIGNATURE OF FUNERAL SERVICE LICENSEE OR OTHER AGENT | 23. LICENSE NUMBER (Of Licensee)

ITEMS 24-28 MUST BE COMPLETED BY PERSON WHO PRONOUNCES OR CERTIFIES DEATH | 24. DATE PRONOUNCED DEAD (Mo/Day/Yr) | 25. TIME PRONOUNCED DEAD

26. SIGNATURE OF PERSON PRONOUNCING DEATH (Only when applicable) | 27. LICENSE NUMBER | 28. DATE SIGNED (Mo/Day/Yr)

29. ACTUAL OR PRESUMED DATE OF DEATH (Mo/Day/Yr) (Spell Month) | 30. ACTUAL OR PRESUMED TIME OF DEATH | 31. WAS MEDICAL EXAMINER OR CORONER CONTACTED? □ Yes □ No

CAUSE OF DEATH (See instructions and examples)

32. PART I. Enter the chain of events–diseases, injuries, or complications–that directly caused the death. DO NOT enter terminal events such as cardiac arrest, respiratory arrest, or ventricular fibrillation without showing the etiology. DO NOT ABBREVIATE. Enter only one cause on a line. Add additional lines if necessary.

Approximate interval: Onset to death

IMMEDIATE CAUSE (Final disease or condition resulting in death) → a. _____ Due to (or as a consequence of):

Sequentially list conditions, if any, leading to the cause listed on line a. Enter the UNDERLYING CAUSE (disease or injury that initiated the events resulting in death) LAST

b. _____ Due to (or as a consequence of):

c. _____ Due to (or as a consequence of):

d. _____

PART II. Enter other significant conditions contributing to death but not resulting in the underlying cause given in PART I | 33. WAS AN AUTOPSY PERFORMED? □ Yes □ No

34. WERE AUTOPSY FINDINGS AVAILABLE TO COMPLETE THE CAUSE OF DEATH? □ Yes □ No

35. DID TOBACCO USE CONTRIBUTE TO DEATH? □ Yes □ Probably □ No □ Unknown | 36. IF FEMALE: □ Not pregnant within past year □ Pregnant at time of death □ Not pregnant, but pregnant within 42 days of death □ Not pregnant, but pregnant 43 days to 1 year before death □ Unknown if pregnant within the past year | 37. MANNER OF DEATH □ Natural □ Homicide □ Accident □ Pending Investigation □ Suicide □ Could not be determined

38. DATE OF INJURY (Mo/Day/Yr) (Spell Month) | 39. TIME OF INJURY | 40. PLACE OF INJURY (e.g., Decedent's home; construction site; restaurant; wooded area) | 41. INJURY AT WORK? □ Yes □ No

42. LOCATION OF INJURY: State: | City or Town: | Street & Number: | Apartment No.: | Zip Code:

43. DESCRIBE HOW INJURY OCCURRED: | 44. IF TRANSPORTATION INJURY, SPECIFY: □ Driver/Operator □ Passenger □ Pedestrian □ Other (Specify)

45. CERTIFIER (Check only one):
□ Certifying physician-To the best of my knowledge, death occurred due to the cause(s) and manner stated.
□ Pronouncing & Certifying physician-To the best of my knowledge, death occurred at the time, date, and place, and due to the cause(s) and manner stated.
□ Medical Examiner/Coroner-On the basis of examination, and/or investigation, in my opinion, death occurred at the time, date, and place, and due to the cause(s) and manner stated.

Signature of certifier:

46. NAME, ADDRESS, AND ZIP CODE OF PERSON COMPLETING CAUSE OF DEATH (Item 32)

47. TITLE OF CERTIFIER | 48. LICENSE NUMBER | 49. DATE CERTIFIED (Mo/Day/Yr) | 50. FOR REGISTRAR ONLY- DATE FILED (Mo/Day/Yr)

51. DECEDENT'S EDUCATION-Check the box that best describes the highest degree or level of school completed at the time of death.
□ 8th grade or less
□ 9th - 12th grade; no diploma
□ High school graduate or GED completed
□ Some college credit, but no degree
□ Associate degree (e.g., AA, AS)
□ Bachelor's degree (e.g., BA, AB, BS)
□ Master's degree (e.g., MA, MS, MEng, MEd, MSW, MBA)
□ Doctorate (e.g., PhD, EdD) or Professional degree (e.g., MD, DDS, DVM, LLB, JD)

52. DECEDENT OF HISPANIC ORIGIN? Check the box that best describes whether the decedent is Spanish/Hispanic/Latino. Check the "No" box if decedent is not Spanish/Hispanic/Latino.
□ No, not Spanish/Hispanic/Latino
□ Yes, Mexican, Mexican American, Chicano
□ Yes, Puerto Rican
□ Yes, Cuban
□ Yes, other Spanish/Hispanic/Latino (Specify) _____

53. DECEDENT'S RACE (Check one or more races to indicate what the decedent considered himself or herself to be)
□ White
□ Black or African American
□ American Indian or Alaska Native (Name of the enrolled or principal tribe) _____
□ Asian Indian
□ Chinese
□ Filipino
□ Japanese
□ Korean
□ Vietnamese
□ Other Asian (Specify) _____
□ Native Hawaiian
□ Guamanian or Chamorro
□ Samoan
□ Other Pacific Islander (Specify) _____
□ Other (Specify) _____

54. DECEDENT'S USUAL OCCUPATION (Indicate type of work done during most of working life. DO NOT USE RETIRED.)

55. KIND OF BUSINESS/INDUSTRY

NAME OF DECEDENT — For use by physician or institution

To Be Completed/ Verified By: FUNERAL DIRECTOR:

To Be Completed By: MEDICAL CERTIFIER

To Be Completed By: FUNERAL DIRECTOR

REV. 11/2003

FIGURE 6.3

APPENDIX 6C: MODEL BIRTH CERTIFICATE

U.S. STANDARD CERTIFICATE OF LIVE BIRTH

BIRTH NUMBER:

LOCAL FILE NO.

C H I L D

1. CHILD'S NAME (First, Middle, Last, Suffix)	2. TIME OF BIRTH (24 hr)	3. SEX	4. DATE OF BIRTH (Mo/Day/Yr)

5. FACILITY NAME (If not institution, give street and number)	6. CITY, TOWN, OR LOCATION OF BIRTH	7. COUNTY OF BIRTH

M O T H E R

8a. MOTHER'S CURRENT LEGAL NAME (First, Middle, Last, Suffix)	8b. DATE OF BIRTH (Mo/Day/Yr)

8c. MOTHER'S NAME PRIOR TO FIRST MARRIAGE (First, Middle, Last, Suffix)	8d. BIRTHPLACE (State, Territory, or Foreign Country)

9a. RESIDENCE OF MOTHER-STATE	9b. COUNTY	9c. CITY, TOWN, OR LOCATION

9d. STREET AND NUMBER	9e. APT. NO.	9f. ZIP CODE	9g. INSIDE CITY LIMITS? □ Yes □ No

F A T H E R

10a. FATHER'S CURRENT LEGAL NAME (First, Middle, Last, Suffix)	10b. DATE OF BIRTH (Mo/Day/Yr)	10c. BIRTHPLACE (State, Territory, or Foreign Country)

CERTIFIER

11. CERTIFIER'S NAME: _____ TITLE: □ MD □ DO □ HOSPITAL ADMIN. □ CNM/CM □ OTHER MIDWIFE □ OTHER (Specify)_____	12. DATE CERTIFIED ___/___/___ MM DD YYYY	13. DATE FILED BY REGISTRAR ___/___/___ MM DD YYYY

INFORMATION FOR ADMINISTRATIVE USE

M O T H E R

14. MOTHER'S MAILING ADDRESS: 9 Same as residence, or: State:	City, Town, or Location:
Street & Number:	Apartment No.:	Zip Code:

15. MOTHER MARRIED? (At birth, conception, or any time between) □ Yes □ No IF NO, HAS PATERNITY ACKNOWLEDGEMENT BEEN SIGNED IN THE HOSPITAL? □ Yes □ No	16. SOCIAL SECURITY NUMBER REQUESTED FOR CHILD? □ Yes □ No	17. FACILITY ID. (NPI)

18. MOTHER'S SOCIAL SECURITY NUMBER:	19. FATHER'S SOCIAL SECURITY NUMBER:

INFORMATION FOR MEDICAL AND HEALTH PURPOSES ONLY

M O T H E R

20. MOTHER'S EDUCATION (Check the box that best describes the highest degree or level of school completed at the time of delivery)	21. MOTHER OF HISPANIC ORIGIN? (Check the box that best describes whether the mother is Spanish/Hispanic/Latina. Check the "No" box if mother is not Spanish/Hispanic/Latina)	22. MOTHER'S RACE (Check one or more races to indicate what the mother considers herself to be)
□ 8th grade or less	□ No, not Spanish/Hispanic/Latina	□ White
□ 9th - 12th grade, no diploma	□ Yes, Mexican, Mexican American, Chicana	□ Black or African American
□ High school graduate or GED completed	□ Yes, Puerto Rican	□ American Indian or Alaska Native (Name of the enrolled or principal tribe)_____
□ Some college credit but no degree	□ Yes, Cuban	□ Asian Indian
□ Associate degree (e.g., AA, AS)	□ Yes, other Spanish/Hispanic/Latina	□ Chinese
□ Bachelor's degree (e.g., BA, AB, BS)	(Specify)_____	□ Filipino
□ Master's degree (e.g., MA, MS, MEng, MEd, MSW, MBA)		□ Japanese
□ Doctorate (e.g., PhD, EdD) or Professional degree (e.g., MD, DDS, DVM, LLB, JD)		□ Korean □ Vietnamese □ Other Asian (Specify)_____ □ Native Hawaiian □ Guamanian or Chamorro □ Samoan □ Other Pacific Islander (Specify)_____ □ Other (Specify)_____

F A T H E R

23. FATHER'S EDUCATION (Check the box that best describes the highest degree or level of school completed at the time of delivery)	24. FATHER OF HISPANIC ORIGIN? (Check the box that best describes whether the father is Spanish/Hispanic/Latino. Check the "No" box if father is not Spanish/Hispanic/Latino)	25. FATHER'S RACE (Check one or more races to indicate what the father considers himself to be)
□ 8th grade or less	□ No, not Spanish/Hispanic/Latino	□ White
□ 9th - 12th grade, no diploma	□ Yes, Mexican, Mexican American, Chicano	□ Black or African American
□ High school graduate or GED completed	□ Yes, Puerto Rican	□ American Indian or Alaska Native (Name of the enrolled or principal tribe)_____
□ Some college credit but no degree	□ Yes, Cuban	□ Asian Indian
□ Associate degree (e.g., AA, AS)	□ Yes, other Spanish/Hispanic/Latino	□ Chinese
□ Bachelor's degree (e.g., BA, AB, BS)	(Specify)_____	□ Filipino
□ Master's degree (e.g., MA, MS, MEng, MEd, MSW, MBA)		□ Japanese
□ Doctorate (e.g., PhD, EdD) or Professional degree (e.g., MD, DDS, DVM, LLB, JD)		□ Korean □ Vietnamese □ Other Asian (Specify)_____ □ Native Hawaiian □ Guamanian or Chamorro □ Samoan □ Other Pacific Islander (Specify)_____ □ Other (Specify)_____

Mother's Name

Mother's Medical Record No.

26. PLACE WHERE BIRTH OCCURRED (Check one) □ Hospital □ Freestanding birthing center □ Home Birth: Planned to deliver at home? 9 Yes 9 No □ Clinic/Doctor's office □ Other (Specify)_____	27. ATTENDANT'S NAME, TITLE, AND NPI NAME: _____ NPI:_____ TITLE: □ MD □ DO □ CNM/CM □ OTHER MIDWIFE □ OTHER (Specify)_____	28. MOTHER TRANSFERRED FOR MATERNAL MEDICAL OR FETAL INDICATIONS FOR DELIVERY? □ Yes □ No IF YES, ENTER NAME OF FACILITY MOTHER TRANSFERRED FROM: _____

REV. 11/2003

FIGURE 6.4

MOTHER

29a. DATE OF FIRST PRENATAL CARE VISIT
___/___/___ □ No Prenatal Care
MM DD YYYY

29b. DATE OF LAST PRENATAL CARE VISIT
___/___/___
MM DD YYYY

30. TOTAL NUMBER OF PRENATAL VISITS FOR THIS PREGNANCY
_____ (If none, enter ʌ0".)

31. MOTHER'S HEIGHT
_____ (feet/inches)

32. MOTHER'S PREPREGNANCY WEIGHT
_____ (pounds)

33. MOTHER'S WEIGHT AT DELIVERY
_____ (pounds)

34. DID MOTHER GET WIC FOOD FOR HERSELF DURING THIS PREGNANCY? □ Yes □ No

35. NUMBER OF PREVIOUS LIVE BIRTHS (Do not include this child)

35a. Now Living
Number _____
□ None

35b. Now Dead
Number _____
□ None

36. NUMBER OF OTHER PREGNANCY OUTCOMES (spontaneous or induced losses or ectopic pregnancies)

36a. Other Outcomes
Number _____
□ None

37. CIGARETTE SMOKING BEFORE AND DURING PREGNANCY
For each time period, enter either the number of cigarettes or the number of packs of cigarettes smoked. IF NONE, ENTER ʌ0".

Average number of cigarettes or packs of cigarettes smoked per day.

	# of cigarettes		# of packs
Three Months Before Pregnancy	_____	OR	_____
First Three Months of Pregnancy	_____	OR	_____
Second Three Months of Pregnancy	_____	OR	_____
Third Trimester of Pregnancy	_____	OR	_____

38. PRINCIPAL SOURCE OF PAYMENT FOR THIS DELIVERY
□ Private Insurance
□ Medicaid
□ Self-pay
□ Other (Specify) _____

35c. DATE OF LAST LIVE BIRTH
___/___
MM YYYY

36b. DATE OF LAST OTHER PREGNANCY OUTCOME
___/___
MM YYYY

39. DATE LAST NORMAL MENSES BEGAN
___/___/___
MM DD YYYY

40. MOTHER'S MEDICAL RECORD NUMBER

MEDICAL AND HEALTH INFORMATION

41. RISK FACTORS IN THIS PREGNANCY (Check all that apply)

Diabetes
□ Prepregnancy (Diagnosis prior to this pregnancy)
□ Gestational (Diagnosis in this pregnancy)

Hypertension
□ Prepregnancy (Chronic)
□ Gestational (PIH, preeclampsia)
□ Eclampsia

□ Previous preterm birth

□ Other previous poor pregnancy outcome (Includes perinatal death, small-for-gestational age/intrauterine growth restricted birth)

□ Pregnancy resulted from infertility treatment-If yes, check all that apply:
□ Fertility-enhancing drugs, Artificial insemination or Intrauterine insemination
□ Assisted reproductive technology (e.g., in vitro fertilization (IVF), gamete intrafallopian transfer (GIFT))

□ Mother had a previous cesarean delivery
If yes, how many _____

□ None of the above

42. INFECTIONS PRESENT AND/OR TREATED DURING THIS PREGNANCY (Check all that apply)
□ Gonorrhea
□ Syphilis
□ Chlamydia
□ Hepatitis B
□ Hepatitis C
□ None of the above

43. OBSTETRIC PROCEDURES (Check all that apply)
□ Cervical cerclage
□ Tocolysis

External cephalic version:
□ Successful
□ Failed
□ None of the above

44. ONSET OF LABOR (Check all that apply)
□ Premature Rupture of the Membranes (prolonged, ∃12 hrs.)
□ Precipitous Labor (<3 hrs.)
□ Prolonged Labor (∃ 20 hrs.)
□ None of the above

45. CHARACTERISTICS OF LABOR AND DELIVERY (Check all that apply)
□ Induction of labor
□ Augmentation of labor
□ Non-vertex presentation
□ Steroids (glucocorticoids) for fetal lung maturation received by the mother prior to delivery
□ Antibiotics received by the mother during labor
□ Clinical chorioamnionitis diagnosed during labor or maternal temperature ≥38°C (100.4°F)
□ Moderate/heavy meconium staining of the amniotic fluid
□ Fetal intolerance of labor such that one or more of the following actions was taken: In-utero resuscitative measures, further fetal assessment, or operative delivery
□ Epidural or spinal anesthesia during labor
□ None of the above

46. METHOD OF DELIVERY

A. Was delivery with forceps attempted but unsuccessful?
□ Yes □ No

B. Was delivery with vacuum extraction attempted but unsuccessful?
□ Yes □ No

C. Fetal presentation at birth
□ Cephalic
□ Breech
□ Other

D. Final route and method of delivery (Check one)
□ Vaginal/Spontaneous
□ Vaginal/Forceps
□ Vaginal/Vacuum
□ Cesarean
If cesarean, was a trial of labor attempted?
□ Yes
□ No

47. MATERNAL MORBIDITY (Check all that apply) (Complications associated with labor and delivery)
□ Maternal transfusion
□ Third or fourth degree perineal laceration
□ Ruptured uterus
□ Unplanned hysterectomy
□ Admission to intensive care unit
□ Unplanned operating room procedure following delivery
□ None of the above

NEWBORN INFORMATION

NEWBORN

Mother's Name _____
Mother's Medical Record No. _____

48. NEWBORN MEDICAL RECORD NUMBER

49. BIRTHWEIGHT (grams preferred, specify unit)
_____
9 grams 9 lb/oz

50. OBSTETRIC ESTIMATE OF GESTATION:
_____ (completed weeks)

51. APGAR SCORE:
Score at 5 minutes: _____
If 5 minute score is less than 6,
Score at 10 minutes: _____

52. PLURALITY - Single, Twin, Triplet, etc.
(Specify) _____

53. IF NOT SINGLE BIRTH - Born First, Second, Third, etc. (Specify) _____

54. ABNORMAL CONDITIONS OF THE NEWBORN (Check all that apply)
□ Assisted ventilation required immediately following delivery
□ Assisted ventilation required for more than six hours
□ NICU admission
□ Newborn given surfactant replacement therapy
□ Antibiotics received by the newborn for suspected neonatal sepsis
□ Seizure or serious neurologic dysfunction
□ Significant birth injury (skeletal fracture(s), peripheral nerve injury, and/or soft tissue/solid organ hemorrhage which requires intervention)
9 None of the above

55. CONGENITAL ANOMALIES OF THE NEWBORN (Check all that apply)
□ Anencephaly
□ Meningomyelocele/Spina bifida
□ Cyanotic congenital heart disease
□ Congenital diaphragmatic hernia
□ Omphalocele
□ Gastroschisis
□ Limb reduction defect (excluding congenital amputation and dwarfing syndromes)
□ Cleft Lip with or without Cleft Palate
□ Cleft Palate alone
□ Down Syndrome
□ Karyotype confirmed
□ Karyotype pending
□ Suspected chromosomal disorder
□ Karyotype confirmed
□ Karyotype pending
□ Hypospadias
□ None of the anomalies listed above

56. WAS INFANT TRANSFERRED WITHIN 24 HOURS OF DELIVERY? 9 Yes 9 No
IF YES, NAME OF FACILITY INFANT TRANSFERRED TO: _____

57. IS INFANT LIVING AT TIME OF REPORT?
□ Yes □ No □ Infant transferred, status unknown

58. IS THE INFANT BEING BREASTFED AT DISCHARGE?
□ Yes □ No

FIGURE 6.5

REFERENCES

Addiss DG, Shaffer N, Fowler BS, Tauxe RV. The epidemiology of appendicitis and appendectomy in the United States. Am J Epidemiol 1990; 132: 910–925.

Ajani UA, Ford ES. Has the risk for coronary heart disease changed among U.S. adults? J Am Coll Cardiol 2006; 48:1177–1182.

Barbaresi WJ, Katusic SK, Colligan RC, Weaver AL, Jacobsen SJ. The incidence of autism in Olmsted County, Minnesota, 1976–1997: results from a population-based study. Arch Pediatr Adolesc Med 2005; 159:37–44.

Bellazzini MA, Minor KD. ED syndromic surveillance for novel H1N1 spring 2009. Am J Emerg Med 2011; 29:70–74.

Boswell J. The life of Samuel Johnson. New York: Penguin, 1791.

Boyko EJ, Koepsell TD, Gaziano JM, Horner RD, Feussner JR. US Department of Veterans Affairs medical care system as a resource to epidemiologists. Am J Epidemiol 2000; 151:307–314.

Boyle CA, Decoufle P. National sources of vital status information: extent of coverage and possible selectivity in reporting. Am J Epidemiol 1990; 131: 160–168.

Buescher PA. Diabetes prevalence and risk factors among North Carolina adults: 2001. NC Med J 2003; 64:68–69.

Caban-Martinez AJ, Lee DJ, Fleming LE, Arheart KL, Leblanc WG, Chung-Bridges K, et al. Dental care access and unmet dental care needs among U.S. workers: the National Health Interview Survey, 1997 to 2003. J Am Dent Assoc 2007; 138: 227–230.

Centers for Disease Control and Prevention. Risk factors for short interpregnancy interval—Utah, June 1996–June 1997. MMWR Morb Mortal Wkly Rep 1998; 43: 930–934.

Centers for Disease Control and Prevention. Reporting of chlamydial infection–Massachusetts, January–June 2003. MMWR Morb Mortal Wkly Rep 2005; 54:558–560.

Centers for Disease Control and Prevention. Update: influenza activity—United States, 2009–10 season. MMWR Morb Mortal Wkly Rep 2010; 59:901–908.

Centers for Disease Control and Prevention. Office-related antibiotic prescribing for persons aged ≤ 14 years—United States, 1993–1994 to 2007–2008. MMWR Morb Mortal Wkly Rep 2011; 60: 1153–1156.

Centers for Disease Control and Prevention. http://wonder.cdc.gov/ 2012.

Centers for Disease Control and Prevention. Summary of notifiable diseases, United States—2010. MMWR 2012; 59:1–116.

Chung WM, Buseman CM, Joyner SN, Hughes SM, Fomby TB, Luby JP, et al. The 2012 West Nile encephalitis epidemic in Dallas, Texas. JAMA 2013; 310:297–307.

Cohen BB, Pokras R, Meads MS, Krushat WM. How will diagnosis-related groups affect epidemiologic research? Am J Epidemiol 1987; 126: 1–9.

Correa-Villaseñor A, Cragan J, Kucik J, O'Leary L, Siffel C, Williams L. The Metropolitan Atlanta Congenital Defects Program: 35 years of birth defects surveillance at the Centers for Disease Control and Prevention. Birth Defects Res A Clin Mol Teratol 2003; 67:617–624.

Cowper DC, Kubal JD, Maynard C, Hynes DM. A primer and comparative review of major US mortality databases. Ann Epidemiol 2002; 12: 462–468.

Cram P, Rosenthal GE, Vaughan-Sarrazin MS. Cardiac revascularization in specialty and general hospitals. N Engl J Med 2005; 352:1454–1462.

Daling JR, Weiss NS, Klopfenstein LL, Cochran LE, Chow WH, Daifuku R. Correlates of homosexual behavior and the incidence of anal cancer. JAMA 1982; 247:1988–1990.

Diez-Roux AV, Link BG, Northridge ME. A multilevel analysis of income inequality and cardiovascular disease risk factors. Soc Sci Med 2000; 50: 673–687.

DiGiuseppe DL, Aron DC, Ranbom L, Harper DL, Rosenthal GE. Reliability of birth certificate data: a multi-hospital comparison to medical records information. Matern Child Health J 2002; 6: 169–179.

Doyle TJ, Glynn MK, Groseclose SL. Completeness of notifiable infectious disease reporting in the United States: an analytical literature review. Am J Epidemiol 2002; 155:866–874.

Dunbar R, van Hest R, Lawrence K, Verver S, Enarson DA, Lombard C, et al. Capture-recapture to estimate completeness of tuberculosis surveillance in two communities in South Africa. Int J Tuberc Lung Dis 2011; 15:1038–1043.

Fisher ES, Baron JA, Malenka DJ, Barrett J, Bubolz TA. Overcoming potential pitfalls in the use of Medicare data for epidemiologic research. Am J Public Health 1990; 80:1487–1490.

Fisher ES, Baron JA, Malenka DJ, Barrett JA, Kniffin WD, Whaley FS, et al. Hip fracture incidence and mortality in New England. Epidemiology 1991; 2:116–122.

Fishman PA, Wagner EH. Managed care data and public health: the experience of Group Health Cooperative of Puget Sound. Annu Rev Public Health 1998; 19:477–491.

Fleming C, Fisher ES, Chang CH, Bubolz TA, Malenka DJ. Studying outcomes and hospital utilization in the elderly. The advantages of a merged data base for Medicare and Veterans Affairs hospitals. Med Care 1992; 30:377–391.

Foege WH, Millar JD, Lane JM. Selective epidemiologic control in smallpox eradication. Am J Epidemiol 1971; 94:311–315.

Fredrickson DS. The field trial: some thoughts on the indispensable ordeal. Bull NY Acad Med 1968; 44:985–993.

Friede A, Reid JA, Ory HW. CDC WONDER: A comprehensive on-line public health information system of the Centers for Disease Control and Prevention. Am J Public Health 1993; 83:1289–1294.

Gittelsohn A, Royston PN. Annotated bibliography of cause-of-death validation studies, 1958–80. National Center for Health Statistics. Vital and Health Statistics 2(89), 1982.

Greb AE, Pauli RM, Kirby RS. Accuracy of fetal death reports: comparison with data from an independent stillbirth assessment program. Am J Public Health 1987; 77:1202–1206.

Grubesic TH, Matisziw TC. On the use of ZIP codes and ZIP code tabulation areas (ZCTAs) for the spatial analysis of epidemiological data. Int J Health Geogr 2006; 5:58.

Harter L, Starzyk P, Frost F. A comparative study of hospital fetal death records and Washington State fetal death certificates. Am J Public Health 1986; 76:1333–1334.

Hauser WA, Annegers JF, Kurland LT. Incidence of epilepsy and unprovoked seizures in Rochester, Minnesota: 1935–1984. Epilepsia 1993; 34:453–468.

Helms CM. A pseudo-epidemic of septicemia among Medicare patients in Iowa. Am J Public Health 1987; 77:1331–1332.

Hennessy S, Leonard CE, Palumbo CM, Newcomb C, Bilker WB. Quality of Medicaid and Medicare data obtained through Centers for Medicare and Medicaid Services (CMS). Med Care 2007; 45:1216–1220.

Honein MA, Paulozzi LJ. Birth defects surveillance: assessing the "gold standard". Am J Public Health 1999; 89:1238–1240.

Hook EB, Regal RR. Capture-recapture methods in epidemiology: methods and limitations. Epidemiol Rev 1995; 17:243–264.

Hoyert DL, Kung HC, Xu J. Autopsy patterns in 2003. National Center for Health Statistics. Vital and Health Statistics 20(32), 2007.

Hynes DM, Koelling K, Stroupe K, Arnold N, Mallin K, Sohn MW, et al. Veterans' access to and use of Medicare and Veterans Affairs health care. Med Care 2007; 45:214–223.

Jiang GX, de Pedro-Cuesta J, Fredrikson S. Guillain-Barré syndrome in southwest Stockholm, 1973–1991. 1. Quality of registered hospital diagnoses and incidence. Acta Neurol Scand 1995; 91:109–117.

Jutte DP, Roos LL, Brownell MD. Administrative record linkage as a tool for public health research. Annu Rev Public Health 2011; 32:91–108.

Kircher T, Nelson J, Burdo H. The autopsy as a measure of accuracy of the death certificate. N Engl J Med 1985; 313:1263–1269.

Klompas M, McVetta J, Lazarus R, Eggleston E, Haney G, Kruskal BA, et al. Integrating clinical practice and public health surveillance using electronic medical record systems. Am J Prev Med 2012; 42:S154–S162.

Konowitz PM, Petrossian GA, Rose DN. The underreporting of disease and physician's knowledge of reporting requirements. Public Health Rep 1984; 99:31–35.

Korn EL, Graubard BI. Epidemiologic studies utilizing surveys: accounting for the sampling design. Am J Public Health 1991; 81:1166–1173.

Korn EL, Graubard BI. Analysis of health surveys. New York: Wiley, 1999.

Lammer EJ, Brown LE, Anderka MT, Guyer B. Classification and analysis of fetal deaths in Massachusetts. JAMA 1989; 261:1757–1762.

Lauderdale DS, Furner SE, Miles TP, Goldberg J. Epidemiologic uses of Medicare data. Epidemiol Rev 1993; 15:319–327.

Lee LM, Teutsch SM, Thacker SB, Louis MES. Principles and practice of public health surveillance (3rd ed.). New York: Oxford University Press, 2010.

Levy PS, Lemeshow S. Sampling of populations: methods and applications (4th ed.). New York: Wiley, 2009.

Lindgren ML, Byers RH Jr, Thomas P, Davis SF, Caldwell B, Rogers M, et al. Trends in perinatal transmission of HIV/AIDS in the United States. JAMA 1999; 282:531–538.

Lumley T. Complex surveys: a guide to analysis using R. New York: Wiley and Sons, 2011.

Lydon-Rochelle MT, Holt VL, Cárdenas V, Nelson JC, Easterling TR, Gardella C, et al. The reporting of pre-existing maternal medical conditions and complications of pregnancy on birth certificates and in hospital discharge data. Am J Obstet Gynecol 2005; 193:125–134.

Marier R. The reporting of communicable disease. Am J Epidemiol 1977; 105:587–590.

Martin JA, Hoyert DL. The national fetal death file. Semin Perinatol 2002; 26:3–11.

Marzuk PM, Tardiff K, Leon AC. Increase in fatal suicidal poisonings and suffocations in the year *Final Exit* was published: a national study. Am J Psychiatry 1994; 151:1813–1814.

Melton LJ. History of the Rochester Epidemiology Project. Mayo Clin Proc 1996; 71:266–274.

Mueller BA, Simon MS, Deapen D, Kamineni A, Malone KE, Daling JR. Childbearing and survival after breast carcinoma in young women. Cancer 2003; 98:1131–1140.

National Center for Health Statistics. Summary of current surveys and data collection systems. Hyattsville, MD: National Center for Health Statistics, 2012.

Pasupathy D, Wood AM, Pell JP, Fleming M, Smith GCS. Time of birth and risk of neonatal death at term: retrospective cohort study. BMJ 2010; 341:c3498.

Psaty BM, Koepsell TD, Siscovick D, Wahl P, Logerfo JP, Inui TS, et al. An approach to several problems in using large databases for population-based case-control studies of the therapeutic efficacy and safety of anti-hypertensive medicines. Stat Med 1991; 10:653–662.

Rasmussen SA, Wong LY, Yang Q, May KM, Friedman JM. Population-based analyses of mortality in trisomy 13 and trisomy 18. Pediatrics 2003; 111:777–784.

Ray WA. Improving automated database studies. Epidemiology 2011; 22:302–304.

Ray WA, Griffin MR. Use of Medicaid data for pharmacoepidemiology. Am J Epidemiol 1989; 129:837–849.

Rhodes JC, Schoendorf KC, Parker JD. Contribution of excess weight gain during pregnancy and macrosomia to the cesarean delivery rate, 1990–2000. Pediatrics 2003; 111:1181–1185.

Rosenberg MJ, Gangarosa EJ, Pollard RA, Wallace M, Brolnitsky O. Shigella surveillance in the United States, 1975. J Infect Dis 1977; 136:458–460.

Roush S, Birkhead G, Koo D, Cobb A, Fleming D. Mandatory reporting of diseases and conditions by health care professionals and laboratories. JAMA 1999; 282:164–170.

Selby JV. Linking automated databases for research in managed care settings. Ann Intern Med 1997; 127:719–724.

Shargorodsky J, Curhan SG, Curhan GC, Eavey R. Change in prevalence of hearing loss in US adolescents. JAMA 2010; 304:772–778.

Smith Sehdev AE, Hutchins GM. Problems with proper completion and accuracy of the cause-of-death statement. Arch Intern Med 2001; 161:277–284.

Speizer FE, Doll R, Heaf P. Observations on recent increase in mortality from asthma. Br Med J 1968; 1:335–339.

St. Sauver JL, Grossardt BR, Yawn BP, Melton LJ 3rd, Rocca WA. Use of a medical records linkage system to enumerate a dynamic population over time: the Rochester Epidemiology Project. Am J Epidemiol 2011; 173:1059–1068.

Steiner C, Elixhauser A, Schnaier J. The Healthcare Cost and Utilization Project: an overview. Eff Clin Pract 2002; 5:143–151.

Tak S, Groenewold M, Alterman T, Park RM, Calvert GM. Excess risk of head and chest colds among teachers and other school workers. J Sch Health 2011; 81:560–565.

Teutsch SM, Churchill RE. Principles and practice of public health surveillance (2nd ed.). New York: Oxford, 2000.

Ton TG, Jain S, Boudreau R, Thacker EL, Strotmeyer ES, Newman AB, et al. Post hoc Parkinson's disease: identifying an uncommon disease in the Cardiovascular Health Study. Neuroepidemiology 2010; 35:241–249.

US Census Bureau. Census 2010: geographic terms and concepts. Washington, D.C.: U.S. Department of Commerce, 2010.

US Census Bureau. Census coverage measurement estimation report: summary of estimates of coverage for persons in the United States. DSSD 2010 Census coverage measurement memorandum series #2010-G-01. Washington, D.C.: U.S. Census Bureau, 2012.

Ventura SJ, Martin JA, Curtin SC, Mathews TJ, Park MM. Births: final data for 1998. National vital statistics reports; vol. 48, no. 3. Hyattsville, MD: National Center for Health Statistics, 2000.

Virnig BA, McBean M. Administrative data for public health surveillance and planning. Annu Rev Public Health 2001; 22:213–230.

Weiss NS. The new world of data linkages in clinical epidemiology: are we being brave or foolhardy? Epidemiology 2011; 22:292–294.

Whitfield K, Kelly H. Using the two-source capture-recapture method to estimate the incidence of acute flaccid paralysis in Victoria, Australia. Bull World Health Organ 2002; 80:846–851.

World Health Organization. International Statistical Classification of Diseases and Related Health Problems—10th revision, edition 2010 (3 volumes). Geneva: World Health Organization, 2011.

EXERCISES

1. For each of the following research topics, suggest a feasible source or sources of existing data on disease occurrence. Assume that the information you need is not available in any published reports. Instead, you need data that you can analyze yourself to address the question(s) of interest, but you do not have the resources to mount your own primary data collection effort.

(a) Trisomy 13 and 18 are rare but clinically serious chromosomal abnormalities usually detected around the time of birth. Although in most cases the disease is rapidly fatal within days, there have been case reports of affected babies living for up to a year or more. Doctors and genetic counselors need reasonably accurate information to advise parents about their child's prognosis. What is the one-year survival for typical babies with one of these defects?

(b) It has been hypothesized that acute appendicitis may sometimes be initiated by an infectious agent. Many infectious diseases exhibit seasonal variations in incidence. How does the incidence of acute appendicitis vary by season of the year?

(c) Relatively short intervals between pregnancies have been associated with increased risk of adverse birth outcomes. Health education and better access to family-planning services have been proposed as preventive strategies. To help guide resources toward women at highest risk, how does the frequency of short interpregnancy intervals vary in relation to maternal age, education, marital status, and Medicaid program participation?

(d) Randomized trials have shown that perinatal transmission of HIV can be significantly reduced by HIV testing during pregnancy and treatment of infected mothers with zidovudine (AZT) before delivery. The U.S. Public Health Service has recommended voluntary screening and AZT treatment since 1994. To what extent has the frequency of perinatally acquired AIDS declined since then?

(e) Some women develop breast cancer during their childbearing years but still want to have children. Little is known about whether the hormonal changes that occur during a subsequent pregnancy may affect the risk of breast cancer recurrence or progression. How does survivorship after a breast cancer diagnosis differ in women who subsequently bear children compared with women who do not?

(f) As an epidemiologist with a state health department, you are interested in estimating the prevalence of diabetes among adults in your state, in determining how the prevalence compares with other states, and in examining how the frequency of diabetes varies among major demographic groups of the state's population. Where might you find this information?

(g) Overuse of antibiotics for minor illnesses is thought to be a major factor contributing to the growing problem of antibiotic-resistant microorganisms. The U.S. Public Health Service has set a goal of reducing the percentage of medically treated ear infections for which antibiotics are prescribed. Where might one best obtain data useful for tracking progress (or lack thereof) toward that goal in pediatric care?

(h) Percutaneous coronary intervention (PCI, including angioplasty and related techniques) and coronary artery bypass grafting (CABG) have become widely used in the health care industry for treatment of coronary heart disease. Both PCI and CABG require an inpatient hospital stay. Much debate has concerned whether performance of these procedures should be concentrated in centers that specialize in them and do them in large numbers, or be performed widely at general hospitals and thus geographically accessible to more of the population. In part because of a strong association between age and coronary heart disease risk, a large percentage of PCI and CABG procedures are performed on older adults. Suppose that you wish to compare the 30-day case fatality after each type of procedure between specialty centers and general hospitals. You want to include a large number of hospitals in each group. Where might you look for suitable data?

(i) In 1991, a book entitled *Final Exit* was published, which provided suggestions for patients with terminal medical illnesses on how to take their own lives. It recommended two methods: self-poisoning with certain prescription medications, and suffocation by plastic bag. Fortuitously, each of these mechanisms of suicide has its own code in the International Classification of Diseases, version 9 (ICD-9), which was then current. Psychiatrists expressed concern that publication of this book might increase the frequency of suicide by these means. What data source could you use to investigate whether those fears were warranted?

(j) Coronary heart disease (CHD) has been the #1 killer in the United States for many years, despite the fact that a great deal is now known about risk factors for CHD. A large study in Framingham, Massachusetts, yielded a "risk equation" that estimates a person's probability of developing CHD in the next 10 years, based on the person's age, gender, smoking status, use of medications for high blood pressure, systolic blood pressure, total cholesterol, and HDL cholesterol. How might you determine whether, among U.S. adults, there has been a change over the last decade in the estimated 10-year risk of developing CHD, based on this risk equation and the characteristics that it uses as inputs?

(k) Socioeconomic disparities in oral health and access to dental care are significant public health issues in the United States. Although some workers get dental health insurance as a benefit of employment, the extent of coverage varies widely among industries and employers. Suppose that you wish to compare the frequency of self-reported unmet need for dental care among workers across a variety of occupations and industries. This information may help in targeting workplace dental health promotion programs where they are most needed. What data source might you consider?

(l) Onset of labor in a pregnant mother and subsequent childbirth can occur (sometimes inconveniently) on any day of the week and at any time of the day or night. Staffing levels on labor and delivery units, and the availability of various hospital diagnostic and treatment services, are often greater during daytime hours on regular workdays than during evenings and weekends. Concern has been raised that limited staff and services during off hours may jeopardize the health of babies born at those times. How might you determine whether the day and time of birth are associated with higher neonatal mortality (death after live birth within the first 28 days of life)?

2. Acute flaccid paralysis (AFP) is a rare neurological condition involving rapid loss of the ability to move one or more limbs or facial muscles. Before widespread vaccination, polio infection was a major cause, and the World Health Organization recommends ongoing surveillance for AFP as one tool for detection of polio outbreaks.

In Australia, all cases of AFP are supposed to be reported by physicians to a national register. As a check on reporting, epidemiologists in the state of Victoria, Australia, also monitored hospital discharge diagnoses for AFP for all pediatric hospitals in the state (Whitfield and Kelly, 2002). Over a three-year period, 14 confirmed new cases of AFP among children under age 15 years were reported to the register

from Victoria state. During the same period, 29 confirmed new cases of AFP among Victoria state residents under age 15 years were identified in hospital discharge records, of whom 10 also appeared in the register. The estimated average population under age 15 years in Victoria state at mid-period was 948,124 persons.

Estimate the incidence rate of AFP for persons under age 15 years in Victoria state during the study period. What other key assumption must be satisfied for your estimate to be accurate?

ANSWERS

1. Each topic has actually been investigated in an epidemiologic study. The data sources that were actually used by the investigators are noted. In some instances, other options would have been possible as well.

(a) Over the years from 1968–1999, 70 children with trisomy 13 and 114 with trisomy 18 were identified in the Metropolitan Atlanta Congenital Defects Program, a population-based registry of children with birth defects. Rasmussen *et al.* (2003) linked these records with Georgia State death certificate data and with the National Death Index to show that about 9% of children with either defect survive to at least 1 year of age. They also used national multiple-cause-of-death death certificate files to determine that about 6% of death certificates listing trisomy 13 or 18 among the conditions contributing to death had died after 1 year of age.

(b) Recognizing that nearly all cases of appendicitis in the United States would require hospitalization, Addiss *et al.* (1990) used National Hospital Discharge Survey data. That survey has since been succeeded by the National Hospital Care Survey, which would provide suitable data if the same study were done today.

(c) CDC epidemiologists used Utah birth certificate data (Centers for Disease Control and Prevention, 1998) to address these questions.

(d) AIDS is legally reportable in all U.S. states and territories. Lindgren *et al.* (1999) used data from this surveillance system, routinely compiled by CDC.

(e) Mueller *et al.* (2003) linked data from three population-based cancer registries in the United States with birth certificate data from the same areas. The three registries were part of the National Cancer Institute's Surveillance, Epidemiology, and End Results (SEER) program, which obtains information on survivorship after diagnosis. Even after accounting for age, stage at diagnosis, calendar year, and region, mortality was found to be about 46% lower among women who bore a child at least 10 months after their breast cancer diagnosis. (Note, however, that an ideal study of the impact of pregnancy after breast cancer on survival would be able to ascertain and adjust for a woman's disease severity, not at the time of diagnosis, but at the time of conception. Because cancer registries generally assess severity at a time close to the original diagnosis, use of registry data alone may not separate the influence of a pregnancy on a woman's subsequent survival from that of her clinical status at the time the pregnancy begins.)

(f) Buescher (2003) used data from the CDC Behavioral Risk Factor Surveillance System (BRFSS) to obtain state-specific information on the prevalence of diabetes. This telephone survey defined a case of diabetes as someone who reported having been told by a doctor that they had diabetes. This method of ascertainment would be subject to reporting error and would have missed persons with diabetes who had not sought medical care for it. However, the BRFSS sample was large enough to give stable state-specific prevalence estimates and to permit an examination of the descriptive epidemiology of diabetes within a state.

(g) CDC epidemiologists used data from the National Ambulatory Care Medical Survey (Centers for Disease Control and Prevention, 2011). They found that the number of antibiotic prescriptions per 1,000 office visits decreased from 300 in 1993–1994 to 229 in 2007–2008. Decreases in antibiotic prescribing were also seen in visits for pharyngitis or for non-specific respiratory infections.

(h) Because a large majority of adults age 65 years or older in the United States are covered by Medicare, a good place to look would be Medicare fee-for-service claims data. Cram et al. (2005) used Medicare inpatient claims data to identify patients who underwent PCI or CABG at one of 15 specialty hospitals or one of 75–82 general hospitals, depending on procedure. The available data captured deaths in the first 30 days. (Linking with the National Death Index would also have been possible as a check on completeness and/or as a source of data on later deaths.) The adjusted risk of dying within 30 days was found to be about 11% lower at specialty hospitals after PCI, and about 16% lower at specialty hospitals after CABG.

(i) Marzuk et al. (1994) obtained unpublished national mortality data from the National Center for Health Statistics, containing ICD-9 codes for the underlying cause of death in each decedent.

They assumed that the population at risk was constant for 1990–1991 and simply compared the number of suicide deaths by ICD-9 code in the relevant categories before and after *Final Exit* was published. They found a 30.8% increase in suicidal asphyxiations by plastic bag, a 5.4% increase in self-poisonings, and little change in suicides by other means or in total suicides.

(j) Although several components of the Framingham risk equation can be obtained by interview, systolic blood pressure and cholesterol would be best measured directly. Fortunately, all of these data items are gathered as part of the National Health and Nutrition Examination Survey (NHANES), which seeks to obtain such data on a representative sample of the U.S. non-institutionalized civilian population. Ajani and Ford (2006) used NHANES data from 1988–1994 and 1999–2002 to compare the estimated 10-year risk of CHD between surveys done about a decade apart. They found no appreciable difference in estimated CHD risk over time and recommended that greater efforts be taken to control known modifiable risk factors such as smoking, hypertension, and high levels of serum cholesterol.

(k) Caban-Martinez et al. (2007) used data from the National Health Interview Survey to address this issue. They combined data from seven annual surveys (1997–2003), which provided interview data on 135,004 employed respondents. One of the main questions of interest was: "During the past 12 months, was there any time when you needed dental care (including check-ups) but didn't get it because you couldn't afford it?" Overall, 11.5% of female and 8.0% of male workers answered yes. Men in health services and food service occupations reported higher levels of unmet need.

(l) Pasupathy et al. (2010), in Scotland, used linked birth and death certificates to address this question. They found that among 1,039,560 full-term singleton births with cephalic presentation and without congenital anomalies, neonatal mortality was about 30% greater among babies born during the evening or on a weekend than among those born during normal working hours on a Monday–Friday.

2. The numerator data given can be organized as in Table 6.5. The table makes it clear that neither the national register nor hospital discharge data identified all AFP cases. Thus it is likely that some additional cases escaped detection by both sources. Under capture-recapture sampling theory, the number of

TABLE 6.5.

Reported to register	Hospitalized for AFP		
	Yes	No	Total
Yes	10	4	14
No	19		
Total	29		

such cases can be estimated if it is assumed that a case's probability of appearance in one data source is statistically independent of the case's probability of appearance in the other data source. Under this assumption, if there are x cases in the lower right cell, then $\frac{10 \times x}{4 \times 19} = 1$. This equation can then be solved for $x = \frac{19 \times 4}{10} = 7.6$ cases.

Under the independence assumption, the estimated incidence rate for AFP over the 3-year period would be $\frac{10 + 4 + 19 + 7.6}{948,124 \times 3}$ ($\times 100,000$) $= 1.43$ cases per 100,000 person-years.

7

Person, Place, and Time

I keep six honest serving-men
(They taught me all I knew);
Their names are What and Why and When
And How and Where and Who...

—RUDYARD KIPLING

ST. ANTHONY'S FIRE

A somber and majestic art work at the Musée d'Unterlinden in the town of Colmar, France, is the *Isenheim Altarpiece* by the 16th-century German artist Matthias Grünewald. It consists of several large painted panels, one showing an emaciated Christ dying on the cross against a black sky, another showing the hermit Saint Anthony being attacked by an army of devils and monsters, and another showing Christ rising triumphantly from the grave and ascending into heaven in a blaze of yellow-orange light. The *Isenheim Altarpiece* is now viewed mainly by museum visitors, but its original purpose was to provide solace and hope to victims of a disease then known as St. Anthony's Fire. The Monastery of St. Anthony in nearby Isenheim, where the work was originally situated, served as a hospital for those afflicted.

Outbreaks of St. Anthony's Fire had occurred in Europe throughout recorded history. It was a horrible disease. Victims lost their mental faculties, becoming paranoid and demented; they developed painful skin sores that made them feel that their body was on fire; fingers, hands, and feet turned black from gangrene and fell off. Most victims either died of complications or were driven to suicide to escape the intractable pain. The *Isenheim Altarpiece* was commissioned to convey a message that although the patients' suffering was great, the suffering of Christ and of St. Anthony had been greater still. The resurrection panel sought to give hope that the suffering would end and that the afterlife would be better.

In 1670, about 160 years after the *Isenheim Altarpiece* was completed, a local French physician named Louis Thuillier began to notice some patterns in the occurrence of St. Anthony's Fire (Carefoot and Sprott, 1967; Bove, 1970). Over the years, he had seen hundreds of cases and was frustrated by how little could be done for them. He noticed, however, that caregivers were often unaffected, even after long exposure to a disease victim, while people who lived in isolation were sometimes stricken. He reasoned that St. Anthony's Fire, unlike other epidemic diseases of the time, such as plague, was probably not spread from person to person. He also noted that the disease was more common among peasants than among the wealthy. Unlike plague, which occurred mainly in cities, where population density was high, St. Anthony's Fire occurred mainly in rural areas. Poring over his records, he also found that he had seen more cases in years of bad weather, when crop yields were low and diets were poor.

Thuillier's observations made him wonder whether something in the diet of rural peasants might be involved. A staple of their diet was rye bread, which he often saw on the table when visiting the houses of patients. While walking through rye fields one day, he recalled that the blue-black cockspurs from a plant fungus that sometimes infected rye had been used by the old alchemists to make powerful medicinal potions. It occurred to him that perhaps eating too much of these cockspurs in contaminated rye could lead to St. Anthony's Fire. It would fit with all the patterns he had seen. He tested his conjecture by showing that feeding cockspurs to animals was fatal.

Dr. Thuillier was thinking like an epidemiologist, observing how the frequency of St. Anthony's Fire varied in relation to personal characteristics, place, and time. And his hypothesis turned out to be correct. The modern name for St. Anthony's Fire is ergotism, now known to be caused by ingesting the pods, or sclerotia, of the fungus *Claviceps purpurea*, which grows on rye. The toxins in these sclerotia include ergot alkaloids, which are such potent vasoconstrictors that they can entirely cut off the blood supply to fingers, hands, and feet and cause gangrene. Other toxins include chemical relatives of LSD, which in sufficient doses can drive people crazy. The sclerotia fall to the ground in autumn and break open the following spring, releasing millions of spores that are spread by wind and especially by fog droplets in bad weather.

Sadly, Thuillier tried in vain to warn peasants about why he thought eating rye bread made from contaminated grain was dangerous. But the peasants had always eaten rye bread, could see no reason to doubt age-old eating habits, had no ready substitute, and saw the disease abating by itself anyway. Two more centuries passed until the life cycle and toxicology of the ergot fungus were worked out well enough to provide overwhelming proof that Thuillier's theory had been correct. The disease is now prevented by careful separation of grain from fungal sclerotia, and by turning over the soil at the end of the growing season deeply enough to bury the sclerotia where they cannot germinate. Even though Thuillier's own intervention efforts proved unsuccessful, his correct reasoning about the cause of St. Anthony's Fire supports the value of epidemiologic methods for identifying opportunities to prevent disease and human suffering.

SEARCHING FOR PATTERNS

If there were one idea that all epidemiologists could agree upon, it would probably be: *diseases do not occur at random*. Every form of human ill health exhibits a pattern of variation in its frequency within populations, between populations, or over time—in a sense, its epidemiologic fingerprint. The simple conceptual framework summarized by the title of this chapter has traditionally been used to organize the many factors with which disease frequency can be associated:

- *Person.* What kinds of people tend to develop the disease, and who tends to be spared? What is unusual about those people?
- *Place.* Where is the disease especially common or rare, and what is different about those places?
- *Time.* How does disease frequency change over time, and what other factors are temporally associated with those changes?

Discovering and characterizing these patterns of variation—that is, *descriptive epidemiology*—can serve several useful purposes, including:

- *Generating hypotheses about underlying causes.* Associations between disease frequency and personal characteristics, place, or time may not necessarily imply that those characteristics cause the disease. But the pattern of associations can often suggest what the underlying causes may be, as illustrated by the history of St. Anthony's Fire and the story of retrolental fibroplasia in Chapter 1.
- *Target efforts at prevention and early detection.* Preventive measures, including screening for occult early disease, almost always involve costs in money and time and can pose risks of their own. Information from descriptive epidemiology can guide the application of preventive interventions to where they can be of greatest benefit in relation to their costs and risks.
- *Assess health disparities.* Social conditions and public policies often play important roles in determining who develops a disease and who among them has a better outcome. In an egalitarian society, unequal distribution of the burden of disease due to these factors can raise concerns about equity and justice.
- *Detect emerging threats to public health.* Early recognition of a disease outbreak can trigger a public health response that minimizes future disease burden.

This chapter seeks to develop the person-place-time framework and illustrates some of its uses through examples.

PERSON

People can be grouped or distinguished from one another on a great many personal characteristics, and

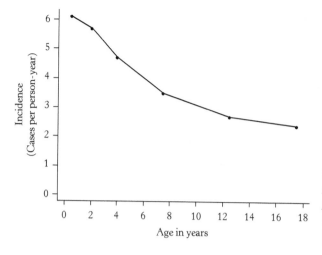

FIGURE 7.1 Incidence of respiratory infections in children by age: Tecumseh, Michigan, 1969–1971. (Based on data from Monto and Ullman [1974])

one might wonder where to begin and end. As a starting point, patterns of disease occurrence are often examined in relation to factors that are routinely ascertained and recorded in available data sources, such as those described in Chapter 6. The scope of information included in these sources is generally limited, often restricted to sociodemographic characteristics such as age, gender, race, and marital status. When additional information is present—for example, birth order or maternal age on a birth certificate, or occupation on a death certificate—it can be considered as well.

Age

Nearly every known disease varies in frequency with age, many to a marked degree. A variety of underlying mechanisms can be responsible, producing quite different patterns of association. For example:

- *Immunity.* A few weeks or months after a baby is born, maternally derived antibodies dissipate and leave the infant susceptible to various common infectious diseases. Figure 7.1 shows how the incidence of acute respiratory infections was found to vary by age among children in the community of Tecumseh, Michigan (Monto and Ullman, 1974). Very high incidence rates for acute respiratory infections were found among children less than one year of age: 6.1 cases *per person-year*. Incidence then declined markedly with age.
- *Human development.* Age can also indicate approximately where someone falls in the maturational sequence of physical, mental,

and behavioral changes that occur over the human lifespan. Figure 7.2 shows how the incidence of traumatic brain injury (TBI) resulting in an emergency-room visit varied by age in King County, Washington (Koepsell *et al.*, 2011). The incidence of TBI due to a fall was much higher among preschoolers than among older children. Being struck by or against an object, often related to play or sports, became more and more common with age. Cycling-related TBI was most common at age 10–14 years, and motor-vehicle-related TBI became common at ages 15–17 when teenagers were old enough to drive. These patterns almost certainly reflect age-related changes in motor skills, ability to perceive danger, and behavior.

- *Slowly progressive disease.* Atherosclerosis can begin in youth, but it generally goes unrecognized until atherosclerotic plaques become large enough to reduce blood flow substantially in major arteries. Many factors influence how rapidly plaques grow—family history, smoking, blood pressure, and lipid levels among them—but the process typically requires several decades before disease becomes clinically apparent. Mortality rates for acute myocardial infarction, which almost always results from atherosclerosis of the coronary arteries, vary in the United States several-thousand-fold from childhood to old age (Figure 7.3)—a pattern that fits with a model of gradual disease pathogenesis.
- *Age-related differences in life style.* Age is also strongly related to the kinds of activities in

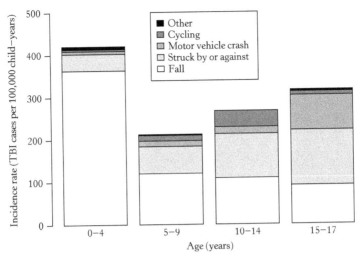

FIGURE 7.2 Incidence of traumatic brain injury by age and mechanism: King County, Washington, 2007–2008. (Based on data from Koepsell *et al.* [2011])

which people engage and the risks they encounter in daily life. For example, mortality rates from motorcycle crashes among U.S. men peak in the young and middle adult years (Figure 7.4). This pattern fits with the ages at which men like to ride motorcycles and with how their driving styles vary with age.

Besides being a personal characteristic, age can also be considered as a time scale on which disease frequency can vary, as discussed later in this chapter.

Gender

Differences in disease frequency between the sexes are also the rule, not the exception. Both biological and non-biological mechanisms can be at play.

- *Biological.* At one extreme, most diseases of the reproductive system occur either only among men (e.g., prostate cancer) or only among women (e.g., uterine cancer, complications of childbirth). Even for some diseases of organs related to reproduction, however, the

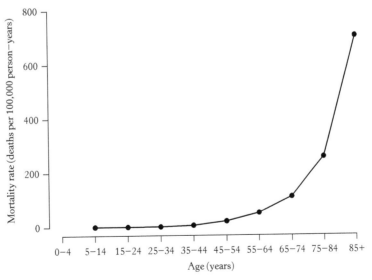

FIGURE 7.3 Mortality from acute myocardial infarction by age: United States, 2009. (Based on data from CDC-WONDER)

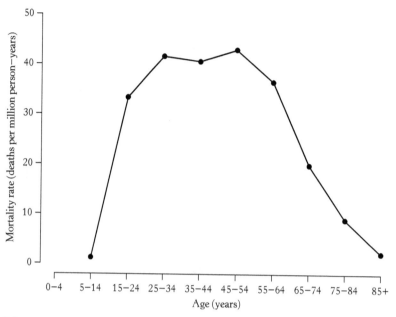

FIGURE 7.4 Mortality from motorcycle crashes among U.S. males by age: 2008–2009. (Based on data from CDC-WONDER)

association with gender is not absolute. The age-adjusted[1] incidence of invasive breast cancer among U.S. *males* in 2009 was 1.4 per 100,000 person-years, not zero (National Program of Cancer Registries, 2012). Yet this rate was about 1% of the rate for U.S. females (122.8 per 100,000 person-years), and it is reasonable to assume that anatomical and hormonal differences between men and women account for a large part of this difference.

Besides diseases of the reproductive system, many other diseases predominate in one gender or the other for reasons that are believed to be biological. Red-green color blindness is inherited as a recessive trait on the X-chromosome and for this reason appears almost entirely in males (Pokorny *et al.*, 1979). In the United States, the prevalence of osteoporosis has been found to be far higher in women than in men (Figure 7.5), which is thought to be explained in part by gender-related hormonal effects on bone physiology (Reeve, 2000).

• *Non-biological.* The major differences in social roles and health-related behavior between men and women almost certainly underlie

many gender differences in disease frequency. Gender serves as a marker for exposure to more proximate disease causes. To revisit the descriptive epidemiology of respiratory infections in Tecumseh, Michigan, Table 7.1 extends the age range of Figure 7.1 into adulthood, revealing a distinctive pattern. High and similar incidence was found in boys and girls during early childhood, declining rapidly with age in both sexes. A growing gap between the incidence for males and for females became evident at older ages, beginning in adolescence. Then secondary peaks in incidence for both genders were seen at about age 20–39 years, occurring a few years earlier for women than for men. These features are very likely related to one another. The secondary peaks occurred at ages when young adults were starting their own families and thus were exposed to respiratory illnesses brought home by their children (who the figure shows to be a high-incidence group). Mothers typically bore a larger share of child-rearing responsibilities, including caring for sick children, which probably contributed to the higher incidence in young adult women. The secondary peak in women occurred a few

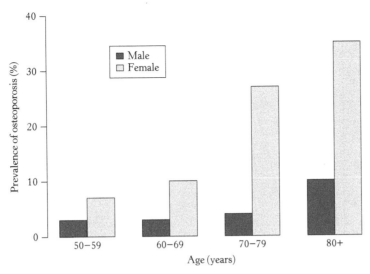

FIGURE 7.5 Prevalence of osteoporosis at the femoral neck or lumbar spine by age and gender: U.S. National Health and Nutrition Examination Survey, 2005–2008.
(Based on data from Looker *et al.* [2012])

TABLE 7.1. MEAN NUMBER OF RESPIRATORY INFECTIONS PER PERSON PER YEAR: TECUMSEH, MICHIGAN, 1965–1971

| Age (years) | Mean number of infections per year | | |
	Females	Males	Difference
0–1	6.0	6.5	−0.5
1–2	5.4	6.1	−0.7
3–4	5.1	4.4	0.7
5–9	3.7	3.4	0.3
10–14	3.1	2.4	0.7
15–19	2.8	2.1	0.7
20–24	3.3	2.1	1.2
25–29	3.1	2.5	0.6
30–39	2.7	1.9	0.8
40–49	1.7	1.3	0.4
50–59	1.6	1.1	0.5
60+	1.2	0.8	0.4

(Based on data from Monto and Ullman [1974])

years earlier than that for men, probably reflecting the tendency for women to marry men a few years older than themselves.

Even larger gender differences have been observed for firearm injury deaths, as shown in Figure 7.6. At ages 15–24 years, firearm mortality in 2009 was more than eight times greater in males than in females. Curves with two or more peaks, such as the curve for males in Figure 7.6, can suggest that what is being examined as a single condition may be disaggregated into two or more component subtypes, each of which has a different descriptive epidemiologic profile. In this instance, the peak in firearm deaths among younger men consists chiefly of homicides, while the peak in older men consists chiefly of suicides.

Race and Ethnicity

Race and ethnicity concern self-perceived membership in groups defined by skin color, ancestral place of residence, language, and cultural heritage. Race and ethnicity are sometimes treated as aspects of a single characteristic and sometimes as separate characteristics. In either case, race/ethnicity is a particularly complicated factor to deal with in epidemiology, as in other fields. There is no consensus that race/ethnicity reflects fundamental biological characteristics, as do age and gender (Lin and Kelsey, 2000; Williams, 1997). Instead, it often serves as a marker for a complex mix of social conditions, cultural traditions, health behaviors, and other nonbiological factors. There is also disagreement about how race/ethnicity should best be categorized, and about the basis for placing a person in a category

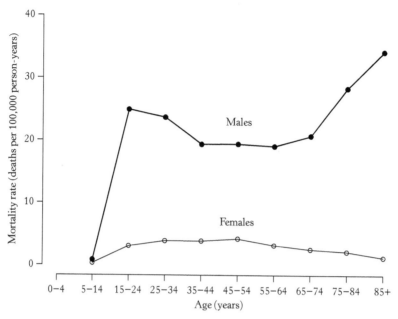

FIGURE 7.6 Mortality rates from firearm injury by age and gender: United States, 2009. (Based on data from CDC-WONDER)

(Hahn *et al.*, 1992; Hahn, 1992). Despite these difficulties, it is indisputable that the frequency of many diseases varies strongly by race and ethnicity, and knowledge of this variation can serve useful purposes, even if the basis for such an association remains uncertain.

Some associations between race/ethnicity and disease frequency almost certainly *are* biologically based. For example, in 2009, the mortality rate from sickle-cell anemia was more than 100-fold greater among blacks in the United States compared to whites. This relationship is surely due to higher prevalence of the hemoglobin S gene among blacks. Being heterozygous for this gene conferred partial resistance to malaria, a leading cause of death in Africa, while being homozygous on the hemoglobin S gene leads to sickle-cell anemia. Higher mortality from sickle-cell anemia in present-day blacks can thus be attributed to the genetic legacy of natural selection pressures that historically operated in part of the world where their ancestors once lived (Allison, 1954). Likewise, dark natural skin pigmentation offered some protection from the adverse effects of prolonged and intense sun exposure, which probably explains why the age-adjusted incidence of malignant melanoma has been found to be more than 20-fold greater in U.S. whites than in U.S. blacks.

However, race and ethnicity are also associated with socioeconomic status, living conditions, dietary habits, cultural background, health behaviors, exposure to discrimination, access to health care, and related factors that can themselves be linked to disease risk. For example, Table 7.2 compares infant mortality rates and the prevalence of low birth weight across five race/ethnicity groups in the United States. To put the observed differences in context, the prevalences of three risk factors related to pregnancy outcomes and infant health are also shown, derived from birth certificate data. Infant mortality and low birth weight were most common in blacks. The data also suggest possible contributing factors at which prevention programs might be directed to help reduce the observed racial disparities in birth outcomes. Oddly, the prevalence of low birth weight was lowest among Hispanic infants, despite the relatively high frequency of teen births, births to unmarried mothers, and late or no prenatal care among Hispanic mothers—a historically consistent finding that has been called the "Hispanic paradox" (de la Rosa, 2002).

As an example of the challenges facing epidemiologists when dealing with race/ethnicity, consider how race-specific infant mortality rates are calculated and interpreted. One issue is how to classify the baby's race when the parents are of different races.

TABLE 7.2. SELECTED BIRTH AND INFANT HEALTH CHARACTERISTICS BY RACE/ETHNICITY OF MOTHER: UNITED STATES, 2005–2007

Characteristic	Non-Hispanic		Hispanic	American Indian or Alaska Native	Asian or Pacific Islander
	White	Black			
Infant mortality rate[a,b]	5.7	13.4	5.5	8.5	4.7
Percent of babies weighing < 2,500 grams[c]	7.2	13.6	6.9	7.5	8.1
Percent of live births with:					
Mother aged <18years[c]	3.0	6.1	5.3	6.3	0.9
Unmarried mother[c]	34.8	71.2	51.3	65.3	16.6
No prenatal care, or only in third trimester	6.5	11.7	9.3	13.1	4.9

[a] Deaths in first year of life per 1,000 births
[b] 2005–2007
[c] 2007
(Based on data from National Center for Health Statistics [2012b])

Before 1989, the National Center for Health Statistics used a complex algorithm, classifying a baby as "white" only if both parents were white. Since 1989, the baby's race has been defined simply as the race of the mother—a change that affects comparability of statistics over time (National Center for Health Statistics, 1994).[2] In 2003, the model birth certificate was updated again, changing the race categories in an attempt at standardization across various federal statistics-gathering systems. A mother could now identify herself as belonging to one, two, or more race categories. Hispanic origin became a separate characteristic that could occur in combination with any race.

Another problem is classifying the race of an infant who dies. Race as recorded on the death certificate (usually by the funeral director) can disagree with race as recorded on the birth certificate. Hahn *et al.* (1992) found that coding inconsistencies were rare for blacks or whites, but that many infants of other races who died were coded as white on the death certificate. Unless this misclassification is corrected by linking birth and death certificates and drawing better race data from the birth certificate, the excess in infant mortality rates among American Indians and Alaska Natives could be underestimated.

Lastly, commonly used race/ethnicity groupings such as those shown in Table 7.2 can obscure large differences within them. For example, a study in King County, Washington, took advantage of disaggregation of the Asian/Pacific Islander category

on birth certificates after 2003 (Centers for Disease Control and Prevention, 2011). Asians (with ancestral origins in the Far East, Southeast Asia, or the Indian subcontinent) were compared to Native Hawaiians or Pacific Islanders (with ancestral origins in Hawaii, Guam, Samoa, or other Pacific Islands) with regard to characteristics recorded on birth certificates. Maternal obesity was much more common in the Hawaiian/Pacific Islander subgroup (49.9% vs. 7.5%), as was smoking during pregnancy (9.8% vs. 1.4%) and late or no prenatal care (15.8% vs. 4.2%), while low birth weight was more common among Asians (7.5% vs. 5.5%).

Socioeconomic Status

Example 7-1. In 1914, a team headed by Dr. Joseph Goldberger of the U.S. Public Health Service was commissioned to investigate pellagra, a disease which had become common in parts of the southeastern United States (Goldberger *et al.*, 1920). Pellagra is characterized by symmetrical skin eruptions; in advanced cases, gastrointestinal and nervous-system symptoms also appear. Earlier small studies had suggested an association between pellagra and poverty.

The research team decided to study seven small cotton-mill villages in South Carolina, each with 500–800 residents, where pellagra was thought to be prevalent. Although local doctors were cooperative, it was felt—and later shown—that many people with pellagra would be missed by relying solely on medical

TABLE 7.3. PERIOD PREVALENCE OF PELLAGRA AND RELATIVE CONSUMPTION OF SELECTED FOODSTUFFS IN SEVEN SOUTH CAROLINA COTTON-MILL VILLAGES

Half-monthly family income per adult male unit	Pellagra cases	Persons	Cases per 1000 persons	Relative consumption[a]			
				Salt pork	Cornmeal and grits	Eggs	Fresh meats
$14.00 and over	1	291	3.4	100	100	100	100
$10.00 – 13.99	3	736	4.1	126	121	97	68
$8.00 – 9.99	10	784	12.8	138	120	75	64
$6.00 – 7.99	27	1037	26.0	144	138	64	45
Under $6.00	56	1312	42.7	138	134	56	40

[a]Relative amount purchased per adult male unit (100 = amount in households with highest economic status)
(Based on data from Goldberger et al. [1920])

records to identify cases. Hence, for several months, biweekly visits were made to every home in which a white cotton-mill worker resided. The field team sought to identify and count pellagra cases according to a standard case definition and to gather data on household composition, income, living conditions, and diet.

Family income information for the preceding half-month was obtained from the female head of household or other responsible family member, supplemented by data from the local cotton mill's payroll. Almost all households proved to have annual family incomes of $700–$1,000. However, the researchers noted that the same family income could result in different standards of living, depending on household size and composition, which were quite variable. Because at least half of most families' income went for food, they chose a measure of family size that weighted each family member in proportion to a previously published scale of food requirements according to age and gender. The weights assigned ranged from 1.0 for an adult male to 0.3 for a child under 2 years of age. Family size was then expressed in "adult male units."

Table 7.3 shows how the period prevalence of pellagra and the consumption of selected food items varied by economic status, measured as half-monthly family income per adult male unit. A striking increase in the frequency of pellagra was found with decreasing economic status. Poorer households were also found to consume more salt pork and cornmeal but fewer eggs and fresh meats. The researchers concluded that poverty was associated with pellagra in this setting and suggested that the association might be due to inability to buy food needed for a balanced diet.

Goldberger et al. (1923) went on to conduct intervention studies in orphanages and sanitariums. Well before the specific nutritional basis for the development of pellagra had been identified, their research indicated that the disease could be prevented by a diet with adequate protein in the form of milk, eggs, or meats. Years later, pellagra was found to result from niacin deficiency. The body can synthesize niacin from the amino acid tryptophan in high-protein foods (Goldsmith, 1965), but the low-protein, high-cornmeal diet that was common among poor Southern cotton-mill workers did not provide an adequate amount of tryptophan.

Goldberger's studies employed a variant of per capita family income, which is still a commonly used index of socioeconomic status. Income, education, and occupational classification (e.g., white-collar, blue-collar, service, farm) are often used individually as indicators of socioeconomic status, each with its own strengths and weaknesses (Galobardes et al., 2006; National Center for Health Statistics, 1998). Summary indices of socioeconomic status have also been developed that combine information from two or more of these variables (Miller, 1991; Krieger et al., 1997).

An individual's own income, education, and/or occupation can influence his or her disease risk through many mechanisms, probably often acting in combination, including safety of living conditions and mode of transportation, quality of diet, access to health care, awareness and practice of healthy behaviors, exposure to health hazards on the job, and others. For example, Figure 7.7 shows a clear trend toward lower prevalence of dental caries with higher family income among U.S. schoolchildren.

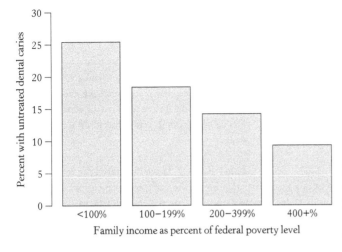

FIGURE 7.7 Prevalence of untreated dental caries among children aged 5–19 years: United States, 2005–8. (Based on data from National Center for Health Statistics [2012b])

Table 7.4 shows a strong gradient in age-adjusted mortality rates from all causes for working-age U.S. adults. In 2005, overall mortality rates varied more than three-fold in relation to education, even when crudely measured using just three broad categories, and by an even larger ratio for selected causes such as injuries. Besides demonstrating health disparities in their own right, such strong associations reinforce the importance of socioeconomic status indicators as potential confounding factors in studies focusing on other exposures.

Indicators of socioeconomic status can also have *contextual* effects. That is, a person's risk of disease may be influenced not only by his or her own education or income, but also by the education or income of others with whom he or she interacts. For example, as Goldberger and colleagues realized, household income should be interpreted in relation to household size and composition. Average income or education levels in the community can serve as indicators of the physical and social environment in which an individual lives or works (Pickett and Pearl, 2001; Von Korff *et al.*, 1992), as will be discussed further in Chapter 16. The amount of *dispersion* in income within a social group—income inequality—may also be associated with differences in health for reasons not yet well understood (Lynch *et al.*, 2000). They may relate to perceptions of disadvantage and/or to deeper features of social structure that favor one subgroup over another (Wagstaff and van Doorslaer, 2000; Kaplan *et al.*, 1996).

Marital Status

Marital status, too, can be associated with disease frequency for many reasons. The incidence of cervical

TABLE 7.4. AGE-ADJUSTED MORTALITY[a] FROM SELECTED CAUSES OF DEATH AMONG ADULTS AGED 25-64 YEARS: SELECTED AMERICAN STATES, 2005

Cause of death	Years of school completed		
	<12	12	13+
All causes	650	478	206
Chronic and non-communicable diseases	484	359	162
Injury	121	92	35
Communicable diseases	44	26	9
HIV infection	14	8	3
Other	30	18	7

[a] Deaths per 100,000 person-years
(Based on data from National Center for Health Statistics [2012a])

cancer was found to be lower in unmarried women than in married women (Leck *et al.*, 1978)—an association now thought to be related to differences in women's likelihood of exposure to sexually transmitted viral agents involved in the etiology of cervical cancer (Trottier and Franco, 2006).

Mother's marital status is routinely recorded on the birth certificate and has proven valuable in perinatal epidemiology. For example, infant mortality in the United States during 2008 was 8.9 per 1,000 liveborn infants among babies of unmarried mothers, vs. 5.1 per 1,000 among babies of married mothers, an association that also held within racial/ethnic groups (Mathews and MacDorman, 2012). In this context, marital status may reflect social support within the household, or instrumental support in the form of income and sharing of child care.

Marital status has often been found to be associated with the frequency of mental illnesses. For example, mortality from suicide has been found to be sharply higher among divorced or separated men compared to married men (Rendall *et al.*, 2011); these associations appear to be much weaker in women (Kposowa, 2000; Baker *et al.*, 1992).

PLACE

Example 7-2. In the late summer of 1854, a particularly terrible outbreak of cholera struck in London, England, with over 500 cholera deaths in ten days (Snow, 1936). What caused cholera epidemics was unknown at that time, but patterns observed during previous outbreaks had suggested an association with living at low elevations. This association spawned various theories about how a person contracted cholera, including a "miasma" hypothesis positing that cholera came from breathing foul air that collected in low-lying areas.

British physician John Snow, who noted that cholera was primarily a gastrointestinal disease, suspected that it might instead arise from ingesting contaminated water, which he thought might be more common in low-elevation areas. He interrupted his work on this theory to investigate the 1854 outbreak. Having obtained from the General Register Office a list of the first 83 deaths ascribed to cholera during the epidemic, he went to the neighborhood where most deaths had occurred. He soon found that nearly all of the fatal cases had lived within a short distance of a public, hand-operated water pump located on Broad Street near the corner of Cambridge Street. In his words:

> There were only ten deaths in houses situated decidedly nearer to another street pump. In five of these cases the families of the deceased persons informed me that they always sent to the pump in Broad Street, as they preferred the water to that of the pump which was nearer. In three other cases, the deceased were children who went to school near the pump in Broad Street. Two of them were known to drink the water; and the parents of the third think it probable that it did so. The other two deaths, beyond the district which this pump supplies, represent only the amount of mortality from cholera that was occurring before the irruption took place....
>
> The result of the inquiry, then, was that there had been no particular outbreak or increase of cholera, in

this part of London, except among the persons who were in the habit of drinking the water of the above-mentioned pump-well.

> I had an interview with the Board of Guardians of St. James's Parish on the evening of Thursday, 7th September, and represented the above circumstances to them. In consequence of what I said, the handle of the pump was removed on the following day....

Later that year, Snow illustrated the results of his investigation of the outbreak using a *spot map* of the area (Figure 7.8), on which each fatal case was shown as a small black bar (Brody *et al.*, 2000). Geographical clustering of cases near the Broad Street pump was clearly evident.

Spot maps like the one Snow constructed remain a useful tool even today in outbreak investigation to suggest spatial clustering of cases. But because they involve simply plotting the place of occurrence of each case, they have much the same limitation as counts do as a measure of disease frequency: namely, they do not account for the distribution of the population at risk. To illustrate, Figure 7.9 shows geographic variation in the frequency of motor-vehicle crash deaths among the 48 contiguous U.S. states, first by *number of deaths* (panel A), then by age-adjusted mortality *rates* (panel B). Panel A is akin to a spot map, showing large numbers of deaths in populous states with large urban centers, such as New York, California, and Illinois. Panel B reveals that the rate of death from a motor-vehicle collision was actually relatively low in those states and much higher in states such as Montana, Wyoming, and North Dakota, where travel distances may be greater and more driving is done on rural roads and highways.

Geographic variability in disease frequency can be due to variations in the physical environment. For example, Figure 7.10 shows age-adjusted mortality rates for malignant melanoma in United States white American males in the late 20th century. Higher rates in the sunnier, warmer southern states agree well with the theory that greater unprotected exposure to sunlight increases the risk of this form of skin cancer (Armstrong and English, 1996). Lyme disease, which results from a spirochetal infection acquired through an *Ixodes scapularis* tick bite, occurs only in parts of the country where environmental conditions favor survival and reproduction of this tick species (Walker, 1998).

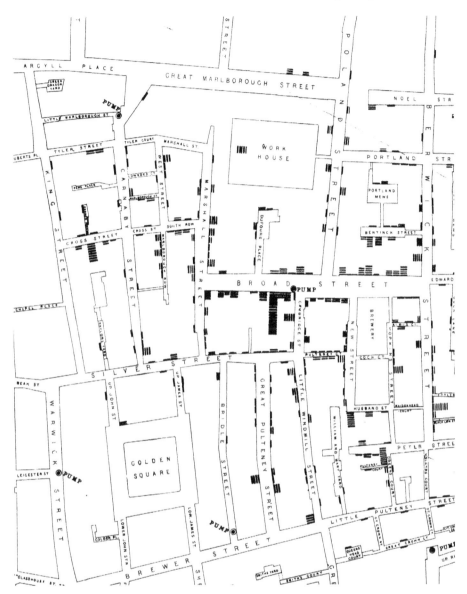

FIGURE 7.8 John Snow's spot map of cholera deaths near the Broad Street pump: London, 1854.
Source: Snow (1936)

Geographic location can also be just a proxy for spatial variation in exposure to disease risk factors that may have little relationship to the natural environment but may instead reflect geographic differences in sociocultural milieu or behavior. For example, Table 7.5 compares selected mortality rates and health habits between Utah and Nevada, two neighboring states that have generally similar climates and topography. The observed disparities almost certainly reflect differences in lifestyle, not in physical environment.

Finally, variation in disease incidence by place can provide clues about important differences in medical practice.

Example 7-3. Ignaz Semmelweis was an obstetrician and teacher at a large public maternity hospital in Vienna during the 1840s (Semmelweis, 1988). At that time, women in labor were admitted to one of two wards at the hospital, depending on the day of the week. For years, despite apparently

(A) By number of deaths

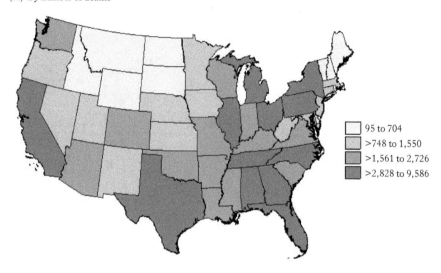

95 to 704
>748 to 1,550
>1,561 to 2,726
>2,828 to 9,586

(B) By age-adjusted mortality rates

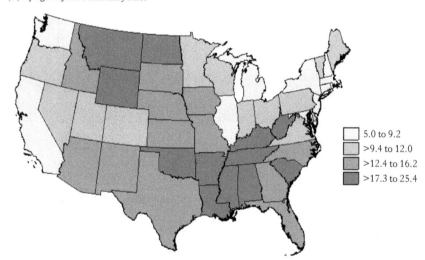

5.0 to 9.2
>9.4 to 12.0
>12.4 to 16.2
>17.3 to 25.4

FIGURE 7.9 Geographic distribution of motor vehicle crash deaths in 48 U.S. states, 2007–2009, by (A) number of deaths, and (B) age-adjusted mortality rates.

similar patient populations, deaths due to puerperal (childbirth-related) fever had been consistently more common among mothers and infants on Ward #1, where Semmelweis worked. He calculated that in 1846, the cumulative incidence of fatal childbirth-related complications was 459/4,010 = 11.4% among mothers on Ward #1, compared to 105/3,754 = 2.8% among mothers on on Ward #2.

Semmelweis noted that medical students received their training on Ward #1, while midwives trained on Ward #2. The medical students and their teachers often participated in autopsies as part of their study of anatomy. When a pathologist was accidentally cut in the finger during an autopsy of a puerperal fever victim and went on to die of a clinically similar disease himself, Semmelweis suspected that transmission of "cadaverous particles" via the hands of students and teachers might be involved in puerperal fever. He noted that other epidemiologic observations also supported this hypothesis, such as rarity of the condition among women who had delivered en route to the hospital and among those who had delivered in past years before the educational emphasis on learning from autopsies. He initiated a policy of regular hand-washing with a chlorinated solution after autopsies and between clinical

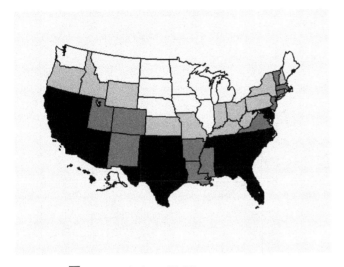

☐ 2.79 - 3.93 deaths per 100,000 person-years

▨ 2.36 - 2.78

▦ 2.16 - 2.35

■ 1.49 - 2.16

FIGURE 7.10 Age-adjusted mortality rates for malignant melanoma: U.S. white males, 1950–1994.

examinations. It was followed by a sharp reduction in the cumulative incidence of fatal complications on Ward #1 to 56/1,841 = 3.0% over the next seven months.

Advances in computing technology and statistics have greatly expanded the accessibility of geographic data and facilitated use of new quantitative techniques for spatial analysis (Jerrett et al., 2010; Boulos et al., 2011; Moore and Carpenter, 1999). Geographic information systems can produce customized maps showing spatial differences in rates, which can be a rich source of hypotheses concerning the underlying factors responsible for the patterns observed (Glass et al., 1995; Becker et al., 1998). Some such systems also incorporate sophisticated statistical tools to test for area-level associations between disease frequency and other factors, or to detect clustering of cases in space and time (Auchincloss et al., 2012).

TABLE 7.5. COMPARISON OF MORTALITY FROM SELECTED DISEASES AND PREVALENCE OF SELECTED BEHAVIORAL RISK FACTORS: UTAH AND NEVADA, 2009

	Utah	Nevada
Age-adjusted mortality[a]		
All causes	658.7	784.8
Cancer of lung, bronchus, or trachea	20.3	52.5
Ischemic heart disease	67.0	100.0
Chronic lower respiratory disease	28.4	52.5
Chronic liver disease and cirrhosis	6.8	11.9
Suicide	17.5	19.1
Homicide	1.9	5.8
Risk factor prevalence[b]		
Current smoking	9.8%	22.0%
Binge drinking	8.8%	17.5%
Heavy alcohol use	3.0%	6.9%
No exercise in past month	17.7%	24.4%

[a] Deaths per 100,000 person-years
[b] Among persons aged 18 years or older
(Based on data from CDC-WONDER and CDC-BRFSS)

TIME

Secular Trends

Patterns of change in disease frequency over periods of calendar time are termed *secular trends*. Figure 7.11 shows the rise and fall of age-adjusted mortality rates for coronary heart disease in the United States during the second half of the 20th century, by race and sex (National Heart, Lung, and Blood Institute,

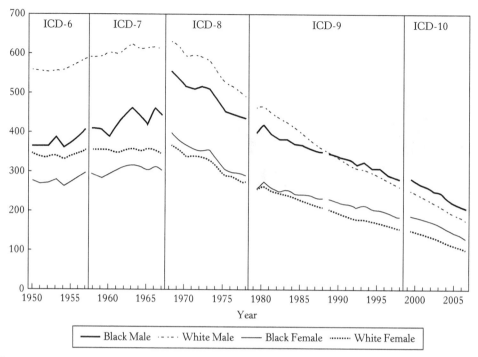

FIGURE 7.11 Age-adjusted secular trend in coronary heart disease mortality: United States, 1950–2006.
Source: National Heart, Lung, and Blood Institute (2009)

2009). Mortality rates peaked in the late 1960s and have been declining ever since—a decline thought to be due to a combination of better control of preventable risk factors and the advent of more effective treatments (Ford *et al.*, 2007). Note particularly the four vertical lines, which indicate when a new version of the International Classification of Diseases (ICD) came into use. The case definition of a coronary heart disease death under ICD evolved during the 57-year period shown, reflecting changes in medical technology and diagnostic practices. Some kinds of deaths that qualified as coronary heart disease deaths under an older version of the ICD no longer qualified under the newer ICD version that replaced it (or vice versa), leading to abrupt discontinuities in the trend lines. Such changes in case definitions must be taken into account when interpreting trends that extend over two or more ICD versions.

An *epidemic* is said to occur when the frequency of a disease has increased over time to exceed the normally expected level (Porta, 2008). This definition is not very specific, and there is no universal method for determining what level is "expected." Often the expected level is simply the historically observed level, and in that sense, any steady rise in disease incidence can qualify as an

epidemic. However, because the term *epidemic* can have dire connotations, the term *outbreak* is sometimes preferred in an acute situation to avoid causing alarm. Short-term disease outbreaks are discussed in Chapter 20.

Cyclical Variation

The incidence of many diseases exhibits a recurring pattern of variation over time periods of a certain length. Some examples are described below.

- *Annual cycles*. Pneumonia and influenza deaths, which are often combined for analysis to minimize the effect of diagnostic misclassification, have historically peaked in the United States during winter and fallen to lower levels in summer (Figure 7.12). In order to gauge whether an epidemic has occurred, the proportion of deaths due to these diseases must be compared to seasonally adjusted expected levels. In Figure 7.12, the epidemic threshold was clearly exceeded in the winters of 2008 and 2011 (Centers for Disease Control and Prevention, 2012).
- *Monthly cycles*. Deaths in the United States have been observed to vary slightly in a

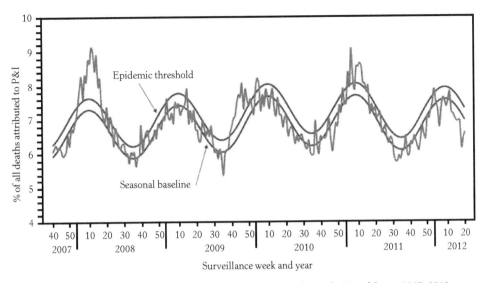

FIGURE 7.12 Proportion of deaths due to pneumonia and influenza, by week: United States, 2007–2012. *Source*: Centers for Disease Central and Prevention (2012).

monthly cycle. Phillips and colleagues (1999) found that deaths due to substance abuse accounted for much of the monthly periodicity and hypothesized an association with the timing of benefit checks from government programs.

- *Weekly cycles.* As was shown in Figure 3.3, the incidence of out-of-hospital cardiac arrest has been found in a European study to vary among the days of the week (Gruska *et al.*, 2005). Contrary to the hypothesis that returning to work after a weekend served as a trigger, the same pattern was observed among retirees. It seems there is an empirical basis for the loathing of Mondays!

- *Diurnal cycles.* Sudden Infant Death Syndrome (SIDS) cases have been found to be most likely to occur—or at least to be discovered—between 6:00 AM and noon (Figure 7.13) (Bergman *et al.*, 1972). This association with time of day served as a clue to investigate factors related to sleep, including sleeping position, as possible contributing causes.

Time Relative to a Salient Event

Another way to consider time-related variation in disease occurrence is to examine when cases occur relative to some event that might have special importance for the disease in question.

- In the summer of 2006, the World Cup soccer matches were held in Munich, Germany. On the seven days when Germany's team played, emergency-department visits for cardiac chest pain, myocardial infarction, or cardiac arrhythmias bore a clear relationship to the starting time of the match (Figure 7.14). The highest incidence was during the two hours after a game began, especially among men with pre-existing coronary heart disease (Wilbert-Lampen *et al.*, 2008).

- Over a five-year period ending in June 1980, some 38 Wisconsin residents were hospitalized for an illness with high fever, low blood pressure, a diffuse red skin rash, peeling of skin on the palms and soles, and failure of internal organs, including the liver, kidneys, or nervous system. The disease came to be known as *toxic-shock syndrome.* Of those 38 cases, 37 were women, all in the age range from 13–52 years. Suspecting a connection with female reproduction, the investigating epidemiologists gathered data about when each girl or woman's first symptoms of toxic-shock syndrome had begun, relative to her most recent menstrual period. Figure 7.15 shows clustering of cases 2–5 days after onset of menses. Further studies revealed a strong association with use of super-absorbent tampons that had recently come on the market. These tampons turned out to provide

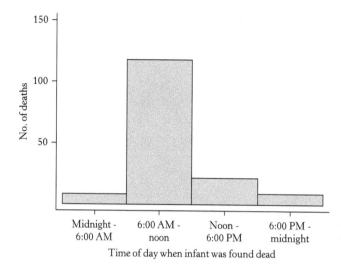

FIGURE 7.13 Incidence of sudden infant death syndrome by time of day when infant was found dead: King County, Washington, 1965–1968.

(Based on data from Bergman *et al.* [1972])

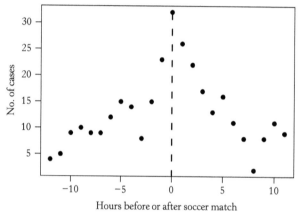

FIGURE 7.14 Emergency department visits for cardiac symptoms in relation to time before or after a World Cup soccer match: Munich, Germany, 2006.

(Based on data from Wilbert-Lampen *et al.* [2008])

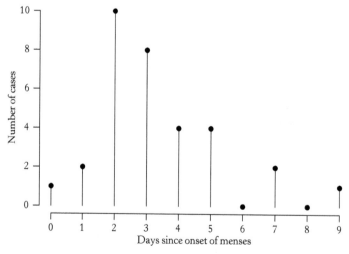

FIGURE 7.15 Number of toxic-shock syndrome cases with symptom onset on days following onset of menses: Wisconsin, 1975–1980.

(Based on data from Davis *et al.* [1980])

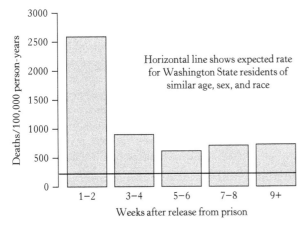

FIGURE 7.16 Mortality rate among recently discharged former prison inmates, relative to mortality rate in all state residents of similar age, sex, and race: Washington State, 1999–2003. (Based on data from Binswanger *et al.* [2007])

a good culture medium for *Staphylococcus aureus*, leading to the release of bacterial toxins into the bloodstream (Davis *et al.*, 1980).

- Prison inmates receive free health care while incarcerated, which terminates abruptly upon release from prison. Using the National Death Index, Binswanger *et al.* (2007) determined the mortality rate among men discharged from a Washington state prison in relation to time since release. Figure 7.16 shows that their mortality rate was well above the expected level based on mortality rates for all state residents of comparable age, sex, and race. The first two weeks after release were a particularly high-risk period, with many of the excess deaths recorded as due to drug overdose, homicide, or suicide.

Age, Period, and Birth Cohort

Consider Table 7.6, which shows mortality rates from lung cancer for several age groups of U.S. women in 1975, 1985, and 1995. Based on this arrangement of rates in rows and columns, two kinds of comparisons immediately come to mind:

- Rates can be compared horizontally within each row to see how lung cancer mortality rates in a particular age group varied over calendar time. The rates were fairly stable in the youngest two age groups, but in women age 55 years or older, the rates climbed steadily from 1975 to 1995.
- Rates can be compared vertically within each column to see how lung cancer mortality rates in a particular calendar year varied by age.

TABLE 7.6. MORTALITY FROM LUNG CANCER AMONG U.S. WOMEN BY AGE, IN 1975, 1985, AND 1995

| Age (years) | Mortality rate[a] | | |
	1975	1985	1995
35–44	7.3	5.7	5.1
45–54	28.1	36.0	30.0
55–64	58.3	94.3	104.5
65–74	67.6	144.9	204.5
75–84	70.8	134.9	244.5
85+	71.5	103.7	186.8

[a]Deaths per 100,000 person-years

Suppose that we are mainly interested in describing how lung cancer mortality rates vary by age among U.S. women, perhaps to help target use of a new screening procedure. We can first scan down the column of rates that were observed in 1975. The rates rose sharply with age up to about age 55, then increased more gradually for each older age group, with the highest rate seen among women 85+ years old. Looking down the 1985 column of rates, however, a different pattern is seen. In that year, the rates rose rapidly with age to peak in the 65–74 age group, then declined for the 75–84 age group and fell even lower for the 85+ age group. Looking down the 1995 column, yet another pattern is seen, with rates rising to a peak in the 75–84 age group and then falling for women age 85 or older. Thus, depending on which calendar year is considered, a different pattern of variation in rates with age is seen, giving three different answers as to which age group has the highest rate. The three patterns are shown graphically in Figure 7.17.

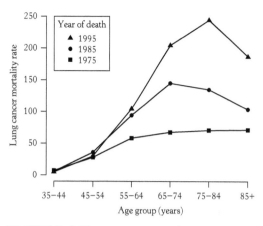

FIGURE 7.17 Lung cancer mortality rates in U.S. women, 1975–1995, connecting rates observed in the same calendar year.

Age (years)	Mortality rate[a]		
	1975	1985	1995
35–44	7.3	5.7	5.1
45–54	28.1	36.0	30.0
55–64	58.3	94.3	104.5
65–74	67.6	144.9	204.5
75–84	70.8	134.9	244.5
85+	71.5	103.7	186.8

[a]Deaths per 100,000 person-years

FIGURE 7.18

But there is another, less obvious, time scale also at play. Note that the age groups were set up to be ten years apart—the same time interval that separates adjacent columns of Table 7.6. As a result, the women who experienced the lung cancer mortality rate of 7.3 in 1975 at ages 35–44 were largely the same women who, ten years later in 1985, had reached ages 45–54 and then had a rate of 36.0. By 1995, this population of women had reached ages 55–64 and had a rate of 104.5. All of these women were born during the ten-year period from 1931–1940 and thus composed a *birth cohort*. Their experience over time is chronicled along a diagonal path in the table, as marked with arrows in the version shown in Figure 7.18. Other birth cohorts trace out other parallel diagonal paths in the table, either above or below that of the 1931–1940 birth cohort. For

example, the 1921–1930 birth cohort experienced the rates shown in the diagonal path one row lower.

Given that information about different birth cohorts also lurks in this same set of data, an alternative approach to examining variation in lung cancer mortality by age is to compare the rates at different ages *within each birth cohort*. To do so, rates are compared along each diagonal path shown in Figure 7.18. This pattern is shown graphically in Figure 7.19. Viewed in this way, the pattern is quite consistent and easy to describe: within each birth cohort, lung cancer mortality rates rose steadily with age. Note that Figures 7.17 and 7.19 show exactly the same data points, but they connect the points differently—one by the calendar year in which the mortality rate was calculated and the other by the birth cohort to which each rate pertains.

But why should a woman's year of birth matter at all here, when the rates being examined pertain to late adulthood? Actually, year of birth is merely a convenient way to identify people who belong to a certain generation. For example, people born shortly after the end of World War II are often referred to as "baby boomers," some of their offspring as "Generation X," and so on. Members of the same generation march through history together as a cohort, often sharing experiences by virtue of being about the same age when various world events and cultural shifts occur. Some of these common experiences can have long-lasting effects on their future risk of developing certain diseases.

For lung cancer, tobacco smoking is now known to be a strong risk factor, as several landmark epidemiologic studies in the 1950s and 1960s helped to establish (Doll and Hill, 1950; Wynder and Graham, 1950; Doll and Hill, 1964). Among U.S. women, smoking became more and more common through much of the early 20th century. Thus, women in later birth cohorts were more likely to have adopted smoking at any given age than were their counterparts in earlier birth cohorts. For example, about 44% of women in the 1921–1930 birth cohort were current smokers by the time they reached age 25 years, compared with about 37% of the 1911–1920 birth cohort when *they* were 25, and only about 18% of the 1901–1910 birth cohort (Burns *et al.*, 1997). The higher prevalence of smoking during early adulthood affected the incidence of lung cancer in later birth cohorts throughout the remainder of women's lives, partly because smoking is a persistent habit and partly because it affects not only current risk but also future risk of lung cancer.

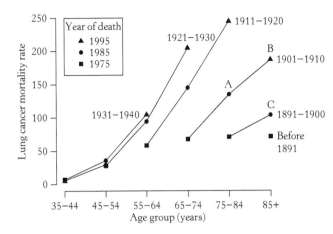

FIGURE 7.19 Lung cancer mortality rates in U.S. women, 1975–1995, connecting rates observed in the same birth cohort and labelling the time path for each birth cohort. (Points A, B, and C are referred to in the text.)

To understand why the relationship between age and lung cancer mortality appears different between Figures 7.17 and 7.19, consider the data point labelled *A* in Figure 7.19. It pertains to the rate observed for women in the 1901–1910 birth cohort in calendar year 1985, at which time they were 75–84 years old. In Figure 7.19, point *A* is connected to point *B*, which pertains to the same birth cohort after they had aged another ten years. The rate for point *B* was thus observed in calendar year 1995. In Figure 7.17, point *A* was connected to point *C*, inasmuch as both *A* and *C* pertain to mortality in the same calendar year, 1985. But moving from point *A* to point *C* involves two other changes: (1) women at point *C* were ten years older than those at point *A*, and (2) they were members of an earlier birth cohort. In this instance, the effect of "dropping down" to an earlier birth cohort outweighs the effect of "sliding up" to an older age group. An age effect is mixed with a birth cohort effect.

More broadly, age, birth cohort, and calendar year (sometimes called *period*) are three conceptually separate time scales, each of which can influence disease frequency by different mechanisms. But the three time scales are also intimately related, because:

$$(\text{Calendar year}) - (\text{age}) = (\text{year of birth})$$

Once any two of these three quantities have been specified, the third is fully determined and cannot vary. Among statisticians, this analytic problem is termed one of *non-identifiability*: it is impossible to isolate the separate contributions of three factors when fixing any two of them automatically fixes the third (Holford, 1991; Clayton and Schifflers, 1987; Weinkam and Sterling, 1991). More details about

the implications of this constraint for statistical modeling of age, period, and birth-cohort effects are discussed by Robertson and Boyle (1998) and by Holford (1991).

Among epidemiologists, alternative ways of displaying the same set of rates, often graphically, have proven helpful in the search for structure, simplicity, and agreement with other observations. For example, Figure 7.17 focuses on age and calendar year, leaving birth cohort in the background. Figure 7.19 focuses on age and birth cohort, leaving calendar year in the background. In this instance, the simplicity and regularity apparent in Figure 7.19 are compelling reasons to think of lung cancer mortality chiefly in terms of age and birth cohort. Tuberculosis (Frost, 1939), testicular cancer (Liu *et al.*, 1999), and malignant melanoma (Dennis *et al.*, 1993) are other diseases for which examining trends in mortality or incidence in terms of birth cohorts has provided useful new insights.

NOTES

1. Age-adjusted rates will be formally covered in Chapter 11, as an example of how bias due to a potential confounding factor can be minimized. For now, one can think of age-adjusted rates as being rates that would be observed if the groups being compared had the same age distribution.

2. And incidentally, by the post-1989 rule, the United States still has never had a black president!

REFERENCES

Allison AC. The distribution of the sickle-cell trait in East Africa and elsewhere, and its apparent relationship to the incidence of subtertian malaria. Trans R Soc Trop Med Hyg 1954; 48:312–318.

Armstrong BK, English DR. Cutaneous malignant melanoma. Chapter 59 in: Schottenfeld D, Fraumeni JF Jr. Cancer epidemiology and prevention (2nd ed.). New York: Oxford University Press, 1996.

Auchincloss AH, Gebreab SY, Mair C, Diez Roux AV. A review of spatial methods in epidemiology, 2000–2010. Annu Rev Public Health 2012; 33:107–122.

Baker SP, O'Neill B, Ginsburg MJ, Li G. The injury fact book (2nd ed.). New York: Oxford University Press, 1992.

Becker KM, Glass GE, Brathwaite W, Zenilman JM. Geographic epidemiology of gonorrhea in Baltimore, Maryland, using a geographic information system. Am J Epidemiol 1998; 147:709–716.

Bergman AB, Ray CG, Pomeroy MA, Wahl PW, Beckwith JB. Studies of the sudden infant death syndrome in King County, Washington. 3. Epidemiology. Pediatrics 1972; 49:860–870.

Binswanger IA, Stern MF, Deyo RA, Heagerty PJ, Cheadle A, Elmore JG, et al. Release from prison—a high risk of death for former inmates. N Engl J Med 2007; 356:157–165.

Boulos DNK, Ghali RR, Ibrahim EM, Boulos MNK, AbdelMalik P. An eight-year snapshot of geospatial cancer research (2002–2009): clinico-epidemiological and methodological findings and trends. Med Oncol 2011; 28:1145–1162.

Bove FJ. The story of ergot. New York: S. Karger, 1970.

Brody H, Rip MR, Vinten-Johansen P, Paneth N, Rachman S. Map-making and myth-making in Broad Street: the London cholera epidemic, 1854. Lancet 2000; 356:64–68.

Burns DM, Lee L, Shen LZ, Gilpin E, Tolley HD, Vaughn J, et al. Cigarette smoking behavior in the United States. Chapter 2 in: Burns DM, Garfinkel L, Samet JM (eds). Changes in cigarette-related disease risks and their implication for prevention and control. Bethesda, MD: National Cancer Institute, 1997.

Carefoot GL, Sprott ER. Famine on the wind: man's battle against plant disease. New York: Rand McNally, 1967.

Centers for Disease Control and Prevention. Maternal, pregnancy, and birth characteristics of Asians and Native Hawaiians/Pacific Islanders—King County, Washington, 2003–2008. MMWR Morb Mortal Wkly Rep 2011; 60:211–213.

Centers for Disease Control and Prevention. Update: influenza activity—United States, 2011–12 season and composition of the 2012–13 influenza vaccine. MMWR Morb Mortal Wkly Rep 2012; 61: 414–420.

Clayton D, Schifflers E. Models for temporal variation in cancer rates: I. Age-period and age-cohort models. Stat Med 1987; 6:449–467.

Davis JP, Chesney PJ, Wand PJ, LaVenture M. Toxic-shock syndrome: epidemiologic features, recurrence, risk factors, and prevention. N Engl J Med 1980; 303:1429–1435.

de la Rosa IA. Perinatal outcomes among Mexican Americans: a review of an epidemiological paradox. Ethn Dis 2002; 12:480–487.

Dennis LK, White E, Lee JAH. Recent cohort trends in malignant melanoma by anatomic site in the United States. Cancer Causes Control 1993; 4: 93–100.

Doll R, Hill AB. Smoking and carcinoma of the lung: preliminary report. Br Med J 1950; 2:739–748.

Doll R, Hill AB. Mortality in relation to smoking: ten years' observations of British doctors. Br Med J 1964; 1:1399–1410.

Ford ES, Ajani UA, Croft JB, Critchley JA, Labarthe DR, Kottke TE, et al. Explaining the decrease in U.S. deaths from coronary disease, 1980–2000. N Engl J Med 2007; 356:2388–2398.

Frost WH. The age selection of mortality from tuberculosis in successive decades. Am J Hygiene 1939; 30:91–96.

Funatogawa I, Funatogawa T, Nakao M, Karita K, Yano E. Changes in body mass index by birth cohort in Japanese adults: results from the National Nutrition Survey of Japan 1956–2005. Int J Epidemiol 2009; 38:83–92.

Galobardes B, Shaw M, Lawlor DA, Davey Smith G, Lynch J. Indicators of socioeconomic position. Chapter 3 in: Oakes JM, Kaufman JS (eds.). Methods in social epidemiology. New York: John Wiley and Sons, 2006.

Glass GE, Schwartz BS, Morgan JM, Johnson DT, Noy PM, Israel E. Environmental risk factors for Lyme disease identified with geographic information systems. Am J Public Health 1995; 85:944–948.

Goldberger J, Waring CH, Tanner WF. Pellagra prevention by diet among institutional inmates. Public Health Rep 1923; 38:2361–2368.

Goldberger J, Wheeler GA, Sydenstricker E. A study of the relation of family income and other economic factors to pellagra incidence in seven cotton-mill villages of South Carolina in 1916. Public Health Rep 1920; 35:2673–2714.

Goldsmith GA. Niacin: antipellagra factor, hypocholesterolemic agent. Model of nutrition research yesterday and today. JAMA 1965; 194:167–173.

Gruska M, Gaul GB, Winkler M, Levnaic S, Reiter C, Voracek M, et al. Increased occurrence of out-of-hospital cardiac arrest on Mondays in a community-based study. Chronobiol Int 2005; 22:107–120.

Hahn RA. The state of federal health statistics on racial and ethnic groups. JAMA 1992; 267:268–271.

Hahn RA, Mulinare J, Teutsch SM. Inconsistencies in coding of race and ethnicity between birth and death in U.S. infants. JAMA 1992; 267:259–263.

Holford TR. Understanding the effects of age, period, and cohort on incidence and mortality rates. Annu Rev Public Health 1991; 12:425–457.

Jerrett M, Gale S, Kontgis C. Spatial modeling in environmental and public health research. Int J Environ Res Public Health 2010; 7:1302–1329.

Kaplan GA, Pamuk ER, Lynch JW, Cohen RD, Balfour JL. Inequality in income and mortality in the United States: analysis of mortality and potential pathways. BMJ 1996; 312:999–1003.

Kipling R. In: Rudyard Kipling's verse. Inclusive edition. London: Hodder and Stoughton, 1933.

Koepsell TD, Rivara FP, Vavilala MS, Wang J, Temkin N, Jaffe KM, *et al.* Incidence and descriptive epidemiologic features of traumatic brain injury in King County, Washington. Pediatrics 2011; 128:946–954.

Kposowa AJ. Marital status and suicide in the National Longitudinal Mortality Study. J Epidemiol Community Health 2000; 34:254–261.

Krieger N, Williams DR, Moss NE. Measuring social class in US public health research: concepts, methodologies, and guidelines. Annu Rev Public Health 1997; 18:341–378.

Leck I, Sibary K, Wakefield J. Incidence of cervical cancer by marital status. J Epidemiol Community Health 1978; 32:108–110.

Lin SS, Kelsey JL. Use of race and ethnicity in epidemiologic research: concepts, methodological issues, and suggestions for research. Epidemiol Rev 2000; 22:187–202.

Liu S, Wen SW, Mao Y, Mery L, Rouleau J. Birth cohort effects underlying the increasing testicular cancer incidence in Canada. Can J Public Health 1999; 90:176–180.

Looker AC, Borrud LG, Dawson-Hughes B, Shepherd JA, Wright NC. Osteoporosis or low bone mass at the femur neck or lumbar spine in older adults: United States, 2005–2008. NCHS Data Brief 2012; 93:1–8.

Lynch JW, Smith GD, Kaplan GA, House JS. Income inequality and mortality: importance to health of individual income, psychosocial environment, or material conditions. BMJ 2000; 320:1200–1204.

Lyon JL, Wetzler HP, Gardner JW, Klauber MR, Williams RR. Cardiovascular mortality in Mormons and non-Mormons in Utah, 1969–1971. Am J Epidemiol 1978; 108:357–366.

Mathews TJ, MacDorman MF. Infant mortality statistics from the 2008 period linked birth/infant death data set. Natl Vital Stat Rep 2012; 60:1–28.

Miller DC. Handbook of research design and social measurement (5th ed.). Newbury Park, CA: Sage Publications, 1991.

Monto AS, Ullman BM. Acute respiratory illness in an American community. The Tecumseh Study. JAMA 1974; 227:164–169.

Moore DA, Carpenter TE. Spatial analytical methods and geographic information systems: use in health research and epidemiology. Epidemiol Rev 1999; 21:143–161.

National Center for Health Statistics. Effect on mortality rates of the 1989 change in tabulating race. Vital Health Stat Series No. 21 (25), Pub. No. (PHS) 94-1853. Hyattsville, MD: National Center for Health Statistics, 1994.

National Center for Health Statistics. Health, United States, 1998 with socioeconomic status and health chartbook. Hyattsville, MD: National Center for Health Statistics, 1998.

National Center for Health Statistics. Health, United States, 2008 with special feature on socioeconomic status and health. Hyattsville, MD: National Center for Health Statistics, 2012a.

National Center for Health Statistics. Health, United States, 2011 with special feature on socioeconomic status and health. Hyattsville, MD: National Center for Health Statistics, 2012b.

National Heart, Lung, and Blood Institute. Morbidity and mortality: 2009 chart book on cardiovascular, lung, and blood diseases. Bethesda, MD: National Heart, Lung, and Blood Institute, 2009.

National Program of Cancer Registries. 1999–2009 incidence, CDC WONDER on-line database. Atlanta, GA: Centers for Disease Control and Prevention and National Cancer Institute, 2012.

Phillips DP, Christenfeld N, Ryan NM. An increase in the number of deaths in the United States in the first week of the month. An association with substance abuse and other causes of death. N Engl J Med 1999; 341:93–98.

Pickett KE, Pearl M. Multilevel analyses of neighbourhood socioeconomic context and health outcomes: a critical review. J Epidemiol Community Health 2001; 55:111–122.

Pokorny J, Smith VC, Verriest G. Congenital color defects. Chapter 7 in Pokorny J, Smith VC, Verriest G, Pinckers AJLG. Congenital and acquired color vision defects. New York: Grune & Stratton, 1979.

Porta M (ed.) A dictionary of epidemiology (5th edition). New York: Oxford University Press, 2008.

Reeve J. How do women develop fragile bones? J Steroid Biochem Mol Biol 2000; 74:375–381.

Rendall MS, Weden MM, Favreault MM, Waldron H. The protective effect of marriage for survival: a review and update. Demography 2011; 48:481–506.

Robertson C, Boyle P. Age-period-cohort analysis of chronic disease rates. I: Modelling approach. Stat Med 1998; 17:1305–1323.

Robinson KA, Baughman W, Rothrock G, Barrett NL, Pass M, Lexau C, et al. Epidemiology of invasive *Streptococcus pneumoniae* infections in the United States, 1995–1998. JAMA 2001; 285:1729–1735.

Samelson EJ, Zhang Y, Kiel DP, Hannan MT, Felson DT. Effect of birth cohort on risk of hip fracture: age-specific incidence rates in the Framingham Study. Am J Public Health 2002; 92:858–862.

Semmelweis I. The etiology, concept, and prophylaxis of childbed fever. In: Buck C, Llopis A, Najera E, Terris M (eds.). The challenge of epidemiology. Issues and selected readings. Washington, D.C.: Pan American Health Organization, 1988.

Snow J. Snow on cholera. New York: Commonwealth Fund, 1936.

Trottier H, Franco EL. The epidemiology of genital human papillomavirus infection. Vaccine 2006; 24 Suppl 1:S1–S15.

Von Korff M, Koepsell T, Curry S, Diehr P. Multi-level analysis in epidemiologic research on health behaviors and outcomes. Am J Epidemiol 1992; 135:1077–1082.

Wagstaff A, van Doorslaer E. Income inequality and health: what does the literature tell us? Annu Rev Public Health 2000; 21:543–567.

Walker DH. Tick-transmitted infectious diseases in the United States. Annu Rev Public Health 1998; 19:237–269.

Weinkam JJ, Sterling TD. A graphical approach to the interpretation of age-period-cohort data. Epidemiology 1991; 2:133–137.

Wilbert-Lampen U, Leistner D, Greven S, Pohl T, Sper S, Völker C, et al. Cardiovascular events during World Cup soccer. N Engl J Med 2008; 358:475–483.

Williams DR. Race and health: basic questions, emerging directions. Ann Epidemiol 1997; 7:322–333.

Wynder EL, Graham EA. Tobacco smoking as a possible etiologic factor in brohiogenic carcinoma: a study of six hundred and eighty-four proved cases. JAMA 1950; 143:329–336.

Yeh RW, Sidney S, Chandra M, Sorel M, Selby JV, Go AS. Population trends in the incidence and outcomes of acute myocardial infarction. N Engl J Med 2010; 362:2155–2165.

EXERCISES

1. *Streptococcus pneumoniae* is a common cause of community-acquired pneumonia, meningitis, and bacteremia. Vaccines have now been developed against many specific strains of *S. pneumoniae*. To help quantify the burden of disease caused by this pathogen on the United States population, Robinson et al. (2001) used data from a nine-state laboratory-based surveillance system to estimate the number of cases and deaths from invasive *S. pneumoniae* infection in the United States in a certain year. Table 7.7 shows the distribution of these events by age.

    To what extent can these data be used to assess which age groups are burdened disproportionately by invasive *S. pneumoniae* in the United States?

2. Mortality from cardiovascular disease in Utah has been found to be among the lowest in the United States. Lyon et al. (1978) studied mortality from cardiovascular disease within Utah, comparing rates in Mormons and non-Mormons. Such a study was possible because, since 1941, the Mormon Church has maintained centralized records of all church members (alive or dead), which could be matched to Utah death records. Table 7.8 shows results for ischemic heart disease, which accounted for a large majority of cardiovascular deaths, expressed in terms of *standardized mortality ratios* (SMRs). The SMR can be interpreted here as the ratio of the cause-specific mortality rate *observed* in a particular study group to the rate that would be *expected* if the age- and sex-specific mortality rates for that cause from the United States as a whole were applied to that study group, given its age and sex composition.

    (a) To what extent do these results appear to help explain why cardiovascular mortality rates in Utah were relatively low compared to the United States as a whole?

    (b) What hypotheses might you advance to account for the difference in rates between Mormons and non-Mormons?

3. Suppose that a large population-based cohort study of women involved ascertaining new cases of hip fracture over a follow-up period of nearly 50 years, up to the time of this data analysis. Figure 7.20 shows four curves. Three of them show the incidence of hip fracture, by age, among study women in each of three birth cohorts: 1901–1910, 1911–1920, and 1921–1930. The fourth curve shows similar data for women in all three birth cohorts combined.

    (a) Identify the group of women to which each curve pertains.

    (b) From these results, the investigators have concluded that projections that fail to account for the differences in hip fracture incidence rates among birth cohorts could underestimate the future public health impact of hip fracture in women. Do you agree? Explain briefly.

4. Myocardial infarction (= MI = "heart attack") is an important form of both fatal and nonfatal heart disease. It results from partial or complete blockage of

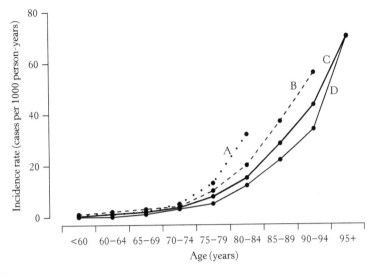

FIGURE 7.20

TABLE 7.7.

Age (years)	Cases	Deaths
<2	12,560	110
2–4	4,020	0
5–17	1,980	50
18–34	4,740	210
35–49	10,150	1,150
50–64	8,840	1,150
65–79	11,890	1,890
80+	8,660	1,520

that ST elevation may sometimes be absent in MI, and that the presence or absence of this finding is associated with differences in clinical course and prognosis. For this reason, MIs are often subclassified as either *ST-elevation MI* (STEMI) or *non-ST-elevation MI* (NSTEMI).

- *Blood tests.* These tests detect proteins that are released into the bloodstream by dying myocardial cells. A relatively new such test measures the level of troponin-I. The troponin-I test has been found to be more sensitive than other tests: that is, it can detect milder degrees of heart damage.

an artery supplying the heart muscle (myocardium). Factors associated with higher risk of MI include older age, male gender, high blood pressure (hypertension), elevated serum cholesterol, diabetes, and smoking.

The diagnosis of MI is based on:

- *Symptoms,* typically crushing chest pain, often radiating to the left arm or shoulder.
- *Electrocardiogram.* The classic finding is called *ST-segment elevation.* However, it is now known

TABLE 7.8. STANDARDIZED MORTALITY RATIO FOR ISCHEMIC HEART DISEASE[a]

Mormons	Non-Mormons	All Utah residents
0.644	0.963	0.737

[a] Relative to 1970 U.S. rates

Therapy includes supportive medical care and treatment of complications, such as arrhythmias or heart failure. In recent years, attempts at revascularization soon after MI have become common: *angioplasty* to open up a blocked vessel with a catheter inserted through a major artery, or *coronary artery bypass grafting* to reroute blood around a blockage via a surgically attached auxiliary vessel. Revascularization is more often attempted after STEMI.

A study examined time trends in the incidence and short-term outcomes of MI over a 10-year period for enrollees aged 30 years or older in a large prepaid health plan in northern California. A summary of results appears in Table 7.9. (Missing numbers were not reported in the published paper.)

For present purposes, assume that only first MIs were studied. Also assume that the true prevalence of hypertension and of elevated levels of serum cholesterol in the enrolled population remained

TABLE 7.9.

	1999	2002	2005	2008
Mid-year enrolled population age 30+	1,055,949	1,288,333	1,530,213	1,878,038
Proportion of population:				
With diagnosed high blood pressure[a]	25.8%	39.3%	45.4%	43.0%
On statin treatment[b]	6.6%	13.1%	19.3%	20.2%
No. of MI cases:				
STEMI	1,987	2,027	1,203	933
NSTEMI	2,240	2,935	3,609	3,135
30-day case fatality after:				
STEMI	11.1%			8.5%
NSTEMI	10.0%			7.6%
Proportion of MI cases receiving:				
Troponin-I test	53%		84%	84%
Revascularization				
STEMI	50%	58%	66%	68%
NSTEMI	33%	38%	38%	40%

[a] Such a diagnosis normally leads to antihypertensive therapy
[b] Used to reduce elevated serum cholesterol levels
(Based on data from Yeh et al. [2010])

about the same throughout the 10-year study period.

(a) Calculate appropriate estimates of the incidence of STEMI, NSTEMI, and all MI in each study year. Briefly describe the time trends in incidence and case fatality.

(b) Which of the following factors could explain the observed time trend in the incidence of (first) MI? Explain briefly.

- More aggressive detection and treatment of high blood pressure
- More frequent treatment of high cholesterol with statins
- Increasing use of the troponin-I test
- Growing popularity of revascularization

(c) Which of the four changing factors mentioned above were likely contributors to the observed time trend in case fatality? Explain briefly.

5. In Japan, a National Nutritional Survey has been done annually for over 50 years. Each year the survey obtains anthropometric data on a random sample of Japanese adults. Figure 7.21 shows mean body weight (in kilograms) among Japanese men in relation to age and survey decade (Funatogawa et al., 2009). Data from ten consecutive annual surveys were combined into each of the five survey decades identified on the right side of the figure.

On the basis of these results, would you expect that a typical 35-year-old Japanese man will weigh more or less ten years from now than he weighs today? Explain your answer briefly.

6. The (real) data shown in Table 7.10 describe an epidemic that occurred over a short period of time:

(a) Summarize the descriptive epidemiologic features.

(b) Based on your answer to part (a), can you suggest what the "mystery epidemic" might have been?

ANSWERS

1. The table shows only numerator data. It provides no information about the size of the population at risk in each age group. (The age groups also span different numbers of years.) When Robinson and colleagues combined this information with denominator estimates obtained from the Census, the incidence rates shown in the Table 7.11 were obtained. There was a clear U-shaped pattern of variation in incidence by age, with infants and older adults at far higher risk than were older children or younger adults. Individuals in the age group that included the mean and median age of cases were in fact at relatively low overall risk. This illustrates how the mean or median age of cases can be misleading as guides to which age group is most commonly affected.

On the other hand, data in the original table are sufficient to allow calculation of age-specific case fatality, a measure of prognosis in afflicted persons. As

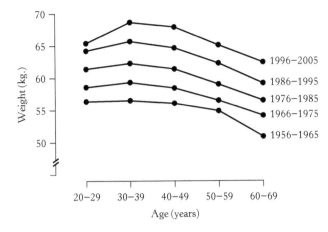

FIGURE 7.21

TABLE 7.10.

Social class	Adult males N[a]	Cumulative mortality	Adult females N	Cumulative mortality	Children N	Cumulative mortality	Total population N	Cumulative mortality
High	173	66.5%	144	3.5%	5	0.0%	322	37.3%
Middle	160	91.9%	93	16.1%	24	0.0%	277	58.5%
Low	454	87.9%	179	45.3%	76	71.1%	709	75.3%
Unknown	875	78.4%	23	8.7%	0	.	898	76.6%
TOTAL	1662	81.0%	439	23.5%	105	51.4%	2206	68.2%

[a] Number at risk

TABLE 7.11.

Age (years)	Incidence[a]	Case fatality
<2	166.9	0.9%
2–4	35.2	0.0%
5–17	3.9	2.5%
18–34	7.4	4.4%
35–49	16.0	11.3%
50–64	23.0	13.0%
65–79	46.4	15.9%
80+	98.5	17.6%

a Cases per 100,000 person-years
(Based on data from Robinson *et al.* [2001])

shown above, older adults were much more likely to die of invasive *S. pneumoniae* infection if they developed it, supporting the notion that the elderly may be a high-priority group for preventive efforts, including vaccination.

2. (a) The SMRs for Utah as a whole confirmed that ischemic heart disease mortality was indeed about 25–27% lower in Utah than expected from U.S. rates. Among non-Mormons, however, the SMRs were very close to 1.0, suggesting that residence in Utah per se had little association with ischemic heart disease mortality.

(b) Lifestyle differences between Mormons and non-Mormons would be a strong possibility. Cigarette smoking is a known strong risk factor for ischemic heart disease, and the Mormon church advocates abstention from tobacco use. Differences in socioeconomic status, access to health care, and other behavioral risk factors for heart disease could also play a role.

3. (a) The shortest curve (A) must refer to women born most recently, in 1921–1930, who had not yet lived beyond 80–84 years of age at the time of this data analysis. Similarly, curve B must refer to the 1911–1920 birth cohort, who had not yet lived beyond 90–94 years of age. Of the two remaining curves, one refers to the 1901–1910 birth cohort only, while the other curve refers to all three birth cohorts combined. Within a given age group, the rates for women from all birth cohorts combined would be a weighted average of the age-specific rates from the three birth cohorts. Hence the curve for all women must fall somewhere between the three cohort-specific

curves. Thus the thick black curve (C) must be the curve for all women combined. By exclusion, the rightmost curve (D) must be the curve for the 1901–1910 birth cohort.

(b) The conclusion is most likely correct. The figure shows that the age-specific incidence of hip fracture was higher in each later birth cohort than in earlier birth cohorts. This pattern suggests that in the future, as women from these more recent birth cohorts age into older age groups, their age-specific rates will be higher than those in effect today. Failure to account for this probable future increase in age-specific rates would lead to underestimation of the future burden of hip fractures among women, at least in this setting.

(This question was based on Samelson *et al.* [2002], although the data were altered for present purposes.)

4. (a) Enrollees in the health plan constituted an open population, so incidence *rates* are needed. Ideally, we would also know the proportion of enrollees age 30+ years who had previously had an MI (and thus were not at risk for a *first* MI). In this study, that information was unavailable, but the proportion of such enrollees was thought to be small, so the mid-year number of enrollees in each calendar year was used as an estimate of the mean number of enrollees at risk for MI in that year. Multiplying each population estimate by 1 year gives the number of person-years for the incidence of STEMI, NSTEMI, and all MIs in that year. For example, the estimated incidence rate of STEMI in 1999 was $1,987/1,055,949 \times 100,000 = 188$ per 100,000 person-years. The complete set of rates is:

TABLE 7.12. INCIDENCE RATE[a]

	1999	2002	2005	2008
STEMI	188	157	79	50
NSTEMI	212	228	236	167
All MI	400	385	315	216

[a] MI cases per 100,000 person-years

The results show steady decline in the incidence of STEMI and of all MIs. In contrast, the incidence of NSTEMI increased gradually from 1999–2005, but then declined to a value well below the rate in 1999.

The 30-day case fatality declined for both STEMI and NSTEMI from 1999 to 2008.

(b) Increases in the proportion of enrollees diagnosed with hypertension and in the proportion receiving statins could represent more aggressive detection and treatment of modifiable risk factors, which could lead to a decrease in incidence of first MIs. Increasing use of the troponin-I test would probably *increase*, not decrease, the apparent incidence of first MI by increasing detection of mild cases that might otherwise have been missed. Revascularization is applied only after an MI has occurred, so changes in its use would not explain changes in the incidence of first MI.

(c) More aggressive control of risk factors for MI (hypertension, elevated cholesterol) should chiefly act to reduce MI incidence; they would be less likely to affect MI outcomes. Increasing use of the troponin-I test could result in increased detection of NSTEMIs (which are not detected by electrocardiograms) and of milder MIs, which would probably have a better prognosis and lower case fatality. Increasing use of revascularization could also reduce 30-day case fatality to the extent that these procedures succeed in preventing further death of myocardium.

(This question was based on Yeh *et al.* [2010]. The numerical results reported therein differ somewhat from those calculated here because their incidence and case fatality results were age- and sex-adjusted, using methods to be covered in future chapters.)

5. The lines in the original figure connect data points that were obtained during the same survey decade. However, men of different ages in the same survey decade also belonged to different birth cohorts. Because the age categories are ten years apart and the survey decades are also ten years apart, the same data points can be reconnected with lines that show the experience of different birth cohorts as they aged.

Figure 7.22 shows that in every birth cohort of Japanese men for whom data are available, mean weight has *increased* from ages 30–39 years to ages 40–49 years. It seems highly likely that this pattern would continue, and that a Japanese man who is 35 years old today can expect to gain weight in the next ten years.

The difference in mean weight between ages 30–39 years and ages 40–49 years along any curve in the original figure represents a combination of two factors operating in different directions: (1) an *increase* in mean weight associated with aging 10 years, plus (2) a *decrease* in mean weight associated with switching from a later birth cohort to an earlier one. The second figure shows that later birth cohorts have almost

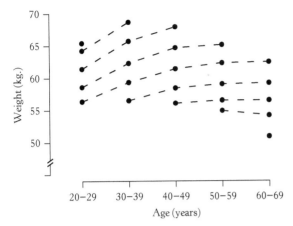

FIGURE 7.22

always had higher mean weight at any given age than earlier birth cohorts.

6. These data concern the sinking of the oceangoing passenger liner *Titanic* in 1912. "Social class" refers to the deck on which passengers had booked their sleeping accommodations, the upper decks having the more expensive staterooms. Most of those of "unknown" social class were single men emigrating to the United States who had not booked staterooms.

When the order came to abandon ship, those on the upper decks had readier access to the lifeboats. The rule was "women and children first," accounting for higher cumulative mortality among men.

8

Inferring a Causal Relation Between Exposure and Disease

Epidemiologists not only measure the occurrence of disease, they seek to identify the causes of disease by interpreting observed patterns of variation in disease occurrence. Epidemiologic research is valued primarily because the causal inferences it generates can inform decisions about prevention of illness. These decisions are faced by:

1. *Individuals on their own.* For example, a middle-aged American man may consider adopting a diet that is relatively low in saturated fat and cholesterol, or high in seafood, with an eye to reducing his risk of a heart attack. Or, a pregnant Kenyan woman who has learned she is seropositive for HIV must decide whether or not to nurse her newborn, balancing the benefits of breast feeding against an increased risk of her child's becoming infected with HIV.
2. *Health care providers on behalf of their patients.* Part of the job of a provider of health care is to advise patients about what they can do to prevent disease. In addition, these providers may have interventions that they can offer directly to reduce disease occurrence. For example, for that same middle-aged man who seeks advice about dietary modification of fat intake, a physician might prescribe a cholesterol-lowering medication.
3. *Society as a whole.* Decisions regarding the prevention of illness and injury are often made collectively. For instance, many communities have chosen to fluoridate their water supplies in an effort to reduce the burden of dental caries. Other communities have not done so, concerned that there may be untoward consequences of fluoridation that would outweigh this benefit.

The information most relevant to these decisions, whoever is making them, is whether a particular exposure (e.g., dietary modification) does or does not give rise to an altered occurrence of illness or injury, and, if so, by how much. These decision makers wish to know whether the exposure in question leads to an increase in risk: that is, but for the presence of the exposure, would some cases of illness or injury not occur (i.e., exposure is causal)? Or, they may wish to know whether the exposure leads to some cases not occurring (exposure is protective). However, epidemiologists may be able to indicate only whether the incidence of illness or injury differs in relation to the presence of a given exposure; i.e., whether an association is present. Associations can be observed in data collected to address a specific question, such as whether the incidence of lung cancer is greater in smokers of cigarettes than in nonsmokers, or whether the prevalence of dental caries is higher in populations whose water supply is not fluoridated than in populations that receive fluoridated water. But, not all observed associations between an exposure or characteristic and disease are causal ones.

Example 8-1. Scurvy had long been recognized as being relatively common among seafarers. Those with scurvy who returned to port often recovered relatively quickly. We now know that these associations were due to the lack of vitamin C in the diets of the men who went to sea. However, prior to the identification of vitamin C, all that was known was that there was something about leaving land that predisposed sailors to scurvy, and something about returning to port that somehow led to its cure. Epidemics of scurvy were not restricted to sailors; they could occur any time when there was nutritional deprivation. One such outbreak occurred during the California gold rush, at the Sonora Mining Camp, where, "In November of 1849 they established a hospital for the destitute sick, of which there were large numbers, with land scurvy being the most prominent disease" (Carpenter, 1986). It was not terribly surprising that scurvy was common then, because the miners' diet "seemed to consist of stewed beans and flapjacks 21 times per week, though the latter was occasionally replaced by flour dumplings and molasses." To address the problem, "Some miners resorted to the old treatment of burial up to the neck in earth. The whole camp would do it at once, except a few who remained out to keep out grizzlies and coyotes." Apparently, "these miners would try to maximize the effect of land by immersing themselves in it." We would not have expected that immersion in land had any influence on the natural history of scurvy (we know of no studies of the efficacy of this treatment!) since the association between not being in proximity to land and the development of scurvy need not be a causal one.

When we are trying to judge whether an association represents a causal influence of an exposure, we run into an immediate impediment: We don't actually observe causes. We do observe associations, and perhaps an apparent temporal sequence of events, but we must infer causes. For instance, most of us have inferred that we can cause a car to start by turning its key in the ignition. How have we made that inference? First, there is a very strong association: Almost all of the time when we turn the key, the car will promptly start, and rarely if ever will it do so when the key is not turned in the ignition. Second, there's a very reasonable mechanism, in terms of the way the car has been built, that underlies this association and would predict that it would be a causal one. Nonetheless, we haven't *seen* causation. Rather, we've noted events, and in our minds we have drawn a connection.

When we attempt to make an inference regarding causes of disease, we have several handicaps that were not present in our automotive example. First, exposure may occur long before disease appears. Taking up cigarette smoking as a teenager probably has little effect on one's risk of lung cancer until well into adulthood. This means that our observations may have to span years or even decades, depending on the nature of the disease and how its occurrence is influenced by the exposure. Also, our ability to infer causation may be impaired by the fact that the same illness can occur due to the action of causes other than the one we happen to be investigating. Smoking may be a cause of lung cancer, but since this disease can occur even in the absence of smoking as a result of other etiologic factors, the association between smoking and lung cancer will be diluted in proportion to the frequency of these factors.

Finally, the lack of a perfect correspondence between the presence of a particular exposure and the occurrence of a particular disease arises when the exposure can exert its influence only in the presence of another factor. Cigarette smoking by itself will not cause lung cancer; most people who smoke cigarettes never develop lung cancer. Whether it is the presence of a genetic characteristic or some other environmental exposure, there have to be reasons why only the occasional cigarette smoker becomes ill with this disease and other smokers do not.

In epidemiology, as in other sciences, we make observations and try to draw inferences from these observations. The inferences take the shape of judgments about the likelihood of the truth or falsity of hypotheses regarding cause and effect. A given hypothesis can stimulate us to make additional observations to test its validity. Some of the hypotheses that are generated, if unrefuted by additional observations, are sufficiently plausible that they are tentatively accepted as valid, and so serve as a guide to decisions about prevention. As an example, the increasing incidence of cancers of the respiratory tract in the first half of the 20th century in Europe and North America followed an increase in cigarette consumption in these populations. This temporal correlation, and the fact that the respiratory tract receives a large, direct exposure to inhaled cigarette smoke, were compatible with the hypothesis that cigarette smoking could cause cancers at this site. This hypothesis has been tested many times in epidemiologic studies, most notably through comparisons of the incidence of respiratory cancer in smokers and nonsmokers who appeared to be similar otherwise. Those comparisons typically have revealed a strikingly higher incidence among smokers. Non-epidemiologic studies have gone on to identify many substances in cigarette smoke whose administration to laboratory animals resulted in an increased incidence of cancer. To most of us, the causal hypothesis remains unrefuted, and so we are willing to tally an increased risk of respiratory cancer as a consequence of cigarette smoking when deciding on the desirability of preventing or modifying cigarette-smoking behavior.

EVIDENCE USED TO DRAW CAUSAL INFERENCES

Beginning in the middle of the 20th century, stimulated by the accumulating data pointing to a possible causal influence of cigarette smoking on lung cancer and other diseases, specific types of evidence have been identified that bear on the plausibility of a causal relation between an exposure and a disease (U. S. Public Health Service, 1964; Hill, 1965). Our version of these types of evidence—they differ slightly from epidemiologist to epidemiologist—is contained in Table 8.1.

Results from Randomized Trials

First, we ask if an association has been observed in one or more randomized trials. As discussed in Chapter 13, trials of this sort involve the recruitment of study participants who allow the investigator to allocate them, using some form of random process, either to receive or to not receive an intervention (or one of several possible interventions). Thus, a difference in the incidence of illness or death between intervention groups, especially a large difference, cannot be readily attributed to other characteristics of persons who received or failed to receive the intervention; on average, those other characteristics will be present to the same extent in both groups. As an example, families living in urban squatter settlements in Karachi, Pakistan, were assigned at random (depending on their neighborhood) to receive either: a supply of soap, as well as an educational program designed to encourage hand washing after

defecation and prior to cooking, eating, and feeding a child; or no intervention (Luby *et al.*, 2004). During the subsequent year, the incidence of diarrhea among the 3,163 children in the intervention neighborhoods was less than half that in the 1,528 children living in the control neighborhoods. The study was large enough that the probability of a difference in incidence of the observed magnitude or greater occurring by chance, given no true influence of the intervention, was extremely small. Because of randomization, the intervention neighborhoods and control neighborhoods would have been expected to be similar with regard to other predictors of the incidence of childhood diarrhea (e.g., parental literacy, number of persons per household), and they were in fact found to be similar. Therefore, there is no other plausible explanation for the association other than a beneficial influence of the intervention itself.

Not every potential causal relationship can be evaluated by means of a randomized trial. Sometimes, the intervention under consideration has one or more known consequences whose importance dwarfs that of the condition whose relationship to the exposure is in question. So, let us say we are interested in the question of whether an induced abortion can predispose a woman to developing breast cancer later in life. One of the ways we would not go about studying this is to ask pregnant women who are considering having an abortion to allow themselves to enter a study in which the luck of the draw would dictate which among them would indeed have the abortion and which ones would attempt to carry their pregnancy to term! In other circumstances, data already available from non-randomized studies may suggest a causal relationship. For example, one reason that no randomized trial has been conducted to examine whether cigarette smoking is an etiologic factor in the occurrence of lung cancer is that this question is seen by most people as having been resolved in the absence of such a trial. As a result, even if a randomized trial of cigarette smoking and health were feasible to undertake, most people would not view it as being ethical.

Inferences from Non-randomized Studies

When the only data available to guide a causal inference come from non-randomized studies, it is necessary to tread particularly carefully so as to sidestep errors that might lead us to make a causal inference when no causation is present, or the reverse. Just as with randomized trials, an association between exposure and illness must be evident in order even to

---

TABLE 8.1. SOURCES OF SUPPORT FOR THE HYPOTHESIS THAT A GIVEN EXPOSURE IS A CAUSE OF DISEASE OR INJURY IN HUMAN BEINGS

1. Data from randomized studies in human beings show an association between the presence of the exposure and disease occurrence
2. Data from non-randomized studies in human beings show an association, and:
   (a) The suspected cause precedes the presence of the disease.
   (b) The association is strong.
   (c) There is:
       i. No plausible non-causal explanation that would account for the (entirety of the) association; and
       ii. A plausible explanation for the association's being a causal one.
   (d) The magnitude of the association is strongest when it is predicted to be so.

consider the possibility of a cause–effect relationship. Generally there will be more than one study available through which to judge whether an association is or is not present, and in this circumstance, the results of each study (along with its size and perceived quality) need to be taken into account so that an overall assessment can be made.

Temporal Sequence of Events

Of course, an association between exposure and disease can only be attributed to the causal influence of the exposure if it is clear that the exposure precedes the disease in time. From the epidemiologic studies in which these associations have emerged, it will generally be straightforward whether the exposure or the disease occurred first. For example, an excess risk of lung cancer among cigarette smokers is not observed until at least a decade after smoking has been initiated. Thus, it is hard to imagine that in some way a person's lung tumor had influenced him or her to begin to smoke cigarettes 10 or more years before it was diagnosed. Nonetheless, the sequence of events may not be so obvious, and special efforts in the study design and analysis may be needed to clarify the situation.

Example 8-2.   Reye's syndrome (RS) is a childhood condition characterized by damage to the liver and central nervous system. The damage may be transient, but in many instances the disease leads to death or retardation. RS typically develops following a bout of chickenpox or influenza, and it was suspected that the use of aspirin to treat the symptoms of these infections predisposed a child to getting RS. The results of an epidemiologic study indicating an increased incidence of RS in children who took aspirin for fever, relative to children in general, could be interpreted in one of two ways:

1. Aspirin use predisposes to RS; or
2. Early in its course, and before it is diagnosed as such, RS gives rise to fever that leads to aspirin use. The association observed may thus reflect the causal influence of RS on aspirin use, rather than the reverse.

Anticipating this possible ambiguity, some epidemiologic studies (Halpin *et al.*, 1982; Hurwitz *et al.*, 1987; Forsyth *et al.*, 1989) confined their study populations to children with a recent episode of chicken pox or flu. Their observation of a substantially higher risk of RS in children with one of these conditions who received aspirin, relative to other children with a similar recent infection who did

not, argues strongly against the second interpretation above, and strongly in favor of the notion that aspirin use did in fact precede the presence of RS.

Strength of the Association

The larger the association between the presence of an exposure and the occurrence of illness or injury, the more likely it is that association reflects a causal influence of the exposure. This is because, the larger the association, the less likely it is that errors in the study, or the presence of other risk factors for the disease that tend to coexist with the one in question, could be responsible for the whole of the association. For example, one of the arguments in support of a causal relationship between cigarette smoking and lung cancer is that the incidence of lung cancer between smokers and nonsmokers is markedly different. In order for one of the correlates of smoking behavior (e.g., alcohol consumption, socioeconomic status, occupation) to entirely explain that large association, it would have to be associated with lung cancer to at least that degree and also be highly correlated with cigarette smoking.

The strength of an association is generally quantified as the ratio of the incidence of disease between exposed and non-exposed individuals; for example, we would describe the strength of the association between smoking and lung cancer by saying that smokers have about a 10-fold greater risk than do nonsmokers. A relative rather than absolute measure is used to characterize "strength," since it is expected that the sources of bias encountered in epidemiologic studies tend to be present to a similar relative degree whether an association is present or absent, strong or weak. One way to think of this is to imagine that we are trying to estimate the passage of time without the benefit of a timepiece. If we erred by one second after the first ten had elapsed, then after 60 seconds it is more likely that would mis-estimate that duration by 6 seconds (one in 10) than by just one second (one in 60). By the same token, absolute measures of the size of an association—the difference in incidence between exposed and non-exposed persons—are strongly influenced by the underlying frequency of the disease being studied, and so do not serve as well as ratio measures for judging whether an association is present beyond the influence of error.

Plausibility of Causal and Non-causal Hypotheses

The stronger the basis for suspecting that an exposure ought to cause a disease or injury, the stronger will be the inference that an association between that exposure and disease or injury is a causal one. Conversely, a compelling alternative explanation can argue against causation. Many different types of evidence, epidemiologic and non-epidemiologic, can provide a basis for suspicion. Cigarette smoke contains many substances that are carcinogenic in the laboratory setting; it comes into direct contact with the bronchi when inhaled; and the incidence of cancers of the bronchi and lung from population to population, and over time within one population, has paralleled the prevalence of cigarette smoking. All of the foregoing strengthen an inference of a causal connection when one is seeking to interpret an observed association, within a population, between cigarette smoking and the incidence of cancers of the bronchi and lung. Similarly, it might be expected that wearing a helmet can provide structural protection against head injury in a bicycle crash, or that wearing a condom can provide a physical barrier against HIV transmission. Because of this, an association between helmet use and a reduced risk of head injury, or between condom use and a reduced risk of acquiring HIV, is widely interpreted as indicating at least some degree of protection.

Many studies of possible exposure/disease associations are able to gather information to assess the plausibility of at least some non-causal explanations for any association that is observed.

Example 8-3.   In a multicenter study in Europe (de Vicenzi, 1994), heterosexual couples of whom only one member had been infected with HIV were followed for approximately two years. The incidence of a new HIV infection in the previously negative partner was monitored in relation to whether or not the couple consistently used a condom during sexual intercourse in those two years. Of 124 couples who consistently used a condom, no instances of transmission occurred, whereas 12 of the 121 previously uninfected members of couples who did not consistently use condoms became HIV-positive.

The investigators sought to uncover other characteristics of couples who did and did not consistently use condoms that might have been responsible for this difference. For example, the efficiency of transmission of HIV is known to be relatively greater from men to women than from women to men. Did the condom-using couples tend to have a relatively low proportion of men as the initially infected partner? No, at least not to any appreciable degree: in 61 percent of the condom-using couples, the index

partner was male, in contrast to 67 percent of the other couples. Did the condom-using couples simply have sexual intercourse relatively less frequently, and for this reason have a low rate of transmission? No, their median frequency of sexual intercourse during the follow-up period actually was higher (twice per week) than that of the other couples (once per week). The distribution of other potential risk factors for HIV transmission similarly did not suggest that anything other than that consistent condom use itself was responsible for the observed difference in the occurrence of HIV.

Pattern of Variation in the Strength of the Association

Often, the risk of a disease among exposed persons is seen to rise steadily as the intensity of exposure increases. In some of these instances, our knowledge of the basis underlying the induction of the disease is complete enough to have predicted the steady rise. For example, we know that exposure to carbon monoxide (CO) gives rise to hypoxia because this molecule competes with oxygen for hemoglobin transport, so we would predict that the occurrence of hypoxic signs and symptoms would rise with increasingly high CO concentrations in inspired air.

Even when our knowledge of the mechanism underlying disease occurrence is less precise, we tend to use the presence of such a "dose–response" relationship as supporting a causal hypothesis. Early in the course of research on this subject, the observed rise in the risk of lung cancer with an increasing number of cigarettes smoked each day was viewed as supporting the hypothesis of a causal influence of smoking on the incidence of this disease.

The intensity of an exposure is only one of several characteristics that can be examined for its possible impact on disease incidence. The risk of endometrial cancer among post-menopausal women who have taken estrogens unopposed by a progestogen appears to be heavily influenced by the duration and recency of use: the longer and more recent the use, the higher the risk of this cancer. In other instances, the interval from the time the exposure first was encountered has a substantial bearing on risk. For example, the inference that receipt of A/New Jersey influenza (swine flu) vaccine predisposed to the occurrence of Guillain-Barré syndrome was enhanced when it was observed that the high risk of this disease was largely confined to the second and third weeks following vaccination (Marks and Halpin, 1980). Since it takes 1–2 weeks for primary immune responses to be mounted, the observed temporal pattern of increased risk is compatible with the hypothesis that, in some way, an immune response to the vaccine was responsible—just as an immune response to various infectious illnesses had been suspected as being responsible for many prior cases of Guillain-Barré syndrome in unvaccinated persons.

The presence of a steady rise in risk with increasing intensity or duration of exposure does not mean that a causal relation must be present. One or more factors might be strongly associated with both exposure and disease to give rise to a pattern of this sort without there being any causal connection between them. For example, while a woman's age at which she first nurses a baby may be directly related to breast cancer risk in a graded way, this association would probably be the result of the strong relationship between age at first birth (whether the woman had breastfed or not) and both age at first breast feeding and breast cancer risk. Similarly, the lack of a steady rise in risk with increasing intensity or duration of exposure by no means precludes a causal relationship. For example, while the risk of thyroid cancer among adults who survived childhood cancer rises steadily with increasing therapeutic radiation dose received during childhood through 30 Gy, the risk declines with doses beyond this (Sigurdson *et al.*, 2005). It is likely that therapeutic radiation can indeed be a cause of thyroid cancer, but another consequence of radiation doses above 30 Gy—death of thyroid cells—limits the development of cancer in that organ. Furthermore, some causal relationships are threshold in nature: squeezing the trigger of a gun can lead to a homicide but, beyond a certain intensity of squeezing, the risk of homicide stays constant!

Yet another way to examine variation in the strength of an association between exposure and disease is according to the presence of other characteristics or other exposures that might be predicted to have an influence. The restriction of the association of tetracycline use to the development of discolored teeth to children under five years of age argues in support of a causal connection, since:

- Tetracyclines chelate with calcium ions; and
- Only in children under five are the crowns of teeth still undergoing calcification.

In the same way, the hypothesis that long-term estrogen use is a cause of endometrial cancer is supported by the observation that such use is strongly associated with cancer risk only when it is not accompanied by a progestogen, since progestogens are known to counter estrogen-stimulated proliferation of endometrial tissue.

In summary, a causal inference is strengthened when the size of an association between exposure and disease varies in a way that could be predicted from other knowledge. The variation may be on the basis of some feature of the exposure itself (e.g., intensity, duration, or recency), or of another characteristic or exposure altogether (Weiss, 1981).

The pattern of associations between a given exposure and *different* outcomes occasionally can inform a causal inference as well (Weiss, 2002; Lipsitch *et al.*, 2010). For example, we believe that screening sigmoidoscopy (endoscopic evaluation of the rectum and lower colon) leads to reduced mortality from tumors arising in the rectum and lower colon because screened persons have: (1) a sharply reduced death rate from those tumors; and (2) *no* reduced death rate from tumors arising in the upper colon, beyond the reach of the sigmoidoscope (Selby *et al.*, 1992). Similarly, a causal inference is strengthened if several related exposures have been evaluated with respect to the occurrence of a single disease, and an association is observed only for the one (or ones) for which an association had been predicted. Thus, the inference that the observed association between the presence of ovarian endometriosis and the subsequent occurrence of ovarian cancer represents a causal relationship is supported by the absence of a similar association for extra-ovarian endometriosis (Brinton *et al.*, 1997). In contrast, the increased risk of stomach cancer in users of cimetidine and of antacids (Schumacher *et al.*, 1990) argues more strongly that as-yet-diagnosed stomach cancer (or an antecedent of stomach cancer) leads to use of the treatments for peptic disease than it does for both agents' acting to cause stomach cancer.

Example 8-4. In March of 2000, a conjugate vaccine that targets seven pneumococcal serotypes was licensed for use in young children in the United States. This vaccine has the potential to affect pneumococcal carriage and transmission, unlike the polysaccharide vaccine for adults that targets 23 serotypes and that has been available for some time. In a United States surveillance area with a population of about 19 million, the incidence of all invasive pneumococcal disease in children under five years fell 75% between 1998–1999 (pre-vaccine) and 2000–2003. To determine whether the beneficial impact of the conjugate vaccine extended to non-vaccinees, Lexau *et al.* (2005) examined incidence trends in adults 50 years of age and above who resided in this same area. For invasive pneumococcal disease resulting from infection from one of the seven serotypes against which the conjugate vaccine was directed, the annual incidence fell from 22.4 per 100,000 in 1998–1999 to 10.2 per 100,000 in 2002–2003 ($p < .001$). The corresponding rates for invasive pneumococcal disease arising from the 16 serotypes contained only in the polysaccharide vaccine were 12.4 per 100,000 and 12.5 per 100,000, respectively ($p = .87$). The *specificity* of this association, with a decreased incidence restricted to that segment of pneumococcal disease hypothesized to be susceptible to the influence of the 7-valent vaccine, argues strongly in support of an extension of the benefit of this form of childhood immunization to the adult population.

APPLICATION OF THE GUIDELINES

A tentative inference regarding the presence or absence of a causal relationship between exposure and disease—such an inference is always tentative, pending the presence of additional data—is made by means of a subjective process in which one judges how many of the above features are present and (especially) the degree to which they are present. In some instances, the process is straightforward—all the evidence supports a causal hypothesis—and nearly all persons considering the issue arrive at the same conclusion: for instance, that cigarette smoke is a cause of lung cancer. In other instances, little or none of the evidence argues in support of causation—such as, in the case of occupational exposure to magnetic fields and cancer, or of silicone breast implants and scleroderma—and most observers feel it is not appropriate to infer an etiologic connection when considering action to modify or remove the exposure in question. Since it is impossible to rule out completely the existence of an effect of exposure on disease occurrence that is weak enough to be below the limits of detection in epidemiologic studies, it is also not surprising that some debate continues regarding the safety of such exposures as occupational magnetic fields and silicone breast implants.

Some of the underpinnings of a particular causal hypothesis may be stronger than others. Years ago, in laboratory studies, aflatoxin (the toxic product of the mold *Aspergillus flavus*) had been found to be an extremely potent carcinogen, but at that time the only relevant data in humans consisted of correlations of liver cancer mortality rates across national populations with differences in estimated aflatoxin intake. While the interpretation of the positive correlations seen in these studies was ambiguous—the populations with the highest rates no doubt differed in relevant ways other than their consumption of aflatoxin—the strength of the laboratory evidence served as a basis for a (very) tentative causal inference. Later, stronger epidemiologic data became available to further support the hypothesis (Qian *et al.*, 1994; Wang *et al.*, 1996). In contrast, the enormously strong association between aspirin and Reye's syndrome observed in epidemiologic studies, along with the lack of any such association with other analgesics (Halpin *et al.*, 1982; Hurwitz *et al.*, 1987; Forsyth *et al.*, 1989), served as an adequate basis for discouraging aspirin use in children in the absence of any precise knowledge of the means by which aspirin use might have caused the occasional child with flu or chicken pox to develop this complication.

COMMON MISPERCEPTIONS OF THE NATURE OF CAUSES OF ILLNESS AND INJURY

Misperception #1: There Are Direct and Indirect Causes of Disease, and the Direct Causes Are More Important

If we accept the definition of a cause of disease as that given previously—but for the presence of an exposure, some additional cases of disease would not occur—then for purposes of causal inference it is not critical that we know where in the sequence of events leading to disease a given exposure has taken place. The psychological and sociological forces that give rise to and sustain cigarette-smoking behavior are just as much causes of lung cancer as smoking itself, if it is inferred that in the absence of these forces, some persons would not become or remain cigarette smokers, and thus would not develop lung cancer. Other cultural and economic forces that have led men to become asbestos miners or women to become commercial sex workers are also causes of asbestosis or AIDS, if it is judged that some additional cases of these illnesses occurred as a result of the victims having worked in those occupations.

In any event, our labeling of a causal agent as "direct" may be due only to our ignorance of the "downstream" consequences of the actions of that agent. For example, cigarette smoking would no longer be considered a "direct" cause of lung cancer once we understood the biochemical and molecular changes produced by the carcinogens in cigarette smoke. The accuracy with which we label cigarette smoking as acting directly or indirectly is not relevant to whether its presence truly does give rise to lung cancer in some individuals.

Misperception #2: In Order to Be Considered a Cause of Disease, an Exposure Must Be Present in Every Case

If the illness or injury in question is defined by the presence of a particular causal agent—e.g., staphylococcal pneumonia, or motor vehicle injury—then of course that causal factor must be present in every case. But many illnesses or injuries are defined by a particular manifestation—e.g., myocardial infarction, or a fracture of the femur—which allows for the possibility of two or more separate pathways that can lead to that disease or injury. The fact that a particular exposure is not a necessary cause of a disease in no way detracts from its potential causal role. Excessive alcohol consumption is not the cause of every motor vehicle injury, but it surely is a cause of some such injuries.

Misperception #3: In Order to Be Considered a Cause of Disease, an Exposure Must Be Capable of Producing That Disease on Its Own

Clearly, this cannot be considered appropriate as a criterion: We acknowledge that infection with the tubercle bacillus is a cause of tuberculosis, but also that only some infected persons—particularly those who are malnourished and/or consume excessive amounts of alcohol—develop the disease. Nonetheless, the issue is at the heart of a controversy exemplified by the question "Do guns kill people, or do people kill people?" A gun by itself cannot commit a homicide; it needs an assailant to pull the trigger. Does the need for an assailant detract from the hypothesis that the availability of a gun is a cause of homicide? No, as long as there is evidence to suggest that, because of the presence of a gun, some homicides occurred that otherwise would not. The nature of such evidence may take the forms described earlier in the chapter—an association between gun availability and homicide occurrence, and non-epidemiologic data regarding possible differences in the ability or inclination of potential assailants to commit a homicide using a gun or using another weapon.

CAUSAL INFERENCE IN PRACTICE: THE EXAMPLE OF SLEEPING POSITION AND SUDDEN INFANT DEATH SYNDROME (SIDS)

In North America and Europe, SIDS (otherwise known as "crib death" or "cot death") is a relatively common cause of death among infants beyond the first several weeks of life. Until the early 1990s, the mortality rate from SIDS had been relatively stable in most parts of the world. Research had been done for several decades to try to determine what the causes were, but little progress was made until the late 1980s and early 1990s when studies examined the possibility that the sleeping position of the infant was somehow involved.

The initial studies (see (Guntheroth and Spiers, 1992; Dwyer and Ponsonby, 1996), for a summary) were conducted in Australia, New Zealand, and several parts of Europe. All but one used a case-control design—that is, a comparison of the last or usual sleeping position between infants who died of SIDS and a control group of healthy infants. In each of the case-control studies, there was a higher proportion of SIDS cases who had been put to sleep in the prone (face down) position. From these results, it was possible to estimate (through means described in Chapter 9) that there was at least a several-fold increase in the incidence of SIDS associated with the prone sleeping position. The temporal sequence of events underlying this consistently observed and strong association was compatible with a causal influence of sleeping position. One additional study addressed the (unlikely) possibility that recall bias had been responsible for the positive association seen in the case-control studies—that parents of recently deceased infants and parents of healthy children had not furnished information about sleeping position with the same degree of accuracy. These Australian investigators (Dwyer *et al.*, 1991) queried parents of some 3,000 5-week-old healthy infants regarding the position in which they laid the child down to sleep. Those infants who had usually been put to sleep prone subsequently had a three-fold increase in the risk of SIDS relative to other infants. Since the magnitude of the increase in risk associated with sleeping prone observed in this study was well within the range of those observed in the case-control studies, the possibility of differential recall between parents of cases and parents of controls as the entire basis for the association could largely be dismissed.

Is there a plausible means by which sleeping prone can lead to SIDS? There are several candidates, including oropharyngeal or nasal obstruction and thermal imbalance. However, when the results of the initial epidemiologic studies appeared, these were no more than candidate hypotheses.

Despite the uncertainty regarding why sleeping prone might be hazardous, most observers made the inference that it indeed was hazardous, at least regarding the risk of SIDS. For example, in 1992 the American Academy of Pediatrics Task Force on Infant Positioning recommended (AAP Task Force on Infant Positioning and SIDS, 1992) that

> healthy infants, when being put down for sleep, be positioned on their side or back.... This recommendation is made with the full recognition that the existing studies have methodologic limitations, and were conducted in countries with infant care practices and other Sudden Infant Death Syndrome risk factors that differ from those in the United States...However, taken as a group the studies are convincing.

The Task Force recommendation took into account not only the data relating sleeping position to the incidence of SIDS, but also the fact that there were no data "even strongly suggesting that sleeping in the lateral or supine position is harmful to healthy infants." Conceivably, the Task Force could have recommended that no action regarding sleeping position be taken until randomized trials had been conducted to address the issue. However, they viewed the data from the non-randomized studies to be compelling, enough so that it would be unethical to ask a parent to allow the sleeping position of his/her child to be decided at random.

The hypothesis that sleeping position can influence an infant's risk of SIDS subsequently has received support from the experience of populations in which large changes have taken place in the proportion of infants who sleep prone. In England, for example, a "Back to Sleep" campaign was mounted beginning in December of 1991 in the wake of the studies mentioned above. This campaign was associated with a decline in prone sleeping: Based on two samples of newborns, the prevalence fell from 21% in mid-1991 to 4% in mid-1992 (Hiley and Morley, 1994). A striking change in mortality from SIDS accompanied the change in sleeping position: There were 912 SIDS deaths in England in 1991, but only 456 in 1992.

Critics of epidemiologic research have argued that epidemiologic studies can raise questions but cannot answer them. The studies of sleeping position and SIDS, the causal inferences drawn from them, and the benefits of the actions that were based on those inferences, would appear to be a good rebuttal to an argument of this sort.

REFERENCES

AAP Task Force on Infant Positioning and SIDS. Positioning and SIDS. Pediatrics 1992; 89: 1120–1126.

Brinton LA, Gridley G, Persson I, Baron J, Bergqvist A. Cancer risk after a hospital discharge diagnosis of endometriosis. Am J Obstet Gynecol 1997; 176:572–579.

Carpenter KJ. The history of scurvy and vitamin C. Cambridge, UK: Cambridge University Press, 1986.

de Vicenzi I. A longitudinal study of human immunodeficiency virus transmission by heterosexual partners. European Study Group on Heterosexual Transmission of HIV. N Engl J Med 1994; 331:341–346.

Dwyer T, Ponsonby AL. The decline of SIDS: a success story for epidemiology. Epidemiology 1996; 7:323–325.

Dwyer T, Ponsonby AL, Newman NM, Gibbons LE. Prospective cohort study of prone sleeping position and sudden infant death syndrome. Lancet 1991; 337:1244–1247.

Forsyth BW, Horwitz RI, Acampora D, Shapiro ED, Viscoli CM, Feinstein AR, et al. New epidemiologic evidence confirming that bias does not explain the aspirin/Reye's syndrome association. JAMA 1989; 261:2517–2524.

Guntheroth WG, Spiers PS. Sleeping prone and the risk of sudden infant death syndrome. JAMA 1992; 267:2359–2362.

Halpin TJ, Holtzhauer FJ, Campbell RJ, Hall LJ, Correa-Villasenor A, Lanese R, et al. Reye's syndrome and medication use. JAMA 1982; 248:687–691.

Hiley CMH, Morley CJ. Evaluation of government's campaign to reduce risk of cot death. BMJ 1994; 309:703–704.

Hill AB. The environment and disease: association or causation. Proc R Soc Med 1965; 58:295–300.

Hurwitz ES, Barrett MJ, Bregman D, Gunn WJ, Pinsky P, Schonberger LB, et al. Public Health Service study of Reye's syndrome and medications. Report of the main study. JAMA 1987; 257: 1905–1911.

Lexau CA, Lynfield R, Danila R, Pilishvili T, Facklam R, Farley MM, et al. Changing epidemiology of invasive pneumococcal disease among older adults in the era of pediatric pneumococcal conjugate vaccine. JAMA 2005; 294:2043–2051.

Lipsitch M, Tchetgen Tchetgen E, Cohen T. Negative controls: a tool for detecting confounding and bias in observational studies. Epidemiology 2010; 21:383–388.

Luby SP, Agboatwalla M, Painter J, Altaf A, Billhimer WL, Hoekstra RM. Effect of intensive handwashing promotion on childhood diarrhea in high-risk communities in Pakistan: a randomized controlled trial. JAMA 2004; 291:2547–2554.

Marks JS, Halpin TJ. Guillain-Barré syndrome in recipients of A/New Jersey influenza vaccine. JAMA 1980; 243:2490–2494.

Orlowski JP, Campbell P, Goldstein S. Reye's syndrome: a case-control study of medication use and associated viruses in Australia. Cleve Clin J Med 1990; 57:323–329.

Qian GS, Ross RK, Yu MC, Yuan JM, Gao YT, Henderson BE, *et al.* A follow-up study of urinary markers of aflatoxin exposure and liver cancer risk in Shanghai, People's Republic of China. Cancer Epidemiol Biomarkers Prev 1994; 3:3–10.

Ray WA, Murray KT, Meredith S, Narasimhulu SS, Hall K, Stein CM. Oral erythromycin and the risk of sudden death from cardiac causes. N Engl J Med 2004; 351:1089–1096.

Schumacher MC, Jick SS, Jick H, Feld AD. Cimetidine use and gastric cancer. Epidemiology 1990; 1:251–254.

Selby JV, Friedman GD, Quesenberry CP Jr, Weiss NS. A case-control study of screening sigmoidoscopy and mortality from colorectal cancer. N Engl J Med 1992; 326:653–657.

Sigurdson AJ, Ronckers CM, Mertens AC, Stovall M, Smith SA, Liu Y, *et al.* Primary thyroid cancer after a first tumour in childhood (the Childhood Cancer Survivor Study): a nested case-control study. Lancet 2005; 365:2014–2023.

U S Public Health Service. Smoking and health. Report of the Advisory Committee to the Suregeon General of the Public Health Service. PHS Pub. No. 1103. Washington, D.C.: U.S. Department of Health, Education, and Welfare, 1964.

Wang LY, Hatch M, Chen CJ, Levin B, You SL, Lu SN, *et al.* Aflatoxin exposure and risk of hepatocellular carcinoma in Taiwan. Int J Cancer 1996; 67:620–625.

Weiss NS. Inferring causal relationships: elaboration of the criterion of "dose-response." Am J Epidemiol 1981; 113:487–490.

Weiss NS. Can the "specificity" of an association be rehabilitated as a basis for supporting a causal hypothesis? Epidemiology 2002; 13:6–8.

EXERCISES

1. The following is excerpted from a letter to the editor of the *New England Journal of Medicine* (1998; 338:921):

> Although the link between sexual behavior, human papilloma virus (HPV) infection, and anogenital cancer is strong, there are clearly other factors of equal or greater importance, because many more people are infected with HPVs than have cancer. To view these malignant conditions as simply being caused by sexually transmitted infections is misleading. In the context of a multi-factorial disease, attributing cause to one recognized infectious step in the process has the potential to confuse clinicians and arouse undue fear in the general population. We would urge caution in the use of terms such as "cause," which can be over-interpreted. We believe public health is best served by the more difficult approach involving education about the multi-factorial nature of risk associated with disease.

(a) When seeking to infer whether or not HPV infection is a cause of anogenital cancer, is it desirable to consider whether:

  i "there are clearly other factors of equal or greater importance..."?

  ii An inference of cause and effect may "confuse clinicians and arouse undue fear in the general population"?

(b) Is inferring a causal relationship between HPV and anogenital cancer inconsistent with "the multi-factorial nature of risk"?

2. The following appeared in the "News" section of the *Lancet* of March 27, 1999:

> Excessive breast self-examination may promote anxiety. A new study of women with a family history of breast cancer adds to evidence that excessive breast self-examination is counterproductive, because it increases anxiety and may make early detection of breast cancer more difficult.
>
> Researchers from the University of Wales College of Medicine, Cardiff, UK, and Sheffield University, UK, surveyed 833 women aged 17–77 years, from families with histories of breast cancer. 18% claimed to examine their breasts daily or weekly, 56% once or twice a month, and 26% rarely. General anxiety and cancer-specific

anxiety were lowest among women who examined themselves least often, and highest among the hypervigilant women—differences that were strongly significant.

What is another plausible interpretation of these data, other than that "excessive" breast self-examination increases a woman's level of anxiety?

3. An Australian study (Orlowski *et al.*, 1990) observed no association between a child's use of aspirin and the occurrence of Reye's syndrome. The authors noted that all prior studies of this issue had found a strong association. The following paraphrases the concluding sentences of their paper:

A different burden of proof is required if one attempts to prove a hypothesis than if one wants to disprove the proposal. This is best understood with a simple analogy. If one observes 100 swans that are all white, one might propose that all swans are white. But only one black swan is needed to prove that not all swans are white. Our study is the black swan that proves that aspirin does not cause Reye's syndrome.

Assume the authors' own study is both large and flawless. Do you agree with their conclusion? If yes, why? If no, why not?

4. Use of the antibiotic erythromycin is associated with the development of cardiac electrophysiological abnormalities, abnormalities that may lead to an arrhythmia and sudden death. This drug is metabolized by cytochrome P-450 3A (CYP3A) isozymes. Since a number of other drugs inhibit CYP3A activity, it has been hypothesized that the concomitant use of erythromycin and one of these drugs may predispose to sudden cardiac death.

The data in the table below are taken from a cohort study of this question (Ray *et al.*, 2004):

TABLE 8.2.

Current drug use			Sudden cardiac death
CYP3A inhibitor	Antibiotic	Person-years	
Yes	Erythromycin	194	3
	None	36,518	116
No	Erythromycin	4,874	7
	None	1,163,087	1,235

(a) Do the above data support the hypothesis that the deleterious impact of erythromycin use on the incidence of sudden cardiac death is aggravated by the concomitant use of a CYP3A inhibitor?

(b) In the same study, use of another antibiotic, amoxicillin (a drug that does not lead to cardiac electrophysiological changes), was not associated with an increased risk of sudden cardiac death, whether in patients taking or not taking a CYP3A inhibitor. Does this bear on your interpretation of the data pertaining to erythromycin? If yes, why? If no, why not?

ANSWERS

1. (a) i Ranking of causal factors serves no purpose here. The fact that other causes of anogenital cancer exist does not detract from an inference that HPV infection does so, too.

   ii The assessment of a possible causal relationship between an exposure, such as HPV infection, and cancer incidence is a separate task from communicating that inference to clinicians and to the population as a whole.

   (b) HPV infection is not sufficient to produce an anogenital cancer; other factors must be involved. But, if it is judged that some persons could be spared developing a cancer by not acquiring an HPV infection, then it would be incorrect not to speak of HPV infection as a cause of cancer.

2. Another interpretation, arguably a more plausible one: Anxiety leads to "excessive" self-examination.

3. From this study, the only hypothesis that can be refuted is that *all* epidemiologic studies will find an association between aspirin and Reye's syndrome. It is true that an inference of cause and effect is strengthened by an association between exposure and disease having been observed consistently across studies. Nonetheless, we recognize that an agent with the capacity to cause disease may not be able to exert its deleterious influence if other necessary factors are not present. The fact that Reye's syndrome was unassociated with aspirin in the authors' study population—perhaps some additional, interacting factor (e.g., a flu epidemic) was absent in that population—does not preclude it from being a cause in another setting.

4. (a) Yes, the data support the hypothesis that the elevated incidence of sudden cardiac death in persons taking erythromycin is largely restricted to persons also taking a CYP3A inhibitor.

(b) The absence of a relationship between the use of a different antibiotic, amoxicillin, and sudden cardiac death suggests that the association between erythromycin and mortality (among persons taking a drug that inhibits CYP3A activity) is a causal one, and not simply the result of an association between the reason for erythromycin use and mortality from this cause.

TABLE 8.3.

Exposure group	Incidence (per 1,000 person-years)	Incidence ratio
CYP3A inhibitor		
Erythromycin	15.46	4.87
No antibiotic	3.18	1
No CYP3A inhibitor		
Erythromycin	1.44	1.35
No antibiotic	1.06	1

9

Measures of Excess Risk

In Tasmania during 1988–1990, information was obtained from the parents of 2,607 1-month-old infants regarding their baby's usual sleeping position (Dwyer *et al.*, 1991). The cumulative incidence of crib death (sudden infant death syndrome) through one year of age in these children was compared between those who were usually put to sleep prone (on their stomach) or in another position (side or back). The results shown in Table 9.1 were obtained.

In order to estimate the occurrence of crib death in relation to sleeping position, the risk in one group can be divided by that in the other. Let us label, arbitrarily, infants who were usually put to sleep prone as "exposed" and the others "non-exposed." The cumulative incidence in the exposed (I_e) is 9/846 = 10.64 per 1000. The cumulative incidence in the non-exposed (I_o) is 6/1761 = 3.41 per 1000. The relative incidence, or *relative risk* (RR) is:

$$RR = \frac{I_e}{I_o} = \frac{10.64}{3.41} = 3.1$$

Alternatively, from studies of this sort, the observed number of exposed persons who develop the illness or injury under study can be divided by the number that would have been "expected"; that is, the number predicted to occur if exposed persons had the same risk as the non-exposed. This represents another way of calculating the relative risk. In this example, there were 9 crib deaths that occurred among infants put to sleep in the prone position. The expected number, based on the risk in the other infants, is $6/1761 \times 846 = 2.88$. The ratio of observed-to-expected deaths, 9/2.88, is 3.1, the same number that was obtained above when dividing I_e by I_o.

To begin to introduce other measures of altered risk, let's consider Table 9.2, which is the generic version of the data table we just produced in the example on crib death.

TABLE 9.1. SLEEPING POSITION AND CRIB DEATH

Usual sleeping position	Crib death? Yes	No	Total
Prone	9	837	846
Other	6	1,755	1,761
Total	15	2,592	2,607

The *difference* in risk between exposed and non-exposed persons would be:

$$I_e - I_o = \frac{a}{a+b} - \frac{c}{c+d}$$

In the example, the risk difference would be:

$$I_e - I_o = 10.64 \text{ per } 1000 - 3.41 \text{ per } 1000$$
$$= 7.23 \text{ per } 1000$$

If the association between exposure and disease is suspected to represent a causal one, then the term

TABLE 9.2. LAYOUT OF DATA RELATING A DICHOTOMOUS EXPOSURE VARIABLE AND A DICHOTOMOUS DISEASE OUTCOME

Exposure	Disease Present	Absent	All persons
Yes	a	b	$a+b$
No	c	d	$c+d$

I_e = cumulative incidence in exposed = $\frac{a}{a+b}$

I_o = cumulative incidence in non-exposed = $\frac{c}{c+d}$

I_t = overall cumulative incidence = $\frac{a+b}{a+b+c+d}$

attributable risk (AR) can be used to describe the difference in risk. It corresponds to the added risk of disease due to the exposure.

The *AR* also can be expressed as a percentage of the incidence in the exposed:

$$\frac{I_e - I_o}{I_e} \times 100\%$$

In the present example, the attributable risk percent (*AR%*) would be:

$$\frac{9/846 - 6/1761}{9/846} \times 100\% = 68.0\%$$

This value is an estimate of the percentage of crib death occurrence among prone-sleeping infants that is due to this sleeping position (assuming an inference has been made that the prone sleeping position is in fact a cause of crib death), and not to other causes of crib death to which all infants are subject.

The *AR%* is commonly used to describe the results of prevention trials (for example, of a vaccine), where it is termed "efficacy." In calculations done using the results of vaccine studies, unvaccinated persons constitute the "exposed" group, vaccinated persons the "non-exposed." For example, in a trial of polio vaccine from the 1950s, the cumulative incidence of polio in unvaccinated children during the several-month duration of the study was 57 per 100,000; the corresponding incidence in vaccinated children was 16 per 100,000. The vaccine efficacy was estimated as:

$$\frac{\text{Incidence (unvaccinated)} - \text{Incidence (vaccinated)}}{\text{Incidence (unvaccinated)}}$$

$$= \frac{57/100,000 - 16/100,000}{57/100,000} \times 100\% = 71.9\%$$

To the extent that vaccination can reduce the degree of transmission of infection in a given study population, the incidence of infection in unvaccinated persons will be less than that expected had no one in the population been vaccinated ("herd immunity"). In such a circumstance, the measured vaccine efficacy will be an underestimate of the true efficacy.

In a population in which there are both exposed and non-exposed individuals, the contribution to overall incidence of a given exposure (the *population attributable risk*, or *PAR*) is calculated as $I_t - I_o$, where I_t = total incidence in the population. In the example on crib death, $I_t = 15/2607$. Thus, the *PAR*

would be:

$$\frac{15}{2607} - \frac{6}{1761} = 2.35 \text{ per } 1000$$

If the association with sleeping position were causal, these data suggest that in Tasmania during the time of the study, 2.35 crib deaths per 1000 infants could be attributed to being put to sleep in the prone position.

Note that in some study designs; e.g., most case-control studies, it will not be possible to calculate I_t directly from the results obtained. In such instances, it may be possible to estimate I_t from information available apart from the study itself.

The *PAR* can also be expressed as a percentage of the total incidence (the *population attributable risk percent*), which in the present example would be:

$$\frac{15/2607 - 6/1761}{15/2607} \times 100\% = 40.8\%$$

That is, about 41% of the incidence of crib death in Tasmania would have been due to sleeping prone.

All of the above terms for expressing an altered *risk* have a counterpart when it is an altered *rate* that is being considered. So, there is a relative rate (or rate ratio), rate difference, attributable rate, attributable rate percent, population attributable rate, and population attributable rate percent. However, it is an unusual epidemiologist who rigorously distinguishes each of these when he/she writes or speaks, from the analogous term that pertains to "risk."

Table 9.3 lists the measures of excess risk, along with: 1) the factors that influence the size of each measure, and 2) the purpose to which each one can be put. As indicated in Chapter 8, the principal use of the *relative risk* is to guide inferences of cause and effect when an association is observed between an exposure and disease occurrence in epidemiologic studies. The *risk difference* quantifies the potential importance of this association in absolute terms: Over a given period of time, how many additional ill or injured persons would there be out of the total number who were exposed? For a relative risk of a given size, the risk difference associated with a given exposure will be larger for a commonly occurring illness than for a rare one. If the condition in question is common enough, even small relative risks can have a relatively large impact on disease occurrence. For example, consider the relationship between cigarette smoking and the incidence of two adverse outcomes among persons with type 2 diabetes: myocardial infarction (MI); and leg amputation or death due to

TABLE 9.3. APPLICATION OF MEASURES OF EXCESS RISK IN EPIDEMIOLOGY

Measure of excess risk	Abbreviation	Formula	Helps answer the question:
Relative risk	RR	I_e/I_o	Does exposure (E) cause disease (D)?
Risk difference (attributable risk to the exposed)	AR	$I_e - I_o$	(If E is believed to cause D): Among persons exposed to E, what amount of the incidence of D is E responsible for? Should anything be done to modify or eliminate E?
Attributable risk (%)	AR%	$\frac{RR-1}{RR} \times 100\%$	(If E is believed to cause D): What proportion of the occurrence of disease in exposed individuals was due to the exposure?
Attributable risk to the population	PAR	$I_t - I_o$	(If E is believed to cause D): Should resources be allocated to controlling E or, instead, to exposures causing greater health problems in the population?
Attributable risk to the population (%)	PAR%	$\frac{I_t - I_o}{I_t} \times 100\%$	(If E is believed to cause D): What portion of D in the population is caused by E? Should resources allocated to combating D be directed toward etiologic research or control of known etiologies (e.g., E)?

I_e = incidence in exposed
I_o = incidence in non-exposed
I_t = incidence in all persons, exposed plus non-exposed

peripheral arterial disease. Diabetics who smoke one pack of cigarettes per day double (approximately) their risk of an MI, but increase their risk of peripheral arterial disease by about a factor of 10 (Weiss, 1972). Both associations probably reflect the causal influence of smoking. The attributable risk (since we have drawn a causal inference, we are "entitled" to use this term instead of "risk difference") related to smoking for each condition is shown in Table 9.4.

Smoking one pack of cigarettes per day makes a greater relative contribution to the incidence of

TABLE 9.4. CIGARETTE SMOKING IN RELATION TO VASCULAR DISEASE IN PERSONS WITH TYPE 2 DIABETES

Condition	Annual incidence per 1000 person-years		RR	AR [a]
	Smokers (I_e)	Nonsmokers (I_o)		
Myocardial infarction	20	10	2	10
Complications of peripheral arterial disease	5	0.5	10	4.5

[a]Rate per 1000 person-years

manifestations of peripheral arterial disease than of MI. Nonetheless, the absolute impact of smoking on the rate of MI—10 per 1000 person-years—actually exceeds that of peripheral vascular disease—4.5 per 1000 person-years—due to the much higher rate of MI in the absence of smoking.

For associations believed to be causal, it is the *AR* (estimated collectively from all available studies) that is used to weigh the adverse and beneficial effects of the exposure on health outcomes. For example, observations in the 1970s of a 4-fold increase in the rate of MI associated with current use of oral contraceptives (OCs) resulted in recommendations against such use for women in their mid-40s. The incidence among women in their mid-40s who did not use OCs was about 10 per million person-years, so the *AR* was about $(4 \times 10) - 10 = 30$ per million person-years. This contrasts with the absence of any such proscription for women under the age of 35, despite the fact that the *RR* for MI was the same in them as for a 45-year-old. In these younger women, whose annual rate of MI in the absence of OC use was only about 0.8 per million, the *AR* for MI associated with OC use was:

$$(4 \times 0.8) - (0.8) = 2.4 \text{ per million person-years.}$$

This figure seemed quite small relative to the health and other benefits that use of OCs was known to provide.

For some persons, the reciprocal of the attributable risk—the number of exposed persons or exposed person-time needed for one additional outcome event to occur—is easier to grasp than the attributable risk itself. So, one would say that among women in their mid-40s in the 1970s, the number of person-years of OC use necessary to produce one additional case of MI was 1/30 per million person-years = 33,333 person-years. The corresponding figure for women under the age of 35 was 1/24 per million person-years = 416,667 person-years. When applied in a clinical setting, this approach to considering the added risk or benefit of an intervention is referred to as the "number needed to treat."

Even in a person who has been exposed to an agent and who has developed the illness that the agent has the capacity to cause, the person's illness might have occurred through other means (unless the agent is a *necessary* cause of the disease). The AR% indicates what fraction of exposed individuals who developed a disease indeed did so because of the causal action(s) of that exposure. Among a group of diseased individuals who had received the exposure, almost never is there the equivalent of a fingerprint left behind by the causal exposure (in the form of a specific illness manifestation), so there is no way to discern which persons became ill specifically because of its effects. Thus, in any one such person, all that can be said is that the AR% for the group translates into his/her likelihood that the disease occurred as a result of his/her exposure to the agent in question. This notion of the likelihood of causation in an ill, exposed individual has application in civil litigation (Weiss, 2005)—though some individuals question the validity of this sort of application in some instances (Greenland, 1999)—since in that setting a typical question is whether, more probably than not, a person's illness occurred because of his/her exposure to an agent. If it has been inferred that exposure to that agent has the capacity to cause the illness, then the AR% would appear to provide the relevant probability.

If it is believed that a given exposure can cause a given illness, it may be useful to calculate the PAR, which quantifies the contribution to the overall incidence of that illness in the population at large that can be attributed to the exposure. The information provided by the PAR can potentially be useful in allocating resources for prevention: a higher priority generally would be given to efforts to eliminate or modify exposures that are believed to produce a large burden of disease in the population (for example, cigarette smoking in most societies) than to exposures whose impact is smaller.

The PAR% is used to address a somewhat different question: What fraction of the population's incidence of a given disease can be accounted for by the presence of a particular causal agent? If that fraction is high, an argument can be made that directing resources towards modifying or eliminating the agent (or the factors with which it interacts to allow it to produce the disease) might be a better investment than trying to identify other causal pathways leading to the same disease. It is likely that the campaigns mounted in many countries beginning in the mid-1990s to have parents place their infants in the supine position were stimulated by the high percentage (in addition to the high absolute rate) of crib death occurrence that was estimated to be attributable to the prone sleeping position.

Sometimes we wish to estimate the reduction in a population's incidence of disease that might occur from the elimination of more than one of its causes. This cannot be accomplished simply by adding the PAR% calculated for each exposure alone: in a person with both exposures, the illness can only be prevented once. What must be done is to obtain a new PAR% associated with the presence of *either* the first or second exposure. For example, assume that among the 1,755 infants in the Tasmanian study of crib death who usually were put to sleep on their back or side—the low-risk position—three events occurred in the 500 who had been passively exposed to cigarette smoke in their home (another risk factor for crib death). The PAR% for the two exposures, the prone sleeping position and exposure to passive smoking, would be estimated as shown in Table 9.5. From this calculation we would conclude that, if the causal actions of prone sleeping and passive smoking on the occurrence of crib death could be blocked or eliminated, the incidence of crib death in Tasmania would diminish by 58.7%.

As indicated in Table 9.3, the size of both the PAR and the PAR% is influenced by the frequency of the exposure: The more common a factor that predisposes to a given disease, the greater amount or percentage of that disease it will be responsible for. Thus, a PAR or PAR% estimated from a study in one population will not accurately characterize the same parameter in a second population if the prevalence of the exposure differs between the two.

Statistical significance is often assessed when a possible association between exposure and disease is investigated. It is not a measure of excess risk. Instead, it assesses the likelihood of observing an association at least as large as the one seen, if in truth no association were present in the population from which the study subjects were drawn. The size of the p-value that is generated in statistical hypothesis testing is heavily dependent on the size of the study population: the larger the number of subjects, the smaller the p value. The size of the study is to some extent arbitrary, so we ought not use the p value for any purpose other than evaluating the role of chance. Similarly, we would not use the *RR* for any purpose beyond that which it could achieve: guidance in an inference of possible cause and effect. And so on for the other measures in Table 9.3: each has a role in answering a particular question from among the several questions that can be posed concerning the influence of an exposure on disease occurrence.

ESTIMATING THE RELATIVE RISK IN SETTINGS WHERE INCIDENCE RATES CANNOT BE CALCULATED

Case-Control Studies

These studies compare antecedent exposures or characteristics of ill or injured persons (cases) with those of persons at risk of the illness or injury (see Chapter 15). Even though incidence rates are typically not obtained, either for exposed or for non-exposed persons, the data gathered often can be used to provide a good estimate of the relative risk. To understand how this can be done, consider a cohort study in which exposed and non-exposed persons are followed for a certain period of time. Table 9.6 summarizes their experience with regard to a particular disease.

The cumulative incidence of the disease in exposed and non-exposed persons over a given period of follow-up is $a/(a + b)$ and $c/(c + d)$, respectively. The relative risk (RR) is defined as:

$$\frac{a/(a+b)}{c/(c+d)}$$

If the incidence of the disease is relatively low during the follow-up period in both exposed and non-exposed persons, then a will be small relative to b, and c will be small relative to d. Therefore

$$RR = \frac{a/(a+b)}{c/(c+d)} \approx \frac{a/b}{c/d} = \frac{a/c}{b/d}$$

The expression $\frac{a/c}{b/d}$ is the *odds ratio (OR)*: the numerator a/c is the odds of exposure in persons who develop the disease, and the denominator b/d is the odds of exposure in persons who remain well. It is important to note that the numerator of the odds ratio can be estimated from a sample of cases, while the denominator can be estimated from a sample of non-cases. Neither estimate is influenced by the proportion of cases among the subjects actually chosen for study.

In the hypothetical example shown in Table 9.7, assume that 100 of 10,000 persons exposed to a particular substance or organism developed a disease, in contrast with 300 of 90,000 non-exposed persons.

If a case-control study including 50% of cases but only 1% of non-cases had been performed, the results shown in Table 9-8 would be expected.

When controls are chosen in this way—from persons who had not developed the disease by the end

---

TABLE 9.5. CALCULATION OF PAR% FOR TWO EXPOSURES ASSOCIATED WITH AN INCREASED RISK OF CRIB DEATH

Exposure status	Crib death?		
	Yes	No	Total
Prone sleeping or passive smoking	$9 + 3 = 12$	$837 + 497 = 1,334$	$846 + 500 = 1,348$
Neither of the above	$6 - 3 = 3$	$1,755 - 497 = 1,258$	$1,761 - 500 = 1,261$
Total	15	2,592	2,607

$$PAR\% = \frac{15/2,607 - 3/1,261}{15/2,607} \times 100\% = 58.7\%$$

TABLE 9.6. DATA LAYOUT FOR A
HYPOTHETICAL COHORT STUDY

Exposed	Disease		Total
	Yes	No	
Yes	a	b	$a+b$
No	c	d	$c+d$

TABLE 9.7. HYPOTHETICAL RESULTS
OF A COHORT STUDY

Exposed	Disease		Total
	Yes	No	
Yes	100	9,900	10,000
No	300	89,700	90,000

$RR = \frac{100/10,000}{300/90,000} = 3.00$

of the same time period during which other persons (the cases) had developed it—the less common the disease in both exposed and non-exposed persons during the period, the better the odds ratio will estimate the ratio of cumulative incidence (Zhang and Yu, 1998). In the previous example, only 1% and 0.33% of exposed and non-exposed persons, respectively, developed the illness, and so the relative cumulative incidence and odds ratio were in close correspondence (3.00 versus 3.02). However, it is also possible to choose controls from persons free of disease only until the corresponding cases have been diagnosed; a person can appear in the study first as a control and later as a case. If this approach is used, the odds ratio will be a valid estimate of the ratio of

TABLE 9.8. EFFECT OF CASE-CONTROL
SAMPLING WITHIN A HYPOTHETICAL
COHORT STUDY

Exposed	Disease	
	Yes	No
Yes	$100 \times 0.5 = 50$	$9,900 \times 0.01 = 99$
No	$300 \times 0.5 = 150$	$89,700 \times 0.01 = 897$

$RR \approx OR = \frac{50/150}{90/897} = 3.02$

incidence rates (i.e., number of cases divided by the person-time at risk) irrespective of the disease frequency (Greenland and Thomas, 1982; Rodrigues and Kirkwood, 1990; Pearce, 1993).

Proportional Mortality (Morbidity) Studies

It may happen that in a particular setting you know the number of exposed individuals who have developed an illness or have died, but you have no means of enumerating either the total number of exposed persons or the person-time from which the illnesses or deaths occurred. Let us say you have available to you records of deaths among members of a particular labor union. While information on cause of death is present in the files—perhaps a death certificate had to be submitted to receive benefits—the union is not able to tell you the size of its membership over time, and so the denominator needed to calculate a death rate for any given cause cannot be determined. Nonetheless, what can be calculated is the proportional mortality—the fraction of all deaths that are due to a particular cause of death. To assess whether this fraction is atypical, it can be compared to the corresponding fraction for demographically comparable persons who died in the geographic population in which the union members resided. So, for example, if five percent of deaths in union members were due to nonmalignant respiratory disease, but only two percent of deaths in population at large were due to this cause, one could estimate the relative risk of death from respiratory disease associated with union membership as being $0.05/0.02 = 2.5$.

The potential limitations of the *proportional mortality ratio* calculated above are evident: Even if the rate of death from respiratory disease among union members were identical to that in the remainder of the population, the *proportion* of deaths from this cause would be elevated if the death rate from all other causes (combined) in union members were relatively low. Or, that proportion would be depressed if the rate of death from other causes in union members were relatively high. Therefore, proportional mortality (or morbidity) ratios must be interpreted cautiously, since their magnitude takes into account more than the one thing we are using them to estimate: i.e., the ratio of the rate of death or illness between exposed and non-exposed persons. (For a more complete discussion of the uses and limitations of the proportional mortality ratio, see Chapter 3.)

ESTIMATING THE ATTRIBUTABLE RISK AND OTHER MEASURES OF EXCESS RISK FROM RESULTS OF CASE-CONTROL STUDIES

Occasionally, a case-control study identifies a large odds ratio relating an exposure and a disease, and for this and other reasons a causal influence of the exposure may be suspected. The decision to seek to limit or eliminate that exposure requires weighing its negative and positive consequences. This weighing must be done in absolute, rather than in relative terms, since the same relative increase (or decrease) in risk is of far greater consequence for common than for rare outcomes. As we have seen, the absolute increase in the risk of disease believed to be due to a dichotomous exposure, the attributable risk $I_e - I_o$, can be obtained directly from studies that directly measure the incidence in (I_e) and non-exposed persons (I_o). Since I_e can be expressed as the relative risk (RR) times I_o, the term $I_e - I_o$ can be rewritten as $(RR \cdot I_o) - I_o$, or as $I_o(RR - 1)$. Since the RR can be estimated from the results of a case-control study by means of the odds ratio, the only additional piece of information needed to estimate the AR is an estimate of I_o. For the population in which the study has been conducted, I_o can be estimated if:

1. The overall incidence (I) of the disease in that population is known or can be approximated; and
2. The frequency of exposure (p_e) in the controls selected for study reasonably reflects that of the population that gave rise to the cases.

Given (1) and (2) above,

$$I = I_e(p_e) + I_o(1 - p_e)$$

$$= I_o \cdot RR(p_e) + I_o(1 - p_e)$$

$$= I_o[p_e(RR - 1) + 1],$$

and so $I_o = \dfrac{I}{p_e(RR - 1) + 1}.$

Thus, $AR = I_o(RR - 1)$

$$= \dfrac{I(RR - 1)}{p_e(RR - 1) + \frac{RR-1}{RR-1}}$$

$$= \dfrac{I}{p_e + \frac{1}{RR-1}}$$

For example, consider a disease with an incidence rate of 10 per 100,000 person-years in a population in which five percent of persons have been exposed during a relevant period of time. The following table summarizes data from a hypothetical case-control study conducted in that population:

TABLE 9.9.

Exposed?	Cases	Controls	OR
Yes	15%	5%	3.35
No	85%	95%	1

The AR that corresponds to the estimated 3.35-fold increase in risk is:

$$AR = \dfrac{I}{p_e + \frac{1}{RR-1}}$$

$$= \dfrac{10}{0.05 + \frac{1}{3.35-1}}$$

$$= 21.0 \text{ per } 100,000 \text{ person-years.}$$

From the results of case-control studies that suggest a causal relationship, it is also possible to estimate the percentage of exposed persons with the disease who developed it because of their exposure, rather than through one or more causal pathways not involving the exposure. This measure, the attributable risk percent ($AR\%$) among exposed persons, was defined earlier as:

$$AR\% = \dfrac{I_e - I_o}{I_e} \times 100\%$$

The terms in the formula for the $AR\%$ can be rearranged as:

$$\dfrac{I_e - I_o}{I_e} = \dfrac{I_e}{I_e} - \dfrac{I_o}{I_e}$$

$$= 1 - \dfrac{1}{RR}$$

$$= \dfrac{RR}{RR} - \dfrac{1}{RR}$$

$$= \dfrac{RR - 1}{RR} \times 100\%$$

Therefore, estimates of the $AR\%$ can be obtained from case-control studies that can estimate the RR, by means of the odds ratio (see Appendix 5A), even if neither I_e nor I_o is known. So, in the hypothetical study that obtained an odds ratio of 3.35, the $AR\%$ could be estimated as:

$$\frac{3.35 - 1}{3.35} \times 100\% = 70.1\%$$

It is also possible to estimate the percentage of a disease's occurrence in the population as a whole that resulted from the actions of given exposure. This measure, the population attributable risk percent ($PAR\%$), is simply the $AR\%$ multiplied by the proportion of cases in that population who were exposed (p_c):

$$PAR\% = AR\%(p_c) \times 100\%$$

$$= \frac{RR - 1}{RR} \times p_c \times 100\%$$

In the present example, the $PAR\% = 70.1\% \times 0.15 = 10.5\%$.

REFERENCES

Braddon WL. The cause and prevention of beri-beri. London: Rebman Ltd., 1907.

Cole P, Monson RR, Haning H, Friedell GH. Smoking and cancer of the lower urinary tract. N Engl J Med 1971; 284:129–334.

Doll R, Hill AB. Smoking and carcinoma of the lung. Br Med J 1950; 2:739–748.

Dwyer T, Ponsonby AL, Newman NM, Gibbons LE. Prospective cohort study of prone sleeping position and sudden infant death syndrome. Lancet 1991; 337:1244–1247.

Greenland S. Relation of probability of causation to relative risk and doubling dose: a methodologic error that has become a social problem. Am J Public Health 1999; 89:1166–1169.

Greenland S, Thomas DC. On the need for the rare disease assumption in case-control studies. Am J Epidemiol 1982; 116:547–553.

Pearce N. What does the odds ratio estimate in a case-control study? Int J Epidemiol 1993; 22:1189–1192.

Ray WA, Murray KT, Hall K, Arbogast PG, Stein CM. Azithromycin and the risk of cardiovascular death. N Engl J Med 2012; 366:1881–1890.

Rodrigues L, Kirkwood BR. Case-control designs in the study of common diseases: updates on the demise of the rare disease assumption and the choice of sampling scheme for controls. Int J Epidemiol 1990; 19:205–213.

Weiss NS. Cigarette smoking and arteriosclerosis obliterans: an epidemiologic approach. Am J Epidemiol 1972; 95:17–25.

Weiss NS. General concepts of epidemiology. In: Faigman D, Kaye D, Saks M, Sanders J (eds.). Modern scientific evidence: the law and science of expert testimony. St. Paul, MN: West, 2005.

Zhang J, Yu KF. What's the relative risk? A method for correcting the odds ratio in cohort studies of common outcomes. JAMA 1998; 280:1690–1691.

EXERCISES

1. You are the epidemiology consultant to a large local factory. Because of some suspicion on the part of physicians who provide care to employees there, you conduct a study of the occurrence of a particular respiratory disease among the workers, and obtain the following results.

   - Incidence of respiratory disease among workers exposed to chemical A = 200 per 100,000 person-years.
   - Incidence of respiratory disease among workers not exposed to chemical A = 20 per 100,000 person-years.
   - Incidence in the general population in which the factory is situated = 21 per 100,000 person-years.

   Assume that no one who works outside of the factory is exposed to chemical A.

   (a) What are the relative rate (RR), attributable rate (AR), and the population attributable rate percent ($PAR\%$) associated with occupational exposure to this chemical?
   (b) How can you account for the low $PAR\%$ in view of the high RR?
   (c) Based on the high RR and other available information, you believe that the association between occupational exposure to chemical A and the incidence of this respiratory disease to be a causal one.

      i. Among exposed workers who developed the respiratory disease, what fraction of them did so as a result of his employment?
      ii. In making your recommendations to management and labor as they consider the benefits and costs of extra protection for the workers, which measure of excess risk would you use? Why?

2. Consider a randomized trial in which the incidence of disease X has been monitored in persons who were and were not vaccinated against the disease. The

incidence in the latter (unvaccinated) group was three times that of the former group.

Is this information adequate to permit an estimate of the efficacy of vaccination against disease X? If yes, what is that estimate? If no, why not?

3. Approximately 12 percent of the deaths in children aged five through nine in the United States in 1987 were due to cancer. In contrast, approximately one-fourth of the deaths at ages 60–64 were due to this condition. Is it correct to say that the risk of death from cancer was approximately twice as great in the older age group? If not, why not?

4. Comment on the following (paraphrased from a letter to the editor of a medical journal):

> Prospective and retrospective studies conducted during the 1950s all concluded that cigarette smoking accounted for only about 20% of lung cancer incidence in women. Therefore, the steady rise in lung cancer in women since that time must have some other cause, and air pollution by carcinogens is the obvious answer. Enthusiasm for the cigarette theory should not be allowed to hold back the thorough investigation of every possible factor.

5. The following data are taken from a study by Braddon (1907) on the epidemiology of beri-beri in Singapore:

TABLE 9.10.

	Hospital admissions (all causes) per 1000 population in 1900	New beri-beri cases per 1000 hospital admissions in 1900
Chinese	62	150
Europeans	310	1.4

Do these data support the hypothesis that the incidence rate of beri-beri was greater among Chinese than European residents of Singapore? If yes, to what degree? If no, why not?

6. The data shown in Table 9.11 were obtained in a study of smoking in relation to the incidence of bladder cancer (Cole *et al.*, 1971). Among women, the relative risk of bladder cancer for each category of intensity or duration of smoking was the same as or slightly higher than the relative risk among men. However:

(a) The population attributable rate percent among men was greater, 39% to 29%. How could this be?

(b) The attributable rate among male smokers was more than double that among female smokers. Why?

TABLE 9.11. INCIDENCE AND ATTRIBUTABLE RATE PER 100,000 PERSON-YEARS AND POPULATION ATTRIBUTABLE RATE PERCENT

	Men	Women
Incidence in smokers	48.0	19.2
Incidence in non-smokers	25.4	9.6
Total incidence	41.8	13.5
Attributable rate in smokers	22.6	9.6
Population attributable rate	16.4	3.9
Population attributable rate percent	39%	29%

TABLE 9.12.

	Daily cigarette consumption				
	None or < 5	5–14	15–24	25–49	50+
Men with lung cancer	26	208	196	174	45
Controls	65	242	201	118	23

7. The data shown above come from a case-control study of cigarette smoking and lung cancer in British men, among the very first on this topic (Doll and Hill, 1950):

(a) Estimate the risk of lung cancer to cigarette smokers in each category of daily consumption relative to the risk of men who never smoked or smoked few than 5 cigarettes per day.

(b) Estimate the proportion of lung cancer among British males in this age group that could have been prevented if no man had ever smoked more than 4 cigarettes per day during his lifetime.

(c) Assuming that the incidence of lung cancer among males in this age group is 80 per 100,000 per year, what is the incidence of lung cancer in smokers of more than 4 cigarettes per day attributable to their smoking?

8. Because of concerns stemming from case reports about short-term cardiovascular toxicity of some antibiotics, a cohort study was done comparing mortality from cardiovascular disease during the five days following the initiation of azithromycin and amoxicillin. The following mortality rates (per 10^6 during the first 5 days) are stratified according to the underlying risk of cardiovascular death, as estimated from clinical information regarding a history of cardiovascular disease, cigarette smoking, etc.

TABLE 9.13.

	Type of antibiotic		Relative risk
Underlying risk	Azithromycin	Amoxicillin	
High	410	165	2.5
Medium	80	35	2.3
Low	14	5	2.8

(In this study, careful attention was paid to the measurement of and control for confounding variables. For purposes of answering the question below, assume that no confounding was present.)

The authors concluded that in terms of prescribing azithromycin, "there should be more careful attention [paid] to the baseline cardiovascular risk." What do you believe to have been the basis for their recommendation?

ANSWERS

1. (a)

$$RR = 200/20$$

$$= 10$$

$$AR = 200 \text{ per } 100,000 - 20 \text{ per } 100,000$$

$$= 180 \text{ per } 100,000 \text{ person-years}$$

$$PAR\% = \frac{21 - 20}{21} \times 100\%$$

$$= 4.8\%$$

(b) The size of the *PAR%* depends on two things:

- the size of the relative risk; and
- the proportion of the population exposed.

The *PAR%* is low because occupational exposure to chemical A must be relatively uncommon in this population.

(c) i. $AR\% = \frac{200-20}{200} \times 100\% = 90\%$. Only 10% of exposed workers with the respiratory disease would have developed it in the absence of exposure to chemical A.

ii. Attributable rate—it alone describes the extra absolute risk to the workers themselves. In deciding whether exposure to chemical A should continue or not continue, the AR for respiratory disease would be weighed along with the other risks and benefits related to this exposure.

2. Vaccine efficacy can be calculated as follows:

$$\text{Vaccine efficacy} = \frac{I_{unvacc} - I_{vacc}}{I_{unvacc}}$$

$$= \frac{I_{unvacc}}{I_{unvacc}} - \frac{I_{vacc}}{I_{unvacc}}$$

$$= 1 - \frac{1}{3}$$

$$= 66.7\%$$

3. It is not correct to conclude that the risk of death from cancer is twice as great in the older age group. The statement compares the proportional mortality for deaths due to cancer in the 5–9-year-old age group with that for the group 60–64 years of age. Differences in the occurrence of the denominator event, rate of death from other causes, can also influence the size of the proportionate mortality. Since the rate from "other" causes of death is far higher in the older than in the younger age group, the true risk of death from cancer at ages 60–64 years is far more than twice that at ages 5–9 years. To illustrate this, consider the following table that presents approximate death rates for persons in these two age groups:

TABLE 9.14.

	Annual death rate per 100,000		Cancer deaths
Age (years)	Cancer	All causes	÷ total deaths
5–9	6	50	0.12
60–64	750	3,000	0.25

Although the percentage of deaths from cancer at ages 60–64 is about twice that at age 5–9 (0.25 vs. 0.12), the ratio of annual cancer mortality *rates* is far larger: 750 per 100,000 vs. 6 per 100,000, or 125.

4. The figure of 20% is the population attributable risk percent. This measure depends on the size of the relative risk as well as the proportion of the population exposed. If smoking among women had become more frequent over time, it could have led both to an increase in the overall incidence of lung cancer as well as to an increase in the *PAR%* due to smoking.

5. Incidence of beri-beri in 1901:

TABLE 9.15.

Chinese:	$62/1000 \times 150/1000 = 9.3/1000$
Europeans:	$310/1000 \times 1.4/1000 = 0.43/1000$

Relative incidence:

The incidence of beri-beri among Chinese residents of Singapore was 21.6 times that of Europeans.

TABLE 9.16.

Based on cases per 1000 admissions:	$150/1.4 = 107.1$
Based on incidence:	$9.3/.43 = 21.6$

The ratio based on cases per hospital admissions is inflated, due to the relatively low incidence of hospitalization for other reasons among Chinese.

6. (a) The prevalence of smoking among men in this population must be higher than that among women.

 (b) Among nonsmokers, the incidence of bladder cancer in men (25.4 per 100,000 person-years) is greater than in women (9.6). The identical RR associated with smoking will therefore produce a larger added rate in men than in women.

TABLE 9.17.

	Daily cigarette consumption				
	None or < 5	5–14	15–24	25–49	50+
Odds ratio[a]	1.0	2.15	2.44	3.69	4.89

[a] Approximates the relative risk

7. (a) (See Table 9.17)

 (b) $PAR\% = \frac{RR-1}{RR} \times$ (proportion of cases exposed) $\times 100\%$

 $RR = OR = \frac{623/26}{584/65} = 2.67$

 Of the 649 men with lung cancer, 623 had smoked ≥ 5 cigarettes per day so:

$$PAR\% = \frac{2.67-1}{2.67} \times \frac{623}{649} \times 100\% = 60\%$$

 (c) The question asks for the added incidence of lung cancer among men who smoked ≥ 5 cigarettes per day: i.e., the attributable rate.

$$AR = \frac{I}{P_e + \frac{1}{RR-1}}$$

$$= \frac{80}{\frac{584}{649} + \frac{1}{2.67-1}}$$

$$= 53.4 \text{ per } 100,000 \text{ per year}$$

8. The attributable risk of cardiovascular death associated with azithromycin initiation in persons already at an increased underlying risk of death from cardiovascular disease is high ($410 - 165 = 245$ per million), far higher than in persons at a low underlying risk ($14 - 5 = 9$ per million).

 (This problem is based on Ray *et al.* [2012].)

10

Measurement Error

In epidemiology, victories are few and at this point a whole field may be on the verge of propagating pathological science, which means they cannot get good enough resolution to identify the effects they're studying. Epidemiologists may be seeing and reporting that there are canals on Mars because they're looking at Mars through Galileo's telescope. And that's the nature of the field and all the statistical wizardry in the world isn't going to change that.

—G. TAUBES

Although it is likely that few epidemiologists would share Taubes's pessimistic outlook, most would agree that improving the resolution of their measurement tools would allow them to describe more accurately the relationship between exposures and diseases they are studying. This chapter addresses the sources, assessment, and consequences of measurement error. It also gives examples of exposure–disease relationships that, figuratively, were as large as Mars itself, not just its "canals," and that could readily be detected by epidemiologic tools whose accuracy was similar to that of Galileo's telescope.

SOURCES OF MEASUREMENT ERROR

Mismeasurement of *exposure* status or level is present to at least some degree in nearly every epidemiologic study, since nearly every means of ascertaining the presence or level of exposure is imperfect. Interviews or questionnaires can obtain erroneous information: a subject may have been misinformed about his/her exposure status, or may even intentionally misrepresent it. The methods used to make direct measurements on study subjects (e.g., blood pressure by means of a cuff), or on samples taken from them, often contain error. For characteristics that vary over time within an individual, such as blood pressure, the problem is compounded if (as is often the case) an opportunity exists to make measurements on each subject on only a single occasion, since the value obtained on that occasion may not correspond to

the person's longer-term average value. Records that might contain information on past exposures or on correlates of these—such as employment, medical, or vital records—not only have the potential limitations given above, they may be incomplete or not faithfully transcribed.

Error in measurement of health *outcomes* can occur in epidemiologic studies as well. For example:

- Current diagnostic technology may not be applied to all persons who might meet the criteria for being a "case": for example, the prevalence of gallstone disease or endometriosis would be substantially underestimated if reliance were placed exclusively on a positive result on a particular diagnostic test, since so many persons with these conditions are asymptomatic and are not given the test.
- The available diagnostic technology may be limited in its ability to discriminate subgroups, within a larger group of ill persons, who have experienced a similar pathophysiological process. For example, among all persons with arthritis, there will be some in whom it will be uncertain whether or not they have a particular type, such as rheumatoid arthritis.
- Even when the appropriate diagnostic tests have been used in the care of a particular individual, the results of those tests may not be available to those conducting the epidemiologic study in which that individual is a subject. For example, in a large study of the

efficacy of pneumococcal vaccine that relied exclusively on computerized data available on Medicaid recipients, the investigators (Gable *et al.*, 1990) compared the incidence of pneumonia between persons who had and had not been vaccinated. Though they would have preferred to study pneumococcal pneumonia *per se*, the computerized records could only specify the broader outcome—pneumonia— irrespective of its microbiologic etiology. This probably led to a substantial degree of misclassification in this study, since pneumococcal pneumonia typically constitutes less than a third of all pneumonia.

ASSESSING MEASUREMENT ERROR

As used here, the terms *measure* and *test* refer broadly to almost any way of capturing data on a certain characteristic of study subjects. The underlying characteristic itself can be anything: disease status, exposure status, a potential confounder or effect modifier, and so on. The data-gathering method may be by self-administered questionnaire, personal interview, physical examination, laboratory test, extraction of information from medical records, direct observation of behavior, or other approaches.

Regardless of the characteristic or data-collection method, there is a *true* value of the characteristic being measured for each study subject. For example, each study subject has a certain true body weight at a certain time. The true value for each subject may be unknown; only the measured value may be available, such as body weight as self-reported to a telephone interviewer. Any discrepancy between the true value and the measured value is measurement error.

The consequences of measurement error depend on how much of it is present, so ways of quantifying it are needed. Quantitative indices of measurement error can be useful when choosing among different measures of the same characteristic during the study-design phase, for detecting data quality problems during staff training and data collection, and for gauging how large a role measurement error may have played in determining study results during data analysis. This section offers a brief introduction to indices of measurement error, a topic that has been studied extensively. Good sources for more information include White *et al.* (2008); Fleiss *et al.* (2003); Zhou *et al.* (2011); and Pepe (2003).

In broad terms, two properties are desirable in any measure:

- *Reliability.* A good measure should yield the same value if applied repeatedly under conditions in which the true characteristic is believed to remain the same.
- *Validity.* A good measure method should yield the *correct* value. Being consistent is not enough if the results are consistently wrong.

Reliability and validity apply broadly to any kind of measurement, but the approach to quantifying them depends on the *scale* of measurement. Those of greatest importance in epidemiologic research include:

1. *Continuous.* The measure can in principle take on any numerical value, including fractional values, over a defined range. For example, body weight can be almost any positive real number, depending on the units in which it is expressed. For practical reasons, continuous measures are recorded to a fixed number of digits of precision, but this choice is arbitrary and not an intrinsic property of the measure.

2. *Categorical*

   (a) *Ordinal.* Three or more discrete values are possible, which fall into a natural sequence according to how much of the characteristic being measured is present. For example, disease severity can be mild, moderate, or severe.

   (b) *Nominal.* Two or more discrete values are possible, but there is no particular ordering among them. For example, marital status can be currently married, never married, divorced, separated, or widowed.

   Sometimes only two values are possible, and the nominal scale is referred to as *binary*. For example, a certain disease can be either present or absent; gender can be either male or female.

Measurement error on a categorical measure is commonly termed *misclassification*.

The above list of measurement scales is itself ordered from "fine" to "coarse." A relatively fine measurement can often be converted to a coarser one by grouping values together. For example, age can be converted from a continuous variable to an ordinal one by assigning each person to one of several age groups based on the original age value. Marital status can be converted from a nominal variable to a binary one (currently married or not, say). Degrading the scale of measurement in this way may be done for convenience in data collection, analysis, or presentation, although some information is lost in the process.

Reliability

Reliability concerns agreement among replicate measurements. Reliability is also termed *reproducibility* or *consistency*. Adjectives are sometimes applied to it to indicate how the replicate measurements are related. For example, *intra-observer* reliability refers to agreement among measurements made by the same observer, while *inter-observer* reliability refers to agreement among measurements taken by different observers. *Test-retest* reliability refers to agreement among measurements on the same subjects at different times. Similar approaches to quantifying reliability are used in all these situations.

Concordance (Percent Agreement)

Concordance applies to categorical measures. Suppose that a certain categorical measurement is obtained twice under similar circumstances on each of several study subjects. Concordance is simply the proportion of all tested subjects for whom both measurements are the same. Expressed as a percentage, this quantity is also termed the *percent agreement*. Either way, it is easy to calculate and to grasp, which probably explains why it continues to appear in the literature.

Unfortunately, concordance has a serious limitation: it fails to account for the level of agreement that chance alone could produce. For example, say that the measurement of interest is binary, and that two independent measurements are made on every study subject. Each result is either positive or negative. The results can be organized as in Table 10.1: *a*, *b*, *c*, and *d* are the number of subjects with each combination of results, and N is the total number of people tested. The observed concordance is $(a + d)/N$.

Now suppose that the underlying characteristic being measured is truly present in 10% of people. Suspecting this, two lazy data collectors could simply record "+" for a random 10% of tested subjects and "–" for the rest, without ever doing any

TABLE 10.1. DATA LAYOUT FOR RELIABILITY ASSESSMENT ON A BINARY MEASURE

Measurement #1	Measurement #2 +	–	Total
+	a	b	a + b
–	c	d	c + d
Total	a + c	b + d	N

TABLE 10.2. EXPECTED RESULTS IF TWO OBSERVERS EACH ASSIGN A POSITIVE RESULT TO A RANDOM 10% OF STUDY SUBJECTS

Observer #1	Observer #2 +	–
+	1	9
–	9	81

real observations. The expected results would be as shown in Table 10.2. The lazy observers would have recorded the same result for 82% of subjects. This might naïvely be interpreted as an impressive degree of concordance, but in truth it merely reflects agreement by chance.

Because of this problem, concordance alone is of rather limited value as an index of reliability. However, it is used in calculation of a better index, *kappa*.

Kappa

Kappa (κ) is a widely used measure of reliability for categorical measures that is designed to correct for chance agreement (Fleiss *et al.*, 2003; Cohen, 1960). It is defined as:

$$\kappa = \frac{P_o - P_e}{1 - P_e} \qquad (10.1)$$

where P_o is the observed concordance, and P_e is the concordance expected by chance. P_e is based only on the row and column totals—that is, on the distribution of results for each observer (or measurement occasion) considered separately. For a binary variable, using the notation of Table 10.1,

$$P_o = \frac{a + d}{N}$$

$$P_e = \left[\frac{(a + b)(a + c)}{N} + \frac{(c + d)(b + d)}{N} \right] / N$$

The expression in brackets for P_e can be seen to be the sum of two terms, each of which is the expected number of observations in one of the two cells on the main (concordant) diagonal in Table 10.1 if measurements #1 and #2 were independent of each other. For example, the overall proportion of positive results on measurement #1 is $(a + b)/N$. If measurements #1 and #2 were independent, then this same proportion would apply regardless of the value of measurement #2—that is, within each column of

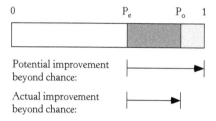

FIGURE 10.1 Graphical interpretation of kappa.

the table. One would thus expect $\dfrac{(a+b)}{N}(a+c)$ subjects to fall into the upper left cell. By similar logic, one would expect $\dfrac{(c+d)}{N}(b+d)$ subjects in the lower right cell. (Readers familiar with the χ^2 test may recognize these two terms as the expected values of a and d under the null hypothesis of no association between measurements #1 and #2.) The final expression for P_e sums those two expected counts and divides by N to express the result as a proportion of all subjects. P_o and P_e are thus similar, one being based on observed cell frequencies and the other on expected cell frequencies.

Figure 10.1 sketches the idea behind kappa. As with any proportion, concordance can range from 0 to 1. P_e is the concordance expected by chance, so $1 - P_e$ can be thought of as the amount of potential "room for improvement" between P_e and perfect agreement. Kappa represents the amount by which the observed concordance (P_o) exceeds that expected by chance (P_e), expressed as a proportion of the potential improvement beyond chance.

Kappa normally falls between 0 and 1, but it can become negative if $P_o < P_e$, indicating that agreement is even worse than chance alone could produce. Landis and Koch (1977) proposed the adjectives listed in Table 10.3 for interpretation of kappa.

TABLE 10.3. GUIDELINES FOR INTERPRETATION OF KAPPA

Kappa	Interpretation
>.80	Almost perfect
.61–.80	Substantial
.41–.60	Moderate
.21–.40	Fair
.00–.20	Slight
<.00	Poor

(Based on Landis and Koch [1977])

Example 10-1. In many epidemiologic studies, disease-specific mortality is a key outcome that requires classifying each death as to whether it was or was not due to a disease of interest. Often this adjudication is done by a clinical expert or a panel of experts, rather than depending on death certificate data alone. In a population-based study of stroke in Corpus Christi, Texas, Brown *et al.* (2007) investigated the reliability of cause-of-death classification for 186 deaths among persons who had been identified through the surveillance system as having had an ischemic stroke or transient ischemic attack. All available medical records and nursing-home records were compiled into a dossier about each decedent. These dossiers were then given to two different neurologists, each of whom was asked to classify each patient's death as due to stroke or due to another cause. The two neurologists worked separately and had no knowledge of each other's judgments. The resulting cause-of-death attributions were:

TABLE 10.4.

Neurologist #1	Neurologist #2		
	Stroke	Other	Total
Stroke	94	16	110
Other	17	59	76
Total	111	75	186

The observed concordance was $(94 + 59)/186 = 0.823$, seemingly quite high, but chance alone would lead to concordance of:

$$\left(\frac{110 \times 111}{186} + \frac{76 \times 75}{186}\right)/186 = 0.518$$

Kappa was $(0.823 - 0.518)/(1 - 0.518) = 0.632$, still representing "substantial" agreement beyond chance.

More complex variants of kappa have been developed to quantify reliability for categorical variables with more than two levels, either ordered or unordered, as described in Appendix 10A. Fleiss *et al.* (2003) describe other variants of kappa that accommodate more than two repeated measurements on each subject, and they describe how to estimate confidence limits for kappa.

The value of kappa depends in part on the true prevalence of the characteristic being measured. Thompson and Walter (1988) described the mathematical basis for this relationship, showing that kappa declines as prevalence approaches 0 or 1. This property should be kept in mind when comparing kappas among populations in which the prevalence of the characteristic under study differs substantially.

Kappa can be useful in the interpretation of study results, especially when there is concern that an observed association may be seriously attenuated by error in measurement of disease or exposure. Thompson (1990) derived a mathematical relationship between kappa, sensitivity and specificity (discussed below), and the amount of bias in an observed odds ratio, under certain assumptions. As kappa approaches zero, attenuation of the odds ratio becomes severe, and a true exposure–disease association may go undetected due to measurement error.

Intraclass Correlation Coefficient

For continuous measures, reliability can be quantified using the *intraclass correlation coefficient* (ICC), which is based on the analysis of variance. The simplest situation is when two separate measurements of the same characteristic have been made on each person in a group of study subjects. The two measurements on each person may have been made by two different observers, say, or using two different measuring instruments, or at two different times. For example, suppose that in a study of dietary sodium intake, urine specimens have been obtained from each of 50 people. To determine the reliability of the urinary sodium assay, two separate aliquots of urine are extracted from each person's original specimen, and the assay is run on all 100 resulting aliquots. For any particular person, the aliquots are interchangeable: it would not matter which aliquot is labelled #1 and which #2. The total variance among the $50 \times 2 = 100$ observations can then be partitioned statistically into two components, *between*-person variance (σ_B^2) and *within*-person variance (σ_W^2), such that total variance $= \sigma_B^2 + \sigma_W^2$. Intuitively, reliability of the measurement technique would be high if almost all of the variance is between-person and very little is within-person. The intraclass correlation coefficient expresses this idea quantitatively:

$$\text{ICC} = \frac{\sigma_B^2}{\sigma_B^2 + \sigma_W^2}$$

In words, the ICC is the fraction of the total variance that is due to between-person variation. ICC = 1 if all of the variation is between people—that is, if the two urinary sodium measurements for each person agree exactly. ICC = 0 if $\sigma_B^2 = 0$, which occurs if the means of the two measurements on each person are no more variable than if the 100 urine samples had simply been grouped at random into 50 pairs.

Even for this simple situation, the computing formula for the ICC is fairly complex (see White et al. (2008); Rosner (2006); Fleiss (1986)), but nowadays the calculations would usually be done by computer using statistical software to obtain both a point estimate and a confidence interval for the ICC. The numerical value of the ICC can be interpreted using the same descriptors as for kappa, as shown in Table 10.3.

There are several other forms of the ICC for more elaborate reliability studies, based on different analysis of variance models. The models differ according to whether the replicate observations on each subject are considered interchangeable; and if not, which statistical model best captures the sources of variation likely to affect an observed value (White et al., 2008; Fleiss, 1986).

Validity

Validity concerns the degree to which a measurement reflects the truth. To evaluate the validity of a measure, it must thus be possible to ascertain a study subject's true status on the characteristic being measured. This need is usually met by a separate *criterion measure* whose validity is already established or that can be safely assumed, often called a *gold standard*. For example, the gold standard for presence or absence of Alzheimer's disease might be the verdict of a competent neuropathologist after microscopic examination of brain tissue. But in many situations, applying a gold standard test routinely to everyone may be too risky, invasive, time-consuming, or costly, which motivates a search for more feasible alternative measures.

Sensitivity and Specificity

In epidemiology, the true characteristic of interest is often binary, such as the presence or absence of a certain disease or a certain exposure. Suppose that the characteristic is indeed the presence or absence of a certain disease, and that a gold standard test for true disease status has been applied to a set of study subjects. Some subjects prove to have the condition according to this gold standard; others prove not to have it. Now suppose that a new test for the condition yields a binary result, positive or negative, and is

TABLE 10.5. DATA LAYOUT FOR ASSESSING THE VALIDITY OF A BINARY TEST

Test result	True disease status	
	Present	Absent
+	a	b
−	c	d
Total	$a+c$	$b+d$

where:

a = number of *true positives*
b = number of *false positives*
c = number of *false negatives*
d = number of *true negatives*

TABLE 10.6. RESULTS OF THE SINGLE-PRIMER POLYMERASE CHAIN REACTION (PCR) TEST FOR CYTOMEGALOVIRUS (CMV) IN RELATION TO VIRAL CULTURE, THE GOLD STANDARD

PCR result	Viral culture	
	+	−
+	17	4
−	43	11,343
Total	60	11,347

(Based on data from Boppana *et al.* [2010])

$$\text{Sensitivity} = 17/(17+43) = 0.283$$
$$\text{Specificity} = 11,343/(4+11,343) = 0.9996$$

also applied to the same people. The correspondence between the new test result and true disease status (according to the gold standard) can be summarized as in Table 10.5.

Two key aspects of the test's validity can be defined as:

$$\text{Sensitivity} = a/(a+c)$$
$$\text{Specificity} = d/(b+d)$$

Sensitivity answers the question: When the disease is truly present, how often does the test detect it? Here there are $a + c$ true cases, and the test yields a positive result on a of them, so sensitivity is $a/(a + c)$. *Specificity* answers the question: When the disease is truly absent, how often does the test so indicate by giving a negative result? Here there are $b + d$ true non-cases, and the test is negative on d of them, so its specificity is $d/(b + d)$. Keep in mind that in other situations, the characteristic being measured may be something other than disease status—e.g., whether a subject has or has not been exposed to a certain drug—but the same ideas and definitions still apply.

Example 10-2.   Boppana *et al.* (2010) sought to evaluate a new test for detecting congenital cytomegalovirus (CMV) infection in newborns. The gold standard method is viral culture on a saliva or urine sample, but viral culture is costly and requires tissue-culture facilities, which are unavailable in many settings. A new test based on single-primer polymerase chain reaction (PCR) laboratory methods was developed to detect CMV DNA in a

dried blood spot, which is already widely obtained on newborns to screen for other congenital diseases. Both viral culture and the new PCR test were applied to 11,407 newborns at seven U.S. medical centers, with results shown in Table 10.6.

These results showed that the new PCR test had low sensitivity: when CMV was truly present as indicated by viral culture, the PCR test was positive only 28.3% of the time—that is, it would fail to detect 71.7% of the cases. For that reason, the investigators judged that it would be of limited value in screening newborns for congenital CMV infection. On the other hand, the PCR test was highly specific: when a newborn was *not* infected with CMV, the test was negative 99.96% of the time.

High sensitivity and high specificity are both desirable, but neither can be considered in isolation. For example, a test that always yields a positive result has perfect sensitivity (1.0) and would detect every case. But it also has terrible specificity (0.0), giving a false positive result for every non-case. It fails to discriminate between those with and those without the underlying characteristic. In practice, almost every test is imperfect, with sensitivity and specificity falling somewhere between 0 and 1.

Sensitivity and specificity are useful for comparing the performance of competing tests. For example, in their study of congenital CMV infection, Boppana *et al.* (2010) also studied a second, two-primer PCR test. It proved to have sensitivity of 0.344 and specificity of 0.9998—slightly superior to the single-primer PCR test, whose sensitivity was 0.283 and specificity was 0.9996. Thus, regardless of whether a child truly had CMV infection or not, the two-primer test was more likely than the single-primer test to give a correct result. Still, even the two-primer test's sensitivity was judged too low to warrant its routine use in clinical practice.

Statistically, sensitivity and specificity are proportions. Confidence limits for them can thus be obtained as for any proportion, as described in Appendix 4A. Both measures can also be viewed as conditional probabilities: if T_+ and T_- denote positive and negative test results, respectively, and C_+ and C_- denote presence or absence of the underlying characteristic, then sensitivity = $\Pr(T_+|C_+)$, and specificity = $\Pr(T_-|C_-)$. Taken together, sensitivity and specificity are termed the *operating characteristics* of the test.

Sensitivity and specificity are often treated as fixed properties of a test or measure. As can be seen from their computing formulas, sensitivity depends only on how the test performs among those who truly have the characteristic of interest, and specificity depends only on how it performs among those who truly do not have the characteristic. Thus, neither property depends directly on the true prevalence of the characteristic itself.

But in reality, for many tests, sensitivity and specificity do tend to vary somewhat from one observer, target population, case definition, or setting to another (Brenner and Gefeller, 1997; Ransohoff and Feinstein, 1978). For example, in a study of pulse oximetry for detecting congenital heart defects in newborns, Ewer *et al.* (2011) found that pulse oximetry had sensitivity of 0.49 for all such defects, but its sensitivity was 0.75 for "critical" defects, defined as those that were fatal or that required surgery within the first 28 days of life. The more profound physiological abnormalities in newborns with a "critical" defect were probably more likely to yield a positive pulse oximetry test result than the abnormalities in infants with milder defects. In addition, pulse oximetry was found to be more sensitive when applied within six hours after birth than when applied later. So in general, sensitivity and specificity estimates are best interpreted as reflecting how a test performs when applied in a certain way to a certain target population. Methods have been described for obtaining sensitivity and specificity estimates adjusted for patient characteristics and other factors, which in principle may support fairer comparisons of tests that have been evaluated on different populations (Janes and Pepe, 2008; Pepe and Longton, 2005; Coughlin *et al.*, 1992).

Likelihood Ratio

A measure closely related to sensitivity and specificity is the *likelihood ratio*, sometimes called the *diagnostic likelihood ratio* to distinguish it from the statistical concept of the same name (Deeks and Altman, 2004; Gallagher, 1998). It can take a different value for each possible test result, expressing the relative frequency of that result in persons with vs. persons without the underlying characteristic. For a binary test, call the two values LR_+ and LR_-. If, as before, T denotes the test result and C the underlying characteristic, then:

$$LR_+ = \frac{\Pr(T_+|C_+)}{\Pr(T_+|C_-)}$$

$$LR_- = \frac{\Pr(T_-|C_+)}{\Pr(T_-|C_-)}$$

For the single-primer PCR test for cytomegalovirus (Table 10.6), $LR_+ = (17/60) \div (4/11,347) = 803.7$, meaning that a positive PCR result was 803.7 times more likely in infants with CMV infection by viral culture than in infants without CMV infection. In the same data, $LR_- = (43/60) \div (11,343/11,347) = 0.717$, meaning that a negative PCR result was 0.717 times as likely in infants with CMV infection as in infants without CMV infection.

For a binary test, it can be shown algebraically that $LR_+ = $ sensitivity$/(1 - $ specificity$)$ and $LR_- = (1 - $ sensitivity$)/$specificity. Thus, LR_+ and LR_- can be viewed as two numbers that convey the same information contained in sensitivity and specificity, but in a different way. In theory, likelihood ratios also do not depend on prevalence of the underlying condition. However, as with sensitivity and specificity, in practice they can vary in relation to such factors as observer skill, severity of the underlying condition, and setting.

Other Measures

Another important measure of test performance is the *predictive value* associated with a certain test result. Because predictive value is closely related to screening for disease, discussion of it is deferred to Chapter 19, where it will be seen to depend strongly on the prevalence of the underlying condition.

Several other quantitative measures that seek to distill test performance into a single number have also appeared in the medical literature, but most have serious shortcomings (Shapiro, 1999; Zhou *et al.*, 2011). Among them are:

- *Accuracy* refers to the proportion of all test results that agree with the gold standard, or $(a + d)/(a + b + c + d)$ in the notation of Table 10.5. It can be shown to be simply a weighted average of sensitivity and specificity, with weights of prevalence and (1 – prevalence), respectively. In Example 10-2, the accuracy of the single-primer PCR test would be calculated as 0.9959 because truly CMV-noninfected infants were such a large majority of the study sample, obscuring the fact that the test's sensitivity was only 0.283. Another problem is that the same test could be found to have different accuracy in two populations with different prevalences, even if its sensitivity and specificity were the same in both.

- *Youden's index* (J) is sensitivity + specificity − 1. High sensitivity and high specificity are both desirable properties, and both would contribute to a higher value of Youden's index. But it treats false negatives and false positives as equivalent: a test with sensitivity of 0.25 and specificity of 0.9 would have the same Youden's index value as another test with sensitivity of 0.9 and specificity of 0.25. In reality, one type of classification error is almost always more serious than the other—a point to be revisited in the context of screening for disease (Chapter 19).

- The *odds ratio* equals $(ad)/(bc)$ in the notation of Table 10.5. While undeniably useful in etiologic case-control studies, the odds ratio is a measure of association, not of classification accuracy. Pepe *et al.* (2004) have noted that an odds ratio that would ordinarily be regarded as impressively large can be obtained even when a test has serious limitations as a measure of the underlying characteristic. In Example 10-2, the odds ratio for the association between the single-primer PCR test result and true CMV infection status was an eye-popping 1121.1, even though the test failed to detect more than 70% of cases and was judged too insensitive to be useful in practice.

A final caveat about terminology may be in order. The terms "false negative rate" (or "fraction" or "proportion") and "false positive rate" (or "fraction" or "proportion") appear sometimes in the literature on test evaluation. Unfortunately, these terms are not consistently defined and can be dangerously ambiguous (Naeger *et al.*, 2013). "False negative rate," for example, clearly seeks to convey the relative frequency of false-negative test results, and hence its numerator is the number of false negatives (c in Table 10.5). But its denominator is not so obvious. It could be $a + c$, in which case the "false negative rate" equals (1 − sensitivity); or it could be $c + d$, in which case the "false negative rate" equals what will be defined in Chapter 19 as (1 − negative predictive value). The numerical results and their interpretations are completely different, depending on which denominator is used. A similar problem applies to "false positive rate." Unfortunately, different authors have used different definitions of these terms, so the careful reader must look closely at an article's "Methods" section and/or the footnotes to its tables and figures to ferret out the meaning in a particular paper. Authors can usually avoid confusion by sticking with unambiguous, well-defined terms such as sensitivity and, if needed, (1 − sensitivity).

Receiver Operating Characteristic (ROC) Curves

Often in epidemiology, the underlying characteristic of interest is binary, but a test or measure for it may yield a result on an ordinal or continuous scale. How can the validity of such a test be evaluated? A fruitful approach is first to simplify the problem by dichotomizing the test results: any result greater than a particular *cutoff* value is classified as positive, and any result at or below the cutoff value classified as negative. Then sensitivity and specificity of the test are calculated as described earlier. The resulting sensitivity and specificity values will almost always be found to depend on the cutoff value selected. Shifting the cutoff value higher or lower usually involves trading off sensitivity against specificity. If the calculations are carried out for *all possible* cutoff values, the results form a set of (sensitivity, specificity) pairs, one pair for each cutoff value. These results can then be shown as a two-dimensional plot of sensitivity vs. specificity. This is essentially the idea behind a *receiver operating characteristic* (ROC) curve. ROC curves were originally developed to describe and compare the accuracy of radar receivers, which explains their odd name. By convention, sensitivity is plotted on the vertical axis and $(1 - \text{specificity})$, rather than specificity itself, on the horizontal axis.

Example 10-3. The Prostate-Specific Antigen (PSA) test quantifies the concentration in blood of a certain protein antigen in prostate tissue. PSA levels have been found to be elevated in men with prostate cancer. Since the 1990s, the test has been used clinically to screen for prostate cancer in asymptomatic men. Thompson *et al.* (2005) studied performance of the PSA test among 5,587 men in the placebo arm of a prostate cancer prevention trial. All were deemed clinically to be free of prostate cancer at the start of the trial, underwent prostate biopsy at the end of the trial to ascertain presence or absence of prostate cancer, and had had a PSA test within one year prior to the biopsy.

Table 10.7 shows how well the PSA test discriminated between men with and without prostate cancer (according to prostate biopsy, the gold standard) at various cutoff levels reported in the published article. For example, at a cutoff value of 3.1 ng/mL, 394 of the 1,225 men with prostate cancer on biopsy would be classified as having a positive PSA test because their PSA level was greater than 3.1. Of the 4,362 men without prostate cancer on biopsy, 580 of them had a positive PSA test by the same scoring rule.

Thus the sensitivity of the PSA test at a cutoff of 3.1 ng/mL was $394/1,225 = 0.322$, and its specificity at that cutoff was $(4,362 - 580)/4,362 = 0.867$. Comparing vertically across rows, note how the test's sensitivity decreases as the cutoff is shifted higher, while its specificity increases. The first and last rows of Table 10.7 were added in order to enclose the full range of possible PSA test results: all subjects would have PSA values greater than 0 and less than ∞.

An ROC curve corresponding to Table 10.7 is shown in Figure 10.2.

Besides showing an ROC curve for the PSA test based on the data of Thompson *et al.*, Figure 10.2 also shows ROC curves for two other hypothetical tests:

- *Uninformative test.* The diagonal dashed line shows the ROC curve for a test that is utterly unable to discriminate between those with and those without the underlying characteristic: every gain in sensitivity is coupled with an equal loss in specificity, and vice versa. Such a curve would be obtained if the distributions of test values were identical in those with and those without the underlying characteristic.
- *Perfect test.* The dotted line shows a right-angled ROC "curve" for a test that can, at some cutoff value, discriminate perfectly

TABLE 10.7. SENSITIVITY AND SPECIFICITY OF THE PSA TEST FOR PROSTATE CANCER AT DIFFERENT CUTOFF VALUES

Cutoff value (ng/mL)[a]	Number with positive test among:		Sensitivity	Specificity
	Cases[b] ($n = 1,225$)	Noncases ($n = 4,362$)		
0.0	1,225	4,362	1.000	0.000
1.1	1,022	2,665	0.834	0.389
1.6	821	1,802	0.670	0.587
2.1	644	1,200	0.526	0.725
2.6	496	824	0.405	0.811
3.1	394	580	0.322	0.867
4.1	251	270	0.205	0.938
6.1	56	65	0.046	0.985
8.1	21	26	0.017	0.994
10.1	11	13	0.009	0.997
∞	0	0	0.000	1.000

[a] All PSA test results greater than cutoff value regarded as positive
[b] Men with prostate cancer
(Based on data from Thompson *et al.* [2005])

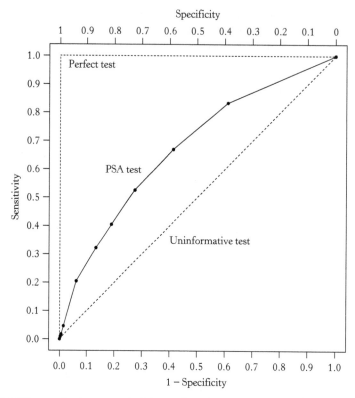

FIGURE 10.2 ROC curves for three tests: the PSA test (based on data in Table 10.7), a hypothetical uninformative test, and a hypothetical perfect test.

between those with and those without the underlying characteristic. That cutoff value would correspond to the point at the extreme upper-left corner, where the test has sensitivity = specificity = 1.0. (The same point might correspond to any cutoff value within a certain range, not just a single value.)

In general, the more accurate a test is, the farther toward the upper left its curve falls in an ROC plot. This rule can be used to discern at a glance which of two tests is more accurate when both ROC curves are shown on the same plot. The rule applies even if the two tests yield results in entirely different units on totally different scales. To see why it works, consider Figure 10.3, showing ROC curves for two hypothetical tests, A and B. Say that point 1 is arbitrarily picked on the ROC curve for test A, at which it has a certain sensitivity and specificity. Test B's sensitivity and specificity can be adjusted up or down by choosing different cutoff values on its own results scale, so let us choose the cutoff that gives test B the same specificity as test A has at point 1. At that specificity, test B's performance is shown by point 2,

directly above point 1. Comparing points 2 and 1, we see that at the same fixed value of specificity, test B has greater sensitivity. Likewise, at the same fixed value of sensitivity, test B has greater specificity (points 3 and 1).

In part because of this convenient graphical property, the *area under the curve* (AUC, also called the C-statistic) is often used in conjunction with ROC curves as a single summary measure of test accuracy. As can be seen in Figure 10.2, for an uninformative test, AUC = 0.5; for a perfect test, AUC = 1.0. For the PSA test, AUC = 0.678 (as calculated from the original ungrouped data). Although it is possible for the ROC curves for two different tests to cross, that situation is not common; accordingly, in most situations the AUC is a useful summary number that allows the discriminating ability of one test to be compared with that of a competing test. Hanley and McNeil (1982) describe methods for obtaining confidence limits for AUC. Methods are also available to determine whether the ROC curves for two tests applied to the same persons differ more than chance alone could easily explain (Hanley and McNeil, 1983).

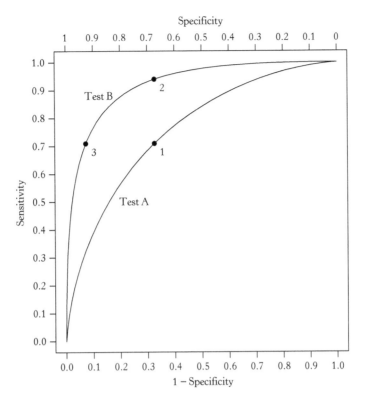

FIGURE 10.3 ROC curves for two hypothetical tests, A (worse) and B (better). At fixed specificity, test B has higher sensitivity (points 1 vs. 2); at fixed sensitivity, test B has higher specificity (points 1 vs. 3).

ROC curve methodology has been extended in a number of ways (Pepe, 2003). The method described above yields an empirical ROC curve, based directly on the data, but methods also exist to generate smoothed, or fitted, ROC curves (Shapiro, 1999), covariate-adjusted ROC curves (Janes and Pepe, 2008; Shapiro, 1999), and summary ROC curves that combine evidence from several test-evaluation studies, using meta-analysis techniques (Jones and Athanasiou, 2005; Harbord *et al.*, 2008; Walter, 2002). Time-dependent ROC curves and AUC can be used when a test is being evaluated as a predictor of some future event (Heagerty *et al.*, 2000; Chambless and Diao, 2006).

Sometimes no suitable gold standard is available for the underlying characteristic of interest. Fairly complex statistical methods have been proposed to permit sensitivity and specificity to be estimated indirectly in this situation (Zhou *et al.*, 2011; Reitsma *et al.*, 2009; Pepe, 2003; Hui and Zhou, 1998). These methods generally require that several imperfect tests be applied to the same study subjects, and they often require making assumptions about independence of measurement error across tests that can be difficult to test.

Continuous Variables

If both the gold standard and the measure being evaluated are continuous variables, the Pearson product-moment correlation can be used to quantify validity—in fact, the correlation between the two is called the *validity coefficient*. When both variables are expressed in the same units, this correlation can be disaggregated statistically into two components: (1) systematic bias, as reflected in a difference between the means; and (2) subject-level error (White *et al.*, 2008). If both the measure and the gold standard are ordinal variables, the Spearman rank correlation can be used to quantify the measure's validity.

CONSEQUENCES OF MEASUREMENT ERROR

The impact of measurement error on the results of a given epidemiologic study depends in part on how the error has arisen. If differential (selective) mismeasurement of exposure status has occurred—that is, when the ascertainment of exposure has been influenced by the presence or absence of disease—then the results can be biased positively or negatively. If, for example, ill persons are better able to recall a prior exposure than well persons who were chosen as a basis for comparison—perhaps the illness has prompted a heightened awareness of events that occurred prior to the onset of that illness—then a positive association between that exposure and illness will be observed in an interview-based case-control study even if none truly was present.

As another example of differential measurement error, the weight of persons after they have been diagnosed with type II diabetes may not reflect their weight during the period of time when the diabetes was developing: Because of the effects of dietary modification, it is often lower. A comparison of weight in persons with type II diabetes (of more than a very short duration) and non-diabetic controls, in order to assess the possible etiologic role of being overweight, could underestimate the size of the true association, since in the controls a corresponding stimulus to weight reduction would not generally have been present.

Similarly, differential misclassification of disease status can give rise to a falsely high or a falsely low estimate of risk associated with a given exposure. Studies that are most susceptible to this type of bias are those of conditions whose recognition can be influenced by knowledge of exposure status.

Example 10-4.   To some extent, Reye's syndrome is a disease of exclusion: there is no pattern of test results that is unequivocally indicative of the presence of this disease. For a number of years before any formal epidemiologic studies of Reye's syndrome were done, there was a widespread suspicion that taking aspirin might predispose to this disease. As a consequence, investigators of the relationship of Reye's syndrome to prior aspirin use had to design their studies to deal with the possibility that some physicians might have incorporated a child's prior use of aspirin as one criterion for diagnosing him or her as having Reye's syndrome. Specifically (Hurwitz et al., 1987), they included only clinically serious cases (in whom it was believed this potential bias was less likely to operate); defined the disease using standardized criteria across collaborating institutions; and had the records of all cases reviewed by

an expert panel whose members were ignorant of the child's prior use of medications.

Had steps not been taken to minimize it, the differential misclassification of outcome in this instance (differential because the likelihood of diagnosing the disease differed depending on exposure status) could have led to a falsely large estimate of the size of the association.

Nondifferential (nonselective) error in measurement of *exposure* is present when errors in assessing a subject's exposure status are similar in frequency and degree between ill and well persons. Nondifferential misclassification of *outcome* is present when errors in assessing a subject's illness or injury status are similar whether that subject has been exposed or not. The presence of nondifferential mismeasurement of exposure, which is ubiquitous in epidemiologic studies, generally leads to an attenuation of the estimated size of a true association between exposure and disease (Thomas, 1995). As an illustration of this point, consider the following hypothetical example:

Example 10-5.   Assume that in a case-control study in which a dichotomous exposure was measured perfectly, the following results would be obtained:

TABLE 10.8.

Exposure	Cases	Controls	Odds ratio
Yes	150	75	
			$\frac{150}{150} \div \frac{75}{225} = 3.0$
No	150	225	
	300	300	

However, if one-third of exposed persons were misclassified as being non-exposed, both among cases and controls, the results would instead look like this:

TABLE 10.9.

Exposure	Cases	Controls	Odds ratio
Yes	$150 - 50^a$	$75 - 25^a$	
			$\frac{100}{200} \div \frac{50}{250} = 2.5$
No	$150 + 50$	$225 + 25$	
	300	300	

^{a} $150 \times 1/3 = 50, 75 \times 1/3 = 25$

The observed odds ratio is now closer to the null value of 1.0.

TABLE 10.10.

Exposure	Cases	Controls	Odds ratio
Yes	$150 - 50 + 30$	$75 - 25 + 45$	
			$\frac{130}{170} \div \frac{95}{205} = 1.65$
No	$150 + 50 - 30^a$	$225 + 25 - 45^a$	
	300	300	

$^a 150 \times 0.2 = 30, 225 \times 0.2 = 45$

The bias towards the null would increase further if some truly non-exposed persons were to be incorrectly classified as having been exposed. Assume this occurs in 20% of truly non-exposed persons, both among cases and controls, as in Table 10.10. This result is even closer to the null, and differs enough from the true odds ratio that the interpretation of the results of the study could well be influenced.

To what extent will a true association be attenuated by the presence of nondifferential misclassification of exposure? The larger the degree of misclassification, the greater the attenuation. As noted earlier, for a dichotomous exposure, misclassification can be thought of as having two components:

1. Some persons with the exposure are falsely labeled as having been nonexposed; that is, the measure being used to assess exposure status has less than 100% *sensitivity*; and
2. Persons without the exposure are falsely labeled as exposed; that is, there is less than 100% *specificity* of the measure.

While either a low sensitivity or a low specificity of the means by which exposure is identified will lead to bias toward the null result, the degree of bias depends on the frequency of exposure in the population from which the study subjects were sampled.

Example 10-6. Let us say that we are comparing the one-year cumulative incidence of a certain illness in persons who do or do not consume food A. Assume there is no error in ascertaining the presence of the illness, which occurs at a rate 10 times higher in consumers of A than the annual incidence of 10 per 10,000 persons who do not eat A. If one in 11 persons in the study population ate food A, the results of a study with perfect ascertainment of A consumption would look as in Table 10.11.

TABLE 10.11. THE TRUTH

Consumption	Illness			Relative
of food A	Yes	No	Total	risk
Yes	10	990	1,000	
				10
No	10	9,990	10,000	

If eating A had been correctly ascertained in only 80% of A consumers (sensitivity = 80%), in both ill and well persons, but all non-eaters of A were correctly classified as such (specificity = 100%), the results would appear as in Table 10.12.

On the other hand, had all A eaters been correctly classified (100% sensitivity), but 20% of A non-eaters had been misclassified as A eaters (80% specificity), the results would instead look as in Table 10.13.

In this instance, because a relatively small proportion (1 of 11) of the population ate food A, the absolute number of misclassified persons was much higher when there was less-than-perfect specificity than where there was less-than-perfect sensitivity. Though the true relative risk of 10 was underestimated in both scenarios where nondifferential misclassification of exposure was present, the degree of underestimation was particularly great in the presence of less-than-100% specificity. If food A had been consumed by the majority of persons, rather than the minority, then the degree of underestimation of the relative risk would be influenced more by the sensitivity of ascertainment than by the specificity, since even a small relative impairment of sensitivity would lead to a relatively larger number of misclassified persons. This topic has been discussed in greater detail elsewhere (Flegal *et al.*, 1986).

The foregoing discussion applies entirely to studies that ascertain exposure status for individual

TABLE 10.12. EXPOSURE STATUS ASCERTAINED WITH 80% SENSITIVITY AND 100% SPECIFICITY

Consumption of food A	Illness			Relative risk
	Yes	No	Total	
Yes	$10(0.8) = 8$	$990(0.8) = 792$	800	
				8.5
No	$10 + 2 = 12$	$9,990 + 198$ $= 10,188$	10,200	

TABLE 10.13. EXPOSURE STATUS ASCERTAINED WITH 100% SENSITIVITY AND 80% SPECIFICITY

Consumption of food A	Illness			Relative risk
	Yes	No	Total	
Yes	$10 + 2 = 12$	$990 + 1,998$ $= 2,988$	3,000	
				4.0
No	$10(0.8) = 8$	$9,990(0.8)$ $= 7,992$	8,000	

subjects within a population. In ecological studies, in which the possible effect of an exposure is estimated by correlating disease rates across groups with differences in their exposure prevalence, nondifferential misclassification of the latter can actually lead to an inflated estimate of the influence of exposure on disease risk (Brenner *et al.*, 1992). An example is given in Chapter 16.

In cohort studies, if ascertainment of *disease status* is incomplete, but is comparably incomplete for exposed and non-exposed persons, then the *ratio* of observed disease incidence between the exposed and the non-exposed (i.e., the relative risk), will be the same as if this type of misclassification had not been present. (In case-control studies this will be true for the odds ratio as well, except when the disease in question occurs with a very high frequency in the study population.) In contrast, to the extent that persons without a disease are falsely labeled as having it, the observed relative risk will be closer to the null than the true value.

Example 10-7. Let us return to the example of illness in relation to consumption of food A, this time assuming that it is illness status and not exposure status that is subject to misclassification. Again, in the absence of any misclassification, the data would look like this:

TABLE 10.14. THE TRUTH

Consumption of food A	Illness			Relative risk
	Yes	No	Total	
Yes	10	990	1,000	
				10
No	10	9,990	10,000	

TABLE 10.15. ILLNESS STATUS ASCERTAINED WITH 90%
SENSITIVITY AND 100% SPECIFICITY

Consumption of food A	Illness			Relative risk
	Yes	No	Total	
Yes	$10(.9) = 9$	$990 + 1 = 991$	1,000	
				10
No	$10(.9) = 9$	$9,990 + 1 = 9,991$	10,000	

TABLE 10.16. ILLNESS STATUS ASCERTAINED WITH 100%
SENSITIVITY AND 99% SPECIFICITY

Consumption of food A	Illness			Relative risk
	Yes	No	Total	
Yes	$10 + 10 = 20$	$990(.99)$ $= 980$	1,000	
				1.82
No	$10 + 100 = 110$	$9,990(.99)$ $= 9,890$	10,000	

If 10% of persons who became ill were not recognized as such (sensitivity = 90%), the numbers shown in Table 10.15 would result. The under-ascertainment of cases has no influence on the denominator of the cumulative incidence in exposed and non-exposed persons, and, since the numerators remain the same *relative* to one another, there is no impact on the size of the relative risk.

In contrast, if specificity in ascertaining illness is less than 100%, the influence on the relative risk can be substantial. Consider the situation in which just one percent of well persons were inadvertently believed to have developed the illness (Table 10.16). The observed relative risk in the presence of less-than-perfect specificity is reduced considerably towards the null value of 1.0, from 10.0 to 1.82.

The minimization of measurement error is, of course, the objective of every epidemiologic study. Whether for exposure or disease, we would like our tools to be reliable—obtaining the same value or result each time we make a measurement—and to be valid—obtaining the true value or result. The means of enhancing reliability and validity depends on just what tool is being used, the setting in which the study is done, and on other factors. This topic is beyond the scope of the present book; an introduction to it can be found in White *et al.* (2008).

Largely because of our inability to accurately measure certain exposures, a number of etiologic questions of great interest have not been satisfactorily addressed in epidemiologic studies. To this day we are unsure of the role of certain types of air and water pollution on health, or of the long-term consequences of certain dietary or occupational exposures, primarily because it is not possible to quantify with great reliability and validity how much exposure to these agents has been received by study participants. Nonetheless, we should not lose sight of the possibility that a potential association we wish to investigate may be so strong that the presence of misclassification, sometimes even a substantial degree of it, will not obscure the entirety of that association.

Example 10-8.   In order to explore the possibility that anal intercourse could in some way predispose to the subsequent occurrence of anal cancer, Daling *et al.* (1982) conducted a case-control study. Men diagnosed with anal cancer in western Washington State during 1974–1979 were compared to controls (men with other cancers) for a history of syphilis, as determined from records of the Washington State Health Department. These investigators knew that for a number of years prior to the time of the study, the majority of men in Washington with a new diagnosis of syphilis reported a history of recent sexual contact with another man. They found eight of 47 men with anal cancer (17.0%) also were listed in health department records as having syphilis, in contrast to only 1–2% of men with the other forms of cancer studied.

Daling *et al.* pursued this lead by comparing the distribution of marital status between men with anal cancer and controls. They reasoned that men who engaged in receptive anal intercourse would be less likely to be married to a woman than would other men. Because marital status is ascertained routinely by cancer registries in the United States, they were able to use data from U.S. registries outside of Washington State as well. The results again supported their hypothesis: 24.4% of men with anal cancer had never been married, in contrast to about 8% of men with colon or rectal cancer (controls). No corresponding difference in the distribution of marital status was present between women with anal cancer and control women.

These registry-based studies were rife with misclassification. In the second study, for example, it is likely that only the minority of never-married men had had anal intercourse, the actual exposure of interest. However, the strong association observed using the misclassified exposure status quickly led to an interview-based case-control study (Daling *et al.*, 1987), which observed an even stronger association: 25.9% of men with anal cancer versus only 1.6% of controls stated they had previously engaged in anal intercourse.

Example 10-9. In Britain, procedures to inactivate live virus in blood products were initiated in 1985. However, screening of blood products for hepatitis B virus began there in 1972. Thus, while hemophiliacs (in whom receipt of blood products is nearly universal) treated in Britain beginning in 1972–1985 would be expected to have become infected with hepatitis C virus (because this infection was probably present in an appreciable proportion of blood samples that were donated), few of them should have been infected with hepatitis B virus.

In an effort to learn of long-term consequences of infection with hepatitis C virus, the mortality from liver cancer and other liver disease was documented among hemophiliacs treated in Britain during 1972–1985 (Darby *et al.*, 1997). Five deaths from liver cancer occurred among members of this cohort, with only 0.90 expected based on mortality rates in demographically similar men. The

corresponding numbers for other liver disease were: 51 deaths observed, versus 3.05 expected.

The investigators did not assess the presence of hepatitis C infection in a single study subject, so it is not known if there were some hemophiliacs who escaped infection with this virus. Also, in the general British male population that served as the basis for comparison, there were certainly a small number of non-hemophiliac men who were infected with hepatitis C. Yet, the presence of what must be a *very* strong association between hepatitis C infection and fatal liver disease, combined with the relatively modest level of exposure misclassification, permitted the study to contribute to our knowledge of some deleterious consequences of hepatitis C infection.

CORRECTING FOR MEASUREMENT ERROR

Because measurement error is such a common and important problem in research, much statistical work has been devoted to quantifying it and addressing it in data analysis. Books by White *et al.* (2008) and Gustafson (2004) discuss several approaches, as do several review articles (Chen, 1989; Thomas *et al.*, 1993; Thürigen *et al.*, 2000; Walter and Irwig, 1988). Just as ways to quantify measurement error depend on the scale of measurement of the variable in question, so do approaches to correcting for measurement error.

Categorical variables play an especially prominent role in epidemiology. Appendix 10B. describes and illustrates at some length a method for evaluating and correcting for misclassification (Barron, 1977; Greenland and Kleinbaum, 1983; Morrissey and Spiegelman, 1999), which can be viewed as a generalization of the approach used in Examples 10-5 to 10-7. The method can be applied when one, two, or more variables are subject to misclassification. Acquaintance with some basic matrix algebra helps in understanding the mathematical basis of the method (as for multiple regression) but is not essential for applying it properly using widely available statistical packages or spreadsheet programs. A major attraction of the method is that it is reversible—that is, it can be used for problems of the following sort:

(Hypothetical true values) + (Misclassification pattern) → (Projected observed values)

or for problems of this sort:

(Observed values) + (Misclassification pattern) → (Estimated true values)

CONCLUDING REMARKS

Although sophisticated statistical tools are available to quantify and correct for measurement error, the adage that "an ounce of prevention is worth a pound of cure" remains wise advice in epidemiologic methods as well as in medicine. Probably the most effective method for dealing with measurement error is to prevent or minimize it in the first place, rather than to rely on complex analysis and untestable assumptions later in an attempt to fix the problem. Minimizing measurement error requires paying careful attention to the choice of measures during study design, and to monitoring and maintaining data quality during study execution.

APPENDIX 10A: VARIANTS OF KAPPA FOR CATEGORICAL VARIABLES WITH THREE OR MORE CATEGORIES

Kappa can also be used to quantify the reliability of nominal measures that can take any of, say, h unordered values. The data for two replicate measurements can be arranged as in Table 10.17, which contains one cell for each possible combination of values. The n's represent the number of subjects in each cell, r's are row totals, and c's are column totals.

The observed concordance is

$$P_o = \frac{\sum_{i=1}^{h} n_{ii}}{N}$$

The concordance expected by chance is

$$P_e = \frac{\sum_{i=1}^{h} r_i \cdot c_i / N}{N} \qquad (10.2)$$

and kappa is calculated as before (Equation 10.1).

The resulting value of kappa depends in part on h, the number of categories, which in turn may reflect a choice made by investigators on how finely or coarsely study subjects are grouped (Maclure and Willett, 1987). Other things being equal, kappa decreases as h increases. For example, kappa measuring agreement between two different sources of information on race is likely to be greater if race is categorized as white / black / other than if race is categorized as as white / black / Native American / Chinese / Japanese / Hawaiian / Pacific Islander / other.

Weighted kappa is a variant of kappa that can be used for ordinal measures. The data layout shown in Table 10.17 still applies, as long as the values defining the rows and columns are arranged in their proper order—e.g., from mild to severe. As before, perfect agreement occurs when all observations fall on the main diagonal from upper left to bottom right. But among the off-diagonal cells, the severity of disagreement depends on how far off the main diagonal a cell lies. Cells that lie just adjacent to the main diagonal, such as the n_{12} and n_{21} cells, contain observations for which the discrepancy between the two measurements was relatively mild—just one category. In contrast, cells farthest from the main diagonal, such as the n_{1h} and n_{h1} cells, contain observations for which the two measurements fell toward opposite ends of the scale, representing serious disagreements.

Weighted kappa is designed to give "full credit" when the two observations for a study subject agree exactly, and "partial credit" if they disagree, depending on how far apart the two measurements are. Various weighting schemes can be used, but a common choice is to give the cell in row i and column j a weight of

$$w_{ij} = 1 - \frac{(i-j)^2}{(h-1)^2} \qquad (10.3)$$

TABLE 10.17. DATA LAYOUT FOR RELIABILITY ASSESSMENT ON A CATEGORICAL MEASURE WITH 3+ POSSIBLE VALUES

First measurement	Second measurement				
	Value 1	Value 2	...	Value h	Total
Value 1	n_{11}	n_{12}	...	n_{1h}	r_1
Value 2	n_{21}	n_{22}	...	n_{2h}	r_2
⋮	⋮	⋮	...	⋮	⋮
Value h	n_{h1}	n_{h2}	...	n_{hh}	r_h
Total	c_1	c_2	...	c_h	N

For example, if $h = 4$, then weights of 1, 0.89, 0.55, and 0 apply to cells representing discrepancies of 0, 1, 2, and 3 categories, respectively. The weighted concordance observed is then

$$P_o = \frac{\sum_{i=1}^{h} \sum_{j=1}^{h} w_{ij} \cdot n_{ij}}{N}$$

The weighted concordance expected by chance is

$$P_e = \frac{\sum_{i=1}^{h} \sum_{j=1}^{h} w_{ij} \cdot r_i \cdot c_j / N}{N}$$

and kappa is again calculated from Equation 10.1. Using the weights above, weighted kappa converges to the intraclass correlation coefficient as N increases (Fleiss et al., 2003). Brenner and Kliebsch (1996) showed that the value of weighted kappa tends to increase with h, which should be borne in mind when comparing measures of the same characteristic but with different numbers of categories. Weighted kappa and other methods of reliability assessment for ordinal data are reviewed by Nelson and Pepe (2000).

Fleiss et al. (2003) give formulas for the approximate standard error of kappa and weighted kappa, which can be used to obtain confidence limits for them. They also describe extensions of kappa to more than two measurements per study subject.

APPENDIX 10B: USING MISCLASSIFICATION MATRICES TO ADDRESS MEASUREMENT ERROR IN CATEGORICAL VARIABLES

Consider a study that involves an exposure E and an outcome Y, both binary variables taking values of $+$ or $-$. The number of study subjects with each possible combination of E and Y can be organized into a 2×2 table:

TABLE 10.18.

	Y_+	Y_-
E_+	Cell #1	Cell #2
E_-	Cell #3	Cell #4

The cells of such a table can be referred to in either of two ways: by specifying a combination of E and Y values (E_+Y_+, E_+Y_-, E_-Y_+, or E_-Y_-); or by cell number (1, 2, 3, or 4). The first way is more descriptive, while the second is more compact. Both ways will prove useful below.

In addressing misclassification, two such tables are of interest: (1) a table **t** that would result if subjects were classified by their *true* status on both variables; and (2) a table **m** that results when subjects are classified by their *measured*, possibly *misclassified*, status on both variables.

Misclassification Matrix

The true table **t** and the measured table **m** can be related to each other through a square *misclassification matrix*, **C**, which has one column for each cell of **t** and one row for each cell of **m**. That is, **C** is a 4×4 matrix with the following layout:

TABLE 10.19.

Measured	True			
	E_+Y_+	E_+Y_-	E_-Y_+	E_-Y_-
E_+Y_+	p_{11}	p_{12}	p_{13}	p_{14}
E_+Y_-	p_{21}	p_{22}	p_{23}	p_{24}
E_-Y_+	p_{31}	p_{32}	p_{33}	p_{34}
E_-Y_-	p_{41}	p_{42}	p_{43}	p_{44}
Total	1	1	1	1

Each cell of **C** contains a probability. Consider the first column. The value p_{11} is the probability that a subject whose true status is E_+Y_+ would have a measured status of E_+Y_+: that is, that he/she would be correctly classified on both variables. One row down, p_{21} is the probability that a subject who is truly E_+Y_+ would be correctly classified on E but misclassified on Y. Next, p_{31} is the probability that a subject who is truly E_+Y_+ would be misclassified on E but correctly classified on Y. Finally, p_{41} is the probability that a subject who is truly E_+Y_+ would be misclassified on both E and Y. In general, p_{ij} is the conditional probability of a subject's having the measured status indicated by row i of **C**, given that the subject's true status is indicated by column j of **C**. Equivalently, p_{ij} is the probability that a subject in cell j of the **t** table would end up in cell i of the **m** table. Regardless of his/her true status, every subject must have a measured status that is one of the four possible combinations of E and Y values, so the probabilities in each column must sum to 1.

The misclassification matrix **C** is somewhat similar to Table 10.5, inasmuch as both involve cross-classifying true status with measured status. However, Table 10.5 concerns only one variable, which could be E or Y, while the **C** matrix concerns both variables together. Also, the cells of Table 10.5 contain counts of subjects, while the cells of **C** contain probabilities.

The values in **C** depend on several factors:

- The sensitivity and specificity of the measure of E
- The sensitivity and specificity of the measure of Y
- Whether the sensitivity and/or specificity of the E measure depend on the true value of Y
- Whether the sensitivity and/or specificity of the Y measure depend on the true value of E
- Whether being misclassified on E is associated with being misclassified on Y.

Table 10.20 shows six examples of possible misclassification patterns and how **C** might look in each case. The examples are discussed in order below.

1. In this example, both E and Y are always measured without error: **C** has 1 on its main diagonal and 0 everywhere else.
2. This example corresponds to Example 10-5 in the main text: E is subject to misclassification with sensitivity $sens_E = 2/3$ and specificity $spec_E = 0.9$. Half of the ps in **C** are zero, because they are in cells that would involve misclassification of Y, which is impossible in this scenario. The fact that the two non-zero ps in column 1 are the same as those in column 2 (albeit in different rows) follows from misclassification of E being *nondifferential* in relation to Y. The non-zero ps in columns 3 and 4 are also the same, for the same reason.
3. This example corresponds to Example 10-7 in the main text: Y is subject to misclassification with sensitivity $sens_Y = 0.9$ and specificity $spec_Y = 1$. More than half of the ps are zero, because: (1) E is never misclassified, and (2) the measure of Y is perfectly specific, which rules out misclassification of Y when the true status is Y_-. The two non-zero ps in column 1 are the same as those in column 3 because misclassification of Y is nondifferential with respect to E.
4. In this example, only E is subject to measurement error, but the misclassification probabilities for E differ between subjects who are truly Y_+ and those who are

truly Y_-. That is, **C** shows *differential* misclassification of E: the non-zero cells in column 1 have values different from those in column 2, and the values in columns 3 and 4 also differ. Such a pattern might be seen in a case-control study of a fatal illness in which exposure data on cases came from proxy respondents who had incomplete knowledge of each case's exposure history, while controls were interviewed on their own behalf.

5. Sometimes empirical estimates of the ps can come from a validation substudy, as noted below. As in this example, these estimates need not follow any simple pattern. However, if the measures of E and Y are any good, there should be relatively high ps along the main diagonal.
6. This example illustrates a pattern that could arise if both E and Y are assumed to be subject to misclassification, but no validation study has been possible to estimate all of the individual ps in **C**. Instead, estimates of the sensitivity and specificity of E and of Y come from external sources. If misclassification of each variable is assumed to be nondifferential, and if the probabilities of misclassification on E and Y are assumed to be statistically independent, then the **C** matrix shown can be calculated from the four operating characteristics of E and Y shown at left. For example, $p_{11} = (0.9)(0.8)$. As shown below (see Example 10-12), there is an easy way to do the necessary calculations to obtain **C** in such situations.

Information to construct **C** can come from several sources. Among the best theoretically is a *validation substudy*, in which a representative sample of study subjects have E and Y measured in two ways: using the standard measures being applied study-wide, and using gold-standard measures that establish true status on E and Y. Cross-tabulation of measured status with true status for all validation substudy subjects provides empirical estimates of the ps. Separate validation studies for E and for Y are also possible but cannot examine whether misclassification of E and of Y operate independently. Alternatively, *external information* about the sensitivity and specificity of the study's measures of E and of Y can be used to fill in **C**. Ideally, external information should come from a setting in which factors that could affect the operating characteristics of the measures—nature of the study population, measurement technique, observer training, etc.—were as similar as possible to those in the current study setting. In the absence of extensive data, assumptions must also be made about whether the pattern of misclassification is differential or nondifferential, and about statistical independence.

TABLE 10.20. EXAMPLES OF MISCLASSIFICATION PATTERNS AND CORRESPONDING MISCLASSIFICATION MATRICES **C**

No.	Misclassification pattern	**C** matrix

1 — No misclassification

Measured	True			
	E_+Y_+	E_+Y_-	E_-Y_+	E_-Y_-
E_+Y_+	1	0	0	0
E_+Y_-	0	1	0	0
E_-Y_+	0	0	1	0
E_-Y_-	0	0	0	1

2 — Nondifferential misclassification of E only:
$sens_E = 2/3$
$spec_E = 0.8$

Measured	True			
	E_+Y_+	E_+Y_-	E_-Y_+	E_-Y_-
E_+Y_+	2/3	0	0.2	0
E_+Y_-	0	2/3	0	0.2
E_-Y_+	1/3	0	0.8	0
E_-Y_-	0	1/3	0	0.8

3 — Nondifferential misclassification of Y only:
$sens_Y = 0.9$
$spec_Y = 1$

Measured	True			
	E_+Y_+	E_+Y_-	E_-Y_+	E_-Y_-
E_+Y_+	0.9	0	0	0
E_+Y_-	0.1	1	0	0
E_-Y_+	0	0	0.9	0
E_-Y_-	0	0	0.1	1

4 — Differential misclassification of E only:
$sens_{E|Y_+} = 0.7$
$sens_{E|Y_-} = 0.95$
$spec_{E|Y_+} = 0.8$
$spec_{E|Y_-} = 0.9$

Measured	True			
	E_+Y_+	E_+Y_-	E_-Y_+	E_-Y_-
E_+Y_+	0.7	0	0.2	0
E_+Y_-	0	0.95	0	0.1
E_-Y_+	0.3	0	0.8	0
E_-Y_-	0	0.05	0	0.9

5 — Possible complex pattern from large validation study

Measured	True			
	E_+Y_+	E_+Y_-	E_-Y_+	E_-Y_-
E_+Y_+	0.86	0.20	0.02	0.00
E_+Y_-	0.04	0.67	0.09	0.10
E_-Y_+	0.07	0.12	0.75	0.14
E_-Y_-	0.03	0.01	0.14	0.76

6 — Nondifferential, independent misclassification of both E and Y (see text):
$sens_E = 0.9$
$spec_E = 0.75$
$sens_Y = 0.8$
$spec_Y = 0.95$

Measured	True			
	E_+Y_+	E_+Y_-	E_-Y_+	E_-Y_-
E_+Y_+	0.720	0.045	0.200	0.013
E_+Y_-	0.180	0.855	0.050	0.237
E_-Y_+	0.080	0.005	0.600	0.038
E_-Y_-	0.020	0.095	0.150	0.712

Application #1: Hypothetical True → Misclassified

Now consider a problem in which the aim is to anticipate the effects of misclassification of E, Y, or both, on results of a study being planned. Preparations for the study have provided information on the expected frequency of E and Y and on the hypothesized association between them, which can be represented in the 2×2 table **t** of hypothetical true results with no misclassification. Meanwhile, the misclassification matrix **C** has been filled in from information sources just mentioned.

To estimate the results that would be expected in the face of misclassification, formulas can written out showing how to calculate each cell of **m** as a function of the relevant cells of **t** and **C**. For example, $m_1 = (t_1 \cdot p_{11}) + (t_2 \cdot p_{12}) + (t_3 \cdot p_{13}) + (t_4 \cdot p_{14})$. In words, cell m_1 will contain the number of subjects in cell t_1 who stay in the same cell of **m**, plus the numbers of subjects who are moved into cell m_1 from each of the other three cells of **t**. Similar formulas are needed for m_2, m_3, and m_4.

Fortunately, the messy proliferation of formulas can be avoided. Matrix multiplication does exactly the computational task required if the **m** and **t** tables are rearranged as four-element column vectors: $\mathbf{m_v} = (m_1, m_2, m_3, m_4)$, and $\mathbf{t_v} = (t_1, t_2, t_3, t_4)$, both arranged vertically as shown in the examples below. In matrix form:

$$\mathbf{m_v} = \mathbf{C} \cdot \mathbf{t_v} \qquad (10.4)$$

The matrix multiplication capability needed to apply Equation (10.4) is built into widely available statistical and spreadsheet programs and online matrix calculators, and it can be invoked using commands not much longer than Equation (10.4) itself. Once $\mathbf{m_v}$ is obtained, its elements can be rearranged into a 2×2 table containing the final results.[1]

Example 10-10. Say that researchers at the U.S. Department of Veterans Affairs are conducting a large cohort study of U.S. veterans to investigate a wide variety of associations between genetic traits and diseases. DNA samples have been obtained on thousands of veterans, each of whom also completed a lengthy health questionnaire upon study enrollment.

As part of this effort, the researchers wish to confirm or refute findings from a German study (Treutlein *et al.*, 2009) that found an association between allele A on the genetic marker rs13160562 and alcohol-use disorders, with an odds ratio of 0.70 (95% CI: 0.59 – 0.83). The German study involved detailed interviews of each study subject by two psychiatrists, yielding presumably error-free classification of subjects on presence or absence of an alcohol-use disorder. In the study of U.S. veterans, however, outcome classification would instead be based on answers to a set of alcohol-related questions in the enrollment questionnaire, which

together make up a scale called the AUDIT-C. A previous validation study in U.S. veterans (Frank *et al.*, 2008) found that the AUDIT-C had sensitivity = 0.96 and specificity = 0.70 for alcohol-use disorders when used in white males, the predominant demographic group in the German study. For present purposes, rs13160562 status is assumed to be classified without error, and misclassification on the outcome is expected to be similar regardless of genotype.

"Allele frequency" in this kind of study refers to the allele distribution in the overall gene pool from cases and that from controls. Each case or control contributes two alleles—one inherited from each parent—to his/her respective gene pool. Assuming that rs13160562 allele frequency in the case gene pool (25.2% allele A) and the control gene pool (32.6% allele A) in the German study were to apply in U.S. veterans, and if the true prevalence of alcohol-use disorders in U.S. veterans were as found in the earlier validation study (15%), the expected distribution of alleles for, say, 500 participants in the U.S. veteran study in the absence of misclassification would be as shown in Table 10.21. Remember that each subject contributes two alleles, and that expected counts, unlike observed counts, need not be integers.

But given the anticipated amount of outcome misclassification, how strong an observed association would be expected in the U.S. veteran study? The appropriate misclassification matrix **C** is shown in Table 10.22.

This matrix reflects nondifferential misclassification of Y and no misclassification of E. Equation (10.4) is then applied as shown in Table 10.23.

The rightmost column vector is $\mathbf{m_v}$, which can be rearranged in tabular form as shown in Table 10.24. In this table, $OR = 0.89$, a fairly substantial degree of attenuation compared to the assumed true OR of 0.70. This result might, in turn, have implications concerning the sample size needed for adequate statistical power to study the issue in U.S. veterans.

TABLE 10.21.

Allele A on rs13160562	Alcohol use disorder	
	$+$	$-$
$+$	37.8	277.1
$-$	112.2	572.9

TABLE 10.22.

Measured	True			
	E_+Y_+	E_+Y_-	E_-Y_+	E_-Y_-
E_+Y_+	0.96	0.30	0	0
E_+Y_-	0.04	0.70	0	0
E_-Y_+	0	0	0.96	0.30
E_-Y_-	0	0	0.04	0.70

TABLE 10.23.

$$
\begin{bmatrix}
0.96 & 0.30 & 0 & 0 \\
0.04 & 0.70 & 0 & 0 \\
0 & 0 & 0.96 & 0.30 \\
0 & 0 & 0.04 & 0.70
\end{bmatrix}
\times
\begin{bmatrix}
37.8 \\
277.1 \\
112.2 \\
572.9
\end{bmatrix}
=
\begin{bmatrix}
119.4 \\
195.5 \\
279.6 \\
405.5
\end{bmatrix}
$$

TABLE 10.24.

Allele A on rs13160562	Alcohol use disorder	
	+	−
+	119.4	195.5
−	279.6	405.5

Application #2: Misclassified → Estimated True

Now consider the opposite problem: given a set of observed results **m**, the aim is to "correct" for misclassification by working back to an estimate of **t**, the true 2 × 2 table that would generate the observed results when combined with a specified pattern of misclassification. A "brute force" approach—constructing a separate formula for each cell of **t**—would be even messier than before. But by premultiplying both sides of Equation (10.4) by $\mathbf{C}^{-1}$, the matrix inverse of **C**, the solution in matrix form is simply:

$$\mathbf{t_v} = \mathbf{C}^{-1} \cdot \mathbf{m_v} \qquad (10.5)$$

which again can be carried out easily using widely available software.[2] The four-element vector $\mathbf{t_v}$ can then be rearranged into a 2 × 2 table to show the final results.

Example 10-11. Elbaz *et al.* (2003) conducted a case-control study to determine the degree to which Parkinson's disease (PD) runs in families. Part of the study involved asking PD cases and controls whether any of their relatives had PD. A concern in such a study is the possibility of *family information bias*, a form of recall bias due to disease cases being more likely than controls to be aware of, and to report having, a relative with the condition of interest (Sackett, 1979). The Elbaz *et al.*, study was conducted in Olmsted County, Minnesota, whose residents receive nearly all of their health care through the Mayo Clinic. For a sample of cases and controls, the researchers reviewed medical records for subjects and their families to determine independently whether any relatives had PD. Using medical record data as the gold standard, they found that the sensitivity of self-report for a family history of PD was 0.68 for cases and 0.45 for controls, while specificity was 0.99 for cases and 0.998 for controls—a pattern consistent with family information bias. Given the study setting, it is probably safe to assume no misclassification of PD status.

Based on the interview data, the main results were:[3]

TABLE 10.25.

Family history of PD	Cases (Y_+)	Controls (Y_-)
+	22	6
−	111	113

In this table, $OR = 3.73$. But might family information bias be responsible for the entire positive

TABLE 10.26.

Measured	True			
	E_+Y_+	E_+Y_-	E_-Y_+	E_-Y_-
E_+Y_+	0.68	0	0.01	0
E_+Y_-	0	0.45	0	0.002
E_-Y_+	0.32	0	0.99	0
E_-Y_-	0	0.55	0	0.998

TABLE 10.27.

$$\begin{bmatrix} 0.68 & 0 & 0.01 & 0 \\ 0 & 0.45 & 0 & 0.002 \\ 0.32 & 0 & 0.99 & 0 \\ 0 & 0.55 & 0 & 0.998 \end{bmatrix}^{-1} \times \begin{bmatrix} 22 \\ 6 \\ 111 \\ 113 \end{bmatrix} = \begin{bmatrix} 30.9 \\ 12.9 \\ 102.1 \\ 106.1 \end{bmatrix}$$

association observed? Equation (10.5) can be used to address this question, using a misclassification matrix **C** as shown in Table 10.26. Exposure misclassification is thought to be differential, leading to different values in columns 1 and 2 and in columns 3 and 4. In Table 10.27, equation (10.5) is then applied to solve for $\mathbf{t_v}$.

Rearranging $\mathbf{t_v}$ into a table yields estimated true results, corrected for differential exposure misclassification:

TABLE 10.28.

Family history of PD	Cases (Y_+)	Controls (Y_-)
+	30.9	12.9
−	102.1	106.1

in which $OR = 2.49$. The comparison of ORs suggests that some, but not all, of the observed association was due to family information bias.

Example 10-12. The U.S. Centers for Disease Control and Prevention (CDC) recommends that adults under age 65 years receive pneumococcal vaccine if they have any of several chronic health conditions, including heart disease. The CDC Behavioral Risk Factor Surveillance System (BRFSS, described in Chapter 6) gathers data on both pneumococcal vaccination status and history of myocardial infarction (MI) on a large sample of U.S. adults each year via telephone interviews. BRFSS data can thus be used to estimate pneumococcal vaccination coverage

for adults with and without a history of MI. Results of the 2012 BRFSS survey for adults aged 60–64 years are shown in Table 10.29, after applying survey weights to obtain estimates for all U.S. adults in that age group.

The results suggest that only about half of adults in this age group with a history of MI had received pneumococcal vaccination. On the other hand, coverage among them was about 21 percentage points higher than in comparably aged adults without such a history.

However, both self-reported history of MI and self-reported receipt of pneumococcal vaccine must be assumed subject to misclassification in a telephone survey. Two studies separate from BRFSS investigated the validity of self-reported history of MI and of self-reported history of pneumococcal vaccination in other settings. Okura *et al.* (2004) compared self-reported history of MI against medical records (the gold standard) for a sample of adult residents of Olmsted County, Minnesota, and found that self-report had sensitivity = 0.895 and specificity = 0.982. In another study, Shenson *et al.* (2005) compared self-reported pneumococcal vaccination status against Medicare claims data for a sample of older adults in a four-county area in the northeastern United States. They found that self-report had sensitivity = 0.75 and specificity = 0.83.

If results of those two validation studies are assumed to hold for BRFSS respondents, two misclassification matrices can be constructed, one for E (call it $\mathbf{C_E}$) and one for Y (call it $\mathbf{C_Y}$). The $\mathbf{C_E}$

TABLE 10.29.

History of MI	Yes (Y_+)	No (Y_-)	Percent vaccinated
+	741,584	658,788	53.0%
−	5,029,022	10,668,621	32.0%

Reported having had pneumococcal vaccination

TABLE 10.30.

$\mathbf{C_E}$ Measured	True E_+Y_+	E_+Y_-	E_-Y_+	E_-Y_-	$\mathbf{C_Y}$ Measured	True E_+Y_+	E_+Y_-	E_-Y_+	E_-Y_-
E_+Y_+	0.895	0	0.018	0	E_+Y_+	0.75	0.17	0	0
E_+Y_-	0	0.895	0	0.018	E_+Y_-	0.25	0.83	0	0
E_-Y_+	0.105	0	0.982	0	E_-Y_+	0	0	0.75	0.17
E_-Y_-	0	0.105	0	0.982	E_-Y_-	0	0	0.25	0.83

TABLE 10.31.

$$\begin{bmatrix} 0.671 & 0.152 & 0.014 & 0.003 \\ 0.224 & 0.743 & 0.005 & 0.015 \\ 0.079 & 0.018 & 0.736 & 0.167 \\ 0.026 & 0.087 & 0.245 & 0.815 \end{bmatrix}^{-1} \times \begin{bmatrix} 741,584 \\ 658,788 \\ 5,029,022 \\ 10,668,621 \end{bmatrix} = \begin{bmatrix} 888,549 \\ 357,297 \\ 4,049,284 \\ 11,802,885 \end{bmatrix}$$

matrix assumes no misclassification on Y, while the $\mathbf{C_Y}$ matrix assumes no misclassification on E. Here, misclassification is also assumed to be nondifferential on both E and Y (see Table 10.30).

If misclassification of E and of Y is further assumed to be statistically independent, then an overall misclassification matrix $\mathbf{C}$ that reflects misclassification of both variables can be computed with matrix multiplication as $\mathbf{C} = \mathbf{C_E} \cdot \mathbf{C_Y}$. The resulting $\mathbf{C}$ is the square matrix shown in Table 10.31. A doubly corrected table of results can then be obtained by applying Equation (10.5) as shown in Table 10.31.

This estimate of $\mathbf{t_v}$ can be rearranged as:

TABLE 10.32.

History of MI	Had pneumococcal vaccination Yes	No	Percent vaccinated
+	888,549	357,297	71.3%
−	4,049,284	11,802,885	25.5%

Compared to the uncorrected results, Table 10.32 suggests somewhat higher true vaccine coverage among adults aged 60–64 with a history of MI, and a larger difference between those with and without such a history.

Comments on the Method

In principle, the misclassification-matrix method described above can be extended to accommodate exposures or outcomes with more than two levels, or simultaneous misclassification of additional variables, such as confounders or effect modifiers (Greenland and Kleinbaum, 1983). The misclassification matrix $\mathbf{C}$ would then have one row and column for each possible combination of E, Y, and possibly other variables. In practice, however, the price paid is that many more p estimates must be supplied and/or many more assumptions made about whether misclassification is differential or nondifferential for each variable and whether the misclassification probabilities are statistically independent.

The method as described above yields only point estimates. Obtaining confidence limits is complicated by the fact that both the original data and the *p*s are subject to sampling error (Greenland, 1988, 2008). Multiple imputation provides another approach to this issue (Cole *et al.*, 2006).

Special care is needed when using the misclassification-matrix method to correct for possible outcome misclassification in case-control studies, because the distribution of *Y* in the study sample differs from that in the source population due to case-control sampling (Jurek *et al.*, 2013). A parallel caveat would also apply when correcting for exposure misclassification in cohort studies in which the distribution of *E* differs from that in the source population due to unequal sampling of exposed and non-exposed persons.

Because the operating characteristics of a measure can vary in relation to many factors, there is often uncertainty about the extent to which external estimates apply in the study at hand. *Sensitivity analysis* (in which "sensitivity" refers to the degree to which results change depending on the values of particular inputs or assumptions that are subject to uncertainty) can be used along with methods for the correction of measurement error (Fox *et al.*, 2005; Lash and Fink, 2003).

NOTES

1. For example, in the public-domain statistical language **R**, one can enter: `mv <- C %*% tv`. In Stata, `matrix mv = C * tv`.
2. In **R**, using the built-in `solve` function: `tv <- solve(C, mv)`. In Stata, `matrix tv = INV(C) * mv`.
3. In actuality, controls were matched to cases, but matching is ignored here because data needed to reconstruct the matched analysis were not reported in the article.

REFERENCES

Barron BA. The effects of misclassification on the estimation of relative risk. Biometrics 1977; 33:414–418.

Boppana SB, Ross SA, Novak Z, Shimamura M, Tolan RW Jr, Palmer AL, *et al.* Dried blood spot real-time polymerase chain reaction assays to screen newborns for congenital cytomegalovirus infection. JAMA 2010; 303:1375–1382.

Brenner H, Gefeller O. Variation of sensitivity, specificity, likelihood ratios, and predictive values with disease prevalence. Stat Med 1997; 16:981–991.

Brenner H, Greenland S, Savitz DA. The effects of nondifferential confounder misclassification in ecologic studies. Epidemiology 1992; 3:456–459.

Brenner H, Kliebsch U. Dependence of weighted kappa coefficients on the number of categories. Epidemiology 1996; 7:199–202.

Brown DL, Al-Senani F, Lisabeth LD, Farnie MA, Colletti LA, Langa KM, *et al.* Defining cause of death in stroke patients: The Brain Attack Surveillance in Corpus Christi project. Am J Epidemiol 2007; 165:591–596.

Chambless LE, Diao G. Estimation of time-dependent area under the ROC curve for long-term risk prediction. Stat Med 2006; 25:3474–3486.

Chen TT. A review of methods for misclassified categorical data in epidemiology. Stat Med 1989; 8:1095–106; discussion 1107–1108.

Cohen J. A coefficient of agreement for nominal scales. Educ Psychol Meas 1960; 20:37–46.

Cole SR, Chu H, Greenland S. Multiple-imputation for measurement-error correction. Int J Epidemiol 2006; 35:1074–1081.

Coughlin SS, Trock B, Criqui MH, Pickle LW, Browner D, Tefft MC. The logistic modeling of sensitivity, specificity, and predictive value of a diagnostic test. J Clin Epidemiol 1992; 45:1–7.

Daling JR, Weiss NS, Hislop TG, Maden C, Coates RJ, Sherman KJ, *et al.* Sexual practices, sexually transmitted diseases, and the incidence of anal cancer. N Engl J Med 1987; 317:973–977.

Daling JR, Weiss NS, Klopfenstein LL, Cochran LE, Chow WH, Daifuku R. Correlates of homosexual behavior and the incidence of anal cancer. JAMA 1982; 247:1988–1990.

Darby SC, Ewart DW, Giangrande PL, Spooner RJ, Rizza CR, Dusheiko GM, *et al.* Mortality from liver cancer and liver disease in haemophilic men and boys in UK given blood products contaminated with hepatitis C. Lancet 1997; 350:1425–1431.

Deeks JJ, Altman DG. Diagnostic tests 4: likelihood ratios. BMJ 2004; 329:168–169.

Elbaz A, McDonnell SK, Maraganore DM, Strain KJ, Schaid DJ, Bower JH, *et al.* Validity of family history data on PD: evidence for a family information bias. Neurology 2003; 61:11–17.

Ewer AK, Middleton LJ, Furmston AT, Bhoyar A, Daniels JP, Thangaratinam S, *et al.* Pulse oximetry screening for congenital heart defects in newborn infants (PulseOx): a test accuracy study. Lancet 2011; 378:785–794.

Flegal KM, Brownie C, Haas JD. The effects of exposure misclassification on estimates of relative risk. Am J Epidemiol 1986; 123:736–751.

Fleiss JL. The design and analysis of clinical experiments. New York: Wiley and Sons, 1986.

Fleiss JL, Levin B, Paik MC. Statistical methods for rates and proportions (3rd ed.). New York: Wiley and Sons, 2003.

Fox MP, Lash TL, Greenland S. A method to automate probabilistic sensitivity analyses of misclassified binary variables. Int J Epidemiol 2005; 34:1370–1376.

Frank D, DeBenedetti AF, Volk RJ, Williams EC, Kivlahan DR, Bradley KA. Effectiveness of the AUDIT-C as a screening test for alcohol misuse in three race/ethnic groups. J Gen Intern Med 2008; 23:781–787.

Gable CB, Holzer SS, Engelhart L, Friedman RB, Smeltz F, Schroeder D, et al. Pneumococcal vaccine. Efficacy and associated cost savings. JAMA 1990; 264:2910–2915.

Gallagher EJ. Clinical utility of likelihood ratios. Ann Emerg Med 1998; 31:391–397.

Greenland S. Variance estimation for epidemiologic effect estimates under misclassification. Stat Med 1988; 7:745–757.

Greenland S. Maximum-likelihood and closed-form estimators of epidemiologic measures under misclassification. J Stat Planning Infer 2008; 138:528–538.

Greenland S, Kleinbaum DG. Correcting for misclassification in two-way tables and matched-pair studies. Int J Epidemiol 1983; 12:93–97. [Correction in Int J Epidemiol 1988; 17:700]

Gustafson P. Measurement error and misclassification in statistics and epidemiology: impacts and Bayesian adjustments. New York: Chapman and Hall, 2004.

Hall MC, Kieke B, Gonzales R, Belongia EA. Spectrum bias of a rapid antigen detection test for group A beta-hemolytic streptococcal pharyngitis in a pediatric population. Pediatrics 2004; 114:182–186.

Hanley JA, McNeil BJ. The meaning and use of the area under a receiver operating characteristic (ROC) curve. Radiology 1982; 143:29–36.

Hanley JA, McNeil BJ. A method of comparing the areas under receiver operating characteristic curves derived from the same cases. Radiology 1983; 148:839–843.

Harbord RM, Whiting P, Sterne JAC, Egger M, Deeks JJ, Shang A, et al. An empirical comparison of methods for meta-analysis of diagnostic accuracy showed hierarchical models are necessary. J Clin Epidemiol 2008; 61:1095–1103.

Heagerty PJ, Lumley T, Pepe MS. Time-dependent ROC curves for censored survival data and a diagnostic marker. Biometrics 2000; 56:337–344.

Hui SL, Zhou XH. Evaluation of diagnostic tests without gold standards. Stat Meth Med Res 1998; 7:354–370.

Hurwitz ES, Barrett MJ, Bregman D, Gunn WJ, Pinsky P, Schonberger LB, et al. Public Health Service study of Reye's syndrome and medications. Report of the main study. JAMA 1987; 257:1905–1911.

Inouye SK, Foreman MD, Mion LC, Katz KH, Cooney LM Jr. Nurses' recognition of delirium and its symptoms: comparison of nurse and researcher ratings. Arch Intern Med 2001; 161:2467–2473.

Janes H, Pepe MS. Adjusting for covariates in studies of diagnostic, screening, or prognostic markers: an old concept in a new setting. Am J Epidemiol 2008; 168:89–97.

Jones CM, Athanasiou T. Summary receiver operating characteristic curve analysis techniques in the evaluation of diagnostic tests. Ann Thorac Surg 2005; 79:16–20.

Jurek AM, Maldonado G, Greenland S. Adjusting for outcome misclassification: the importance of accounting for case-control sampling and other forms of outcome-related selection. Ann Epidemiol 2013; 23:129–135.

Klebanoff MA, Levine RJ, DerSimonian R, Clemens JD, Wilkins DG. Maternal serum paraxanthine, a caffeine metabolite, and the risk of spontaneous abortion. N Engl J Med 1999; 341:1639–1644.

Landis JR, Koch GG. The measurement of observer agreement for categorical data. Biometrics 1977; 33:159–174.

Lash TL, Fink AK. Semi-automated sensitivity analysis to assess systematic errors in observational data. Epidemiology 2003; 14:451–458.

Maclure M, Willett WC. Misinterpretation and misuse of the kappa statistic. Am J Epidemiol 1987; 126:161–169.

Morrissey MJ, Spiegelman D. Matrix methods for estimating odds ratios with misclassified exposure data: extensions and comparisons. Biometrics 1999; 55:338–344.

Naeger DM, Kohi MP, Webb EM, Phelps A, Ordovas KG, Newman TB. Correctly using sensitivity, specificity, and predictive values in clinical practice: how to avoid three common pitfalls. AJR Am J Roentgenol 2013; 200:W566–W570.

Nelson JC, Pepe MS. Statistical description of interrater variability in ordinal ratings. Stat Meth Med Res 2000; 9:475–496.

Okura Y, Urban LH, Mahoney DW, Jacobsen SJ, Rodeheffer RJ. Agreement between self-report questionnaires and medical record data was substantial for diabetes, hypertension, myocardial infarction and stroke but not for heart failure. J Clin Epidemiol 2004; 57:1096–1103.

Pepe MS. The statistical evaluation of medical tests for classification and prediction. New York: Oxford, 2003.

Pepe MS, Janes H, Longton G, Leisenring W, Newcomb P. Limitations of the odds ratio in gauging the performance of a diagnostic, prognostic, or screening marker. Am J Epidemiol 2004; 159:882–890.

Pepe MS, Longton G. Standardizing diagnostic markers to evaluate and compare their performance. Epidemiology 2005; 16:598–603.

Ransohoff DF, Feinstein AR. Problems of spectrum and bias in evaluating the efficacy of diagnostic tests. N Engl J Med 1978; 299:926–930.

Reitsma JB, Rutjes AWS, Khan KS, Coomarasamy A, Bossuyt PM. A review of solutions for diagnostic accuracy studies with an imperfect or missing reference standard. J Clin Epidemiol 2009; 62:797–806.

Rimon E, Levy S, Sapir A, Gelzer G, Peled R, Ergas D, et al. Diagnosis of iron deficiency anemia in the elderly by transferrin receptor-ferritin index. Arch Intern Med 2002; 162:445–449.

Rosner B. Fundamentals of biostatistics (6th ed.). New York: Duxbury Press, 2006.

Sackett DL. Bias in analytic research. J Chronic Dis 1979; 32:51–63.

Shapiro DE. The interpretation of diagnostic tests. Stat Methods Med Res 1999; 8:113–134.

Shenson D, Dimartino D, Bolen J, Campbell M, Lu PJ, Singleton JA. Validation of self-reported pneumococcal vaccination in behavioral risk factor surveillance surveys: experience from the Sickness Prevention Achieved Through Regional Collaboration (SPARC) program. Vaccine 2005; 23:1015–1020.

Stoler MH, Schiffman M. Interobserver reproducibility of cervical cytologic and histologic interpretations. Realistic estimates from the ASCUS-LSIL Triage Study. JAMA 2001; 285:1500–1505.

Taubes G. Epidemiology Monitor 1996; 17:1–14.

Thomas D, Stram D, Dwyer J. Exposure measurement error: influence on exposure–disease relationships and methods of correction. Annu Rev Public Health 1993; 14:69–93.

Thomas DC. Re: "When will nondifferential misclassification of an exposure preserve the direction of a trend?" Am J Epidemiol 1995; 142:782–783.

Thompson IM, Ankerst DP, Chi C, Lucia MS, Goodman PJ, Crowley JJ, et al. Operating characteristics of prostate-specific antigen in men with an initial PSA level of 3.0 ng/ml or lower. JAMA 2005; 294:66–70.

Thompson WD. Kappa and attenuation of the odds ratio. Epidemiology 1990; 1:357–369.

Thompson WD, Walter SD. Variance and dissent. A reappraisal of the kappa coefficient. J Clin Epidemiol 1988; 41:949–958.

Thürigen D, Spiegelman D, Blettner M, Heuer C, Brenner H. Measurement error correction using validation data: a review of methods and their applicability in case-control studies. Stat Methods Med Res 2000; 9:447–474.

Treutlein J, Cichon S, Ridinger M, Wodarz N, Soyka M, Zill P, et al. Genome-wide association study of alcohol dependence. Arch Gen Psychiatry 2009; 66:773–784.

Walter SD. Properties of the summary receiver operating characteristic (SROC) curve for diagnostic test data. Stat Med 2002; 21:1237–1256.

Walter SD, Irwig LM. Estimation of test error rates, disease prevalence and relative risk from misclassified data: a review. J Clin Epidemiol 1988; 41:923–937.

White E, Armstrong BK, Saracci R. Principles of exposure measurement in epidemiology: collecting, evaluating, and improving measures of disease risk factors (2nd ed.). New York: Oxford, 2008.

Zhou XH, Obuchowski NA, McClish DK. Statistical methods in diagnostic medicine (2nd ed.). New York: Wiley and Sons, 2011.

EXERCISES

1. Delirium is a common but often unrecognized problem among hospitalized older adults. Recognizing it can be important for treatment. A study in New Haven, Connecticut, compared assessment of delirium between physicians and nurses on 2,721 older inpatients (Inouye *et al.*, 2001). Each patient was classified by a physician and separately by a nurse as having delirium or not. The results were as follows:

TABLE 10.33.

Nurse	Physician		Total
	Delirium	No delirium	
Delirium	46	105	151
No delirium	193	2,377	2,570
Total	239	2,482	2,721

(a) What percentage of the time did the physicians and nurses agree in their ratings?

(b) Given the overall frequency with which physicians and nurses rated these patients as having delirium, how much agreement would one expect just by chance?

(c) Calculate kappa. How good is this level of concordance after correcting for chance agreement?

TABLE 10.34.

First pathologist's interpretation	Second pathologist's interpretation				
	Negative	ASCUS	LSIL	$\geq$HSIL	Total
Negative	1,325	322	52	8	1,707
ASCUS	568	633	245	27	1,473
LSIL	57	292	908	78	1,335
$\geq$HSIL	14	98	117	204	433
Total	1,964	1,345	1,322	317	4,948

2. As part of a randomized trial of alternative strategies for treatment of low-grade abnormalities on cervical cytology, Stoler and Schiffman (2001) collected a cervical cytology specimen on each of 4,948 women referred to the trial. Monolayer cytology preparations were evaluated independently by two highly trained pathologists. Each pathologist then assigned each specimen to one of four categories:

- Negative
- ASCUS: atypical squamous cells of undetermined significance
- LSIL: low-grade squamous intraepithelial lesion
- $\geq$HSIL: high-grade squamous intraepithelial lesion, or more advanced disease

The results are shown in Table 10.34. How would you summarize quantitatively the reproducibility of the pathologists' interpretations?

3. Iron deficiency anemia can be diagnosed definitively by the absence of iron stores in a bone-marrow aspirate. However, bone marrow aspiration is a painful, fairly invasive procedure. For research purposes, Rimon et al. (2002) obtained bone-marrow aspirates on 63 older adults on a geriatric care unit, 49 of whom proved to have iron deficiency anemia.

On ordinary venous blood samples from the same patients, the investigators also performed three routine tests (serum iron, transferrin saturation, and serum ferritin) and a new test based on a transferrin receptor level assay, the *transferrin receptor–ferritin index* (TR-F index). The correspondence between test results and bone marrow aspirate results was as shown in Table 10.35.

(a) What were the sensitivity and specificity of the new TR-F index using a cutoff value of 1.5? How did they compare with the sensitivity and specificity of the combined three routine tests?

(b) The sensitivity of the composite result of three routine tests was very low. Can you suggest a way

TABLE 10.35.

Test and result	Iron deficiency anemia, by bone marrow aspiration	
	Present	Absent
Composite of routine tests		
Positive[a]	8	0
Negative	41	14
TR-F index		
> 1.5	43	1
$\leq$ 1.5	6	13

[a] All three routine tests abnormal

to increase the sensitivity of the composite result by combining information from the three component tests in a different way?

4. As part of the Collaborative Perinatal Project (a prospective study of pregnancy, labor, and, child development conducted in the United States from 1959 to 1966), serum samples were obtained from approximately 42,000 women at the beginning of their pregnancy. Serum samples from the 591 women who subsequently experienced a spontaneous abortion during that pregnancy, and a matched sample of 2,558 controls, were assayed for levels of paraxanthine (a metabolite of caffeine). The results are summarized in Figure 10.4, based on Klebanoff et al. (1999).

The half-life of paraxanthine in serum is approximately five hours. Therefore, serum paraxanthine is a marker only of short-term caffeine intake, so the values obtained on the samples of these subjects may not mirror those present when the events leading to the spontaneous abortion took place. Had the "relevant" levels of serum paraxanthine been possible to obtain—e.g., long-term levels, or levels closer to the

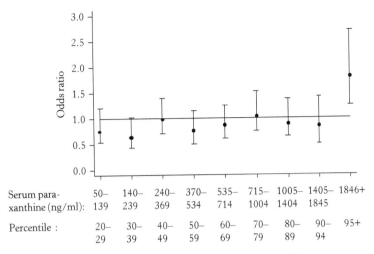

FIGURE 10.4 Odds ratio for spontaneous abortion in relation to serum paraxanthine.

time when the pathology leading to this spontaneous abortion occurred—would you anticipate the odds ratio associated with a value of more than 1845 ng/ml to be greater than, the same as, or less than the odds ratio of 1.9 observed in this study? Why?

5. Group A β-hemolytic streptococcus (GABHS) infection is one of many causes of sore throat in children. Unlike viral sore throat, GABHS infection is treatable with antibiotics. If left untreated, it can evolve into rheumatic fever.

The definitive test for GABHS is a positive throat culture for the organism. However, it takes time for the organism to grow, and the culture result is not normally available until about 48 hours after specimen collection. This time lag creates extra work for clinic staff to track down the parent of a culture-positive child, and it can delay initiation of antibiotic therapy. Accordingly, there has been much interest in developing a test that can correctly identify a child with GABHS infection at the time of the initial clinical evaluation. Two candidates, the Centor score and the Rapid Antigen Detection Test (RADT), were evaluated in a study involving 561 children with sore throat's at a large primary care clinic in Marshfield, Wisconsin (Hall *et al.*, 2004).

(a) The Centor score is based on four clinical features: (1) a history of fever; (2) absence of cough; (3) presence of pharyngeal or tonsillar exudate on examination of the throat; and (4) presence of tender anterior cervical lymph nodes. Each feature is worth 1 point, and a child's Centor score is the total number of points. (In this study, the Centor score was slightly modified to count any mention of cervical lymph node enlargement as positive, with or without tenderness.) The

following table summarizes the modified Centor score results in relation to whether a child was ultimately found to have GABHS:

TABLE 10.36.

Centor score	Final diagnosis	
	GABHS	Not GABHS
0	19	87
1	31	164
2	51	106
3 or 4	51	52
Total	152	409

In this table, a child's final diagnosis was actually based on a combination of evidence from the throat culture and the RADT, as described later. For our purposes, assume that this final diagnosis was error-free. Calculate the sensitivity and specificity of the Centor score at cutoffs of 0, 1, 2, and 3 or 4. Use the rule that any score equal to or greater than the cutoff is considered positive.

(b) The RADT is an immunochromatographic dipstick assay, performed on a swab that has been applied to the back of the throat and both tonsils. If the dipstick turns color, the test is positive. If the dipstick does not change color, the test is negative. According to the manufacturer, the RADT has a sensitivity of 96.0% and a specificity of 97.8%.

At the study clinic, if the RADT was positive, the child was considered to have GABHS infection, and no throat culture was obtained.

If the RADT was negative, another throat swab was obtained and sent for culture. If that throat culture was positive, the child was considered to have GABHS infection despite the initial negative RADT. If the RADT and the throat culture were both negative, the child was considered not to have GABHS infection.

Overall, 117 of the 561 children tested had a positive RADT. Of those with a negative RADT, 35 had a positive throat culture. From these data, can you calculate the sensitivity and specificity of the RADT? If so, do so; if not, explain briefly why not.

6. Assume you have conducted two case-control studies of the efficacy of seat belt use against the incidence of a skeletal fracture among persons involved in an automobile crash. The studies were done a number of years apart, in 1975 and 1990, and the prevalence of seat belt use was greater in the more recent of the two. The "cases" in each study were persons who sustained a fracture in a car crash. "Controls" were persons in crashes that were identical to those in which the cases were involved (in terms of such characteristics as vehicle speed and vehicle type) who did not sustain a fracture and who were similar to the cases in terms of demographic and other characteristics that influence the likelihood of fracture.

Assume that in each of the two studies, in which 1000 cases and 1000 controls had been enrolled, the "correct" data (i.e., those that would have been obtained had there been no misclassification) were as shown in Table 10.37.

(a) What would be the odds ratio for each of the two years relating use of seat belts to fracture risk in the absence of any misclassification?
(b) What would the two odds ratios be if 10% of both cases and controls who were unbelted reported, incorrectly, having worn a seat belt at the time

of the crash (i.e., 90% specificity of the ascertainment modality)?
(c) What would these odds ratios be if misclassification arose exclusively from the ascertainment modality being only 90% sensitive; i.e., if 10% of the cases and controls who truly had worn a belt were labeled as unbelted?

When misclassification of exposure status is present, why do the odds ratios obtained in the study conducted in 1975 differ from the corresponding odds ratios obtained in 1990?

ANSWERS

1. (a) They agreed $\frac{46 + 2,377}{2,721} \times 100\% = 89.0\%$ of the time. Call this proportion P_o.

(b) The proportion expected to agree by chance (P_e) can be calculated as follows:

$$P_e = \frac{\dfrac{151 \times 239}{2,721} + \dfrac{2,570 \times 2,482}{2,721}}{2,721} = 0.866$$

Overall, physicians rated $239/2,721 = 0.088 = 8.8\%$ of patients as having delirium, while nurses rated $151/2,721 = 0.055 = 5.5\%$ of patients as having delirium. Just by chance, then, one would expect $0.088 \times 0.055 \times 2,721 = 13.3$ patients to be rated as having delirium by both the physician and the nurse. Similarly, one would expect $(1 - 0.088) \times (1 - 0.055) \times 2,721 = 2,344.3$ patients to be rated as having delirium by *neither* the physician nor the nurse just by chance. Hence the level of agreement expected by chance would be $(13.3 + 2,344.3)/2,721 = 0.866 = 86.6\%$.

(c) $\kappa = \dfrac{P_o - P_e}{1 - P_e} = \dfrac{0.890 - 0.866}{1 - 0.866} = 0.18$

TABLE 10.37. TRUE ASSOCIATION BETWEEN SEAT BELT USE AND CASE-CONTROL STATUS, BY YEAR

Seat belt use	Correct data, 1975	
	Cases	Controls
Yes	50	100
No	950	900
Seat belt use	Correct data, 1990	
	Cases	Controls
Yes	322	500
No	678	500

Using the descriptor from Table 10.3, this represents only *slight* agreement between physicians and nurses beyond what chance alone could explain.

2. One approach is to treat the pathologists' interpretation as a four-category nominal scale, with no ordering of the categories. The concordance between pathologists was $(1,325 + 633 + 908 + 204)/4,948 = 0.620$, implying that the they agreed with each other's interpretations 62% of the time.

Because some of this agreement could be due to chance, however, kappa would also be appropriate. The concordance expected by chance, obtained using equation 10.2, was 0.296. Kappa can be calculated as $(0.620 - 0.296)/(1 - 0.296) = 0.461$, indicating a moderate level of agreement.

Another reasonable approach is to treat the four-category scale of interpretations as being ordered as to degree of abnormality, from "none" to "highly abnormal". This view of the data lends itself to using weighted kappa. Using the weighting scheme described in Equation 10.3, $p_o = 0.938$, $p_e = 0.790$, and $\kappa_w = 0.705$. The weighted kappa (κ_w) value is higher than the unweighted kappa value because the former gives partial credit for relatively small discrepancies of one or two categories, which were common here.

3. (a) The sensitivity of the TR-F index was $43/49 = 0.878$, compared with $8/49 = 0.163$ for the routine tests. The specificity of the TR-F index was $13/14 = 0.929$, compared with $14/14 = 1.000$ for the routine tests. Hence the new test was much more sensitive than the routine ones for iron deficiency anemia, but a bit less specific.

   (b) The investigators scored the composite test as positive only if *all three* component tests were abnormal. One could almost certainly increase the sensitivity of this composite test by scoring it as positive if *any one* of the three component tests was abnormal. This change in the scoring rule might decrease its specificity, however.

4. If the "relevant" serum levels were correctly classified, one would expect that the resulting OR would be greater than 1.9. The use of the nondifferentially misclassified value of serum paraxanthine for each subject is expected to produce a result spuriously close to the null.

5. (a) It is helpful to create columns showing the number of children who would be classified as positive at each score level, since these numbers are needed to calculate sensitivity and specificity at each score level. The number of positives at a certain score level would be the total number of GABHS cases with that score or

greater—i.e., in or below that row of the original table. The results are shown in Table 10.38.

Finally, the sensitivity for each row is $a/152$, and the specificity is $(409 - b)/409$. See Table 10.39.

TABLE 10.38.

| Cutoff on Centor score | No. with positive test | |
	GABHS (a)	Not GABHS (b)
0	152	409
1	133	322
2	102	158
3 or 4	51	52

(b) Accurate sensitivity and specificity estimates for the RADT cannot be obtained from these results for lack of an independent gold standard result on all children. Here, the gold standard, throat culture, was performed only if the RADT was negative. Consider Table 10.40. Sensitivity is defined as $a/(a+c)$, but we do not have a value for a. (We do know that $a + b = 117$, but we do not know how many of the positive RADTs were true positives and how many were false positives.) Specificity is defined as $d/(b+d)$, but we do not have a value for b, for the same reason.

Although we cannot obtain a good point estimate for sensitivity or specificity, it is nonetheless possible to conclude that the manufacturer's claim of 96.0% sensitivity is too high, at least for the RADT as applied in the study setting. To see this, start with the definition of sensitivity: $a/(a+c)$. We know that $c = 35$, because 35 of the children with a negative RADT had a positive throat culture. We also know that there were 117 positive RADTs, so $a + b = 117$. Thus, $0 \leq a \leq 117$, and sensitivity must fall between $0/(0 + 35) = 0$ and $117/(117 + 35) = 0.77$. Even at the highest possible value compatible with these data (0.77), the RADT's sensitivity falls well below that claimed by the manufacturer.

Now consider specificity = $d/(b+d)$. We know that 117 children had a positive RADT, so the remaining 444 had a negative RADT and hence received a throat culture. Of these, 35 had a positive throat culture, and $444 - 35 = 409$ had a negative throat culture. Thus, $d = 409$. As before, we know that there were 117 positive RADTs overall, so $0 \leq b \leq 117$. Specificity must

TABLE 10.39.

Cutoff on Centor score	No. with positive test		Sensitivity	Specificity
	GABHS	Not GABHS		
0	152	409	1.000	0.000
1	133	322	0.875	0.213
2	102	158	0.671	0.614
3 or 4	51	52	0.336	0.873

TABLE 10.40.

RADT	Throat culture	
	+	−
+	a	b
−	c	d

TABLE 10.41. SEAT BELT USE IN RELATION TO CASE-CONTROL STATUS UNDER MISCLASSIFICATION

Year	Seat belts	Truth		Misclassified exposure status: Sensitivity of interview = 100% Specificity of interview = 90%		Misclassified exposure status: Sensitivity of interview = 90% Specificity of interview = 100%	
		Cases	Controls	Cases	Controls	Cases	Controls
1975	Yes	50	100	$50 + 95 = 145$	$100 + 90 = 190$	$50 - 5 = 45$	$100 - 10 = 90$
	No	950	900	$950 - 95 = 855$	$900 - 90 = 810$	$950 + 5 = 955$	$900 + 10 = 910$
	$OR = \dfrac{50/950}{100/900} = 0.47$			$OR = \dfrac{145/855}{190/810} = 0.72$		$OR = \dfrac{45/955}{90/910} = 0.48$	
1990	Yes	322	500	$322 + 68 = 390$	$500 + 50 = 550$	$322 - 32 = 290$	$500 - 50 = 450$
	No	678	500	$678 - 68 = 610$	$500 - 50 = 450$	$678 + 32 = 710$	$500 + 50 = 550$
	$OR = \dfrac{322/678}{500/500} = 0.47$			$OR = \dfrac{390/610}{450/550} = 0.52$		$OR = \dfrac{290/710}{550/450} = 0.50$	

therefore lie between $409/(117 + 409) = .778$ and $409/(0 + 409) = 1.000$. The manufacturer's claim about specificity falls within this range, so the data do not refute it.

6. The true odds ratio relating seat belt use to skeletal fracture is 0.47 in each year (Table 10.41). If the method of ascertaining seat belt use were 90% *specific*, the odds ratio (OR) observed in the earlier study would be more biased (towards the null) by nondifferential misclassification than the OR in the later study, since the absolute number of misclassified individuals would be greater in the earlier study. The impact of less-than-perfect specificity of the criterion

for exposure leads to a larger number of misclassified subjects when the exposure frequency is low (e.g., seat belt use in 1975) than when it is high (e.g., in 1990). When the *sensitivity* is 90%, the observed odds ratios are relatively close to the true value of 0.47. Nonetheless, the 1990 analysis is more biased than that for 1975, since the absolute number of individuals misclassified regarding seat belt use was greater in 1990.

Moral: The impact of misclassification of exposure status depends not only on the relative degree of misclassification, but on the relative size of that part of the study population in which the misclassification is present.

11

Confounding and Its Control: Basic

Confounding occurs in epidemiologic research when the measured association between an exposure and disease occurrence is distorted by an imbalance between exposed and non-exposed persons with regard to one or more other risk factors for the disease. An example of likely confounding is the association between low blood levels of beta-carotene and an increased incidence of several types of cancer observed in a number of cohort and case-control studies. Persons randomized to receive supplements of beta-carotene do not have a lower incidence of these cancers than persons randomized to receive a placebo (Alpha-Tocopherol, Beta Carotene Cancer Prevention Study Group, 1994; Omenn *et al.*, 1996), so it is likely that the association present in the non-randomized studies is due to confounding. Perhaps one or more nutrients contained in the same foods in which beta-carotene is found protect against the development of the cancers in question, rather than beta-carotene itself.

RATE ADJUSTMENT
Rationale and Mechanics

To see in a quantitative way how confounding operates, as well as one of the ways in which confounding can be dealt with, consider the following hypothetical example. Let us say you have obtained mortality rates for a one-year period for two communities: Community A, located in the developed world, and Community B, located in the developing world. You would like to compare these rates. Characteristic of many communities in the developing world at present, Community B has a young population relative to that of Community A. Reviewing the data shown in Table 11.1, you observe that within each of the three age groups for which data are available, the mortality rates in Community B are exactly double those of Community A.

The rates for persons of all ages combined were obtained by simply dividing the total number of deaths in each community by the size of the total population: 66/9,000 = 7.3 per 1,000 person-years in Community A, and 70/10,000 = 7.0 per 1,000 person-years in Community B. In this example, a comparison of rates obtained in this way—termed "crude" rates—provides what at first glance may be surprising: the overall mortality rate in Community B is not twice that of Community A, as it is for individuals within each of the three age categories. In fact, it is less than that of Community A (7.0 versus 7.3 per 1000 person-years)! The explanation for the disparity between comparisons of crude and age-specific rates lies in:

- The relationsip of age to mortality rates—in both communities these rates rise sharply with increasing age; and
- The difference in the age distribution of the two communities—on average, persons in A are older than those in B.

The crude rates permit the differences in mortality by age to be mixed in with (confound) the community-related differences in mortality. Community A, with its relatively higher proportion of older (and therefore higher risk) persons is "penalized" in the comparison to Community B, so much so that the truly lower mortality rate present in residents of Community A at any given age is not only obscured when considering persons of all ages combined, it is reversed.

Armed with the data in the above table, however, it is possible by means of *adjustment*—also called *standardization*—to nullify the confounding effect of age. One approach to adjustment involves calculating what would have been the overall mortality rates

TABLE 11.1. MORTALITY RATES IN TWO HYPOTHETICAL
COMMUNITIES

| | Community A | | | Community B | | |
Age	No. of deaths	Mid-year population	Rate[a]	No. of deaths	Mid-year population	Rate[a]
Young	1	1,000	1	10	5,000	2
Middle	15	3,000	5	40	4,000	10
Old	50	5,000	10	20	1,000	20
Total	66	9,000	7.3	70	10,000	7.0

[a] Deaths per 1,000 person-years

in A and B if they had had the same age composition. It proceeds as follows:

1. Pick a reference population distribution. One way (of many) to do this is to combine the two populations:

TABLE 11.2.

Young = $1,000 + 5,000 = 6,000$
Middle = $3,000 + 4,000 = 7,000$
Old = $5,000 + 1,000 = 6,000$

2. Apply age-specific rates for each population under study to the reference population, and add up the expected deaths across the age categories. In this instance, one obtains the number of deaths that would be expected if the community's age-specific rates had operated on the reference population's size and age distribution.
3. Divide the number of expected deaths in each group by the reference population:

In the above calculations, the age disparity between the two communities has been eliminated.

TABLE 11.4.

Community A: $101/19,000 = 5.3$ per 1,000 person-years
Community B: $202/19,000 = 10.6$ per 1,000 person-years

The overall rates, now termed *age-adjusted* or *age-standardized rates*, are in the ratio of 2:1, exactly the ratio seen in the comparison of age-specific rates of the communities (Table 11.4).

As was noted in Chapter 4, the crude rate in each community is a weighted average of the age-specific rates in that community. But because in this example the age distributions of Community A and Community B differ, the weights for the age-specific rates also differ. In Community A, the rates for older people get relatively more weight because older people compose a larger proportion of Community A's population. In Community B, the rates for younger people get more weight. It is also possible to think of the adjustment process as the application of a standard set of "weights" to the category-specific rates in the exposure groups to be compared. In the present example, using as before the combined mid-year populations of the two communities to

TABLE 11.3.

| | Community A | | | Community B | | |
Rate[a]	Reference population	Expected deaths	Rate[a]	Reference population	Expected deaths	
1 ×	6,000	= 6	2 ×	6,000	= 12	
5 ×	7,000	= 35	10 ×	7,000	= 70	
10 ×	6,000	= 60	20 ×	6,000	= 120	
	19,000	101		19,000	202	

[a] Deaths per 1,000 person-years

derive the standard weights, the following would be obtained:

TABLE 11.5.

Age group	Standard weights
Young	$\frac{1,000 + 5,000}{19,000} = 0.316$
Middle	$\frac{3,000 + 4,000}{19,000} = 0.368$
Old	$\frac{5,000 + 1,000}{19,000} = 0.316$

Applying this set of weights to the age-specific rates observed in each community would produce the same pair of adjusted rates as before:

TABLE 11.6.

Community A			Community B		
Rate[a]	Weight		Rate[a]	Weight	
1	× 0.316	= 0.316	2	× 0.316	= 0.632
5	× 0.368	= 1.84	10	× 0.368	= 3.68
10	× 0.316	= 3.16	20	× 0.316	= 6.32
		5.3[a]			10.6[a]

[a] Deaths per 1,000 person-years

Choice of a Standard Population

The decision to use the combined mid-year populations of Community A and Community B was an arbitrary one. What would the results of rate adjustment have looked like had another age distribution been used? Here are two other sets of "weights" based on the respective age distributions of Community A and Community B.

TABLE 11.7.

Age	Standard population	
	Community A	Community B
Young	$1,000/9,000 = 0.111$	$5,000/10,000 = 0.50$
Middle	$3,000/9,000 = 0.333$	$4,000/10,000 = 0.40$
Old	$5,000/9,000 = 0.555$	$1,000/10,000 = 0.10$

The age-adjusted rates can be calculated using these weights instead:

TABLE 11.8.

Adjusted rate[a] in:	Standard population	
	Community A	Community B
Community A	7.33	3.5
Community B	14.65	7.0
Ratio (B/A)	2.0	2.0
Difference (B - A)	7.33	3.5

[a] Deaths per 1,000 person-years

The size of the adjusted rate in each community varies depending on the standard population chosen. Using the age distribution of A as the standard produces high absolute rates, (14.65 and 7.33 per 1000 person-years) because of the relatively great weight (0.555) given to the rates in older persons. Conversely, since the choice of B's age distribution as a standard assigns a weight of only 0.10 to the rates in older persons, the absolute rates in this case are smaller (7.0 and 3.5 per 1000 person-years). However, because the ratio of the rates is exactly 2.0 in each age category, the *ratio* of the age-adjusted rates is 2.0 no matter what age distribution is chosen to assign the weights.

In this example, because the difference in rates between the two communities is not constant across age categories, the size of the difference between the adjusted rates will be influenced by the choice of the standard:

- 7.33 per 1000 person-years if the age distribution of A is the standard;
- 3.5 per 1000 person-years if that of B is the standard.

There are situations in which it is desirable to compare lifetime cumulative incidence or lifetime cumulative mortality across populations with different age structures. In these situations, it is also necessary to incorporate adjustment for age to avoid introducing confounding. One approach (Day, 1976) simply involves adding age-specific rates across equal-size age strata to produce (for all but very common illnesses or causes of death) a good approximation of the cumulative incidence of (or mortality from) that condition through a given age, one that is standardized to a uniform age distribution. Another approach provides a "standardized lifetime risk" (Sasieni and Adams, 1999) by weighting the age-specific rates in a given population by the proportion of a standard population that survives until the end of each particular age interval.

Presentation of Results as Observed and Expected Number of Cases

Sometimes data such as those collected to describe mortality rates in Community A and Community B are summarized by: (1) indicating the observed number of deaths that occurred in B; and then (2) comparing that number to the one expected, had the age-specific rates in the comparison population, A, been present in a population of the same size and age distribution as B. The observed number of deaths in Community B is 70. The expected number, adjusted for age, is:

TABLE 11.9.

Mid-year population of B	Rate in A (per 1,000 person-years)	Expected number of deaths in B
5,000	1	5
4,000	5	20
1,000	10	10
		35

The ratio of the observed and expected number of deaths, called the *standardized mortality ratio* (SMR), is 70/35 = 2.0. Note that this calculation of the SMR is very similar to the calculation performed above of the adjusted rate using the age distribution of Community B as the standard population. To make the calculations identical, all that is needed is to divide the observed and expected numbers—70 and 35—by the size of the denominator—10,000 person-years—to arrive at the rates obtained earlier, 7.0 per 1000 person-years in B and 3.5 per 1000 person-years in A.

ADJUSTMENT OF RELATIVE RISKS AND ODDS RATIOS: DEALING WITH NON-UNIFORMITY OF THE SIZE OF THE OBSERVED ASSOCIATION ACROSS STRATA

If it is believed that the measure of interest (e.g., relative risk, risk difference) truly varies from stratum to stratum, it is not useful to obtain a summary estimate of this measure across strata, crude or standardized. Instead, the results should be presented for the individual strata separately. The observation of inter-stratum variation in the measure of interest does not necessarily mean there truly is variation, of course,

since chance can be an explanation for this as well. (A discussion of the bases for regarding observed inter-stratum variability in the size of an exposure–disease association as reflecting genuine effect modification appears in Chapter 18.) If, despite the presence of variation, there is no reason to believe that it is due to more than chance, it is reasonable to summarize across strata and, if necessary, adjust for the variable(s) that define the strata. But now, the choice of weights to be attached to the strata can make a difference in the estimate of the overall size of the association: If large weights are attached to the strata where the association is relatively large, the estimate will be greater than if small weights are chosen. What is a fair way to go about assigning stratum-specific weights in this circumstance?

The standardized mortality (or morbidity) ratio, SMR, often is used as the adjusted relative risk in occupational cohort studies, or in any cohort study in which the rates are to be compared between a relatively small exposed population and a much larger one (e.g., a national population). In calculating the SMR, the "weights" attached to the stratum-specific rates derive from the distribution of the confounding variable(s) in the exposed group. So, in the above example, thinking of residents of Community B as the "exposed" persons, it was their age distribution that served as the standard. This approach has the virtue of attaching the greatest "weights" to the strata that are numerically the largest in the exposed group. It avoids the possibility of having an externally derived set of weights inadvertently giving relatively great emphasis to a stratum with very few observations.

But in other cohort studies, and in virtually all case-control studies, the weights that provide the most statistically stable estimate will be obtained from all persons included in the study, both exposed and non-exposed. Specifically, the weight attached to each stratum should be in proportion to the inverse of its variance. A computationally easy method of approaching this was proposed by Mantel and Haenszel (1959) for case-control studies, and this method has been adapted for cohort studies as well. (For a discussion of other approaches to standardizing relative risks, see Rothman *et al.*, 2008, pp. 270–276.)

To illustrate how this method works, let us consider the data shown in Table 11.10 from three hypothetical studies of the incidence of coronary heart disease (CHD) in women of reproductive age in relation to current use of high-potency oral contraceptives (OCs). One is a study of a closed cohort

TABLE 11.10. DATA LAYOUT IN THREE HYPOTHETICAL STUDIES OF CHD INCIDENCE IN RELATION TO OC USE, BY PHYSICAL ACTIVITY STATUS

A. Example

Physical activity	Cumulative incidence study		Study with person-time data		Case-control study		
	CHD cases	No. of women	CHD cases	No. of person-years	CHD cases	Controls	Total
Sedentary							
OC users	6	29,000	6	29,000	6	29	
OC nonusers	3	44,000	3	44,000	3	44	
		73,000		73,000	9	73	82
Active							
OC users	7	57,000	7	57,000	7	57	
OC nonusers	1	33,000	1	33,000	1	33	
		90,000		90,000	8	90	98

B. General case

Potential confounder	Cases	No. of persons	Cases	Person-time	Cases	Control	Total
Stratum i							
Exposed	a_i	N_{i1}	a_i	T_{i1}	a_i	c_i	
Nonexposed	b_i	N_{i0}	b_i	T_{i0}	b_i	d_i	
		N_i		T_i	$a_i + b_i$	$c_i + d_i$	N_i

of women in which we seek to estimate the cumulative incidence of CHD in OC users relative to that in nonusers. The second deals with person-time data, and seeks to estimate the relative incidence rates. The third is a case-control study in which the odds ratio is to be calculated as an estimate of the relative risk. In each study there is the same confounding factor, physical activity, for which adjustment has to be made.

In the "General case" panel of Table 11-10, in the ith stratum:

a_i = No. of exposed cases

b_i = No. of non-exposed cases

N_{i1} = No. of exposed persons

N_{i0} = No. of non-exposed persons

N_i = Total no. of persons

T_{i1} = Amount of person-time among the exposed

T_{i0} = Amount of person-time among the non-exposed

T_i = Total person-time

c_i = No. of exposed controls

d_i = No. of non-exposed controls

The adjusted relative risk, adjusted relative rate and adjusted relative odds, are calculated as follows:
Cumulative incidence study:

Adjusted relative risk

$$= \frac{\sum_i a_i \cdot N_{i0}/N_i}{\sum_i b_i \cdot N_{i1}/N_i}$$

$$= \frac{6 \cdot 44,000/73,000 + 7 \cdot 33,000/90,000}{3 \cdot 29,000/73,000 + 1 \cdot 57,000/90,000}$$

$$= 3.39$$

Study with person-time data:

Adjusted rate ratio

$$= \frac{\sum_i a_i \cdot T_{i0}/T_i}{\sum_i b_i \cdot T_{i1}/T_i}$$

$$= \frac{6 \cdot 44,000/73,000 + 7 \cdot 33,000/90,000}{3 \cdot 29,000/73,000 + 1 \cdot 57,000/90,000}$$

$$= 3.39$$

Case-control study:

$$\text{Adjusted odds ratio} = \frac{\sum_i a_i \cdot d_i / N_i}{\sum_i b_i \cdot c_i / N_i}$$

$$= \frac{6 \cdot 44/82 + 7 \cdot 33/98}{3 \cdot 29/82 + 1 \cdot 57/98}$$

$$= 3.39$$

UNDER WHAT CONDITIONS WILL CONFOUNDING BE PRESENT?

Earlier it was shown that the comparison of mortality rates in hypothetical communities A and B was confounded by age, since death rates increased with increasing age and the two communities had different age distributions. Only a variable that in some way is related both to exposure and to disease has the potential to act as a confounder. But whether it actually confounds also depends on the nature of these relationships.

Relationship of Potential Confounding Variable to Exposure Status or Level

A characteristic or experience that occurs only as a consequence of a given exposure cannot distort the relationship of that exposure to disease occurrence, so generally it is not treated as a confounding variable. For example, bronchial epithelial changes occur in response to long-term cigarette smoking. Their presence increases the risk of bronchial cancer, but statistical control for these changes (if they could be measured) would not be appropriate when seeking to measure a possible association between cigarette smoking and bronchial cancer. To be a confounding factor, a variable would have to give rise to cigarette smoking or be associated with a characteristic that did—in addition to being related on its own to the incidence of bronchial cancer. Adjustment for a consequence of exposure can only serve to blunt the measured exposure–disease association.

There *are* circumstances in which adjustment is made for a consequence of exposure, but these arise only when there is interest in examining the possibility of an exposure–disease association *beyond* that arising from that specific consequence. For example, most epidemiologic studies seeking to assess whether use of OCs during the teenage years alters a woman's later risk of breast cancer have adjusted for the age at which she gives birth to her first child. They have done so despite the fact that age-at-first-birth does not meet the usual criteria for a confounder: While late age-at-first-birth tends to predict an elevated risk of breast cancer, use of OCs during the teenage years tends to delay a first pregnancy and childbirth, not vice versa. Nonetheless, since these studies are interested in answering the question "Does teenage use of OCs affect breast cancer risk *beyond its ability to delay a first pregnancy?*" an adjustment for this consequence of exposure is warranted.

Temporal sequence aside, how does one judge whether a potential confounder is associated with exposure status? Should one simply look at the data that have been gathered, or consider information external to the study? If, in the underlying population from which the study participants have been drawn, there truly is no association between the exposure and the potential confounding variable, that variable will not be a true confounder. So, if a variable is not credibly related to exposure (e.g., day of the week of birth and cigarette smoking), one would not consider it a confounder. Any association that might be present in the data should be interpreted as having occurred by chance and should be ignored. However, since there are very few variables whose lack of association with exposure status can be claimed with confidence *a priori*, we tend to examine the data that have been gathered to guide this judgment. That examination should not involve an assessment of the role of chance as a possible explanation for any association observed between exposure and potential confounder. A large *p*-value may say as much about the small size of the sample as about the true absence of a relationship in the underlying population from which that sample had been drawn.

Relationship of Potential Confounding Variable to Outcome

No matter how strongly a variable is related to exposure status, if it is not also related to the occurrence of the disease in question, it cannot be a confounder. The nature of that relationship to disease may take one of several forms:

1. The potential confounding variable can be an actual cause of the disease. For example, an imbalance in cigarette-smoking behavior between persons employed in a certain industry and a comparison group would distort the assessment of the association between employment in that industry and the occurrence of lung cancer.

2. The potential confounder can be associated with a cause of the disease that, in the context of the study, cannot be measured. A study of a possibly altered incidence of prostate cancer among white and black men who worked in the above industry would wish to deal with potential confounding by race, given the higher risk of this disease in black men. What would no doubt be ascertained in such a study would be racial phenotype, based on some combination of skin pigment, hair characteristics, etc. *Unmeasured* in the study would be the characteristics of black men—genetic or environmental ones—that actually predispose to prostate cancer. The racial phenotype, which is not a cause of prostate cancer in and of itself, would be used as a surrogate for the genuine cause(s).

3. A variable can be a confounder if it is related to the *recognition* of the outcome in question, even if it has no relationship to the actual occurrence of that outcome. An example of such a variable might be cervical screening, when assessing a potential association between use of OCs and the development of preneoplastic lesions of the uterine cervix. Since: (a) these lesions are asymptomatic and are detected only by means of cervical screening; and (b) OC users generally have a higher frequency of screening than do nonusers, a comparison of the occurrence of cervical preneoplastic lesions between users and nonusers of OCs would be confounded unless efforts were made to "force" (in the design or analysis) the level of screening to be similar between the two groups of women.

STRATEGIES FOR CONTROLLING CONFOUNDING

Confounding can be dealt with not only in the analysis of data gathered in an epidemiologic study, but in the design of those studies. As discussed in Chapter 13, addressing a possible association by means of a *randomized trial* generally achieves good control of confounding since, except in very small trials, the distribution of other factors that influence disease occurrence will be approximately balanced between persons assigned to the intervention and to the control arms of the study.

In non-randomized studies, occasionally it may be possible to select as a study population one in which exposure status is not related to any appreciable degree to other risk factors for the disease.

Example 11-1. During the 1990s, several studies compared the prevalence of HIV infection in men from different ethnic groups in which male circumcision was either almost universally present or almost universally absent. While HIV prevalence was much higher in groups that did not practice circumcision, the interpretation of these observations was obscured by the presence of other differences between them that bear on the acquisition of HIV (e.g., numbers of female sex partners). In an effort to minimize confounding of this sort, Agot *et al.* (2004) conducted a similar study among rural Luo men in Kenya, in whom it was suspected that circumcision status (influenced primarily by membership in particular Africa-instituted churches) would bear little relation to other HIV risk factors. Indeed, in that population, the presence of these risk factors was found to be nearly identical between men who had and had not undergone circumcision.

A commonly used approach to controlling confounding in non-randomized studies is *restriction* of the study population to a segment that is homogeneous with respect to a particular risk factor for disease. For example, nearly all studies of occupational factors in relation to the incidence of breast cancer are restricted to women. The inclusion of men in such studies would: (a) lead to confounding (unless other measures to control confounding were employed), since men have a much lower incidence of breast cancer than women and the patterns of employment differ between sexes; and (b) not add appreciably to the power of the study to detect an association.

In cohort studies, control of confounding can be achieved by *matching* non-exposed subjects to exposed ones for the presence or level of a variable that is related to disease occurrence. For example, in their cohort study of the possible influence of induced abortion on the occurrence of adverse outcomes in a subsequent pregnancy, Daling and Emanuel (1975) matched one pregnant woman who had no history of induced abortion to each pregnant woman who did have such a history for age, number of prior pregnancies, and a history of prior stillbirth or miscarriage. Thus, the comparison of the two groups for the occurrence of fetal or neonatal deaths, prematurity, or congenital malformations in that pregnancy was not distorted by any dissimilarity between them with regard to one or more of the matching characteristics.

In case-control studies, controls can be matched to cases for the presence or level of characteristics (other than the exposure of interest) that predict the occurrence of that illness. However, the primary purpose of matching in this situation is not control of confounding—if the matching variable is related to the exposure in question, it will be necessary to account for it in the analysis in any case if a valid result is to be obtained (see Chapter 15). Rather, the purpose is an increase in study efficiency. For example, if a case-control study of occupational influences on breast cancer did not restrict its subjects to women, almost surely that study would match controls to cases on the basis of sex. Failure to do so would generate a control group of roughly equal numbers of men and women. This would result in: (a) an analysis in which one stratum—that of men—contained a very high ratio of controls to cases; and therefore (b) a study whose power to address the hypothesis would be substantially less than had it attempted to have the ratio of women to men be similar for cases and controls.

Some studies employ multiple strategies to isolate the possible effect of the exposure of interest from other factors related to the disease with which it is correlated.

Example 11-2. In a study conducted in two urban areas of Brazil, Victora *et al.* (1987) compared infants who died of diarrhea or respiratory disease with other infants in terms of breast feeding and other types of dietary intake (as ascertained through interviews with parents) during a period of time prior to the onset of the cases' illnesses. Because a number of correlates of breast feeding practices are themselves related to infant mortality, the authors gave considerable attention to control of possible confounding. First, they *restricted* their study population to singletons of birth weight > 1500 grams who had not been hospitalized for more than two weeks beginning at birth. Prior to the start of the study, it was anticipated that infants excluded by these criteria would be relatively less likely to have been breast-fed through the first year of life and also at increased risk of death from diarrhea or respiratory disease. Also, it was expected that there would be so few of them—especially among exclusive breast feeders—that statistical adjustment might not have been feasible. Later, in the analysis of their data, the authors adjusted for a number of additional characteristics, including interval from preceding birth, maternal education, father's occupation, and neighborhood of residence. (For purposes of efficiency, they had already chosen control infants from the same neighborhoods as the cases.) They also adjusted for one of the characteristics used to restrict their sample—birth weight—in categories of 500 grams, beginning at 1500 grams.

Because of the care with which confounding was addressed in this study, the strong association of mortality with *not* breast feeding that was observed could be interpreted with some confidence as reflecting a genuine protective effect of nursing during the first year of life.

RESIDUAL CONFOUNDING

An effort to control for a variable's confounding influence will be incomplete to the extent that:

- The variable has not been measured accurately; or
- The variable has not been categorized or modeled in such a way as to fully capture the nature of its relationship to disease and/or exposure.

Nondifferential mismeasurement of a confounder generally will lead to an estimate of the size of the exposure–disease association that is falsely close to the unadjusted (crude) estimate (Greenland, 2012). In the extreme case, in which the means of measuring the confounding variable is completely inaccurate, the "adjusted" and crude estimates will be identical.

Example 11-3. To explore the possibility that sexually transmitted infections other than human papillomavirus (HPV) can predispose to cervical cancer, two case-control studies were conducted by investigators at the National Cancer Institute to examine whether a woman's risk of this disease was related to the number of sexual partners she had had. Each study controlled for the presence of cervical HPV DNA, but they used different methods. The first, conducted in 1986–1987, employed Southern blot DNA hybridization, whereas the second (conducted in 1989–1990) used PCR, a more sensitive technique that had only then become available for epidemiologic studies. Evidence of the enhanced ability of the second study to accurately assess HPV status was the much higher odds ratio it obtained for the HPV–cancer association—20.1—than the corresponding odds ratio obtained in the first study—3.7.

Table 11.11 (from Schiffman and Schatzkin, 1994) describes the association between the number of sexual partners and cervical cancer in each study, both with and without adjustment for HPV status.

Adjustment for HPV infection had a large impact on the elevated odds ratios associated with increasing numbers of sexual partners in the second study,

TABLE 11.11. EFFECT OF ADJUSTMENT FOR HPV INFECTION ON THE ASSOCIATION BETWEEN LIFETIME NUMBER OF SEXUAL PARTNERS AND THE RISK OF CERVICAL INTRAEPITHELIAL NEOPLASIA

Lifetime no. of sexual partners	Cases	Controls	Crude odds ratio (95% conf. int.)		Adjusted odds ratio[a] (95% conf. int.)	
Study 1 (1986–1987)						
1	25	69	1.0		1.0	
2	47	61	2.1	(1.2–3.9)	2.2	(1.2–4.0)
3–4	71	79	2.1	(1.2–3.7)	2.0	(1.1–3.6)
5–9	48	89	2.5	(1.4–4.3)	2.4	(1.3–4.3)
10+	48	89	1.5	(0.8–2.7)	1.5	(0.8–2.8)
Study 2 (1989–1990)						
1	40	113	1.0		1.0	
2	34	58	1.7	(0.9–2.9)	1.0	(0.5–1.9)
3–5	127	116	3.1	(2.0–4.8)	1.1	(0.6–1.9)
6–9	116	70	4.7	(2.9–7.5)	1.5	(0.9–2.7)
10+	116	74	4.4	(2.8–7.0)	1.6	(0.9–2.8)

[a] Adjusted for HPV DNA detection

but almost no impact at all in the first study. Misclassification of HPV status in the first study appears to have substantially decreased the ability to adjust for that variable.

If even an accurately measured confounding variable is not categorized appropriately, adjustment will not remove all of its confounding influence. For example, in a study of degree of baldness in relation to the incidence of prostate cancer (perhaps to obtain clues regarding hormonal or genetic influences on this disease), adjustment for age in two groups—perhaps less than 60 years and 60 or greater—would almost certainly lead to the presence of residual confounding. Within each broad category of age, both the degree of baldness and the incidence of prostate cancer rises. Finer stratification on age—perhaps in five-year groups, or using multivariate methods that allow age to be modeled as a continuous variable—would be needed to remove most or all of the confounding.

Sometimes, a potentially confounding variable has a number of dimensions, and residual confounding can occur if some of these dimensions are not considered. For example, in one study (Matukala Nkosi *et al.*, 2012) the associations between several social and economic characteristics and the incidence of lung cancer would have been greatly overestimated by controlling only for

a broadly defined history of cigarette smoking (current, former, never), and not also for the intensity, duration, and recency of smoking.

If a method that requires categorization of a confounder is to be used, how narrow is it necessary to make the categories of the confounding variable? The answer to this question depends on the particulars of the relationship between the confounder and the exposure and disease, respectively. In the hypothetical study of baldness and prostate cancer, it may be necessary to control for race. If the incidence of prostate cancer is similar between Chinese, Japanese, and Filipino men, for example, it would be possible to combine them in a single stratum for analysis (in addition to strata for white and for black men) with no introduction of confounding by race. But there are other instances (e.g., age as a potential confounder of the association between baldness and prostate cancer) in which it is necessary to create relatively fine strata of the confounding variable, so as to prevent its strong relationship to both exposure and disease from distorting the association.

REFERENCES

Agot KE, Ndinya-Achola JO, Kreiss JK, Weiss NS. Risk of HIV-1 in rural Kenya: a comparison of circumcised and uncircumcised men. Epidemiology 2004; 15:157–163.

Alpha-Tocopherol, Beta Carotene Cancer Prevention Study Group. The effect of vitamin E and beta carotene on the incidence of lung cancer and other cancers in male smokers. N Engl J Med 1994; 330:1029–1035.

Daling JR, Emanuel I. Induced abortion and subsequent outcome of pregnancy. Lancet 1975; 2: 170–178.

Dalton SO, Johansen C, Poulsen AH, Norgaard M, Sorensen HT, McLaughlin JK, et al. Cancer risk among users of neuroleptic medication: a population-based cohort study. Br J Cancer 2006; 95: 934–939.

Day NE. A new measure of age-standardized incidence, the cumulative rate. In: Doll R, Payne P, Waterhouse J (eds.), Cancer incidence in five continents, Vol. 3. pp. 443–445 Geneva, Switzerland: International Union Against Cancer Cancer, 1976.

Greenland S. Intuitions, simulations, theorems: the role and limits of methodology. Epidemiology 2012; 23:440–442.

Mantel N, Haenszel W. Statistical aspects of the analysis of data from retrospective studies of disease. J Nat Cancer Inst 1959; 22:719–748.

Matukala Nkosi T, Parent MÉ, Siemiatycki J, Rousseau MC. Socioeconomic position and lung cancer risk: how important is the modeling of smoking? Epidemiology 2012; 23:377–385.

Omenn GS, Goodman GE, Thornquist MD, Balmes J, Cullen MR, Glass A, et al. Effects of a combination of beta carotene and vitamin A on lung cancer and cardiovascular disease. N Engl J Med 1996; 334:1150–1155.

Rothman KJ, Greenland S, Lash TL. Modern epidemiology (3rd ed.). Philadelphia: Lippincott Williams & Wilkins, 2008.

Sasieni PD, Adams J. Standardized lifetime risk. Am J Epidemiol 1999; 149:869–875.

Schiffman MH, Schatzkin A. Test reliability is critically important to molecular epidemiology: an example from studies of human papillomavirus infection and cervical neoplasia. Cancer Res 1994; 54 Suppl:1944s–1947s.

Shapiro JA, Jacobs EJ, Thun MJ. Cigar smoking in men and risk of death from tobacco-related cancers. JNCI 2000; 92:333–337.

Victora CG, Smith PG, Vaughan JP, Nobre LC, Lombardi C, Teixeira AM, et al. Evidence for protection by breast-feeding against infant deaths from infectious diseases in Brazil. Lancet 1987; 2:319–322.

EXERCISES

1. The following questions concern the data presented in Figure 11.1:

   (a) What is the reason for the progressive disparity between crude and age-adjusted death rates?
   (b) For purposes of age-adjustment, can you tell which population was used as a standard? Why, or why not?

2. The data below came from the Surveillance, Epidemiology, and End Results Program, 1990, in which nine geographic areas of the United States were monitored for cancer incidence.

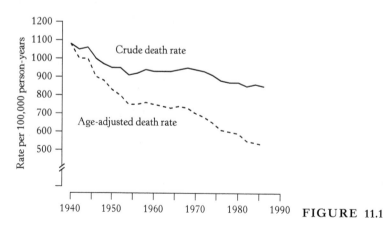

FIGURE 11.1

TABLE 11.12.

Age (years)	White males		Black males	
	No. of bladder cancer cases, 1990	No. of males in survey areas, 1990	No. of bladder cancer cases, 1990	No. of males in survey areas, 1990
0–54	319	7,574,000	20	1,088,000
55–59	253	388,000	10	37,000
60–64	370	382,000	16	34,000
65–69	524	346,000	27	30,000
70–74	550	265,000	20	21,000
75–84	817	288,000	27	21,000

(a) What are the crude incidence rates for bladder cancer for white males and for black males? What is the ratio of these two rates?

(b) What are the age-adjusted incidence rates for bladder cancer for white males and for black males (use the white male population as a standard)? Now, what is the incidence in white males relative to that in black males? Why is it lower than when using crude rates?

3. Below are the results of a (hypothetical) small cohort study of use of hair coloring products in relation to mortality from prostate cancer:

TABLE 11.13.

Age (years)	Use of hair coloring		Non-use of hair coloring	
	Deaths	Man-years	Deaths	Man-years
50–54	0	1,502	1	10,485
55–59	2	1,978	5	21,930
60–64	1	431	22	11,641

Adjusting for age, what is the ratio of the mortality rates from prostate cancer between users and non-users of hair coloring products? What is the corresponding crude mortality rate ratio? Why do the two differ from one another?

4. The data in Figure 11.2 notwithstanding, you would be reluctant to conclude that death rates from cerebrovascular disease in American women of a given age above 85 years are greater than they are for men of that age. What is the basis for your reluctance?

5. The data in the following table describe the median serum creatinine levels obtained 2–5 years prior to diagnosis in persons who developed kidney cancer, and during the corresponding period of time in controls:

TABLE 11.14.

	Cases		Controls	
	No. of subjects	Median serum creatinine[a]	No. of subjects	Median serum creatinine[a]
Men & women combined	180	1.1	435	1.0
Men	114	1.2	173	1.2
Women	66	0.9	262	0.9

[a] mg per dl

The median serum creatinine level was the same for male cases and controls, and also for female cases and controls. However, it was not the same for cases and controls of the two sexes combined. Why?

6. The following is paraphrased from an article published some years ago:

Among persons 25–64 years of age, the annual mortality rate in 1970 from coronary heart disease among edentulous men was 347.6 per 100,000 person-years compared to a rate of 215.1 per 100,000 person-years among men who had at least some teeth left. These data support the hypothesis that under-nutrition and/or lack of mastication play a role in the genesis of coronary heart disease.

Despite the age restriction employed by the authors, it is likely that the comparison made is confounded by age. How can this be? Does the presence of confounding by age exaggerate or minimize whatever true difference may be present?

7. Shapiro *et al.* (2000) examined the association between cigar smoking and death from tobacco-related

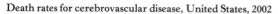

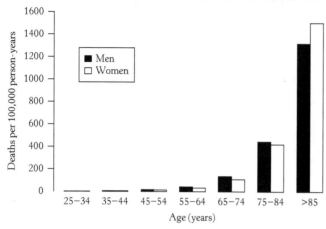

Death rates for cerebrovascular disease, United States, 2002

FIGURE 11.2

cancers in a prospective cohort study. The authors chose to restrict their analysis to the men in the total cohort who had never regularly smoked cigarettes, and so conceded that their results "may not be generalizable to cigar smokers who have previously smoked cigarettes." Nonetheless, there are at least two arguments in support of the authors' decision to exclude men who had smoked cigarettes. First, if the absolute impact of cigar-smoking risk were the same in smokers and nonsmokers of cigarettes, the relative impact would be greater in the latter (who, relative to cigarette smokers, are at lower risk of cancer). What is a second argument?

8. Using data obtained in a prospective cohort study, let us say you observe that the incidence of cancer among persons in the upper fourth of the distribution of serum beta carotene is 60% of that of persons in the lower three-fourths. In that study, the intake of a particular vegetable, V, was ascertained. However, the instrument used to ascertain V did so in but a cursory way. Because V contains nutrients other than beta carotene that might reduce cancer risk, you would like to adjust for intake of V when assessing the association between beta carotene levels and cancer. When you do this, the RR associated with being in the upper fourth of the serum beta carotene distribution is now 0.8 instead of 0.6.

If V intake could have been measured more accurately, and thus confounding by V more completely controlled, would you expect the adjusted RR associated with high serum beta carotene levels to have been:

(a) Less than 0.8
(b) 0.8
(c) Greater than 0.8

Why?

9. In a retrospective cohort study conducted in Denmark (Dalton et al., 2006), the incidence of cancer was monitored in persons who had been prescribed an anti-psychotic drug and compared to the incidence in other persons. While the investigators were unable to ascertain smoking histories on any of the cohort members, they did have information on hospitalization for chronic obstructive pulmonary disease (COPD, a condition related to smoking) that occurred among these persons during the follow-up period. The risk of lung cancer in users of anti-psychotic medications was 1.57 times that of non-users (95% confidence interval 1.40–1.75); after adjustment for hospitalization for COPD, the corresponding relative risk was 1.24 (95% confidence interval 1.10–1.40).

(a) When examining a potential association between exposure and disease, it is generally not advisable to adjust for factors that occur after the exposure has begun. Nonetheless, you believe that the relative risk that better characterizes the relationship between use of an anti-psychotic drug and the incidence of lung cancer is the one that adjusts for hospitalization for COPD. Why?

(b) Had the investigators been able to adjust for smoking history as well as hospitalization for COPD, would you anticipate the relative risk to be larger, smaller, or the same as 1.24? Why?

10. A colleague in the Department of Obstetrics and Gynecology is interested in factors that influence the survival of her patients with endometrial cancer. She has data on several hundred such patients, including estrogen use (both prior to and following diagnosis); stage of disease at diagnosis (e.g., confined to the endometrium, spread to other parts of the uterus, spread beyond the uterus); and survival.

TABLE 11.15.

Age (years)	Age-specific incidence per 1000 person-years, 1990, black males (1)	1990 white male population (thousands) (2)	(1) × (2)
0–54	1.84	7,574	139.23
55–59	.270	388	104.86
60–64	.471	382	179.76
65–69	.900	346	311.40
70–74	.952	265	252.38
75–84	1.29	288	370.29
			1357.92

Under what circumstances, if any, would you advise her to adjust for "stage of disease at diagnosis" when examining:

(a) The relationship between estrogen use *prior to* diagnosis and survival?

(b) The relationship between use *following* diagnosis and survival?

11. Screening for elevated blood glucose is recommended during the 24th–28th week of pregnancy to identify women with gestational diabetes mellitus (GDM), since untreated GDM predisposes to (among other things) respiratory distress syndrome (RDS) in the infant. You are an epidemiologist at a large health maintenance organization (HMO) in which nearly every pregnant female member is screened for blood glucose levels. You would like to do a case-control study of RDS to determine whether, among women with glucose levels below the threshold for a diagnosis of GDM, the risk of RDS rises with increasingly high levels of blood glucose. If you find, for example, that infants of pregnant women just below the presently accepted threshold of blood glucose are at increased risk, an argument could be made for redefining GDM.

Controls for the study will be sampled from members of the organization who delivered a baby without RDS. You are aware that RDS is primarily a condition that affects premature babies. In this study, under what circumstance, if any, would you recommend matching controls to cases on the basis of gestational age at the time of delivery? Explain your recommendation. (Assume that, because of the widespread use of prenatal ultrasound in this health maintenance organization, accurate information on gestational age is available on all pregnancies.)

ANSWERS

1. (a) The relative size of that fraction of the population at highest risk of death—older

people—steadily grew between 1940 and 1986.

(b) The 1940 U.S. population, because it was in that year that the crude and adjusted rates were equal.

2. (a) Crude incidence, 1990:

White males: 2,833/9,243,000
= 0.307 per 1000 person-years
Black males: 120/1,231,000
= 0.0976 per 1000 person-years

Relative incidence = $\frac{0.307}{0.0976}$ = 3.14.

(b) Incidence of bladder cancer in black males, adjusted to the age distribution of white males = 1,358.18/9,243,000 = 0.147 per 1000 person-years.

Ratio of adjusted rates = 0.307/0.147 = 2.09.

The age-adjusted incidence of bladder cancer in black males is higher than the crude incidence, because it is based on a population distribution—that of white males—which is older than that of the black males themselves. Note, for example, that males in the youngest category, 0–54 years, constitute only 7,574,000/9,243,000 = 81.9% of the total in whites, as opposed to 1,086,000/1,229,000 = 88.4% of the total in blacks. Therefore, the ratio of age-adjusted rates will be lower than the ratio of the crude rates (2.09 versus 3.14).

3. Crude mortality rate ratio = $\frac{3/3911}{28/44,056}$ = 1.21.

Age-adjusted mortality rate ratio (see Table 11.10):

$$= \frac{0 \cdot 10,485/11,987 + 2 \cdot 21,930/23,908 + 1 \cdot 11,641/12,072}{1 \cdot 1,502/11,987 + 5 \cdot 1,978/23,908 + 22 \cdot 431/12,072}$$

$$= 2.11.$$

The crude rate ratio was spuriously low because age was a confounding factor:

- Men who used a hair coloring product were younger, on average, than other men, as indicated by the different distributions of person-years across the three age groups; and
- Mortality rates from prostate cancer were seen to increase with increasing age.

Adjustment nullified the mortality advantage of the hair coloring group that resulted from their younger age, leading to an adjusted rate ratio that was higher than the crude one.

4. Residual confounding by age is no doubt at work here. Within the >85-year age stratum, (a) death rates from cerebrovascular disease probably rise rapidly with age (since they rise rapidly with age prior to age 85); and (b) women tend to live to be older than men. This will lead to a "crude" rate in women within the age stratum that, relative to the rate in men, would be higher than an age-adjusted rate.

5. Confounding by gender. Men have higher creatinine levels than women, and the proportion of cases who are men is greater than the proportion of controls.

6. Within the 25–64-year age stratum, there is probably a strong relationship between increasing age and both: (a) being edentulous; and (b) dying from coronary heart disease. Since edentulous men are older, on average, than other men, in the absence of further adjustment for age, their mortality rate from coronary heart disease will be falsely high relative to that in other men.

7. There may be errors in ascertaining cigarette-smoking history, or information may not have been sought about that part of the history which is of greatest etiological relevance. Either of these would allow for the possibility of residual confounding when trying to adjust for differences in cigarette smoking between men who do and do not smoke cigars.

8. The correct answer is c. Incomplete adjustment for the confounding variable, intake of V, will result in an adjusted relative risk that is spuriously close to the crude relative risk. Therefore, since incomplete adjustment led to an increase in the apparent relative risk of cancer associated with high levels of serum beta carotene—from an unadjusted relative risk of 0.6 to 0.8—more complete adjustment would be expected to lead to a relative risk that would be higher still.

9. (a) The COPD-adjusted relative risk is the more valid one because: (i) It is likely that hospitalization for COPD is a result of smoking prior to (as well as after) the receipt of anti-psychotic medications; and (ii) it is much less likely that hospitalization for COPD represents a consequence of use of an anti-psychotic medication (the only circumstance under which it would not be advisable to adjust for this variable).

(b) Adjustment for hospitalization for COPD has almost certainly not entirely removed the confounding effect of smoking. The ability to adjust for smoking as well would almost certainly produce a still smaller estimate of the relative risk relating use of anti-psychotic drugs to the incidence of lung cancer.

10. (a) If use of estrogens were to predispose to the development of relatively non-aggressive endometrial tumors, these probably would be diagnosed at a relatively early stage (e.g., localized to the endometrium). The overall impact of the estrogen use on survival would be estimated best by not "forcing" (by means of adjustment) hormone users and non-users with endometrial cancer to have the same stage distribution, given that early stage at diagnosis is a manifestation of the influence of estrogen. Only if one wanted to assess the impact of estrogen use on survival *beyond* its ability to predispose to early-stage tumors would adjustment for stage of disease at diagnosis be appropriate.

(b) Stage at diagnosis is strongly related to the likelihood of survival from endometrial cancer. Thus, when assessing whether estrogen use following cancer diagnosis is itself related to survival, it would be desirable to adjust for stage at diagnosis if the distribution of stage is associated with estrogen use. Here, unlike Question (10a), estrogen use is not influencing stage of disease at diagnosis, so the stage of disease can act as a confounding factor.

11. Even if it were believed that glucose levels were associated with gestational age at delivery, it would not be appropriate to match on this variable (or to otherwise adjust for it in the analysis). In this study of women without GDM, you are seeking to estimate the association between elevated glucose levels and RDS through whatever means those elevated levels are exerting their influence, including a predisposition to premature delivery. (Only if a different hypothesis were being investigated—the relationship of blood glucose to RDS among infants delivered at a given gestational age—should matching on this variable be considered.)

12

Confounding and Its Control: Advanced

"I can't believe that!" said Alice. "Can't you?" said the Queen in a pitying tone. "Try again: draw a long breath, and shut your eyes." Alice laughed. "There's no use trying," she said, "One can't believe impossible things." "I daresay you haven't had much practice," said the Queen. "When I was your age, I always did it for half-an-hour a day. Why, sometimes I believed as many as six impossible things before breakfast."

—LEWIS CARROLL

THREE VIEWS OF CONFOUNDING

A Modern Fable

Three epidemiologists sat around a table, examining early results from their case-control study of ketchup intake and anxiety among college students. Cases of anxiety disorder had been identified through the campus clinic and counseling service; controls were a random sample of other students at the college. The primary exposure was intake of ketchup, purported to contain natural mellowing agents (Wikipedia, 2012), as assessed by dietary questionnaire. High ketchup intake was considered "exposed", and low ketchup intake was considered "unexposed". Data were also gathered on each respondent's type of diet (vegetarian, fish but no other meat, or omnivore) because of suspicion that it might be a confounding factor. The study was so impeccably designed that it was universally accepted that all participants had been classified without error on all three variables. Here is part of the discussion, which alludes to data in Table 12.1:

Anthony: "I took a first look at the association between ketchup and anxiety, and our hypothesis looks pretty good. The overall odds ratio was 0.40 for high ketchup intake and anxiety. But it's a good thing we collected data on type of diet. In the control group, a lot more meat eaters had high ketchup intake compared to the vegetarians and fish eaters [column (5)]."

Barbara: "Why look at only the controls? Why not everybody?"

Anthony: "Well, I figured the controls were telling us about the relationship between ketchup and diet type in general—at least in the student population—since the controls are pretty much a random sample. And even around here, an anxiety disorder bad enough to seek help for it was fairly rare."

Catherine: "Makes sense. And who'd put ketchup on vegetables or fish? But was there any link between diet type and anxiety?"

Anthony: "Apparently so. I looked at just the people with low ketchup intake in order to focus on the association between diet type and anxiety without having ketchup mixed in. It turned out that the percentage of cases was a lot higher in vegetarians than in fish- or meat-eaters [column (6)]."

Catherine: "Must be the effects of chronic hunger. I'm not sure why meat-eaters had more anxiety than fish-eaters, but you can't argue with the data."

Anthony: "Right. And any way you slice it, diet type was associated with exposure and also with case-control status. Ergo, it's a confounder."

Barbara: "Wait a second. I also checked whether diet type was a confounder, but I did it another way. I just went straight to a comparison of the crude odds ratio and the stratum-specific odds ratios for each diet type [column (7)]. The stratum-specific odds ratios were amazingly close to each other—all three were 0.40—and they were all exactly the same as

TABLE 12.1. RESULTS OF A FICTITIOUS CASE-CONTROL STUDY OF KETCHUP
INTAKE AND ANXIETY

Diet type (1)	Ketchup intake[a] (2)	Anxiety Cases (3)	Anxiety Control (4)	% exposed among controls (5)	% cases among unexposed (6)	Odds ratio (7)
Vegetarian	High	24	16	44%	79%	0.40
	Low	75	20			
Fish	High	8	48	44%	29%	0.40
	Low	25	60			
Omnivore	High	16	32	67%	56%	0.40
	Low	20	16			
All	High	48	96	50%	56%	0.40
	Low	120	96			

[a] High = exposed; low = unexposed

the crude odds ratio. So if the crude and stratum-specific odds ratios are the same, diet type can't be a confounder."

Anthony: "Must be a mistake. Let's recheck the numbers."

They did, and there was no mistake.

Anthony: "Beats me, but I'm sticking with what I was always taught. If it's associated with exposure and with disease and isn't on the causal pathway, it's a confounder. And if it's a confounder, I don't see how we can find that out and then not control for it."

Barbara: "And I'm sticking with what I saw in the data. Whether you control for diet type or not, the odds ratio for ketchup and anxiety is exactly the same. So what's the point of calling it a confounder if it doesn't matter whether you control for it or you don't?"

They looked at each other, then both looked at Catherine. Realizing that she was the tie-breaker, she paused dramatically. Then she glanced briefly at the data table again before pushing it aside with a shrug. "I don't think you can tell from these data whether there's any confounding here or not. We don't really know what would have happened to those high-ketchup eaters if they hadn't eaten so much ketchup."

One thing they all could agree on was that this discussion had made them hungry, so they adjourned for lunch.

The remarks of Anthony, Barbara, and Catherine reflect three different ways of thinking about confounding. As illustrated in this example, based on data published by Whittemore (1978), the three

viewpoints do not necessarily lead to the same conclusion. Still, each perspective provides some unique insights into confounding, sometimes with different implications for what action should be taken.

Below we describe each view and explain why they can disagree. A scenario involving just three variables is considered (see Table 12.2).

1: Comparability View

Under the *comparability* view, C is a confounder of the E-Y association if: (1) the distribution of C differs between the exposed and unexposed groups, and (2) C affects Y in its own right. Under these conditions, the exposed and unexposed groups are not *comparable* with regard to C, which is itself a determinant of Y.

Historically the oldest way of thinking about confounding, the comparability view has also been called

TABLE 12.2.

Symbol	Denotes:
E	A binary exposure: exposed or unexposed
Y	A binary outcome. In etiological studies, Y represents disease status (1 = disease, 0 = no disease); in other contexts it could be a different binary outcome, such as case fatality.
C	A potential confounding factor with k levels, indexed by $i = 1 \ldots k$. C is assumed not to be on a causal path from E to Y.

the *classical* view. Study data can be used to evaluate empirically the extent to which these conditions are met, as shown in Chapter 11. Condition (1) can be evaluated in a full population or in a cohort study by comparing the distribution of C between exposed and unexposed groups (without regard to Y). In a population-based case-control study, if the outcome $Y = 1$ can be assumed to be rare, and if the controls studied are representative of all non-cases, then the C-E association in the control group should approximate that in the source population, and condition (1) can be evaluated in the control group. For condition (2), the C-Y association can be examined among unexposed subjects. Restricting this analysis to the unexposed avoids the possibility that C and Y are found to be associated with each other only because both are associated with E.

In the ketchup study, diet type met both conditions and thus would be considered a confounder under the comparability view. Epidemiologist Anthony's remarks reflect this view.

2: Collapsibility View

The *collapsibility* view focuses on the value of a certain measure of the E-Y association, with and without stratification on C. If that association measure takes the same value within each stratum of C, but the common stratum-specific value differs from the "crude" value obtained without stratification on C, then C is deemed a confounder.

Collapsibility refers to a property of certain multi-way contingency tables (Whittemore, 1978; Newman, 2004). In the current scenario, the study data can be organized as a $2 \times 2 \times k$ table whose cells contain the number of subjects at each possible combination of levels on E, Y, and C. If this table can be *collapsed* into a 2×2 table by summing across levels of C without changing the value of the E-Y association measure, then the 3-way table is said to be *collapsible* over C to a 2-way table, and C is not a confounder.

In the ketchup study, the three 2×2 tables of counts on the left side of Table 12.1 above the solid black line can be viewed as three layers of a single $2 \times 2 \times 3$ table. The 2×2 table below the solid black line is obtained by collapsing that $2 \times 2 \times 3$ table over diet type. In this instance, the measure of association is the odds ratio, and its value is the same with or without stratification on diet type. Hence diet type would not be considered a confounder of the ketchup-anxiety odds ratio. Epidemiologist Barbara's remarks reflect this view.

The collapsibility view requires that two preconditions be met before it addresses confounding by C. First, a particular measure of the E-Y association must be specified at the outset. In principle, one can choose from a wide variety of such measures, several of which are described in Chapter 9. In practice, attention commonly focuses on either a ratio measure (the risk ratio or rate ratio, RR, or the odds ratio, OR, for a case-control study) or a difference measure (the risk difference, or rate difference, RD). The RR, OR, and RD are the three measures considered here. A verdict on whether C confounds the E-Y association under the collapsibility view often depends on which measure of association is used, as shown below.

Second, the collapsibility view addresses confounding by C only when whatever association measure is selected takes the same value in all strata of C. That is, it presupposes no effect modification of the E-Y association by C. When this *homogeneity* condition is met, any reasonable method of adjusting the association measure for C should yield the common stratum-specific value as the adjusted value. (Direct adjustment and the Mantel-Haenszel adjustment methods do so.) Therefore, whenever confounding is evaluated by comparing crude and adjusted measures of association, the collapsibility view is implicitly being adopted. But whether the homogeneity condition is actually met can depend on the measure of E-Y association specified.

Table 12.3 illustrates how the process and outcome of applying the collapsibility view depend on the measure of association. Say that a cohort study of a relatively common outcome has been conducted in a closed population, yielding cumulative incidence in exposed and unexposed groups. Here, C has two levels, which define the strata. The RR, OR, and RD are shown for each stratum and for the collapsed table. (The OR would probably not be of main interest in a cohort study—especially one involving a common outcome—but it is occasionally applied in that context and is shown for illustration.) In this example, the OR takes the same value in both strata, as does the RD, thus satisfying the homogeneity requirement for those measures of association. In contrast, the RR takes different values in the two strata, so C would be considered an effect modifier of the RR, and the collapsibility view of confounding would not apply. For the OR, the value 3.6 in the collapsed table differs from the common stratum-specific value of 6.0, so C would be considered a confounder of the OR. For the RD, the values in the two strata equal the value in

TABLE 12.3. RESULTS OF A HYPOTHETICAL COHORT STUDY, COMPARING STRATUM-SPECIFIC AND POOLED VALUES OF THE RELATIVE RISK (RR), ODDS RATIO (OR), AND RISK DIFFERENCE (RD)

Stratum (C)	Exposure (E)	Outcome $Y = 1$	Outcome $Y = 0$	Outcome Total	Cumulative incidence	RR	OR	RD
1	Exposed	80	120	200	0.40			
	Unexposed	20	180	200	0.10	4.0	6.0	0.30
2	Exposed	90	10	100	0.90			
	Unexposed	60	40	100	0.60	1.5	6.0	0.30
All	Exposed	170	130	300	0.57			
	Unexposed	80	220	300	0.27	2.1	3.6	0.30

(Based on data from Newman [2004])

the collapsed table, so C would not be considered a confounder of the RD.

Under what circumstances is a $2 \times 2 \times k$ table collapsible? The answer again depends on the measure of association (Boivin and Wacholder, 1985; Fleiss *et al.*, 2003; Newman, 2004).

Collapsibility of the RR or RD

For the RR and RD, algebra in Appendix 12A shows that a $2 \times 2 \times k$ table meeting the homogeneity requirement is collapsible over C if and only if:

$$\sum_i w_{ui} \cdot r_{ui} = \sum_i w_{ei} \cdot r_{ui} \qquad (12.1)$$

where w_{ui} is the proportion of unexposed subjects that fall into stratum i, w_{ei} is the proportion of exposed subjects that fall into stratum i, and r_{ui} is the cumulative incidence of the outcome ($Y = 1$) among unexposed subjects in stratum i. The w's are so labelled because they can be regarded as weights, such that $\sum_i w_{ei} = 1$ and $\sum_i w_{ui} = 1$. They describe how the exposed and unexposed subjects are distributed among strata. Interpreted as probabilities, $w_{ei} = \Pr(\text{stratum } i \mid \text{exposed})$, and $w_{ui} = \Pr(\text{stratum } i \mid \text{unexposed})$. By the weighted-average rule presented in Chapter 4, the left side of Equation (12.1) can be seen to be the crude cumulative incidence among unexposed subjects. The right side can be interpreted as the adjusted cumulative incidence in the unexposed group, treating the exposed group as the standard population. Equation (12.1) thus asserts that if the cumulative incidence in the unexposed group is the same whether one adjusts for C

or not, then the table is collapsible, and there is no confounding by C.

To see how collapsibility of the RR or RD relates to the comparability view of confounding, recall that in order for C to be a confounder under the comparability view, it must meet both of the following conditions: (1) C must be associated with E, and (2) C must be associated with Y among the unexposed. Now consider Equation (12.1) in relation to these two conditions:

- If C and E are unassociated, then C cannot be a confounder under the comparability view. Absence of a C-E association implies that $w_{ei} = w_{ui}$ in every stratum, which implies that Equation (12.1) holds, which implies that the RR or RD is collapsible over C, which implies that C is not a confounder under the collapsibility view.
- If C and Y are unassociated among the unexposed, then C cannot be a confounder under the comparability view. Absence of a C-Y association among the unexposed implies that r_{ui} is constant across strata of C, which implies that both sides of equation (12.1) are weighted averages of this constant and must therefore be equal, which implies that the RR or RD is collapsible over C, which implies that C is not a confounder under the collapsibility view.

Thus, if C is not a confounder of the RR or RD under the comparability view, it cannot be a confounder under the collapsibility view, either.

When C has only two categories, an even stronger statement can be made about agreement between the two views. Equation (12.1) can then be reduced to $(w_{u1} - w_{e1})(r_{u1} - r_{u2}) = 0$. This simpler equation implies that the RR or RD is collapsible over C in a $2 \times 2 \times 2$ table if *and only if* either $w_{u1} = w_{e1}$, or $r_{u1} = r_{u2}$, or both. Happily, those are exactly the conditions that lead to absence of confounding under the comparability view. Thus, when C is dichotomous, the comparability and collapsibility views always lead to exactly the same verdict on whether C is a confounder of the RR or RD.

Unfortunately, however, when C has more than two levels, the comparability and collapsibility views do not always agree about whether C is a confounder of the RR or RD. In particular, $2 \times 2 \times k$ tables exist in which the comparability view classifies C as a confounder while the collapsibility view does not. Appendix 12B shows two such examples, one for the RR and one for the RD. In each instance, there is a C-E association and a C-Y association among the unexposed, yet the data satisfy Equation (12.1) and the table is collapsible over C. How common such examples are in practice is hard to know, but in principle, an infinite number exist.

For the RR and RD, disagreements in the other direction cannot occur: if C is a confounder under the collapsibility view, it will always be a confounder under the comparability view as well. This follows from the demonstration above that absence of confounding under the comparability view implies absence of confounding under the collapsibility view. Mathematically, then, the set of situations in which C is a confounder of the RR or RD under the collapsibility view is a strictly smaller subset of the set of situations in which C is a confounder under the comparability view.

To summarize for the RR and RD:

- The collapsibility view presupposes homogeneity across strata, which the comparability view does not. When that precondition is met, both views apply. Assuming homogeneity …
- When C has just two categories, both views always reach the same verdict about whether C is a confounder.
- When C has three or more categories, the two views can reach different verdicts. In particular, C can be a confounder under the comparability view and a non-confounder

under the collapsibility view. The reverse cannot occur.

Collapsibility of the OR

The conditions required for collapsibility of the OR in a $2 \times 2 \times k$ table differ from the conditions for collapsibility of the RR or RD. As shown in Appendix 12A, the OR is collapsible over C if and only if:

$$\sum_i w'_{ui} \cdot \psi_{ui} = \sum_i w'_{ei} \cdot \psi_{ui} \qquad (12.2)$$

where w'_{ui} is the proportion of unexposed *controls* (i.e., those with $Y = 0$) that belong to stratum i; w'_{ei} is the proportion of exposed *controls* that belong to stratum i; and ψ_{ui} is the odds of being a case (i.e., having $Y = 1$) among unexposed persons in stratum i. Equation (12.2) is similar in structure to Equation (12.1), in that both compare weighted averages. But the weights in (12.1) refer to proportions in the full study sample, while the weights in (12.2) refer to the controls alone. Also, (12.1) concerns weighted averages of proportions, while (12.2) concerns weighted averages of odds.

We saw earlier that when C has only two categories, the comparability and collapsibility views always agree on whether C is a confounder of the RR or RD (assuming homogeneity across strata). Agreement between views is not guaranteed for the OR, however, even when C is dichotomous. The reason concerns the difference between the weights in Equation (12.1) and those in Equation (12.2). Under the comparability view, if C and E are unassociated in the study population as a whole, then C cannot be a confounder. As noted earlier, this condition corresponds to $w_{ei} = w_{ui}$ for all i in Equation (12.1). But the C-E association *in the study population as a whole* may be different from the C-E association *among the controls alone*. Algebraically, $w_{ei} = w_{ui}$ for all i in Equation (12.1) does not imply that $w'_{ei} = w'_{ui}$ for all i in Equation (12.2), or vice versa. Table 12.3 shows an example in which C and E are unassociated in the full study population but are associated in the controls alone. The data satisfy Equation (12.1) but not Equation (12.2); hence, the OR is not collapsible in that table.

When C has just two categories, it is possible to "resurrect" complete agreement between the comparability and collapsibility views for the OR by modifying one of the conditions required for confounding under the comparability view. Rather than requiring a C-E association in the overall study population in order for C to be a confounder, a C-E association can be required among the controls alone. This modification can be further motivated by noting that a primary use of the *OR* is to quantify the *E-Y* association in case-control studies—a design often selected because of its efficiency for studying rare outcomes. In a population-based case-control study of a rare outcome, the *C-E* association among controls estimates the *C-E* association in the source population from which cases and controls were drawn. Recall that epidemiologist Anthony invoked this rationale in the ketchup study example, noting that if anxiety was rare in the study setting, then the diet–anxiety association in controls should resemble that in the university student population from which study subjects were drawn. With this modification, logic similar to that used earlier for the *RR* and *RD* can be used to show that the *modified* comparability and collapsibility views always render the same verdict about whether *C* is a confounder of the *OR* when *C* is dichotomous (and assuming homogeneity).

But even with that modification to the comparability view, when *C* has three or more categories, the comparability and collapsibility views can still yield differing verdicts about whether *C* is a confounder of the *OR*. In particular, $2 \times 2 \times k$ tables exist in which the *OR* is collapsible over *C*, even if *C* is associated with *E* among the controls and is also associated with *Y* among the unexposed. The ketchup study data in Table 12.1 provided one such example.

To summarize for the *OR*:

- The collapsibility view presupposes homogeneity of the *OR* across strata, which the comparability view does not. When that precondition is met, both views apply. Assuming homogeneity…
- If the comparability view is applied by examining the *C-E* association in the full study population (without regard to *Y*), then the two views can reach different verdicts about whether *C* is a confounder of the *OR*, regardless of how many categories *C* has. Discordant verdicts can occur in either direction. The key reason is that collapsibility of the *OR* depends on the *C-E* association in controls (i.e., conditional on *Y*), which may be different from the *C-E* association the full study population.
- If the comparability view is modified to focus on the *C-E* association only among controls, then the circumstances under which the modified comparability and collapsibility

views agree mimic those for the *RR* and *RD*. That is, the views always agree when *C* is dichotomous; but when *C* has more than two categories, *C* may be deemed a confounder under the modified comparability view even if it is not deemed a confounder under the collapsibility view.

The Homogeneity Assumption, Revisited

The collapsibility view is unique in presupposing homogeneity before it can be used to address confounding. In contrast to the made-up examples presented so far, stratum-specific values of a measure of association are rarely exactly equal in real study data. For the *RR*, *RD*, and *OR*, statistical methods exist to test a null hypothesis of homogeneity in the source population from which study subjects were sampled (Breslow and Day, 1980; Rosner, 2006; Newman, 2001). Tests of this null hypothesis can also be carried out using interaction tests in regression models described later in this chapter. If the *p*-value from such a test does not lead to rejecting this null hypothesis, it is common practice to make a working assumption of homogeneity and proceed to address confounding. With very large sample sizes, even statistically significant heterogeneity among strata may be too small to be of practical importance, in which case homogeneity may still be accepted as a reasonable approximation (Newman, 2001).

Some studies involve an *a priori* hypothesis that an exposure–outcome association will be stronger in certain strata than in others. For example, a larger effect of taking a vitamin supplement might be expected in people with vitamin deficiency than in those with adequate dietary intake of the vitamin. When such heterogeneity has been hypothesized in advance, stratifying on *C* is necessary to address this research question, even if the results do not support the hypothesis.

Whether heterogeneity is hypothesized in advance or is simply discovered during data analysis, once a decision has been made to stratify on *C*, the possibility of confounding by *C* becomes largely irrelevant. Within strata of *C*, subjects are similar on *C*, so it cannot be a confounder. However, if the levels of *C* represent coarse groupings of a continuous variable such as age, or of a finely-categorized variable such as occupation, residual confounding may still be present within strata and require control.

3: Counterfactual View

A model of causal inference based on *counterfactuals* was introduced in Chapter 5. Although the concept of counterfactuals is centuries old (Greenland and Morgenstern, 2001; Maldonado and Greenland, 2002; Höfler, 2005), a connection with confounding was made only in the mid-1980s by Greenland and Robins (1986).

Imagine a "thought experiment" in which each person in a target population of interest is subjected to *each* possible level of a certain exposure, under otherwise identical conditions. A particular person might experience the same outcome at all exposure levels, or his/her outcome could be different at different exposure levels. Whatever outcome this person would experience if subjected to a certain exposure level is called his/her *potential outcome* at that level. With a binary exposure, let Y_{ej} denote the outcome that person j would experience if exposed, and let Y_{uj} denote the outcome that this same person would experience if unexposed, under otherwise identical conditions.[1]

In actuality, at the particular time and under conditions specified by the protocol of a real study, person j is either exposed or unexposed, but not both, so only one of his/her potential outcomes is observable. The other potential outcome is *counterfactual*—an outcome that did not actually occur and thus could not be observed, but that would have occurred if person j's exposure status had been the opposite of what it actually was. Table 12.4 illustrates this situation for several hypothetical study subjects.

TABLE 12.4. EXPOSURE STATUS AND POTENTIAL OUTCOMES FOR SEVERAL HYPOTHETICAL STUDY SUBJECTS, SHOWING WHICH POTENTIAL OUTCOME WOULD BE OBSERVABLE (UNSHADED) AND WHICH WOULD BE COUNTERFACTUAL (SHADED)

Subject	Exposure status	Y_e	Y_u
1	Exposed	0	0
2	Unexposed	1	0
3	Unexposed	0	0
4	Exposed	1	1
5	Unexposed	1	1
⋮	⋮	⋮	⋮

Suppose now that the listing partially shown in Table 12.4 is sorted by exposure status, and the separate listings for exposed and unexposed subjects are set side by side, as in Table 12.5. (Subjects have been renumbered sequentially within exposure groups.) Let N = number of exposed subjects and M = number of unexposed subjects. N and M may differ, so the two listings, if shown in full, could have different lengths. To help distinguish between observable and unobservable quantities, an asterisk (*) henceforth signifies an unobservable one.

The total number of cases (i.e., subjects with $Y = 1$) in each column is obtained by summing the column. Then each case count is divided by the

TABLE 12.5. OBSERVED AND COUNTERFACTUAL OUTCOMES FOR SEVERAL SUBJECTS IN THE EXPOSED AND UNEXPOSED GROUPS, AND CUMULATIVE INCIDENCES CALCULATED FROM THEM. (UNOBSERVABLE QUANTITIES ARE INDICATED BY * AND SHADING.)

	Exposed			Unexposed		
Subject	Y_e	Y_u^*		Subject	Y_e^*	Y_u
1	0	0		1	1	0
2	1	1		2	0	0
3	1	1		3	1	1
4	0	1		4	0	0
5	1	0		5	0	1
⋮	⋮	⋮		⋮	⋮	⋮
N	1	1		M	0	0
No. of cases:	n_e	n_u^*			m_e^*	m_u
Cumulative incidence:	$r_e = \frac{n_e}{N}$	$r_u^* = \frac{n_u^*}{N}$			$r_e^* = \frac{m_e^*}{M}$	$r_u = \frac{m_u}{M}$

corresponding group size to obtain a cumulative incidence. In the exposed group, r_e is the cumulative incidence actually observed, and r_u^* is the cumulative incidence that would have resulted in that group if no members had been exposed. In the unexposed group, r_u is the cumulative incidence actually observed, and r_e^* is the cumulative incidence that would have resulted in that group if all members had been exposed.

This formulation clarifies the relationship between exposure effects on individuals and exposure effects on outcome frequency in groups. If $r_e > r_u^*$, then the exposure increased cumulative incidence in the exposed group. To do so, exposure must also have caused the outcome in at least some individual group members (such as exposed-group subject #5), although it may have had no effect on many others (such as subjects #1, #2, and #3) and may even have prevented the outcome in still other individuals (such as subject #4). On the other hand, if $r_e = r_u^*$, implying no effect of exposure on cumulative incidence in the exposed group, it is possible that the number of members for whom exposure was causative (e.g., subject #5) was exactly offset by an equal number of members for whom exposure was preventive (e.g., subject #4).

Analytic epidemiologic studies are generally designed to estimate exposure effects on outcome frequency in populations and/or defined subpopulations, rather than exposure effects in individual people.[2] Consistent with that aim, the counterfactual view of confounding chiefly concerns inferences about exposure effects on population outcome frequency, which can also be interpreted as the average of individual-level outcomes.

The causal effect of exposure on cumulative incidence in the exposed group would ideally be inferred by comparing r_e with r_u^*. This effect could be quantified as a single number in familiar ways: as a ratio (r_e/r_u^*), as a difference $(r_e - r_u^*$, sometimes termed the *average causal effect among the exposed* because it is also the mean value of $Y_e - Y_u^*$ in exposed-group members), as an odds ratio, or in other ways. Unfortunately, however, r_u^* is not observable. What *is* available for comparison with r_e is r_u, the observed cumulative incidence in the unexposed group. Under the counterfactual view of confounding, an observed exposure–outcome association is confounded if and only if:

$$r_u^* \neq r_u \qquad (12.3)$$

This strikingly simple definition of confounding has several noteworthy features:

- It brings into sharp focus the role played by the unexposed group: namely, to provide a substitute for the unobservable counterfactual outcomes in the exposed group. If $r_e = r_e^*$ and $r_u = r_u^*$, the groups are said to be *exchangeable*: the results would be the same regardless of which group is actually exposed (Greenland and Robins, 1986; Hernán and Robins, 2006a).
- In a properly conducted randomized trial, the groups formed by random assignment are exchangeable by design; therefore $r_u^* = r_u$ and $r_e^* = r_e$, at least in expectation.
- Inequality (12.3) does not require advance specification of a particular measure of association, nor does it require homogeneity of any measure of association across strata.
- Inequality (12.3) addresses whether the E-Y association is confounded, but it does not identify the source of any confounding that may be present. In particular, it does not implicate any particular third variable (e.g., C) as a confounder.
- Which exposure level is called "exposed" is at the discretion of the investigator. An equivalent symmetrical argument could be made if the labelling were reversed, or if the unexposed group were chosen instead as the target population (i.e., seeking to estimate the cumulative incidence that would have been observed in the unexposed group had its members been exposed).

In observational studies, there is no randomization of exposure to render the exposed and unexposed groups exchangeable by design. Moreover, there is no way to confirm or refute from study data whether $r_u^* = r_u$, because r_u^* is unobservable.

Table 12.6 illustrates this conundrum. It shows results of a hypothetical cohort study in a closed population. The observed cumulative incidence is the same in the exposed and unexposed groups: $r_e = 150/(150 + 1,350) = 0.10$ and $r_u = 300/(300 + 2,700) = 0.10$, suggesting no effect of exposure. The shaded rows show three possible sets of unobserved potential outcomes for exposed-group members (Y_u^*) had they not been exposed. All three possibilities would be compatible with the observed number of cases in the exposed group. (Possible

TABLE 12.6. THREE POSSIBLE SETS OF COUNTERFACTUAL
OUTCOMES FOR EXPOSED-GROUP MEMBERS THAT COULD
LEAD TO THE SAME OBSERVED RESULTS IN A
HYPOTHETICAL COHORT STUDY

	Exposed				Unexposed	
Observed	$Y_e = 1$		$Y_e = 0$		$Y_u = 1$	$Y_u = 0$
	150		1,350		300	2,700
Counterfactual	$Y_u^* = 1$	$Y_u^* = 0$	$Y_u^* = 1$	$Y_u^* = 0$		
Possibility #1:	150	0	0	1,350		
Possibility #2:	90	60	60	1,290		
Possibility #3:	90	60	210	1,140		

counterfactual outcomes for the unexposed group are not shown because they are not needed in subsequent calculations, which focus on exposure effects in the exposed group.)

- Under possibility #1, exposure had no effect at all: every subject in the exposed group had the same outcome that he/she would have had if unexposed. Hence $r_u^* = (150 + 0)/1,500 = 0.10 = r_u$, implying no confounding.
- Under possibility #2, exposure actually *did* affect outcome for 120 individuals in the exposed group: in 60, exposure was causative, while in 60 others, it was preventive. But for the exposed group as a whole, those opposing effects of exposure exactly cancelled, so that $r_u^* = (90 + 60)/1,500 = 0.10 = r_u$, implying no confounding.
- Under possibility #3, exposure was causative for 60 exposed-group members, but it was preventive for 210. In this instance, $r_u^* = (90 + 210)/1,500 = 0.20 \neq r_u$, implying confounding. Under this possibility, the cumulative incidence among persons in the exposed group would have been 0.20—twice as high—had these same individuals not been exposed. But the actual unexposed group had a cumulative incidence of only 0.10, in this instance providing a poor substitute for the counterfactual cumulative incidence in the exposed group.

Under the counterfactual view of confounding, any interpretation of $r_e \neq r_u$ as a causal effect of exposure requires an assumption that disease frequency in the unexposed group correctly reflects what disease

frequency would have been in the exposed group had its members not been exposed. This assumption cannot be empirically verified; its acceptance rests on subject-matter knowledge and, to some extent, on faith.

Fortunately, the counterfactual view does allow a way by which the burden of reliance on faith may be lightened somewhat: namely, by replacing a strong assumption of (unconditional) exchangeability between exposed and unexposed groups with a hopefully weaker assumption of *conditional* exchangeability. The idea is that if $r_u \neq r_u^*$, then other causes of Y among unexposed individuals must be differently distributed between the exposed and unexposed groups. And if study subjects are stratified by one or more of these other causes, then *within strata*, the required assumption that $r_u = r_u^*$ may be more likely to be satisfied than without such stratification. This argument may sound familiar: it is, essentially, the comparability view. The assumption of conditional exchangeability replaces inequality (12.3) with:

$$r_u^* \neq \sum_i w_{ei} \cdot r_{ui} \qquad (12.4)$$

as the necessary and sufficient requirement for confounding of the exposure–outcome association, where, as before, w_{ei} is the proportion of exposed-group members that belong to stratum i, and r_{ui} is the cumulative incidence among unexposed subjects in stratum i. The expression on the right side can be seen to be the cumulative incidence in the unexposed group, directly adjusted to the distribution of the stratification factor(s) in the exposed group.

As another cautionary lesson, however, consider Table 12.7, which builds on the hypothetical data in Table 12.6. Say that the investigators are surprised by the apparent absence of an exposure effect $(r_e = r_u)$ in the study behind Table 12.6, and they are concerned that dissimilarities between the exposed and unexposed groups may have resulted in a true effect of exposure being masked by confounding. After a search for stratification variables that might render the exposed and unexposed groups more comparable within strata, a factor C has been found. It behaves like a confounder: its distribution differs between the exposed and unexposed groups, and it is associated with Y within the unexposed group. Within each stratum of C, $RR = 1.50$, which differs from the unstratified value of $RR = 1.00$, thus also meeting the criteria for being a confounder of the RR under the collapsibility view. But, as before, many possible sets of counterfactual outcomes could be compatible with the observed data. Three such sets are shown in Table 12.7, and relevant summary statistics calculated from them are shown in Table 12.8.

- Possibility #1 is the hoped-for ideal. In the pooled data, $r_u = 0.100$, while $r_u^* = 0.067$, implying confounding. But within each stratum, $r_u = r_u^*$, implying no confounding. A true association between exposure and outcome had indeed been masked in Table 12.6 due to confounding by C, as the investigators suspected. Happily, all of that confounding was successfully removed by stratifying on C: the stratum-specific RR's and RR_{adj} all equal the true value (RR^*) of 1.50.

- Possibility #2 shows an apparent paradox. As with Possibility #1, confounding is present in the pooled data $(r_u \neq r_u^*,$ and $RR \neq RR^*)$. But in this case, the stratum-specific estimates of association are also confounded: within each stratum, $r_u \neq r_u^*$, and $RR \neq RR^*$. Yet surprisingly, adjustment for C yields $RR_{adj} = 1.50 = RR^*$, which is unconfounded. The reason is that in the $C = 0$ stratum, r_u *under*estimated r_u^*, while in the $C = 1$ stratum, r_u *over*estimated r_u^*. When information from the two strata was combined to get RR_{adj}, these estimation errors ultimately cancelled each other out. The counterfactual view points out that this kind of thing can happen.

TABLE 12.7. THREE POSSIBLE SETS OF COUNTERFACTUAL OUTCOMES FOR EXPOSED-GROUP MEMBERS, WITHIN STRATA OF C, EACH OF WHICH COULD LEAD TO THE SAME OBSERVED RESULTS

Stratum $C = 0$

	Exposed				Unexposed	
	$Y_e = 1$		$Y_e = 0$		$Y_u = 1$	$Y_u = 0$
Observed:	60		1,020		45	1,170
Counterfactual:	$Y_u^* = 1$	$Y_u^* = 0$	$Y_u^* = 1$	$Y_u^* = 0$		
Possibility #1	30	30	10	1,010		
Possibility #2	40	20	20	1,000		
Possibility #3	60	0	0	1,020		

Stratum $C = 1$

	Exposed				Unexposed	
	$Y_e = 1$		$Y_e = 0$		$Y_u = 1$	$Y_u = 0$
Observed:	90		330		255	1,530
Counterfactual:	$Y_u^* = 1$	$Y_u^* = 0$	$Y_u^* = 1$	$Y_u^* = 0$		
Possibility #1	50	40	10	320		
Possibility #2	20	70	20	310		
Possibility #3	90	0	0	330		

TABLE 12.8. SUMMARY OF STATISTICS COMPUTED FROM RESULTS SHOWN IN TABLE 12.7 (WHERE SHADING INDICATES UNOBSERVABLE QUANTITITES)

Quantity[a]	Stratum		
	$C=0$	$C=1$	Pooled
r_e	0.056	0.214	0.100
r_u	0.037	0.143	0.100
RR	1.50	1.50	1.00
RR_{adj}			1.50
Possibility #1:			
r_u^*	0.037	0.143	0.067
RR^*	1.50	1.50	1.50
Possibility #2:			
r_u^*	0.056	0.095	0.067
RR^*	1.00	2.25	1.50
Possibility #3:			
r_u^*	0.056	0.214	0.100
RR^*	1.00	1.00	1.00

[a] Definitions:
$RR = r_e/r_u$
$RR^* = r_e/r_u^*$
$RR_{adj} = r_e / \sum_i w_{ei} \cdot r_{ui}$

w_{ei} = proportion of exposed subjects that fall into stratum i
r_{ui} = cumulative incidence among unexposed in stratum i

Even though the stratum-specific RRs were biased, RR_{adj} was not, because its denominator, $\sum_i w_{ei} \cdot r_{ui}$, correctly estimated the cumulative incidence that would have been observed in the overall exposed group had they not been exposed.

- Possibility #3 is alarming. It shows that the observed data also could be obtained even if exposure actually had no effect on anyone: every person's outcome would have been exactly the same if his/her exposure status had been reversed. Thus, in truth $RR^* = 1.00$. Nonetheless, in the observed data, C looks for all the world like a confounder. The investigators would almost certainly regard $RR_{adj} = 1.50$ as closer to the truth than the unadjusted $RR = 1.00$—which, unfortunately, would be flatly incorrect. Under possibility #3, the *crude RR* correctly estimated the true effect of exposure, while the

adjusted RR_{adj} was confounded. The underlying problem is that confounding from other sources besides C, and with which C was associated, has not been identified and controlled. Adjusting for C alone not only failed to reduce bias, it actually did more harm than good by *introducing* bias.

The counterfactual view thus shows that a wide range of possibilities can be compatible with the observed data in a non-randomized study. It confronts us with the limits of what can be inferred with confidence about causation from observational data. In stark terms, we cannot tell for sure when confounding is present, cannot tell for sure when it has been adequately controlled, and cannot even be sure whether controlling for an apparent confounder has reduced or increased confounding. Epidemiologist Catherine in the ketchup study alluded to these bleak conclusions when she declared agnosticism about whether diet type was a confounder.

Practical Implications

Confounding is a subtle phenomenon. Each of the three views helps sharpen our understanding of it.

The counterfactual view grounds confounding in a broader theory of causation. It clarifies the link between exposure effects on individuals and effects on outcome frequency in populations. It also identifies the specific conditions that must be met in order for measures of association computed from epidemiologic data to reflect accurately the causal effects of exposure. In so doing, it reinforces the special importance of randomized trials, which offer the best chance of satisfying those conditions. The counterfactual view has also led to useful new analytic approaches to thorny problems, such as causal inference in randomized trials with non-compliance, and certain longitudinal studies wherein a variable can be both a confounder and a mediator. The main limitation of the counterfactual view, however, is those pesky asterisks. Key quantities that we would love to know in order to quantify the extent of confounding are defined clearly enough, but they are not observable and thus not available to guide analysis and inference on real epidemiologic data. To the extent that the counterfactual view uses study data to guide decisions about whether to control for a potential confounder, it does so largely by falling back on the comparability view.

The comparability and collapsibility views are more empirical in orientation, identifying features in data that suggest confounding. The comparability view specifies necessary conditions for a confounder, which in turn imply a strategy of screening potential confounders for their association with exposure, and for their association with outcome among the unexposed. A strength of this approach is that it reveals the direction and strength of the two associations that any confounder must have, thus clarifying the underlying mechanism. However, further analysis must typically follow to determine whether the data suggest effect modification by the potential confounder, and whether the extent of bias due to confounding is of practical importance. There are circumstances in which the comparability criteria for confounding are met, yet no bias results.

Ultimately, the collapsibility view leads to what is arguably the most practical and efficient approach for using study data to screen potential confounders and help decide whether to control for them. To be sure, it requires advance specification of a measure of association; but that choice should almost always be made *a priori* anyway, based on the research goal and study design. Once a measure of association has been chosen, the collapsibility view keeps attention focused on the main analytic goal: to obtain as unbiased and precise an estimate of that measure as possible. A preliminary step normally involves testing the required assumption that the chosen measure of association be homogenous across strata, a step that is useful in its own right for detecting unexpected effect modification.

So in the end, we side with epidemiologist Barbara in opting not to control for diet type in the ketchup study. There was no evidence that confounding due to diet type biased the ketchup–anxiety association of main interest.

Two other important aspects of confounding have received little attention in the foregoing discussion because all three views agree on them. First, the conceptual relationships among exposure, outcome, and other key variables must be specified *a priori* before confounding can be addressed properly. These conceptual relationships cannot be inferred from study data alone; structure must be imposed based on subject-matter knowledge. One facet of this issue is that if a variable C is on a causal pathway from exposure to outcome, it cannot be a confounder, but this cannot be determined empirically.

Second, whether a given variable is an important source of confounding depends on which *other* variables have been controlled. The research scenario addressed so far in this chapter has considered only a single potential confounder, C. But for many outcomes of public health importance—e.g., coronary heart disease, low birth weight, or all-causes mortality—many risk factors are already well known, and they can be considered potential confounders when evaluating a new exposure.

Fortunately, another research tool is available that can be used to codify subject-matter knowledge and to identify important potential sources of confounding of a particular exposure-outcome relationship: namely, *causal diagrams*, described in the next section.

CAUSAL DIAGRAMS

Conceptual models of factors influencing a given health outcome have been represented pictorially for many years, often as words in boxes connected by arrows. The idea of a "web of causation" posited a network of causal factors that act in concert to produce disease (Krieger, 1994). The initial purpose of these diagrams was simply to aid communication—a purpose for which they remain very useful ("A picture is worth a thousand words."). But Greenland *et al.* (1999a), building on work by Pearl (1995), showed that if these diagrams are constructed according to certain rules, they can also provide a rigorous way to address important aspects of confounding. A correctly drawn causal diagram can be used to determine whether controlling for a certain combination of variables would be sufficient to remove confounding of an exposure–outcome association. Equally important, causal diagrams can be used to identify variables that should *not* be controlled, or that need not be controlled.

More recently, causal diagrams have been shown to aid understanding of selection bias (Hernán *et al.*, 2004), measurement bias (Shahar, 2009), and mediation analysis (Shpitser and VanderWeele, 2011). In keeping with the topic of this chapter, the discussion below focuses on confounding.

Construction and Terminology

Much of the terminology related to causal diagrams is inherited from graph theory, a branch of mathematics. A causal diagram consists of *nodes* (also called *vertices*), usually shown pictorially as boxes; and *directed edges* (also called *arcs*), shown as arrows leading from one box to another. Nodes represent variables. These typically include an exposure of interest, an outcome of interest, and other relevant variables, some of which may be potential confounders. For now, we will ignore the substantive roles played by different variables, since the rules for diagram construction do not depend on them. Each node is labelled with a letter and/or a variable name. An example is:

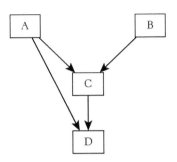

FIGURE 12.1

When an arrow goes from, say, node **X** to node **Y**, then **X** and **Y** are said to be *adjacent* nodes, **X** is called a *parent* of **Y**, and **Y** is called a *child* of **X**. In the above diagram, **A** and **B** are parents of **C**; **C** is a child of **A** and **B**; **D** is a child of **A** and **C**; and so on. When a sequence of one or more arrows leads from **X** to **Y**, *following the direction of the arrows*, then **X** is said to be an *ancestor* of **Y**, and **Y** is a *descendant* of **X**. *Parent* is thus a special case of *ancestor*, and *child* is a special case of *descendant*. In the above diagram, **A**, **B**, and **C** are ancestors of **D**; **C** and **D** are descendants of **A**; **C** and **D** are descendants of **B**; and so on.

A diagram constructed from these components qualifies as a *directed acyclic graph*—a *DAG*, for short—if: (1) all edges are *directed* edges—i.e., each edge is an arrow that points in one direction only; and (2) no node is a descendant of itself. For example, consider the two diagrams in Figure 12.2.

Diagram **A** in Figure 12.2 is a DAG. Diagram **B** is not, because each node is a descendant of itself. However, sometimes a diagram such as **B** can be "unwound" and re-expressed as a DAG by being more explicit about the temporal sequence, as in Figure 12.3.

Strictly speaking, a DAG is a general mathematical construct that can represent many non-epidemiologic systems, such as steps in a manufacturing process, travel routes from one city to another, etc. A *causal diagram* is a special type of DAG that meets the following additional conditions:

- Nodes represent variables.
- An arrow denotes a *direct causal effect*: that is, **X** → **Y** implies that, with all other variables held constant, changing **X** would change **Y**. Thus *parent* and *ancestor* nodes represent *causes*, while *child* and *descendant* nodes represent *effects*.
- If any two variables share a common ancestor (cause), that ancestor is included in the causal diagram. To satisfy this requirement, a causal diagram can include variables that are unmeasured and possibly even unknown, often labelled **U**. If there are several such variables, they may be labelled **U**₁, **U**₂, etc.

A *path* from **X** to **Y** is a route consisting of a series of jumps between adjacent nodes starting at **X** and ending at **Y**, *ignoring the directionality of the arrows*, and without revisiting any node that is already part of the path. There may be multiple paths between two nodes. In Figure 12.4, there are four paths from **A** to **E**: **A-B-C-E**, **A-C-D-E**, **A-B-C-D-E**, and **A-C-E**.

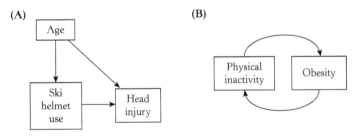

FIGURE 12.2

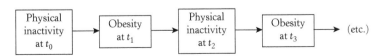

FIGURE 12.3

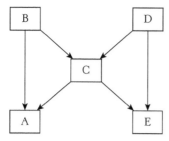

FIGURE 12.4

Along a given path, if two arrowheads converge at node **X**, then **X** is said to be a *collider*; otherwise, **X** is a *non-collider*. In other words, a collider is a shared child of two parent nodes on that path. Note that **X** may be a collider on one path and a non-collider on another. In the above diagram, **C** is a non-collider on the **A-B-C-E** path, but **C** is a collider on the **A-B-C-D-E** path.

Conditioning on a variable **X** essentially means *controlling for* **X**—conceptually, "holding **X** constant." Common ways of conditioning on, or controlling for, **X** include:

- *Restriction*: confining the analysis to subjects who all have the same value of **X**—e.g., restricting a study to women, where **X** is gender.
- *Stratification*: making all comparisons within levels (strata) of **X**.
- *Matching*: making all comparisons within pairs or small sets in which each subject in one group is linked to one or more subjects in the other group who are similar on **X**.
- *Covariate adjustment*: using regression analysis (introduced later in this chapter) or a related statistical technique to account for possible differences on **X** when making comparisons.

(The above list may look familiar: these are standard epidemiologic methods to control confounding by **X**.) Shading of a node is used henceforth to indicate conditioning on that variable—for example:

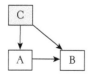

FIGURE 12.5

indicates controlling for **C**.

How an Association Between Two Variables Can Arise

In the absence of measurement error, an association between any two variables **X** and **Y** can arise in five ways (adapted from Glymour, 2006):

1. *Chance*. Even if **X** and **Y** are unassociated in the source population from which study subjects are drawn, they may be associated in the study sample due to sampling variability. Associations due to chance alone are not causal and are not explicitly shown in causal diagrams.
2. *X causes Y*. If **X** is the exposure and **Y** is the outcome, this mechanism corresponds to what is usually the main study hypothesis. However, the same mechanism can apply to any other pair of variables as well. The simplest appearance of this mechanism in a causal diagram would be:

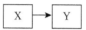

FIGURE 12.6

although **Y** could also be a descendant of **X** via two or more paths, and other intermediate variables could lie on a causal path from **X** to **Y**.

3. *Y causes X*. Nothing in the structure of a causal diagram identifies which node the investigator considers to represent an exposure of main interest, or which node represents the outcome of main interest. A cause–effect relationship in either direction can produce an association between two variables. Hence comments about the previous mechanism apply. If **Y** causes **X** but the investigator mistakenly regarded **X** as the exposure and **Y** as the outcome, this mechanism could be considered reverse causation.
4. *Shared ancestor*. **X** and **Y** may have one or more ancestors in common, resulting in an **X-Y** association. If **X** is the exposure and **Y** is the outcome, this mechanism represents confounding of the main association of interest. The simplest appearance of this mechanism in a causal diagram would be:

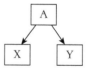

FIGURE 12.7

but more elaborate versions of the same phenomenon can occur—e.g., there may be intermediate variables between **A** and **X** or between **A** and **Y**, and **X** and **Y** may have two or more shared ancestors on the same path or different paths.

5. *Control for a shared descendant*. Even if **X** and **Y** are otherwise unassociated, controlling for a shared

descendant of **X** and **Y** can create an association between them. The simplest appearance of this mechanism in a causal diagram would be:

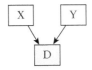

FIGURE 12.8

although, again, intermediate variables could lie on the path from **X** to **D** or from **Y** to **D**, and/or the variable being controlled could be a descendant of **D** rather than **D** itself.

Mechanism #5 is probably the least familiar and least intuitive, but causal-diagram theory has led to greater appreciation of its importance. To illustrate it, consider the non-epidemiologic example in Table 12.9. Suppose that a prestigious private school, Lofty University, uses two main factors in deciding whether to admit an applicant: (1) his/her aptitude test score, and (2) whether a parent of the applicant had attended Lofty U. Panel A describes the overall applicant pool, showing no association between test score and having a parent who attended Lofty U. Panel B shows the percentage of applicants accepted at each possible combination of characteristics. Applicants with a high test score had a 20 percentage-point advantage, those with a parent who attended Lofty U. had a 10 percentage-point advantage, and each factor had the same effect irrespective of the other factor. Panel C shows the characteristics of those accepted to Lofty U. Each cell of panel C is the product of the corresponding cells from panels A and B.

Despite the lack of association between test score and parental alumnus status in the overall applicant pool, Panel C shows that the two factors were associated *among those accepted*: 1/4 of those with a high test score had a parent who was an alumnus, compared to 1/3 of those with a low test score. Panel C results from *conditioning on* acceptance, here by restricting the table to accepted applicants. (An association can also be found in rejected applicants.) In causal-diagram form, see Figure 12.9.

Mechanism #5 involves controlling for a *collider* (or a descendant of a collider), which is why colliders are distinguished from non-colliders along paths in a causal diagram. It is also why mechanism #5 is sometimes called *collider-stratification bias* (Greenland, 2003).

TABLE 12.9. HYPOTHETICAL EXAMPLE ILLUSTRATING ASSOCIATION MECHANISM #5

A: Distribution of characteristics in overall applicant pool

| | Parent went to Lofty U. | |
Test score	Yes	No
High	200	800
Low	200	800

B: Percent of applicants accepted

| | Parent went to Lofty U. | |
Test score	Yes	No
High	40%	30%
Low	20%	10%

C: Distribution of characteristics in *accepted* applicants

| | Parent went to Lofty U. | |
Test score	Yes	No
High	80	240
Low	40	80

As an aside, a form of selection bias known as *Berkson's bias* results from mechanism #5 (Westreich, 2012). Berkson (1946) noticed that diabetes and gallbladder disease, two diseases that occur approximately independently in the population at large, could nonetheless appear to be negatively associated with one another in a sample of hospitalized patients. Each disease can cause hospitalization, and examining their association in a sample of hospitalized patients thus involves conditioning on a common effect. Figure 12.10 portrays the situation in causal-diagram form.

Other examples of mechanism #5 are described by Cole *et al.* (2010); Glymour (2006); Whitcomb *et al.* (2009).

Except for mechanisms #2 and #3, the five mechanisms described above are not mutually exclusive. The overall magnitude of the **X-Y** association can result from several of the mechanisms acting in combination. And that, in essence, is the problem: typically, the main study goal is to isolate the causal effect of an exposure on an outcome (mechanism #2), and other mechanisms influencing that exposure–outcome association are nuisances. Tests of statistical significance can be used to help evaluate whether chance (mechanism #1) could be the sole explanation for an association. Confidence limits

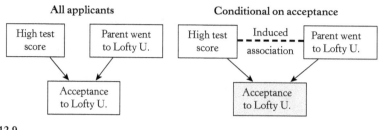

FIGURE 12.9

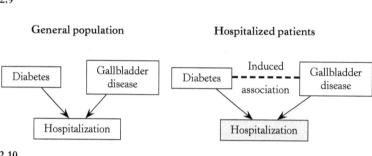

FIGURE 12.10

place probabilistic bounds on where the true association may lie and can also be used to help judge whether chance alone could plausibly have produced the observed association. Reverse causation (mechanism #3) can sometimes be ruled out by subject-matter knowledge about temporal sequence (e.g., occurrence of a disease cannot influence an afflicted person's prior family history), or by the study design. Causal diagrams can guide the approach to eliminating mechanism #4—confounding of the causal component of the exposure–outcome association due to their having shared ancestors—by helping the investigator decide which variables need to be controlled. But mechanism #5 implies that controlling for a variable can also have side effects, inducing or altering associations among that variable's ancestors. These side effects must be taken into account when fashioning a strategy to control confounding.

Application to Control of Confounding
Four examples are discussed below, followed by description of a general algorithm for addressing confounding with causal diagrams. Each example concerns a realistic research scenario, but the causal diagram in each case is deliberately kept simple to focus on a particular issue. A more elaborate causal diagram including other variables would probably be needed in an actual study of each example.

Example 12-1.   Consider a study that aims to determine whether owning a bicycle helmet prevents

having a bicycling-related head injury. If only those two variables were considered, they would be likely to be *positively* associated in the population at large—people who own a bike helmet being more likely to have a biking-related head injury—because both owning a bike helmet and the risk of experiencing a biking-related head injury are associated with owning a bike. In causal-diagram form:

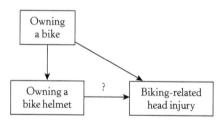

FIGURE 12.11

The study hypothesis is indicated by the arrow with a question mark. But owning a bike would almost certainly increase a person's likelihood of owning a bike helmet, and owning a bike would also make it more likely that a person actually rides a bike and is thus more likely to experience a biking-related head injury. Without controlling for bike ownership, it could appear that owning a bike helmet increases the risk of a biking-related head injury. *Among bike owners*, however, wearing a bike helmet may well *prevent* head injury while biking (e.g., Thompson *et al.* [1989]). A true preventive effect of bike helmet use is confounded by bike ownership in the general population. In causal-diagram terms, bike ownership is a shared ancestor of bike helmet ownership and bike-related head injury. The confounding could be removed by controlling for bike ownership—e.g., by restricting the study to bike owners, or by stratifying on bike ownership.

This simple example shows that confounding appears in a causal diagram as an *unblocked backdoor path* from exposure to outcome. Recall that a *path* from exposure to outcome is a sequence of jumps along a series of adjacent nodes, ignoring the directionality of the arrows between them, that starts at exposure and ends at outcome (without revisiting any node). *Backdoor* refers to the fact that the first jump on a path of interest is from exposure to a *parent* of exposure—in this case, from owning a bike helmet to owning a bike. The backdoor path then leads from the parent of exposure to the outcome. In this example, the rest of the path from the parent of exposure to the outcome involves only one more jump. In other situations, the rest of the path could involve several jumps along a series of adjacent nodes, which could be either ancestors or descendants of the parent of exposure, eventually reaching the outcome. Unblocked backdoor paths, including the one in this example, can be thought of as a separate "chain of associations" that mixes with the causal effect of exposure to produce the overall exposure–outcome association. The backdoor path can be *blocked* in this case by controlling for bike ownership.

Example 12-2. The initial example of confounding described in Chapter 11 concerned mortality in Communities A and B, which differed in their age structure. An appropriate causal diagram might be:

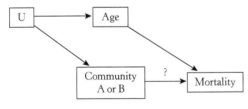

FIGURE 12.12

Although there are known age differences between communities, it is not necessary to posit that age is a *cause* of the community in which a person resides. Manipulating a person's age (were that possible) would not necessarily cause him/her to move from one community to another. Still, other factor(s) must be responsible for the fact that the communities

have different age structures—e.g., historical factors related to migration, or differential survival. These factors, which remain unspecified and unmeasured, are designated **U** in the causal diagram. **U** is included to allow for a non-causal association between age and community. That association is implicit in the structure of the diagram—age and community have a shared ancestor—but it is not shown as a direct link between age and community, because only arrows are allowed in causal diagrams, and they denote direct causation.

Apart from including **U**, this example is similar to the previous one in that there is a single backdoor path from exposure to outcome. Because **U** is unmeasured, there is no way to control for it. However, the backdoor path on which **U** is situated can be blocked by controlling for age, and doing so would remove the confounding.

Example 12-3. Next consider a study that aims to determine the degree to which deployment of an airbag in a vehicular crash affects the risk of death. Assume that airbags were mandated by law in vehicles made after a certain year. Two other probable determinants of whether a crash is fatal are vehicle model year, which reflects other vehicle-design features that affect safety (e.g., braking systems, frame design); and vehicle speed just before a crash. A suitable causal diagram involving these variables would be:

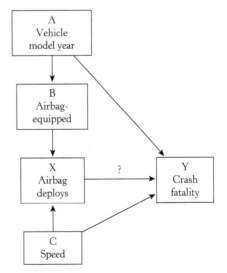

FIGURE 12.13

The exposure, airbag deployment, is assumed to depend on whether an airbag is present, and on vehicle speed at crash time. Presence of an airbag is presumed not to affect crash fatality unless the airbag actually deploys. In this example, three other variables besides exposure are involved, but there are only two backdoor paths. The **X-C-Y** path can be blocked only by controlling for **C**. The **X-B-A-Y** path can be blocked by controlling for **A**, for **B**, or for both **A** and **B**. The causal diagram shows that there is no real need to control for both **A** and **B**, however, to remove confounding; controlling for either **A** or **B** would suffice.

This example shows that causal diagrams focus on *backdoor paths*, not on individual variables as confounders. Often the number of intermediate variables that are shown along a given causal path is at the discretion of the causal diagram's creator. For example, imagine a study to determine whether some new exposure is a cause of myocardial infarction. A backdoor path might involve elevated serum cholesterol. The causal diagram could be shown Figure 12.14, or as Figure 12.15.

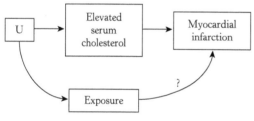

FIGURE 12.14

The version in Figure 12.15 makes the causal diagram busier, but it does not necessarily complicate the problem of controlling confounding. There are more variables, but there are no more paths. In fact, rather than adding several more potential confounders that may need to be evaluated and controlled, sometimes a more detailed version may actually facilitate the task of controlling confounding by offering new opportunities for blocking a path in question. Controlling for any one of the non-colliders along a path suffices to block it.

Example 12-4. It has been hypothesized that traumatic brain injury in early life may increase the risk of developing Alzheimer's disease years later. Alzheimer's disease is also known to be more likely to develop in someone who carries the genetic trait ApoE4, which is present in about 10–15% of people and can be inherited from either parent. Yet another known risk factor is a low educational level. Consider the causal diagram in Figure 12.16.

A low educational level in a child's mother could be a marker of low socioeconomic status, which in turn has been found to be associated with increased risk of child head injury. This association may be due in part to a more hazardous environment and/or to suboptimal parental supervision. Low maternal education would also increase the mother's own risk of developing Alzheimer's disease. If the mother carries the ApoE4 allele, she would be at increased risk for Alzheimer's disease herself and could pass the allele on to her child, affecting the child's risk of Alzheimer's disease in later life.

Admittedly, a more elaborate causal diagram including other variables would probably be needed for a real study of this issue. But focusing on the simplified causal diagram at hand, which of the variables shown must be controlled in order to avoid confounding of the causal effect (if any) of childhood head trauma on the risk of developing Alzheimer's disease in later life?

It is tempting at first glance to see a single backdoor path from **X** to **Y** and to suppose that controlling for any variable along that path would block it. But in reality, the path is already blocked. **C** is a collider. The seductive metaphor that *any* backdoor path represents a chain of associations breaks down when the path contains a collider. In this case, **A** and **B** would be expected to be independent: neither causes the other, and they have no ancestors in common. The ApoE4 genotype in subjects' mothers should be about equally common across all levels of maternal education. Just because **A** and **B** have a descendant in common does

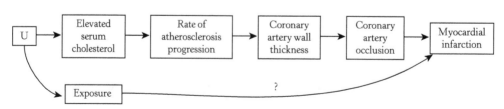

FIGURE 12.15

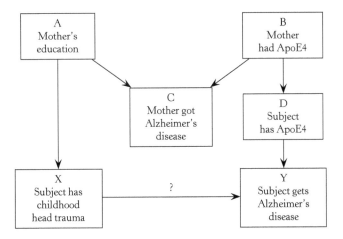

FIGURE 12.16

not imply that **A** and **B** themselves are associated. Table 12.9 concerning admission to Lofty University provided one such example. Only when one *controls for* a common descendant of two variables **X** and **Y** is an **X-Y** association induced or altered. Otherwise, a collider blocks the path on which it is located.

Causal-diagram theory asserts that, in this instance, it actually would be a mistake to control for **C** by itself. Doing so would unblock the backdoor path by creating an association between **A** and **B** that did not previously exist. That would create a **X-A-B-D-Y** chain of associations that could confound the causal effect of **X** on **Y**. This phenomenon has been called *M-bias*, based on the shape of the causal diagram (Greenland, 2003). Note, however, that the new backdoor path created by controlling for **C** could be blocked by controlling for **A**, **B**, or **D** in addition to **C**.

Causal-diagram theory thus leads to a very different assessment of the role played by variables like **C** than do traditional views of confounding. Under the comparability view, **C** looks like a confounder: it is associated with **X** (by virtue of having a common ancestor, **A**), it is associated with **Y** (by virtue of having a common ancestor, **B**), and it does not lie on a causal path from **X** to **Y**. But the causal-diagram view places **C** in context as a collider on a backdoor path from **X** to **Y**. It shows that an investigator would be justified in *not* controlling for **C**; and if it were controlled, other steps would be needed to deal with the side effects of doing so. Theoretical work (Greenland, 2003; VanderWeele and Robins, 2007a) and simulation studies (Liu *et al.*, 2012) have shown that

bias can indeed result from controlling for a collider such as **C** that lies on a backdoor path from exposure to outcome. The size of the bias depends on the strength of other associations along the path in question.

Table 12.10 presents a general algorithm for determining whether controlling for all variables in a given set, **S**, would be sufficient to eliminate confounding of an exposure–outcome effect, assuming a correctly drawn causal diagram. This method, known technically as the *d-separation algorithm* (Pearl, 2000), has been described in several different ways in the literature on causal diagrams (Greenland *et al.*, 1999b; Pearl, 2000; Hernán *et al.*, 2002; Glymour, 2006). Note that:

- The algorithm is not designed to produce a single, unique set **S** of variables that must be controlled. Instead, it takes as input a candidate set **S** of potential control variables proposed by the investigator and yields a binary verdict on whether controlling all variables in **S** would or would not be sufficient to control confounding.
- Often any one of several sets of variables (possibly with overlapping membership) would be sufficient to control confounding. If so, the investigator can choose among these sets, based on such factors as how many variables are in each set and how difficult or costly it would be to obtain data on them.
- Sometimes the empty (null) set passes the sufficiency test specified by the algorithm, in which case no variables need to be controlled.

TABLE 12.10. GENERAL ALGORITHM TO DETERMINE WHETHER CONTROLLING FOR ALL VARIABLES IN A SPECIFIED SET S WOULD BE SUFFICIENT TO REMOVE ALL CONFOUNDING OF THE CAUSAL EFFECT OF EXPOSURE ON OUTCOME, ASSUMING A CORRECTLY DRAWN CAUSAL DIAGRAM

1. Set S must not contain any descendants of the exposure or of the outcome.
2. Identify all backdoor paths from exposure to outcome, and classify each path as either *blocked* or *unblocked*. A path is blocked if it contains:
   (a) A non-collider that is in S; or
   (b) A collider that is *not* in S and
        that has no descendants in S.
   Otherwise the path is unblocked.
3. The causal effect of exposure on outcome is confounded if, and only if, an unblocked backdoor path exists from exposure to outcome.

• For some causal diagrams, no set may exist that suffices to control all confounding; or some variables in a set S that passes the sufficiency test may be unmeasured, making it impossible to apply S in practice.

The algorithm in Table 12.10 is explicit enough that it can be (and has been) codified into a computer program. The larger challenges for the investigator are to create a satisfactory causal diagram in the first place, to find one or more sets of variables that pass the sufficiency test specified by algorithm, and to choose the most feasible set among those that pass the test. Developing a causal diagram depends heavily on subject-matter knowledge, and there are few general rules beyond those that define requirements for a legally constructed causal diagram. Draft causal diagrams can themselves be useful tools for focusing discussion and debate among investigators and subject-matter experts. When there is uncertainty about how parts of the diagram should be specified, it can be informative to apply the algorithm to more than one version of the diagram and compare the results. Recognizing the plight of investigators who struggle with causal-diagram construction, VanderWeele and Shpitser (2011) proposed a generic strategy for confounder selection that requires

less-detailed prior specification of the causal relationships among potential confounders. Using causal-diagram theory, they showed that controlling for *all* variables that are ancestors of either exposure or outcome (or both) should remove all confounding. However, the resulting set may be far from the most efficient set that would remove all confounding. Moreover, controlling for a large number of variables may be feasible only with relatively large sample sizes, and it may sacrifice precision.

Contrasts with Traditional Approaches to Confounding

Causal-diagram theory has helped to refine thinking about confounding in several ways:

• Traditional approaches tend to focus on classifying individual variables: Is C a confounder? Causal-diagram theory focuses instead on causal paths and sets of variables that relate to them: Which paths must be blocked to control confounding, and which sets of control variables would be sufficient to block those paths?
• Traditional approaches assert that a variable cannot be a confounder if it lies on a causal pathway from exposure to outcome. Causal-diagram theory broadens this criterion a bit: any variable that is a descendant of exposure or of outcome should not be controlled.
• Traditional approaches can foster a "more is better" philosophy: the more potential confounders one can control for, the less biased the final estimate of exposure effect will be. Causal-diagram theory encourages and justifies a more selective approach: once a given backdoor path is blocked, controlling for other variables along it is unnecessary. Also, in some cases, there can be pitfalls in controlling for a variable if it is a collider or a descendant of a collider along one or more paths (Schisterman *et al.*, 2009).

Directionality of Confounding Bias

With a little embellishment, causal diagrams can sometimes also be used to predict the direction in which confounding due to a certain unblocked backdoor path would shift the exposure–outcome association compared to the true (unconfounded) association (VanderWeele *et al.*, 2008). The key idea is to attach a sign (+ or –) to each arrow along the backdoor path from exposure to outcome. The sign for each arrow should reflect the direction in which the child variable would change if the parent variable were increased. (For binary variables, a possibly arbitrary choice may be needed as to which of its two levels is "greater" than the other. For categorical variables with three or more unordered categories, no meaningful sign may be possible.) The exposure–outcome association can be expected to be shifted by confounding in the direction indicated by the product of the resulting signs along the backdoor path.

To illustrate, the causal diagram in Example 12-1 can be embellished as:

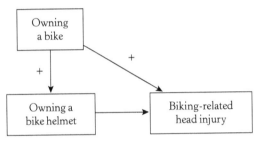

FIGURE 12.17

Bike ownership should be positively associated with bike helmet ownership, and bike ownership should also be positively associated with risk of sustaining a biking-related head injury. The product (+) × (+) is positive, so one would expect the overall association between bike helmet ownership and biking-related head injury to be biased in a positive direction by uncontrolled confounding along that path. More complex situations are discussed by VanderWeele *et al.* (2008). This approach can be useful in gauging the directionality of possible bias due to inability to control a known but unmeasured confounder.

Note that *directionality of bias* in this context refers to where the confounded association lies in relation to the true association on the real number line. Risk ratios, rate ratios, and odds ratios can range from 0 to ∞; the risk difference from –1 to +1; and the rate difference from $-\infty$ to $+\infty$. For the *RR*, say, bias in a positive direction means that $RR_{confounded} > RR_{true}$, while bias in a negative direction means that $RR_{confounded} < RR_{true}$, and likewise for the other measures. The null value (1 for ratio measures, 0 for difference measures) plays no role,

and it is therefore not conceptually correct to think of confounding as creating a bias toward or away from the null. Confounding causes the biased estimate to fall either above or below the true value.

Limitations of Causal Diagrams

Causal diagrams provide a useful tool for representing relationships among key variables, and they provide a rigorous, non-quantitative way to help decide which variables to control. Their limitations include:

- Knowledge and/or assumptions are required about the role played by each variable. However, such assumptions must be made anyway to permit proper data analysis, and often these assumptions are hidden from view. The same data can be consistent with several different causal models, with quite different implications about which variables should be controlled and which should not (Robins, 2001; Hernán *et al.*, 2002; Joffe *et al.*, 2012). Causal diagrams provide a conceptual framework to guide analysis, and they make key assumptions explicit.
- Arrows do not show the strength of associations. Causal diagrams are essentially non-quantitative, and inspection alone cannot distinguish backdoor paths that are important from those that are negligible. However, evidence in study data can help fill this gap and allow testing some of the assumptions implicit in a causal diagram: e.g., the presumed unrelatedness of certain pairs of variables.
- There is no generally accepted way to represent effect modification in a causal diagram. Several suggestions have been made, however (VanderWeele and Robins, 2007b; Weinberg, 2007), and work on the problem continues.

MULTIVARIABLE ANALYSIS

If the number of confounding variables in a study is not too large, and they do not have too many levels, then stratification can work well as a method to control confounding during data analysis. A single confounding variable **C** can be defined in such a way as to have one level for each unique combination on several factors that require control. For example, if there are three age groups (young, middle-aged, and old) and two genders, then **C** could represent age group *and* gender by having six levels: young males, middle-aged males, old males, young females, middle-aged females, and old females.

But in some situations, stratification has serious limitations:

- For many health outcomes, multiple risk factors are already known or suspected by the time a new study begins. Causal-diagram analysis or other approaches to assessing confounding may thus lead to a fairly long list of variables that need to be considered as possible sources of confounding. Stratifying on many variables at once can be problematic. Some study subjects may be lost from the analysis altogether. This happens when: (1) all subjects in a certain stratum have the exposure of interest, or none do; or (2) all subjects in a stratum have the outcome, or none do. An exposure–outcome association cannot be estimated in such strata. These kinds of non-informative strata become more and more common as the number of strata increases, spreading data thinner and thinner. Non-informative strata are, in effect, ignored by the Mantel-Haenszel analysis methods described in Chapter 11, because they contribute zero to sums in both the numerator and denominator. Rate standardization can also become stalled: one or more of the required stratum-specific rates may be 0/0, which is undefined (not zero!).
- All potential confounders and exposures must be analyzed as categorical variables. Confounding factors that are customarily measured on a continuous scale must nonetheless be converted into categorical form in order to stratify by them. Age, for example, must be split into a set of age groups in order to carry out age adjustment. When making this conversion, it is tempting to define many narrow categories in order to maximize comparability within strata and prevent residual confounding. But the resulting large number of strata complicates the problem of non-informative strata just described. Also, categorizing a continuous variable produces a model in which risk changes abruptly when a boundary between categories is crossed. Usually a more plausible model is that risk varies smoothly in relation to the underlying continuous variable in question.

Other traditional approaches for dealing with confounding also break down when many variables must be controlled at once. Restricting on many variables can result in small samples of narrow scope and limited generalizability. Attempts to match on many variables at once can lead to a difficult and costly search for unusual combinations of matching factors and can ultimately leave some subjects stranded without suitable matches, requiring that they be dropped from analysis.

Multivariable analysis[3] includes a set of powerful statistical techniques that are less subject to these limitations. Multivariable methods have become important tools for control of confounding, and most epidemiologists will want to become familiar with their use. This section provides only an introduction, but more extensive coverage can be found in many books: e.g., Vittinghoff *et al.* (2012); Kleinbaum and Klein (2012); Selvin (2011); Kleinbaum and Klein (2010); Fleiss *et al.* (2003); Jewell (2004); Breslow and Day (1987, 1980).

Basic Theory

Multivariable analysis in epidemiology is based on the idea that a person's risk of experiencing a given health outcome can depend on multiple characteristics about him or her. In an analytic epidemiologic study, one such characteristic is an exposure of main interest; others may include potential confounding variables and/or effect modifiers. Collectively, these subject characteristics are often called *predictors*, *explanatory variables*, or *covariates*. Conceptually,

$$\text{Outcome} = f(\text{Subject characteristics}) \quad (12.5)$$

While the number of possibilities for the function $f()$ is infinite in principle, in practice most forms of multivariable analysis in epidemiology are subtypes of *generalized linear models*. These models are mathematically tractable, flexible, and convenient: efficient ways exist to fit them to data, and the results have a straightforward interpretation. Linear regression, logistic regression, log-binomial regression, and Poisson regression all belong to this broad family.

A generalized linear model can be expressed as:

$$g(\hat{y}_j) = \beta_0 + \beta_1 x_{1j} + \beta_2 x_{2j} + \cdots + \beta_k x_{kj}$$

$$= \beta_0 + \sum_{i=1}^{k} \beta_i x_{ij} \quad (12.6)$$

The various parts of this equation—the predictor x-variables, the β-coefficients, the response variable y, and the link function $g()$—are defined and explained below.

Predictor X-Variables

The right-hand side of Equation (12.6) imposes a certain form on the function $f()$ in Equation (12.5). That form is what makes the model a linear one. The expression on the right-hand side of Equation (12.6) is commonly called the *linear predictor*. To see why, recall from basic geometry that a straight line can be represented as $y = a + bx$, where a is the intercept and b is the slope. For example, temperature in degrees Fahrenheit (y) is linearly related to temperature in degrees Centigrade (x) by the equation $y = 32 + (9/5)x$. While that particular linear relation is always exact, linear models can also be used to summarize observed relationships between variables in empirical studies by allowing for inexact agreement between the model and the data. For example, suppose that body weight is assessed in two ways for each of ten study subjects, who are indexed by $j = 1 \ldots 10$. One weight value for subject j is obtained by direct measurement on a scale (y_j), and another is obtained by self-report (x_j). The relationship between x and y is likely to be approxi-

mately linear, as represented by the regression line in Figure 12.18, but with error. In this case, the linear model would be $y_j = a + bx_j + e_j$, where e_j = error, which can vary from subject to subject. By including e_j, this model allows for a discrepancy between each person's actual measured body weight $(y_j$, the vertical position of subject j's data point) and what the best-fitting regression line would predict $(\hat{y}_j$, the vertical position of the regression line directly above or below that data point).

The right-hand side of Equation (12.6) expands the idea of a linear model further by including several x-variables—k of them in all, indexed by $i = 1 \ldots k$. The x-variables numerically encode different characteristics of study subjects, such as age, sex, exposure status, etc. Because the value of any given x-variable can vary across study subjects, the x-variables carry a second subscript, j, which indexes study subjects.

This kind of statistical model requires all input data to be numerical. To meet that requirement, the original data—which may include categorical variables such as female, low ketchup intake, and vegetarian diet—must be coded as numerical values of x-variables. Once coding is complete, there may be more x-variables than there were original subject characteristics, because some characteristics may require more than one x-variable to represent

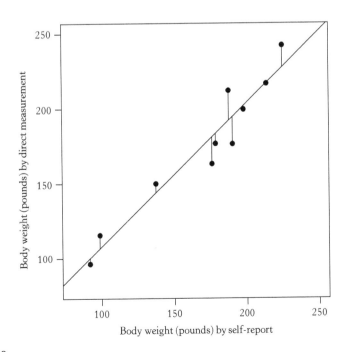

FIGURE 12.18

the information in them. The approach to coding depends on the measurement scale of each original variable:

- *Continuous.* If a characteristic is normally expressed as a number on a continuous scale, the characteristic may simply be used "as is." For example, a subject's age in years might simply be relabelled as one of the x-variables.

    Other options for continuous variables involve transforming the original numerical value in some way, then assigning the transformed value to an x-variable. This is usually done to try to improve the fit of the model to the data. For example, the analyst may define $x_1 = $ (age in years), and $x_2 = $ (age in years)^2 in order to allow for a wider range of possible shapes of the relationship between age and risk. Splines or fractional polynomials can also be used (Greenland, 1995; Royston and Sauerbrei, 2008; Royston *et al.*, 1999). Yet another option is simply to convert a continuous variable into a categorical one by defining a set of cutpoints on it, as when age is broken up into several age groups. The categorical variable is then handled as described below.

- *Binary.* If a characteristic has two categories—such as exposed and unexposed, or male and female—an *indicator* x-variable is typically defined and assigned the value 0 for one category and 1 for the other. For exposed and unexposed, a convenient coding is 0 for unexposed and 1 for exposed. For gender, the coding of one sex as 0 and the other as 1 could be arbitrary.

- *Categorical with three or more categories.* A characteristic that has, say, m levels is typically represented as a set of $m - 1$ indicator x-variables. For example, diet type in the ketchup study had three levels: vegetarian, fish-only, and omnivore. This information could be coded into two x-variables as shown in Table 12.11.

    Here, vegetarian was arbitrarily selected as the *reference* level, for which $x_1 = x_2 = 0$. Each of the x-variables then represents the property of having a diet type other than the default or reference level. Because the three diet types are mutually exclusive, no subject would ever have the combination $x_1 = x_2 = 1$, because a

TABLE 12.11.

Diet type	x_1	x_2
Vegetarian	0	0
Fish-only	1	0
Omnivore	0	1

subject cannot have both a fish-only and an omnivore diet. Note that a binary variable is, in a sense, a special case of the same rule: there are $m = 2$ categories, so $2 - 1 = 1$ indicator variable is needed to capture the information.

Most statistical packages come with built-in tools that can code binary and categorical variables into the required number of indicator x-variables easily or even automatically.

As illustrated later, additional x-variables may be defined as products of those in the initial set of x-variables, in order to allow modeling of interaction effects, such as modification of an exposure's effect by another covariate.

β-Coefficients

The β-coefficients in Equation (12.6) generalize the slope b in the simpler model that includes only a single x-variable. The intercept, denoted a in the simpler model, is now denoted β_0. The value of a given β-coefficient—β_i, say—is assumed to be constant for all subjects. Hence, β-coefficients carry only a single subscript.

The statistical model-fitting problem is to estimate the values of $\beta_0 \ldots \beta_k$ that maximize agreement between the observed data and the model's predictions. The resulting estimates are often denoted as such by adding a "hat" or circumflex: $\hat{\beta}_i$ is the estimate of the slope parameter β_i. The estimates are usually obtained by maximum-likelihood estimation. When there are multiple x-variables and β-coefficients, the solution requires matrix calculus, details of which are beyond the scope of this book. Fortunately, the calculations are almost always carried out by statistical computer software, which spares users from the computational details.

Response Variable, y

On the left-hand side of Equation (12.6), y is a *response* variable. In epidemiologic applications, y would typically be:

TABLE 12.12. FEATURES OF FOUR TYPES OF GENERALIZED LINEAR MODELS COMMONLY USED IN EPIDEMIOLOGY

Type of regression	y represents	Link function	Model form[a]	Interpretation of β_i [b]
Logistic	Occurrence of an outcome event	Logit	$\log\left(\frac{\hat{y}}{1-\hat{y}}\right) = LP$	$\exp(\beta_i)$ = adjusted odds ratio for a 1-unit increase in x_i
Log-binomial	Occurrence of an outcome event	Log	$\log(\hat{y}) = LP$	$\exp(\beta_i)$ = adjusted risk ratio for a 1-unit increase in x_i
Poisson	Number of cases	Log	$\log(\hat{y}) = LP$	$\exp(\beta_i)$ = adjusted rate ratio for a 1-unit increase in x_i
Linear	Continuous outcome	Identity	$\hat{y} = LP$	β_i = adjusted increase in y for a 1-unit increase in x_i

[a] LP = linear predictor = $\beta_0 + \sum \beta_i x_i$
[b] Adjustment is for all other x-variables in the model.

- An indicator variable representing whether a certain binary outcome occurs, such as occurrence of a disease of interest; or
- The number of cases in a specified amount of person-time that corresponds to a certain combination of values on the x-variables. For example, in a cohort study of ketchup intake, y could be the number of anxiety cases among, say, vegetarians with low ketchup intake; or
- The value of a health outcome that is measured on a continuous scale, such as systolic blood pressure or body weight.

The hat on $\hat{y}_j$ denotes that what appears on the left-hand side of Equation (12.6) is the *predicted* (not observed) value of y for subject j, as estimated by the statistical model (which explains the absence of an error term).

Less commonly, y represents an outcome with three or more unordered categories (e.g., different histological types of a malignancy), or with several ordered categories (e.g., stages of a disease). Since those situations are more specialized and involve added statistical complexity, they are not discussed here (see Hosmer *et al.* (2013); Harrell (2001); Ananth and Kleinbaum (1997)).

Link Function, g()

The function $g()$, commonly called the *link* function, serves to transform $\hat{y}$ in such a way that it can reasonably be modeled as a linear function of the x-variables. It links the expected value of the response variable y with the linear predictor.

One purpose served by the link function is to reconcile the range of possible values of the linear predictor (theoretically, $-\infty$ to $+\infty$) with the range of possible values of y. If $\hat{y}$ represents a probability, it can range only from 0 to 1. If $\hat{y}$ represents an expected number of cases, it can range from 0 to $+\infty$. If y is a continuous outcome variable, its range depends substantively on what it measures and on the choice of measurement units. For example, body weight cannot be negative or infinite, but its value could be large if measured in milligrams or small if measured in metric tons. In any event, there are no statistical constraints on the values that a continuous y-variable can take. Another purpose of the link function is to render the results of model-fitting—chiefly, estimates of the β-coefficients—interpretable in epidemiologically meaningful terms.

The type of multivariable analysis that applies to a particular problem depends on what y represents and on the link function. Table 12.12

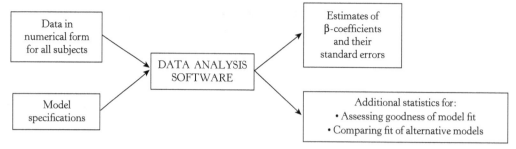

FIGURE 12.19

summarizes several of the most commonly used multivariable methods in epidemiology. A fifth method, *proportional-hazards regression*, is technically not a member of the generalized linear model family, but it has many similar features and is also discussed below.

Overview of Applying Multivariable Analysis

An important early step is checking for and correcting data errors, becoming familiar with the data set through descriptive statistics, and deciding how best to code the original data into numeric form. This step should result in a "clean" data set that includes an observed outcome (y) and values on relevant x-variables for each study subject. The overall process of conducting multivariable analysis then proceeds as sketched in Figure 12.19.

An indispensable tool is computer software that can fit the kinds of multivariable models needed for the task at hand. Several such statistical packages are available, including both commercial products and public-domain software, with similar capabilities but different command languages for manipulating data and for specifying models to be fitted.

Regardless of the form of multivariable analysis or the statistical package used to conduct it, key results are estimates of the β-coefficients and their standard errors. Three properties of the β-coefficient estimates should be noted:

- Each β-coefficient estimate reflects the size of the association between the corresponding x-variable and y, *after accounting for the contributions of all of the other x-variables*. In other words, a β-coefficient reflects the "incremental" effect of a certain x-variable, after adjusting statistically for the effects of the other x-variables.

As shown in Table 12.12, the estimated β-coefficient for the exposure variable can be converted fairly easily into an adjusted estimate of the exposure–outcome association in epidemiologically meaningful terms, such as an adjusted odds ratio, risk ratio, rate ratio, or difference in a continuous outcome. Evaluating confounding with multivariable analysis thus involves comparing the size of that estimated exposure–outcome association across two or more models. A model that includes the exposure as the only x-variable yields a *crude* or *unadjusted* estimate of the exposure–outcome association. A model that includes the exposure and other x-variables as covariates yields an estimate of the exposure–outcome association that is adjusted for those other x-variables. The extent of confounding can then be gauged by comparing the size of the exposure–outcome association with and without adjustment for the suspected confounder(s), in much the same way that one compares measures of exposure–outcome association before and after direct standardization. This strategy can be seen to be an application of the collapsibility view.

- The estimated size of β_i reflects the amount by which a *one-unit* increase in x_i changes the value of the linear predictor. As a special case, if x_i is an indicator variable, coded as 1 when a certain characteristic is present and as 0 when it is absent, then the size of β_i reflects the amount of change in the linear predictor in relation to presence of that characteristic. This property also carries over to an adjusted odds ratio, risk ratio, rate ratio, or change in a continuous outcome that is derived from β_i. Thus, in interpreting β_i or other association measures derived from it, one must keep in mind the units in which x_i is expressed.

- If the estimated value of β_i is zero or nearly zero, this finding implies that x_i evidently contributes little toward predicting the outcome after accounting for the effects of other x-variables in the model. This is because if $\beta_i = 0$, then $\beta_i x_{ij} = 0$, and the term involving x_{ij} makes no net contribution to the linear predictor. It might just as well be omitted from the statistical model altogether. Such a result may signal an opportunity to simplify the statistical model by omitting a relatively unimportant x-variable. As noted above, however, β_i must always be interpreted in relation to the units in which the corresponding x-variable is expressed. If x_i represents annual household income in dollars, a 1-unit increase would reflect a rather small increment, and even a β_i value close to zero might be consistent with an important effect of household income on y.

Statistical analysis programs also produce other statistics that are useful for assessing the model's goodness of fit to the data and for comparing the fit of alternative models. One such statistic is the *deviance* (defined technically as $-2\log[\text{likelihood}]$), which is used in likelihood ratio tests of whether adding one or more additional covariates to a given model yields a statistically significant improvement in fit. Another statistic is the Akaike Information Criterion

(AIC), defined as $2m + \text{deviance}$, where m is the number of model parameters. AIC quantifies goodness of fit while imposing a penalty for the number of parameters that must be estimated, a reflection of model complexity (Vittinghoff *et al.*, 2012; Lindsey and Jones, 1998).

Five Multivariable Analysis Methods

Table 12.12 summarized four types of generalized linear models that are commonly used in epidemiology. Now we take a closer look at each of them, plus a fifth related method, *proportional-hazards regression*.

Logistic Regression

Logistic regression models a binary outcome as a linear function of the x-variables, using a *logit* (also called *log-odds*) link function (Hosmer *et al.*, 2013; Kleinbaum and Klein, 2010). In epidemiology, logistic regression is typically used to obtain adjusted odds ratios, which are appropriate measures of exposure–outcome association in case-control studies. Logistic regression has also historically been used for analysis of cohort studies in closed populations when the outcome event of interest is rare, because then the odds ratio approximates the risk ratio. A variant, *conditional* logistic regression, is used for analysis of matched case-control studies (Breslow *et al.*, 1978). *Unconditional* logistic regression, used for unmatched studies, is the form described above.

Figure 12.20 shows what the logit link function does. Solving the logistic-model equation

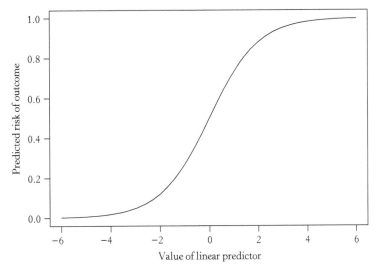

FIGURE 12.20

TABLE 12.13. SUMMARY OF RESULTS FROM APPLYING LOGISTIC REGRESSION TO KETCHUP STUDY DATA IN TABLE 12-12

| | Odds ratios | | | |
| | Model 1 | | Model 2 | |
Predictor	Point estimate	(95% CI)	Point estimate	(95% CI)
High ketchup intake	0.40	(0.26–0.62)	0.40	(0.24–0.66)
Diet type				
Fish-only			0.11	(0.06–0.19)
Omnivore			0.33	(0.18–0.60)

$\log\left(\dfrac{\hat{y}}{1-\hat{y}}\right) = LP$ for $\hat{y}$, we see that *any* value of the linear predictor $(-\infty$ to $+\infty)$ maps to a value of $\hat{y}$ between 0 and 1. This guarantees that $\hat{y}$ will fall within a numerical range that can be interpreted as a probability.

To understand the interpretation of the β-coefficients in logistic regression, say that x_1 is the indicator variable that represents exposure status: $0 =$ unexposed and $1 =$ exposed. Other x-variables represent confounding factors. Consider the logistic regression equations for two individuals who differ on exposure status but who have identical values on all of the other x-variables. Here, $\hat{y}_u$ denotes predicted outcome risk in the unexposed person, and $\hat{y}_e$ denotes predicted outcome risk for the exposed person:

$$\log\left(\frac{\hat{y}_e}{1-\hat{y}_e}\right) = \beta_0 + \beta_1(1) + \beta_2 x_2 + \cdots + \beta_k x_k$$

$$\log\left(\frac{\hat{y}_u}{1-\hat{y}_u}\right) = \beta_0 + \beta_1(0) + \beta_2 x_2 + \cdots + \beta_k x_k$$

Subtracting the second equation from the first and applying properties of logarithms gives:

$$\log\left(\frac{\hat{y}_e}{1-\hat{y}_e}\right) - \log\left(\frac{\hat{y}_u}{1-\hat{y}_u}\right) = \beta_1$$

$$\log\left[\frac{\hat{y}_e/(1-\hat{y}_e)}{\hat{y}_u/(1-\hat{y}_u)}\right] = \beta_1$$

$$\log(OR) = \beta_1$$

$$OR = \exp(\beta_1)$$

Thus, $\exp(\beta_1)$ is the odds ratio for exposure, conditional on (adjusted for) the remaining x-variables. Models fitted to data yield an *estimate* of β_1, denoted

$\hat{\beta}_1$, and its estimated standard error (*se*). Approximate 95% confidence limits for the adjusted *OR* would then be $\exp(\hat{\beta}_1 \pm 1.96 \cdot se)$.

Table 12.13 summarizes the results of applying logistic regression to the ketchup study data in Table 12.1. (Appendix 12C shows more details.) Each predictor listed in Table 12.13 is simply a descriptive label for an indicator x-variable. The extent of confounding by diet type can be assessed by comparing the odds ratio estimates for high ketchup intake from Model 1 (unadjusted) and Model 2 (adjusted for diet type). The point estimates are the same, suggesting no confounding. The confidence limits are slightly wider in Model 2. Point estimates and confidence limits for the odds ratios for fish-only and omnivore diet types (relative to vegetarian, the reference category) are also produced by Model 2 as a by-product.

A third model, shown only in Appendix 12C, added (ketchup intake) × (diet type) interaction terms to Model 2 in order to test for possible effect modification. Based on a comparison of model deviances, this third model showed no statistically significant improvement in fit over Model 2, suggesting no significant modification of the ketchup–anxiety association by diet type.

Log-Binomial Regression

Log-binomial regression also models a binary outcome as a linear function of the x-variables, but it uses the log link function rather than the logit link function. In epidemiology, log-binomial regression is typically used to obtain adjusted risk ratios in cohort studies involving closed populations, particularly when the outcome event of interest is common. An advantage of log-binomial regression over logistic regression in that context is that it produces results in terms of risk ratios without having to depend on an odds-ratio approximation and a rare-outcome assumption (McNutt *et al.*, 2003). A disadvantage is that for very large values of the linear predictor, the predicted outcome $\hat{y}$ can exceed 1.0, which is not interpretable as a probability. The interpretation of $\hat{\beta}_i$ and calculation of confidence limits for it are similar to those of logistic regression, except that risk ratio replaces odds ratio.

Poisson Regression

Poisson regression models the number of cases of a certain outcome as a linear function of the x-variables, using a log link function. In epidemiology, Poisson regression is used to obtain adjusted rate ratios in cohort studies in which person-time may vary among study subjects. With individual-level data, each subject could experience either 0 or 1 outcome events. Poisson regression can also be used when aggregate person-time at risk is available only for subgroups of subjects but not for individuals.

To see why log(number of cases) rather than log(rate) is used on the left side of the regression equation, say that $\hat{c}_i$ is the number of cases expected in a certain subgroup, T_i is the amount of person-time at risk experienced by that subgroup, and *LP* is the linear predictor computed from x-variable values specific to that subgroup. Then:

$$\log(\hat{c}_i/T_i) = LP$$

$$\log(\hat{c}_i) - \log(T_i) = LP$$

$$\log(\hat{c}_i) = \log(T_i) + LP$$

In other words, $\log(T_i)$ is moved to the right side of the regression equation as a so-called *offset* term: no β-coefficient is estimated for it. This formulation asserts that, other things being equal, the expected number of cases is assumed to be proportional to the amount of person-time at risk. The $\hat{c}_i$ that remains on the left side is the quantity that is assumed to follow a Poisson distribution, from which the method gets its name. The interpretation of $\hat{\beta}_i$ and calculation of confidence limits for it are the same as in log-binomial regression. *Conditional* Poisson regression is a closely related variant that can be used for analysis of matched cohort studies (Cummings *et al.*, 2003).

Linear Regression

Linear regression models a continuous outcome as a linear function of the x-variables. Historically the oldest form of regression, it is less often used in epidemiology because binary or case-count response variables are more common in epidemiologic research. Nonetheless, it can be used to model such response variables as birth weight, systolic blood pressure, or other continuous outcomes for which the error terms follow an approximately normal (Gaussian) distribution. $\hat{\beta}_i$ can be interpreted as the expected change in y with a 1-unit increase in x_i, adjusted for the other x-variables in the model.

Proportional-Hazards Regression

Proportional-hazards regression models the hazard rate of a certain outcome as a function of the x-variables (Cox, 1972). It can be considered a multivariable form of survival analysis. The regression model has the form

$$h(t) = h_0(t) \cdot \exp(\beta_1 x_1 + \beta_2 x_2 + \cdots + \beta_k x_k)$$

where $h(t)$ is the hazard rate at time t for a person with a specified combination of x-variable values, and $h_0(t)$ is a *baseline* hazard function representing how the hazard varies over time in a (possibly hypothetical) person for whom all x-variables equal 0. An attraction of the model is that the form of the $h_0(t)$ function need not be specified as a prerequisite to estimating the β-coefficients. In epidemiology, proportional-hazards regression is used in cohort studies or randomized trials in which detailed individual-level data are available on time at risk and the times at which outcome events occur. It can be shown that $\exp(\hat{\beta}_i)$ estimates the adjusted *hazard ratio* for a 1-unit increase in x_i.

Proportional-hazards regression has many similarities with the previously described forms of multivariable analysis in how x-variables are specified and combined, how the β-coefficients can be interpreted in epidemiologically meaningful terms, and how the method can be used to assess and control confounding. Nonetheless, proper use of the method involves dealing with a number of special issues and subtleties, including choice among alternative time scales; the option of allowing different baseline hazard functions for different strata; special diagnostics for testing the proportional-hazards assumption; and the ability to accommodate *time-dependent covariates*, or x-variables whose values change within a subject over time. These and other aspects of applying this powerful analytic tool are discussed by Kalbfleisch and Prentice (2002); Kleinbaum and Klein (2012); Harrell (2001); Hosmer and Lemeshow (2008).

Two Goal-Driven Approaches to Model-Building

A critical aspect of applying any multivariable model is deciding which covariates to include. Two general approaches of particular relevance to epidemiology are described and contrasted here.

- *Exposure-focused.* An analytic epidemiologic study, by definition, seeks to determine whether a certain exposure causes a certain outcome. In that context, the goal of multivariable analysis is to obtain an estimate of the exposure–outcome association that is as unbiased and precise as possible. Causal-diagram analysis can be useful in identifying potential confounding variables that may be candidates for inclusion in such a model, and it provides a principled basis for excluding other variables. Even if a full causal diagram is not worked out in detail, certain underlying principles still apply. In particular, the analyst must decide which other variables would qualify conceptually as potential sources of confounding. Variables that are causally downstream from exposure or outcome would not.

  Not all potential confounding variables turn out to be important sources of confounding. As noted in the earlier section on causal diagrams, a certain backdoor path may turn out to be important, or it may turn out to be negligible because the combination of associations along the path is weak. Multivariable analysis can be used to determine empirically whether blocking a backdoor path by controlling for at least one variable on that path produces a meaningful change in the estimated exposure–outcome association. This strategy is essentially an application of the collapsibility view of confounding. While the counterfactual view of confounding reminds us that data-driven strategies can be fallible, being guided by the extent of change in the estimated exposure–outcome association is in the end a theoretically defensible and pragmatic approach for deciding which variables to include in an exposure-focused multivariable model (Maldonado and Greenland, 1993; Greenland, 1989). Still, this approach requires judgments by the analyst as to what constitutes a negligible change in the estimated exposure–outcome association.

- *Prediction-focused.* In other epidemiologic applications of multivariable models, the goal is to obtain as accurate a prediction of the outcome as possible, using information in a set of predictor variables. Among the predictors, no one variable is singled out as the exposure of main interest for which an *a priori* causal hypothesis is to be tested. Instead, the predictors are of more or less equal importance. Moreover, the causal and conceptual relationships among the predictors are relatively unimportant. For some applications, even the temporal relationship between the predictors and the response may be immaterial. What matters most is the predictive power of the model, without regard to whether the associations on which it is based are causal or not.

  One epidemiologic application of prediction-focused multivariable models is in selecting individuals or subgroups who may be good candidates for a screening test. As discussed in Chapter 19, both the yield of screening, and the proportion of persons with a positive screening test who actually turn out to have the disease in question, are greater when the test is applied to people with a relatively high probability of having the disease. Factors such as race, type of insurance coverage, or past medical history may not truly be causes of the disease in question, but if they are readily available and can accurately identify a high-risk person, they can deserve inclusion in a prediction-focused multivariable model.

  Another application of prediction-focused multivariable models arises in dealing with missing data. One step in applying the technique of *multiple imputation* is to develop a multivariable model that predicts as accurately as possible what a missing value on some key variable might have been, based on other information that is known about the study subject (White *et al.*, 2011; Raghunathan, 2004; Donders *et al.*, 2006; Little and Rubin, 2002). Whether predictors in this imputation model are truly causes of the variable with missing data is immaterial. For example, knowing that someone had visited an oncologist might be a very good predictor of whether he/she had cancer, even though seeing an oncologist would be an effect, not a cause, of cancer.

The goal of a prediction-focused multivariable model leads to different criteria for whether a certain variable is included on the right side of a model equation. In general, if including the variable improves the model's predictive accuracy, after accounting for the number of degrees of freedom consumed by adding it, then the variable is included; otherwise, it is not. Measures of goodness of fit such as the Akaike Information Criterion (AIC) are often used to guide selection of a prediction-focused multivariable model. Other statistical approaches to selecting the optimal prediction-focused model have also been described, and there is no universal consensus on the best method (Vittinghoff *et al.*, 2012; Hosmer *et al.*, 2013; Harrell, 2001; Royston and Sauerbrei, 2008).

Under both model-building approaches, a decision about whether or not to include a candidate variable often depends heavily on what other variables are already included.

While each approach provides an appealing rationale for model-building, the two approaches can lead to different decisions. Under an exposure-focused approach, all multivariable models would of course include the exposure, even if it proved to be unassociated with the outcome after controlling for other covariates. The absence of an exposure–outcome association would be answering the primary research question, possibly refuting the study hypothesis. Whether a covariate is included in an exposure-focused multivariable model depends on its conceptual role and on the extent to which including it affects the point estimate of the exposure–outcome association (which addresses bias) and the width of the confidence interval around that point estimate (which addresses precision). As noted earlier in discussing the comparability view of confounding, a covariate–outcome association is a necessary but not sufficient requirement for bias in the exposure–outcome association due to confounding by that covariate. A covariate can be a good predictor of the outcome without necessarily being an important confounder. Under a prediction-focused approach, no one candidate predictor is more important than any other, and no variable

qualifies *a priori* for automatic inclusion in the model.

As a simple example in which the two approaches lead in different directions, consider Models 1 and 2 in Table 12.13. Which model should be preferred? If the goal is to obtain as unbiased and precise an estimate as possible of the ketchup–anxiety association, then Model 1 must be declared the winner. Model 2, which adds diet, produces no change at all in the ketchup–anxiety odds ratio, so there is no evidence of confounding by diet. Moreover, the confidence limits around the ketchup–anxiety odds ratio are narrower in Model 1, when diet is omitted.

But to extend the fictional ketchup-study example, suppose that the goal of multivariable modeling were different. Say that campus mental-health officials, wanting to make the best use of scarce counseling resources, sought to identify students at high risk of developing anxiety during the school year, based on their responses to the questionnaire they completed on entry. For that purpose, Model 2 would be preferred over Model 1, because including information on diet type improves the ability to predict anxiety accurately, as shown both by likelihood ratio tests and by AIC comparisons in Appendix 12C.

Statistical texts on multivariable analysis often address the issue of variable selection from an implicitly prediction-focused viewpoint. Epidemiologists must keep in mind that when multivariable models are used to assess and control confounding, the goal is different, and the basis for variable selection may thus justifiably differ as well.

Concluding Remarks on Multivariable Analysis

In broad terms, multivariable analysis methods are like power tools: one can do bigger, more complicated jobs with them than would otherwise be possible, but they can also wreak havoc if used improperly. One danger is that the user has a relatively detached perspective on the data. The analyst cannot always detect from a computer-generated table of regression coefficients that sample sizes in a critical subgroup were exceedingly small, or that an implausible data value is the real explanation for some striking finding. Experienced analysts use multivariable analysis in tandem with simpler methods, such as descriptive statistics and cross-tabulations, to stay in close touch with the data. Multivariable methods also rely on assumptions that need to be be kept in mind and that can sometimes be checked.

DATA-REDUCTION APPROACHES

Multivariable methods allow more confounding variables to be controlled simultaneously than would be feasible using traditional methods such as stratification, matching, and restriction. Still, multivariable analysis methods have limits on how many covariates they can accommodate. If the number of covariates exceeds the number of outcome events, it may be mathematically impossible to fit a multivariable model of outcomes to the data. Even when the problem is not quite so severe, but the number of outcome events is less than about 5–10 times the number of predictor variables, simulation studies have suggested that the β-coefficient estimates from logistic and proportional-hazards regression can be quite biased, and confidence intervals for them may no longer have the desired coverage probabilities (Vittinghoff and McCulloch, 2007; Peduzzi et al., 1996, 1995; Concato et al., 1995).

One way of coping with an overabundance of covariates is through *data reduction*. The basic idea is to conduct the analysis in two stages: (1) distill the confounding effects of multiple covariates into a summary variable; and (2) keep the main exposure–outcome analysis simple by controlling only for the summary variable.

Two main variants of this approach are: (1) *propensity score* methods, which base the summary score on relationships between the exposure and the covariates; and (2) *disease risk score* methods, which base the summary score on relationships between the disease (or other outcome) and the covariates. Similar approaches have been used to construct summary scores for smaller sets of related variables, such as comorbidity scores to reflect the influence of past or present illnesses (Charlson et al., 1987).

Propensity Scores

A propensity score is defined as the probability of exposure, conditional on a set of covariate values (Rosenbaum and Rubin, 1983). For a binary exposure, the propensity score is typically estimated via logistic regression, using exposure status as the response variable and the covariates as predictors. Once that model has been fitted, a predicted probability ("propensity") of being exposed is estimated

for each study subject, based on his/her covariate values and the estimated β-coefficients. Note that a subject's propensity score and his/her actual exposure status are two different characteristics.

A properly developed propensity score has a rather remarkable balancing property: given a sufficiently large number of subjects who differ on exposure status but who have the same propensity score, all of the covariates that entered into calculation of the propensity score will tend to be balanced evenly between the exposed subjects and the non-exposed subjects (Rosenbaum and Rubin, 1983, 1984). By breaking the links between exposure and all of the covariates, controlling for the propensity score alone simultaneously controls for confounding by all of the covariates.

Example 12-5. Over a nine-year period, 6,174 patients at a large academic medical center underwent a stress echocardiography test for evaluation of suspected coronary artery disease. Before the test, data were gathered from each patient about sociodemographics, past medical history, and use of medications, including aspirin. Gum et al. (2001) sought to evaluate whether daily or alternate-day use of aspirin was associated with all-cause mortality, as ascertained from the Social Security Death Index. A total of 2,310 patients were regular aspirin users. In the full cohort, 276 patients died during follow-up averaging 4.1 years.

Combining the pre-test questionnaire data with test results, 34 potential confounding factors were identified. These were used to estimate each patient's probability of being a regular aspirin user—i.e., his/her propensity score. Among patients who reported using regular aspirin, 1,351 could be matched to a non-user with a similar propensity score. The remaining 959 aspirin users were omitted from the propensity-score analyses because no suitable match could be found for them.

In the unadjusted comparison, mortality was nearly identical between all aspirin users and all non-users. However, many risk factors for mortality differed substantially between users and non-users, with a trend toward greater disease severity and comorbidity among aspirin users. By contrast, the exposed and unexposed subgroups formed by matching on propensity score were shown to be similar on all covariates. In proportional-hazards regression on the two matched groups, the hazard ratio for death in relation to regular aspirin use was 0.53 (95% CI:

0.38–0.74). The findings thus suggested that a possible beneficial effect of regular aspirin use had been masked by confounding in the unadjusted analysis.

Luo *et al.* (2010) summarize several other examples from major medical journals of studies using propensity scores.

Propensity-score methods are particularly attractive for cohort studies involving relatively rare outcomes. In that setting, there may be relatively few outcome events but plenty of exposed and unexposed subjects, as well as data on multiple potential confounders. A better statistical model with many covariates can be developed for the common exposure than for the rare outcome. Simulation studies suggest that when the ratio of cases to covariates is less than about eight, propensity-score methods tend to outperform multivariable modeling of the outcome (Cepeda *et al.*, 2003). Also, cohort studies often involve several outcome variables but a single exposure. Once developed, the same propensity score can be re-used when analyzing effects of that exposure on many different outcomes. Both simulation studies (Cook and Goldman, 1989) and reviews of studies in which both propensity score methods and multivariable outcome models were used (Shah *et al.*, 2005) suggest that the two approaches yield similar results when direct comparison is possible.

In developing the propensity-score model, an inclusive approach for variable selection has been recommended, especially when working with large databases (Schneeweiss *et al.*, 2009; Robins *et al.*, 1992). The ultimate goal, however, is not to predict exposure as accurately as possible, but to control confounding. For that reason, both theory and simulation results favor including covariates that may be strongly related to outcome, even if they are only weakly associated with exposure (Rubin and Thomas, 1996; Brookhart *et al.*, 2006). By contrast, covariates that are strongly associated with exposure but not with outcome tend to sacrifice precision in the final estimate of the exposure–outcome association without reducing bias (Brookhart *et al.*, 2006).

Once a propensity-score model has been developed, it can be checked by examining whether the covariates have similar distributions between exposed and unexposed subjects with similar propensity scores. If not, the propensity-score model may need refinement, possibly by transforming certain continuous covariates to accommodate nonlinear associations with exposure, or by including interaction terms among the covariates.

In principle, the main exposure–outcome analysis can involve controlling for the propensity score by any of the usual methods: matching, stratification, covariate adjustment, or inverse-probability weighting (described later in this chapter) (Glynn *et al.*, 2006; D'Agostino, 1998). However, matching has particular appeal in part because it serves to "trim off" the tails of the propensity-score distribution, excluding subjects for whom exposure was virtually certain and those for whom exposure was virtually impossible (Rosenbaum and Rubin, 1983). This approach is in keeping with the eventual goal of inferring exposure effects among those who might have been either exposed or unexposed. For example, if the exposure were use of a certain drug, it would be pointless to try to estimate the drug's effects in patients for whom it would be absolutely contraindicated.

Despite their ability to balance many covariates at once, which is seductively reminiscent of randomization, propensity score methods do nothing to control for confounding by unmeasured, poorly measured, or omitted variables. Propensity scores can also be awkward to apply when studying multiple exposures, exposures with many levels, or time-varying exposures. Lastly, propensity score methods make it difficult to evaluate effect modification by individual variables that enter the propensity score.

Disease Risk Scores

A disease risk score is defined as the probability of disease (or other outcome), conditional on being unexposed and on a set of covariate values (Glynn *et al.*, 2012; Arbogast and Ray, 2009). The disease risk score has been aptly called the "prognostic analogue" of the propensity score (Hansen, 2008). It focuses on outcome–covariate associations rather than on exposure–covariate associations, both of which are necessary for confounding by the covariates. For a binary outcome, the disease risk score is often estimated by fitting a logistic regression in unexposed persons, using outcome status as the response variable and the covariates as predictors. Other approaches have also been proposed that use data on both exposed and unexposed subjects for model-building, including in the model an indicator variable for exposure that is later set to zero when estimating the disease risk score (Miettinen, 1976; Hansen, 2008; Arbogast and Ray, 2011). Once a model has been fitted, a predicted probability of experiencing the outcome, conditional on being unexposed, is estimated for each study subject based on his/her covariate values and the estimated β-coefficients. This strategy amounts to estimating each subject's potential outcome if unexposed. However, the disease risk score is calculated for both exposed subjects (whose potential outcome in the absence of exposure is unobserved) and for unexposed subjects (whose outcome in the absence of exposure is observed). The disease risk score is then treated as a single confounding variable in the main exposure–outcome analysis, using methods similar to those used with propensity scores (Stürmer *et al.*, 2005).

Like propensity scores, properly developed disease risk scores also have a desirable balancing property: among unexposed subjects with similar disease risk scores, the covariates will tend to be similarly distributed between cases and non-cases (Hansen, 2008). This balancing property can only be checked directly in unexposed subjects.

Disease risk scores can be an attractive technique for control of confounding when exposure is rare, the outcome event is common among unexposed persons, and many confounders require control. One such setting is when a new treatment has just been introduced for a relatively common disease (Glynn *et al.*, 2012). Another attraction is that the same disease risk score can be re-used for several exposures. Although use of a disease risk score can complicate assessment of effect modification by individual covariates, sometimes estimated disease risk itself can be of interest as a potentially important effect modifier (Hayward *et al.*, 2006; Kent and Hayward, 2007). Glynn *et al.* (2012) give a detailed example of applying disease risk scores to evaluation of statin therapy after myocardial infarction.

INVERSE PROBABILITY WEIGHTING

Let us revisit the method of direct adjustment, as described in Chapter 11. Suppose that a binary exposure is studied in a closed population in relation to a binary outcome Y taking the values 0 or 1. Say also that at least one confounding factor requires control. Directly adjusting the cumulative incidence of $Y = 1$ involves grouping subjects into strata defined by the confounder(s). Each stratum may represent a category on a single confounder (e.g., an age group) or a certain combination of levels on two or more confounders (e.g., an age-gender group). Let there be k strata in all, indexed by $i = 1 \ldots k$. For stratum i, the notation is as shown in Table 12.14.

TABLE 12.14.

	Outcome		
	$Y = 1$	$Y = 0$	Total
Exposed	a_i	b_i	m_i
Unexposed	c_i	d_i	n_i
Total			t_i

The total size of the population under study is $T = \sum_i t_i$.

If the total population is selected as the reference (standard) population to which the cumulative incidences for the exposed and unexposed groups are to be standardized, then the directly-adjusted cumulative incidence for the exposed group is:

$$\frac{\sum_i \left(\frac{a_i}{m_i} \right) \cdot t_i}{T}$$

The numerator is the projected total number of cases if the stratum-specific cumulative incidences in the exposed group were applied to the total study population stratum by stratum. The numerator can be rearranged as:

$$\sum_i \left(\frac{a_i}{m_i} \right) \cdot t_i = \sum_i a_i \cdot \left(\frac{t_i}{m_i} \right)$$

$$= \sum_i a_i \cdot \left(\frac{m_i}{t_i} \right)^{-1} \quad (12.7)$$

The quantity m_i/t_i is the proportion of subjects in stratum i who were exposed, which can also be viewed as the probability of being exposed for each subject in stratum i, which can also be viewed as a simple propensity score based on a single predictor variable (namely, stratum).

With this realization, Equation (12.7) can be reworked to calculate the directly adjusted cumulative incidence using data on individual study subjects. Let the subscript j index individual subjects, and define a variable *PS* (for propensity score) whose value for subject j is $PS_j = m_i/t_i$, where m_i/t_i is the proportion exposed in whichever stratum subject j belongs to. All subjects in stratum i thus have the same value of *PS*.

The observed total number of exposed cases is:

$$\sum_i a_i = \sum_{exposed} Y_j$$

so expression (12.7) becomes:

$$\sum_{\text{exposed}} Y_j \cdot (PS_j)^{-1} \qquad (12.8)$$

This shows that the numerator of the directly adjusted cumulative incidence for the exposed group—that is, the projected total number of cases that would be observed in the standard population—can be calculated by weighting each exposed subject's outcome Y by the inverse of his/her probability of being exposed.

The adjusted cumulative incidence for the exposed group would be expression (12.8) divided by T. But T itself can be expressed in terms of inverse propensity scores as $T = \sum_{j} (PS_j)^{-1}$. For example, in the stratified analysis, within stratum i, each of the m_i exposed subjects has $PS_j = m_i/t_i$, so $\sum_{j} (PS_j)^{-1} = m_i \cdot (t_i/m_i) = t_i$, and summing over all strata gives $\sum_{i} t_i = T$. The adjusted cumulative incidence for the exposed group can thus be written as:

$$\frac{\sum_{\text{exposed}} Y_j \cdot (PS_j)^{-1}}{\sum_{\text{exposed}} (PS_j)^{-1}} \qquad (12.9)$$

Similar algebra shows that the directly adjusted cumulative incidence in the unexposed group is:

$$\frac{\sum_{\text{unexposed}} Y_j \cdot (1 - PS_j)^{-1}}{\sum_{\text{unexposed}} (1 - PS_j)^{-1}} \qquad (12.10)$$

For a binary exposure, the quantity $(1 - PS_j)$ is subject j's probability of *not* being exposed. Expressions (12.9) and (12.10) are thus two special cases of a more general rule: in calculating the adjusted cumulative incidence for a given exposure group, each subject's weight is the inverse of his/her probability of being in that exposure group, conditional on his/her covariate values. Hence the method is known as *inverse probability weighting* (Robins et al., 2000; Hernán and Robins, 2006a; Schmoor et al., 2011). Other labels sometimes used are *inverse probability of exposure weighting*, or *inverse probability of treatment weighting* if the exposure is an intervention.

To illustrate the method, Table 12.15 adjusts for age in the hypothetical comparison of cumulative mortality between Communities A and B from Chapter 11. Community A was arbitrarily chosen to represent "exposed."

Beyond being just another interesting way to do direct adjustment, inverse probability weighting provides a way to generalize direct adjustment to accommodate more adjustment variables, without having to require that all variables be categorical (Rosenbaum, 1987; Robins et al., 2000). This is done by developing a multivariable model, typically with logistic regression, for each subject's probability of being in his/her actual exposure group as a function of his/her covariate values. The process is almost the same as that described earlier for propensity score analysis, except that the response variable is different: for propensity scores, one models the probability of being exposed, while for inverse probability weighting, one models the probability of being in each subject's actual exposure group. Sato and Matsuyama (2003) give other expressions for weights that can be used to adjust to standard populations other than the total study population. Robins et al. (2000) describe how to obtain confidence limits using standard statistical software.

As noted in the earlier section on propensity scores, inverse probability weighting is one of several options for using propensity scores to deal with confounding by many covariates (Schmoor et al., 2011; Lunceford and Davidian, 2004). Inverse probability weighting also plays a key role in application of marginal structural models, described below, to deal with time-dependent confounding (Robins et al., 2000; Cole and Hernán, 2008). In that context, the rightmost column in Table 12.15 can be regarded as an imaginary *pseudopopulation*, in this case twice as large as the original study population, in which confounding by the adjustment factors is gone. That is, the cumulative incidence among exposed persons in the pseudopopulation equals the adjusted cumulative incidence for the exposed group calculated from the original data, and similarly for the unexposed. Disease frequency measures calculated directly from that pseudopopulation can then be used to obtain various measures of exposure–outcome association, including risk differences, risk ratios, or odds ratios, without a need for further adjustment. Inverse probability weighting can also be used to try to minimize bias due to differential censoring (Robins et al., 2000).

When inverse probability weights are estimated with multivariable modeling, more assumptions about model form are needed than with ordinary stratification-based direct adjustment. Also, the

TABLE 12.15. EXAMPLE OF DIRECT ADJUSTMENT WITH INVERSE-PROBABILITY WEIGHTING

Age group	Community	Deaths	Population	Cumulative mortality[a]	PS[b]	IPW[c]	Projected in standard population Deaths	Projected in standard population Population
Young	A	1	1,000	1	0.167	6.000	6	6,000
Young	B	10	5,000	2	0.167	1.200	12	6,000
Middle	A	15	3,000	5	0.429	2.333	35	7,000
Middle	B	40	4,000	10	0.429	1.750	70	7,000
Old	A	50	5,000	10	0.833	1.200	60	6,000
Old	B	20	1,000	20	0.833	6.000	120	6,000

[a] Deaths per 1,000

[b] PS = Propensity score = stratum-specific probability of being in Community A

[c] IPW = Inverse-probability weight: $1/PS$ if Community A, or $1/(1 - PS)$ if Community B

	Cumulative mortality[d]	
Community	Crude	Age-adjusted
A	$\dfrac{1+15+50}{1,000+3,000+5,000}(\times 1,000) = 7.33$	$\dfrac{6+35+60}{6,000+7,000+6,000}(\times 1,000) = 5.32$
B	$\dfrac{10+40+20}{5,000+4,000+1,000}(\times 1,000) = 7.00$	$\dfrac{12+70+120}{6,000+7,000+6,000}(\times 1,000) = 10.63$

[d] Deaths per 1,000

weights can become very large for covariate combinations in which exposure is estimated to be very rare, leading to unduly influential observations and unstable estimates of an exposure–outcome association. Alternative methods for computing "stabilized" weights have been described that are less prone to this problem (Robins *et al.*, 2000; Xiao *et al.*, 2010).

INSTRUMENTAL VARIABLES

Consider the causal diagram shown in Figure 12.21. Say that the study goal is to determine the extent to which an exposure E affects an outcome Y. Confounding by measured factors C could be removed in any of several ways—stratification, matching, restriction, multivariable analysis, or the data-reduction methods described above—but confounding by other unmeasured factors U is not controllable by those methods.

Instrumental variables offer a way to avoid confounding by both C and U—a property hitherto reserved for randomized trials (Grootendorst, 2007; Martens *et al.*, 2006; Hernán and Robins, 2006b; Greenland, 2000). To work this miracle, the instrumental variable IV must satisfy certain conditions that are implicit in the causal diagram in Figure 12.21:

1. IV must affect E.
2. IV must otherwise be unrelated to Y. In particular:

   (a) IV may not affect Y in any other way except through E. That is, Y may be a descendant of IV only via pathways that include E.
   (b) The IV-Y association must also be unconfounded. That is, no unblocked backdoor paths may exist from IV to Y.

An instrumental variable can be viewed as an unconfounded proxy for exposure. Use of instrumental variables has a long history in economics (Newhouse and McClellan, 1998), but their application in the health sciences is relatively recent.

Appendix 12D derives the following formula, which expresses the unconfounded causal effect of exposure in terms of risk difference. It applies to binary Y, E, and IV:

$$RD = \frac{r_1 - r_0}{p_1 - p_0} \qquad (12.11)$$

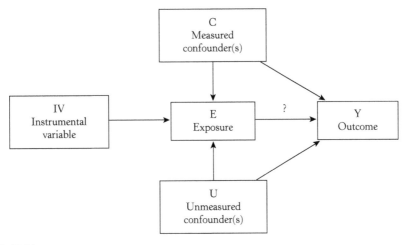

FIGURE 12.21

where RD = unconfounded causal risk difference, r_1 = cumulative incidence among those with $IV = 1$, r_0 = cumulative incidence among those with $IV = 0$, p_1 = proportion exposed in group with $IV = 1$, and p_0 = proportion exposed in group with $IV = 0$. Informally, conditions 2(a) and 2(b) in the list above imply that the *only* reason (besides chance) for a difference in outcome frequency between groups with $IV = 0$ versus $IV = 1$ is the difference in exposure frequency produced by IV. That effect of exposure is "diluted" by the imperfect correlation between IV and E, and the denominator corrects for that dilution. Appendix 12D also provides references to generalizations and extensions of Equation (12.11) to other forms of regression.

The denominator of Equation (12.11) can be interpreted as the *strength* of the instrumental variable—the extent to which exposure status is affected by IV. Strength matters because the estimate of RD is based on scaling up the observed difference in cumulative incidence between the $IV = 1$ and $IV = 0$ groups by the difference in exposure proportions between those groups.

Randomized Trials with Imperfect Compliance

One of the most successful applications of instrumental-variable theory is in estimating the efficacy of an intervention in a randomized trial when not all subjects receive the treatment to which they were randomly assigned.

Example 12-6. Over a 29-month period, 67,800 British men aged 64–74 years were randomized to receive either: (1) an invitation to be screened for an abdominal aortic aneurysm (AAA), or (2) no such invitation (Ashton *et al.*, 2002). Men who accepted the invitation and then screened positive were evaluated for possible elective surgery, in order to prevent catastrophic rupture of the AAA. After a follow-up period averaging 4.1 years, the following results were obtained:

TABLE 12.16.

Group	No. of AAA deaths	No. of men	Deaths per 1,000 men
Invited	65	33,839	1.92
Screened	43	27,147	1.58
Not screened	22	6,692	3.29
Control	113	33,961	3.33

(Based on data from Ashton *et al.* [2002])

The overall reduction in AAA cumulative mortality attributable to the invitation-to-be-screened program is easily obtained as $3.33 - 1.92 = 1.41$ fewer deaths per 1,000 men. However, the investigators also wished to determine the effect of screening among men who were actually screened. Note that a simple comparison of AAA mortality between the screened and not-screened subgroups of the invited group could be confounded by whatever factors led some men to decide to accept the screening invitation while others did not, such as the priority they placed on maintaining their health. Instead, the instrumental variable was each man's randomly assigned treatment; the exposure of interest was actually being screened. Randomized treatment assignment clearly met condition 1 for an instrumental variable: $27,147/33,839 = 80.2\%$ of men invited to be screened actually were screened, compared to none in the control group. Condition 2(a) was almost certainly met because it is highly unlikely that simply being invited for screening would affect AAA mortality in any other way except through actually being screened (and the follow-up care triggered by it). Condition 2(b) was also met because random treatment assignment, by design, would be statistically unrelated to any other measured or unmeasured characteristics except by chance. Hence the use of Equation (12.11) seemed fully justified, and it yielded an estimate of $\dfrac{65/33,839 - 113/33,961}{27,147/33,839} = -0.00175 = 1.75$ fewer deaths per 1,000 men screened. (An alternative approach to this aspect of randomized-trial analysis is described in Chapter 13 and gives the same result.)

Examples in Non-randomized Studies

Probably the biggest challenge in using instrumental-variable methods in non-randomized studies is finding a good instrumental variable. One key feature is *strength*—the magnitude of the *IV-E* association—which is empirically quantifiable. Just as important is *validity*—the extent to which *IV* and *Y* are independent except through *E*—which is only partly verifiable. Associations between *IV* and known, measured risk factors for *Y* can be examined in data, and a valid instrument should be essentially unrelated to them. But unfortunately, there is no way to test whether *IV* is independent of unmeasured or unknown determinants of *Y*. Whether criteria 2(a) and 2(b) are fully met thus ultimately depends on subject-matter knowledge and faith.

One application of instrumental-variable methods that is analogous to the randomized-trial situation has been termed *Mendelian randomization* (Davey Smith and Ebrahim, 2005; Bochud and Rousson, 2010). Many genetic variants are thought to segregate essentially at random at conception, such that a child is equally likely to inherit an allele from either parent. If an allele is a strong determinant of some potentially modifiable personal or environmental characteristic, then genotype may qualify as an instrumental variable to prevent confounding when evaluating the effects of that modifiable characteristic on a health outcome. For example, Trompet *et al.* (2009) used apolipoprotein E (ApoE) genotype

in a Mendelian-randomization analysis of whether low plasma cholesterol is a cause of cancer. In a large cohort study, the incidence of cancer among participants with plasma cholesterol in the lowest tertile was nearly twice as great as in those with plasma cholesterol in the highest tertile. But carriers of the ApoE2 genotype, which was associated with relatively low plasma cholesterol compared to those with the ApoE4 genotype, actually had slightly *lower* cancer incidence, contrary to the hypothesis. The investigators concluded that the initial association between low cholesterol levels and cancer may therefore have been due to confounding. On the other hand, confidence limits for the hazard ratios relating ApoE genotype to cancer incidence (HR = 0.86, 95% CI: 0.50–1.47) and mortality (HR = 0.70, 95% CI: 0.30–1.60) were quite wide, probably due in part to a relatively weak link between genotype and cholesterol level, and indicated that the results would be compatible with both positive and negative true associations. Accordingly, an alternative interpretation (also noted by the investigators) was that the study may have had low statistical power—a drawback of many Mendelian randomization studies—and could not rule out the possibility that low cholesterol levels really do cause cancer.

The search for good instrumental variables in other areas of observational epidemiology has led to a number of creative suggestions. Chen and Briesacher (2011) grouped the instrumental variables used in 26 pharmacoepidemiologic studies into several categories: frequency of prescribing a target drug in a patient's geographic region, or at his/her health care facility, or by his/her physician; patient's past medical history or type of insurance coverage; and calendar time. These authors and others (Davies *et al.*, 2013) have found considerable variability in the extent to which the required conditions for an instrumental variable had been empirically tested when possible, and uncertainty remains about their validity (Martens *et al.*, 2006; Hernán and Robins, 2006b; Rassen *et al.*, 2009a; Bosco *et al.*, 2010).

Concluding Remarks on Instrumental Variables

Instrumental variables currently offer the only alternative to randomization as a way to control confounding by unknown or unmeasured factors. But stiff requirements must be met for an instrument to be valid enough to avoid bias and strong enough to yield a reasonably precise estimate of the unconfounded exposure–outcome association. The demanding necessary assumptions are only partly testable empirically. Equation (12.11) implies that any uncontrolled confounding of the exposure–outcome association can be magnified, sometimes greatly, by a relatively weak IV–exposure association. Moreover, estimates of the unconfounded exposure–outcome association from instrumental-variable methods are often much less precise than estimates obtained by other means (Martens *et al.*, 2006). Thus, the strongest case for their use can be made when large samples are available and the instrumental variable is based on randomization or its near-equivalent.

TIME-DEPENDENT CONFOUNDING

Studies that involve repeated assessments of the same study subjects over time, with possible changes in their status on exposure or other variables, pose special challenges because the same variable may play more than one conceptual role. For example, consider a study that seeks to evaluate the effectiveness of a new treatment (E) for preventing adverse outcomes (Y) among patients with a certain chronic disease. Treatment choices by clinicians are guided in part by a patient's status on a certain biomarker B of disease severity. The study involves periodic measurements of B and E. The causal diagram in Figure 12.22 depicts key features of the situation, showing B and E at just two time points for simplicity.

The study goal is to determine the overall effect of E on Y. A more complete causal diagram might include other measured and unmeasured potential confounders, some of which may change over time. Consider the biomarker measurement B_1. It is affected by prior treatment status E_0 and thus

lies on a causal pathway from E_0 to Y. From that standpoint, B_1 is a mediator of E and should not be controlled. But B_1 also affects subsequent treatment status E_1 and, as a measure of disease severity, B_1 affects Y in its own right. From that standpoint, B_1 is a confounder of E and requires control.

The biomarker in this situation is an example of a *time-dependent confounder*: a characteristic whose value can change over time and that affects both the outcome of interest and subsequent exposure status. Often, as in this example, a time-dependent confounder is also affected by past exposure. Traditional methods for control of confounding generally require choosing whether or not to control for B_1, and either choice can lead to a biased estimate of the effect of E (Robins *et al.*, 2000; Cole *et al.*, 2003).

One approach to the problem is to apply *marginal structural models* (Robins *et al.*, 2000). *Marginal* means that the method seeks to estimate effect measures based on the population-averaged outcomes that would be observed under alternative exposure histories, rather than individual-level causal effects of exposure. *Structural* means that the method models potential (possibly counterfactual) outcomes rather than observed outcomes. Inverse probability weighting is of central importance: confounding is addressed by assigning different analytic weights to different subjects, rather than by including covariates in regression models for outcomes. Each subject's weight is estimated as a function of his/her exposure and covariate history up to each time point at which exposure status may change. An additional weighting factor can be incorporated to correct for differential censoring. Once subjects' weights have been estimated, the main analysis model is kept relatively simple by relying on weighting to control

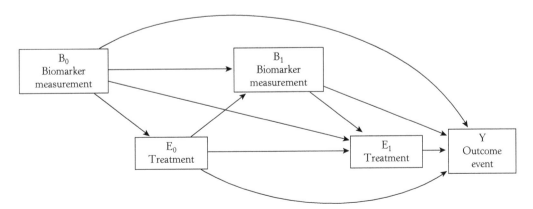

FIGURE 12.22

confounding rather than by including many covariates in the main model. While marginal structural models deal with the complexities of time-dependent confounding and time-varying exposure status, the validity of results still depends on the key assumption of no confounding by unmeasured variables.

Details regarding the implementation and statistical basis for marginal structural models are beyond the scope of this text. However, Bodnar *et al.* (2004) have provided a step-by-step description of applying marginal structural models in a study of prenatal iron supplements in relation to anemia at childbirth, using a design roughly matching the generic example given above. A classic early application evaluated the effect of the anti-retroviral drug zidovudine on survivorship among HIV-positive men, combining marginal structural models with proportional-hazards regression (Hernán *et al.*, 2000). Suarez *et al.* (2011) have summarized several studies comparing results from marginal structural models and more conventional analysis methods. Daniel *et al.* (2013) provided a tutorial on marginal structural models and the related technique of *g*-estimation for the statistically minded.

CONCLUDING REMARKS

Control of confounding is of critical importance in drawing valid conclusions about causation from observational epidemiologic studies. The scope of topics introduced in this chapter attests to the extensive attention that has been devoted to confounding by methodologists in search of ever more powerful and flexible tools to minimize bias. But even with the most sophisticated methods, an assumption of negligible unmeasured confounding remains necessary in order to draw causal inferences from non-randomized studies. Even instrumental variables in non-randomized studies require this assumption a

layer deeper by assuming no confounding between the instrumental variable and the outcome. Because this is ultimately an untestable assumption, the best epidemiologic studies devote considerable effort to thinking about how confounding might arise in a specific context, obtaining good data for addressing possible biases, investigating and controlling confounding during data analysis, and interpreting results with balance and due humility.

APPENDIX 12A: CONDITIONS FOR COLLAPSIBILITY OF THE RISK RATIO, RISK DIFFERENCE, AND ODDS RATIO

Notation consistent with that in the main text is summarized in Table 12.17.

All summations below are over $i = 1 \ldots k$.

Risk Ratio (RR)

Let RR_{ss} denote the common stratum-specific RR, such that $r_{ei}/r_{ui} = RR_{ss}$ for all i. By the weighted-average rule (Chapter 4):

$$RR_{overall} = \frac{\sum w_{ei} \cdot r_{ei}}{\sum w_{ui} \cdot r_{ui}}$$

$$= \frac{\sum w_{ei} \cdot (r_{ui} \cdot RR_{ss})}{\sum w_{ui} \cdot r_{ui}}$$

$$= RR_{ss} \cdot \left(\frac{\sum w_{ei} \cdot r_{ui}}{\sum w_{ui} \cdot r_{ui}} \right)$$

which implies that $RR_{overall} = RR_{ss}$ if and only if $\sum w_{ei} \cdot r_{ui} = \sum w_{ui} \cdot r_{ui}$.

Risk Difference (RD)

Let RD_{ss} denote the common stratum-specific RD, such that $r_{ei} - r_{ui} = RD_{ss}$ for all i. Again applying the

TABLE 12.17.

C (stratum)	Exposed		Unexposed	
	Proportion in stratum	Cumulative incidence	Proportion in stratum	Cumulative incidence
1	w_{e1}	r_{e1}	w_{u1}	r_{u1}
⋮	⋮	⋮	⋮	⋮
k	w_{ek}	r_{ek}	w_{uk}	r_{uk}
Total	1.0		1.0	

weighted-average rule:

$$RD_{overall} = \sum w_{ei} \cdot r_{ei} - \sum w_{ui} \cdot r_{ui}$$

$$= \sum w_{ei} \cdot (r_{ui} + RD_{ss}) - \sum w_{ui} \cdot r_{ui}$$

$$= RD_{ss} \cdot \sum w_{ei}$$

$$+ \left(\sum w_{ei} \cdot r_{ui} - \sum w_{ui} \cdot r_{ui} \right)$$

$$= RD_{ss} + \left(\sum w_{ei} \cdot r_{ui} - \sum w_{ui} \cdot r_{ui} \right)$$

which implies that $RD_{overall} = RD_{ss}$ if and only if $\sum w_{ei} \cdot r_{ui} = \sum w_{ui} \cdot r_{ui}$. This condition is the same as that for collapsibility of the *RR*.

The same algebra holds for the rate ratio and rate difference, inasmuch as the weighted-average rule also applies to person-time incidence rates. However, Greenland (1996) showed that the above collapsibility condition does not necessarily hold if person-time at risk is itself affected by exposure.

Odds Ratio (*OR*)

Building on notation used in the main text, for stratum i, define a_i, b_i, c_i, and d_i as the number of subjects in each cell of the following table:

TABLE 12.18.

	Outcome	
	$Y = 1$	$Y = 0$
Exposed	a_i	b_i
Unexposed	c_i	d_i

Also denote sums across strata as $a. = \sum a_i$, and likewise for b, c, and d. Collapsibility of the *OR* implies that, for some constant k:

$$\frac{(a.)(d.)}{(b.)(c.)} = k \qquad (12.12)$$

and for all i:

$$\frac{a_i d_i}{b_i c_i} = k \qquad (12.13)$$

By (12.13):

$$a_i = k \left(\frac{b_i c_i}{d_i} \right)$$

$$a. = \sum a_i = k \sum \frac{b_i c_i}{d_i} \qquad (12.14)$$

By (12.12):

$$k(b.)(c.) = (a.)(d.)$$

Substituting for $(a.)$ from (12.14):

$$k(b.)(c.) = k \left(\sum \frac{b_i c_i}{d_i} \right)(d.)$$

$$(b.)(c.) = \left(\sum \frac{b_i c_i}{d_i} \right)(d.)$$

Dividing both sides by $(b.)(d.)$:

$$\frac{c.}{d.} = \frac{\left(\sum \frac{b_i c_i}{d_i} \right)}{b.}$$

$$\sum \frac{c_i}{d.} = \sum \frac{b_i}{b.} \cdot \frac{c_i}{d_i}$$

$$\sum \frac{d_i}{d.} \cdot \frac{c_i}{d_i} = \sum \frac{b_i}{b.} \cdot \frac{c_i}{d_i} \qquad (12.15)$$

Equation (12.15) is equivalent to Equation (12.2) in the main text, inasmuch as $w'_{ui} = \frac{d_i}{d.}$, $w'_{ei} = \frac{b_i}{b.}$, and $\psi_{ui} = \frac{c_i}{d_i}$.

APPENDIX 12B: ADDITIONAL EXAMPLES OF 2 × 2 × 3 TABLES THAT ARE COLLAPSIBLE OVER C, EVEN THOUGH C MEETS COMPARABILITY-VIEW CRITERIA AS A CONFOUNDER

TABLE 12.19.

A: Risk ratio (RR)

Stratum	Exposure	Outcome $Y = 1$	$Y = 0$	Total	Percent exposed	Cumulative incidence in unexposed	RR
1	Exposed	24	1,576	1,600	44.4%	0.0375	0.40
	Unexposed	75	1,925	2,000			
2	Exposed	8	4,792	4,800	44.4%	0.0042	0.40
	Unexposed	25	5,975	6,000			
3	Exposed	16	3,184	3,200	66.7%	0.0125	0.40
	Unexposed	20	1,580	1,600			
All	Exposed	48	9,552	9,600	50.0%	0.0125	0.40
	Unexposed	120	9,480	9,600			

B: Risk difference (RD)

Stratum	Exposure	Outcome $Y = 1$	$Y = 0$	Total	Percent exposed	Cumulative incidence in unexposed	RD
1	Exposed	20	980	1,000	66.7%	0.010	0.010
	Unexposed	5	495	500			
2	Exposed	30	470	500	50.0%	0.050	0.010
	Unexposed	25	475	500			
3	Exposed	30	970	1,000	20.0%	0.020	0.010
	Unexposed	80	3,920	4,000			
All	Exposed	80	2,420	2,500	33.3%	0.022	0.010
	Unexposed	110	4,890	5,000			

APPENDIX 12C: LOGISTIC REGRESSION ANALYSIS APPLIED TO THE KETCHUP STUDY DATA

Input Data

Given the small number of variables to be analyzed, an efficient way to input the data in Table 12.1 would be in *grouped* form. The grouped data set shown in Table 12.20 contains five variables, each shown as a column: two indicator (0/1) variables represent diet (Fish and Omnivore; vegetarian diet thus becomes the reference diet category), one represents ketchup intake, one represents anxiety status, and the variable *n* specifies how many subjects had each combination of values on the first four variables. The data set has

one row for each of the 12 possible combinations of values on the first four variables.

Three Logistic Regression Models

Three logistic regression models are of main interest (see Table 12.21). Anxiety is the response variable in all three models. Model 1 will yield an unadjusted OR estimate for high ketchup intake. Model 2 will yield a diet-adjusted OR estimate for high ketchup intake, which can be compared with the OR estimate from Model 1 to gauge the extent to which diet type confounds the ketchup–anxiety OR. Model 3 adds the two possible (ketchup intake) × (diet type) interaction terms, in order to assess possible modification of the ketchup–anxiety OR by diet type.

TABLE 12.20.

Fish	Omnivore	Ketchup	Anxiety	n
0	0	1	1	24
0	0	1	0	16
0	0	0	1	75
0	0	0	0	20
1	0	1	1	8
1	0	1	0	48
1	0	0	1	25
1	0	0	0	60
0	1	1	1	16
0	1	1	0	32
0	1	0	1	20
0	1	0	0	16

- The residual *deviance*, defined as $-2\log(\text{likelihood})$, from which a likelihood-ratio statistic can be calculated to test whether one model fits significantly better than another.[4]
- The number of residual *degrees of freedom (df)* for the model, which is a function of the number of observations and the number of β-coefficients estimated.
- The *Akaike Information Criterion (AIC)*, defined as $2m +$ deviance, where m is the number of β-coefficients estimated (including β_0, the intercept, not shown above). AIC quantifies the model's goodness of fit while imposing a penalty for the number of parameters that need to be estimated. In general, for prediction-focused multivariable models, models with lower AIC are preferred.

These results for the three models are:

TABLE 12.21.

Model	Predictor variables included
1	Ketchup
2	Ketchup, Fish, Omnivore
3	Ketchup, Fish, Omnivore, Ketchup × Fish, Ketchup × Omnivore

TABLE 12.23.

Model	Deviance	df	m	AIC
1	480.08	10	2	484.08
2	411.11	8	4	419.11
3	411.11	6	6	423.11

The specific commands needed to fit these models to the above data depend on the analytic software being employed. The variable n is often called a *frequency weight*. All commonly used software produces, at a minimum, estimates of the β-coefficients and their estimated standard errors. The results are shown in Table 12.22. Other statistics on each model produced by most analytic software include:

Interpretation

Interpreting the results in epidemiologic terms is aided by converting the β-coefficients and their estimated standard errors to odds ratio estimates and their 95% confidence intervals. Recall that $\hat{OR} = \exp(\hat{\beta})$, its lower 95% confidence limit $\approx \exp(\hat{\beta} - 1.96 \cdot se(\hat{\beta}))$, and its upper 95% confidence limit $\approx \exp(\hat{\beta} + 1.96 \cdot se(\hat{\beta}))$. Most analysis

TABLE 12.22.

Variable	Model 1 $\hat{\beta}$	Model 1 s.e.	Model 2 $\hat{\beta}$	Model 2 s.e.	Model 3 $\hat{\beta}$	Model 3 s.e.
Ketchup	−0.9163	0.2236	−0.9163	0.2519	−0.9163	0.4093
Fish			−2.1972	0.2843	−2.1972	0.3464
Omnivore			−1.0986	0.3038	−1.0986	0.4193
Ketchup × Fish					0.0000	0.6083
Ketchup × Omnivore					0.0000	0.6114

TABLE 12.24.

Variable	Model 1 OR	Model 1 (95% CI)	Model 2 OR	Model 2 (95% CI)	Model 3 OR	Model 3 (95% CI)
Ketchup	0.40	(0.26–0.62)	0.40	(0.24–0.66)	0.40	(0.18–0.89)
Fish			0.11	(0.06–0.19)	0.11	(0.06–0.22)
Omnivore			0.33	(0.18–0.60)	0.33	(0.15–0.76)
Ketchup × Fish					1.00	(0.30–3.29)
Ketchup × Omnivore					1.00	(0.30–3.31)

programs can apply these formulas internally and display results in terms of ORs and their confidence limits, either by default or as an option. The results are shown in Table 12.24.

Comparing Models 1 and 2, the two estimated ORs for Ketchup—one unadjusted and the other adjusted for diet type—are exactly the same, implying no confounding by diet type. As a by-product, Model 2 also yields estimated ORs and their confidence intervals for fish and omnivore diets, both relative to vegetarian diet.

Comparing Models 2 and 3, a key issue is whether adding the two (ketchup intake) × (diet type) interaction terms yields a statistically significant improvement in model fit. The difference in deviances $411.11 - 411.11 = 0.00$ can be interpreted as a likelihood-ratio χ^2 statistic with $8 - 6 = 2$ degrees of freedom, which yields a p-value of 1.00. This result implies that Model 3 does not fit the data statistically significantly better than does Model 2. In fact, for these data, the estimated β-coefficients for the two interaction terms both equal 0.0000, implying no effect modification of the ketchup–anxiety OR by diet type.

APPENDIX 12D: HOW INSTRUMENTAL-VARIABLE METHODS CAN YIELD AN UNCONFOUNDED ESTIMATE OF EXPOSURE EFFECT

A relatively informal derivation of Equation (12.11) is given here, followed by references to more formal treatments. For simplicity, consider a cohort study in a closed population. Say that exposure E, outcome Y, instrumental variable IV, and a single unmeasured confounder U are all binary variables taking the values 0 or 1. Assume also that the expected outcome for person i is given by:

$$\hat{Y}_i = \beta_0 + \beta_1 E_i + \beta_2 U_i$$

That is, Y depends on both E and U in a linear probability model with coefficients β_0, β_1, and β_2. The expected cumulative incidence r of $Y = 1$ in a given subgroup can be obtained by averaging terms in the above equation over all subgroup members:

$$r = \beta_0 + \beta_1 \cdot \Pr(E = 1) + \beta_2 \cdot \Pr(U = 1)$$

The study goal is to obtain an unconfounded estimate of β_1, the causal effect of E. If E and U are associated and $\beta_2 \neq 0$, then a simple comparison of cumulative incidence between exposed and non-exposed groups would be confounded by U. Equivalently, omitting the term involving U from the above linear model would yield a confounded estimate of β_1.

Now let IV enter the picture, meeting the standard conditions for an instrumental variable as described in the main text: (1) IV affects E; (2a) IV may not affect Y in any other way except through E; and (2b) the IV-Y association must also be unconfounded by U or any other factor. Additional notation is as shown in Table 12.25.

By condition (1), $p_1 \neq p_0$.

Among persons with $IV = 0$, the expected cumulative incidence would be:

$$r_0 = \beta_0 + \beta_1 p_0 + \beta_2 q_0 \tag{12.16}$$

and among persons with $IV = 1$, the expected cumulative incidence would be:

$$r_1 = \beta_0 + \beta_1 p_1 + \beta_2 q_1 \tag{12.17}$$

TABLE 12.25.

Symbol	Mathematical definition	Description
p_1	$\Pr(E = 1|IV = 1)$	Proportion exposed among those with $IV = 1$
p_0	$\Pr(E = 1|IV = 0)$	Proportion exposed among those with $IV = 0$
q_1	$\Pr(U = 1|IV = 1)$	Proportion with $U = 1$ among those with $IV = 1$
q_0	$\Pr(U = 1|IV = 0)$	Proportion with $U = 1$ among those with $IV = 0$

By condition (2a), no other variables that are affected by IV need be included, because they do not affect Y. Subtracting (12.16) from (12.17) gives:

$$r_1 - r_0 = \beta_1(p_1 - p_0) + \beta_2(q_1 - q_0)$$

But by condition (2b), the IV-Y association cannot be confounded by U. This implies that either $\beta_2 = 0$ or $q_1 = q_0$, and the second term drops out, giving:

$$r_1 - r_0 = \beta_1(p_1 - p_0)$$
$$\beta_1 = \frac{r_1 - r_0}{p_1 - p_0}$$

More formal derivations and extensions can be found in Angrist *et al.* (1996); Martens *et al.* (2006); Hernán and Robins (2006a); Grootendorst (2007). The above estimator can be generalized to continuous Y, E, and IV and for an arbitrary number of other confounders. Condition 2(b) can also be relaxed somewhat by including other measured covariates, so that the IV-Y association is assumed unconfounded after controlling for those covariates. Estimates and standard errors for β_1 are normally obtained from a two-stage modeling process: (1) model $\hat{E}$ as a function of IV, and (2) model $\hat{Y}$ as a function of $\hat{E}$. Non-linear functional forms may be used at either stage (Rassen *et al.*, 2009b).

NOTES

1. Henceforth, the subscript j is sometimes dropped for simplicity, but Y_e and Y_u can always have different values for different individuals.

2. Exceptions would include *n*-of-1 trials, and possibly crossover trials and case-crossover studies, both of which involve aggregating within-individual estimated effects.

3. The adjective *multivariate* has also been used instead of *multivariable*. However, some statisticians reserve *multivariate* for situations in which there are two or more outcome variables. *Multivariable* always refers to situations in which there can be two or more predictor variables.

4. Technically, the two models being compared must be *nested* models, meaning that all predictors in one of the models must be a subset of the predictors in the other model.

REFERENCES

Ananth CV, Kleinbaum DG. Regression models for ordinal responses: a review of methods and applications. Int J Epidemiol 1997; 26: 1323–1333.

Angrist JD, Imbens GW, Rubin DB. Identification of causal effects using instrumental variables. J Am Stat Assoc 1996; 91:444–455.

Arbogast PG, Ray WA. Use of disease risk scores in pharmacoepidemiologic studies. Stat Methods Med Res 2009; 18:67–80.

Arbogast PG, Ray WA. Performance of disease risk scores, propensity scores, and traditional multivariable outcome regression in the presence of multiple confounders. Am J Epidemiol 2011; 174:613–620.

Ashton HA, Buxton MJ, Day NE, Kim LG, Marteau TM, Scott RAP, *et al.* The Multicentre Aneurysm Screening Study (MASS) into the effect of abdominal aortic aneurysm screening on mortality in men: a randomised controlled trial. Lancet 2002; 360:1531–1539.

Berkson J. Limitations of the application of fourfold table analysis to hospital data. Biometrics 1946; 2:47–53.

Bochud M, Rousson V. Usefulness of Mendelian randomization in observational epidemiology. Int J Environ Res Public Health 2010; 7:711–728.

Bodnar LM, Davidian M, Siega-Riz AM, Tsiatis AA. Marginal structural models for analyzing causal effects of time-dependent treatments: an application in perinatal epidemiology. Am J Epidemiol 2004; 159:926–934.

Boivin JF, Wacholder S. Conditions for confounding of the risk ratio and of the odds ratio. Am J Epidemiol 1985; 121:152–158.

Bosco JLF, Silliman RA, Thwin SS, Geiger AM, Buist DSM, Prout MN, *et al.* A most stubborn bias: no adjustment method fully resolves confounding by indication in observational studies. J Clin Epidemiol 2010; 63:64–74.

Breslow NE, Day NE. Statistical methods in cancer research. Volume I: The analysis of case-control studies. Lyon, France: International Agency for Research on Cancer, 1980.

Breslow NE, Day NE. Statistical methods in cancer research. Volume II: The design and analysis of cohort studies. Lyon, France: International Agency for Research on Cancer, 1987.

Breslow NE, Day NE, Halvorsen KT, Prentice RL, Sabai C. Estimation of multiple relative risk functions in matched case-control studies. Am J Epidemiol 1978; 108:299–307.

Brookhart MA, Schneeweiss S, Rothman KJ, Glynn RJ, Avorn J, Stürmer T. Variable selection for propensity score models. Am J Epidemiol 2006; 163:1149–1156.

Carlson KF, Gerberich SG, Church TR, Ryan AD, Alexander BH, Mongin SJ, et al. Tractor-related injuries: a population-based study of a five-state region in the Midwest. Am J Ind Med 2005; 47:254–264.

Carroll L. Through the looking-glass. London: Macmillan, 1968.

Cepeda MS, Boston R, Farrar JT, Strom BL. Comparison of logistic regression versus propensity score when the number of events is low and there are multiple confounders. Am J Epidemiol 2003; 158:280–287.

Charlson ME, Pompei P, Ales KL, MacKenzie CR. A new method of classifying prognostic comorbidity in longitudinal studies: development and validation. J Chronic Dis 1987; 40:373–383.

Chen Y, Briesacher BA. Use of instrumental variable in prescription drug research with observational data: a systematic review. J Clin Epidemiol 2011; 64:687–700.

Cole SR, Hernán MA. Constructing inverse probability weights for marginal structural models. Am J Epidemiol 2008; 168:656–664.

Cole SR, Hernán MA, Robins JM, Anastos K, Chmiel J, Detels R, et al. Effect of highly active antiretroviral therapy on time to acquired immunodeficiency syndrome or death using marginal structural models. Am J Epidemiol 2003; 158:687–694.

Cole SR, Platt RW, Schisterman EF, Chu H, Westreich D, Richardson D, et al. Illustrating bias due to conditioning on a collider. Int J Epidemiol 2010; 39: 417–420.

Concato J, Peduzzi P, Holford TR, Feinstein AR. Importance of events per independent variable in proportional hazards analysis. I. Background, goals, and general strategy. J Clin Epidemiol 1995; 48:1495–1501.

Cook EF, Goldman L. Performance of tests of significance based on stratification by a multivariate confounder score or by a propensity score. J Clin Epidemiol 1989; 42:317–324.

Cox DR. Regression models and life tables (with discussion). J R Stat Soc B 1972; 34:187–220.

Cummings P, McKnight B, Greenland S. Matched cohort methods for injury research. Epidemiol Rev 2003; 25:43–50.

D'Agostino RB Jr. Propensity score methods for bias reduction in the comparison of a treatment to a non-randomized control group. Stat Med 1998; 17:2265–2281.

Daniel RM, Cousens SN, De Stavola BL, Kenward MG, Sterne JAC. Methods for dealing with time-dependent confounding. Stat Med 2013; 32:1584–1618.

Davey Smith G, Ebrahim S. What can Mendelian randomisation tell us about modifiable behavioural and environmental exposures? BMJ 2005; 330:1076–1079.

Davies NM, Smith GD, Windmeijer F, Martin RM. Issues in the reporting and conduct of instrumental variable studies: a systematic review. Epidemiology 2013; 24:363–369.

Donders ART, van der Heijden GJMG, Stijnen T, Moons KGM. Review: a gentle introduction to imputation of missing values. J Clin Epidemiol 2006; 59:1087–1091.

Fleischer NL, Diez Roux AV. Using directed acyclic graphs to guide analyses of neighbourhood health effects: an introduction. J Epidemiol Community Health 2008; 62:842–846.

Fleiss JL, Levin B, Paik MC. Statistical methods for rates and proportions (3rd ed.). New York: Wiley and Sons, 2003.

Glymour MM. Using causal diagrams to understand common problems in social epidemiology. Chapter 16 in: Oakes JM, Kaufman JS (eds.). Methods in social epidemiology. San Francisco, CA: Jossey-Bass, 2006: pp. 393–428.

Glynn RJ, Gagne JJ, Schneeweiss S. Role of disease risk scores in comparative effectiveness research with emerging therapies. Pharmacoepidemiol Drug Saf 2012; 21 Suppl 2:138–147.

Glynn RJ, Schneeweiss S, Stürmer T. Indications for propensity scores and review of their use in pharmacoepidemiology. Basic Clin Pharmacol Toxicol 2006; 98:253–259.

Greenland S. Modeling and variable selection in epidemiologic analysis. Am J Public Health 1989; 79:340–349.

Greenland S. Dose-response and trend analysis in epidemiology: alternatives to categorical analysis. Epidemiology 1995; 6:356–365.

Greenland S. Absence of confounding does not correspond to collapsibility of the rate ratio or rate difference. Epidemiology 1996; 7:498–501.

Greenland S. An introduction to instrumental variables for epidemiologists. Int J Epidemiol 2000; 29:722–729.

Greenland S. Quantifying biases in causal models: classical confounding vs collider-stratification bias. Epidemiology 2003; 14:300–306.

Greenland S, Morgenstern H. Confounding in health research. Annu Rev Public Health 2001; 22:189–212.

Greenland S, Pearl J, Robins JM. Causal diagrams for epidemiologic research. Epidemiology 1999a; 10:37–48.

Greenland S, Robins JM. Identifiability, exchangeability, and epidemiological confounding. Int J Epidemiol 1986; 15:413–419.

Greenland S, Robins JM, Pearl J. Confounding and collapsibility in causal inference. Stat Sci 1999b; 14:29–46.

Grootendorst P. A review of instrumental variables estimation of treatment effects in the applied health sciences. Health Serv Outcomes Res Method 2007; 7:159–179.

Gum PA, Thamilarasan M, Watanabe J, Blackstone EH, Lauer MS. Aspirin use and all-cause mortality among patients being evaluated for known or suspected coronary artery disease: A propensity analysis. JAMA 2001; 286:1187–1194.

Hansen BB. The prognostic analogue of the propensity score. Biometrika 2008; 95:481–488.

Harrell FE Jr. Regression modeling strategies, with applications to linear models, logistic regression, and survival analysis. New York: Springer, 2001.

Hayward RA, Kent DM, Vijan S, Hofer TP. Multivariable risk prediction can greatly enhance the statistical power of clinical trial subgroup analysis. BMC Med Res Methodol 2006; 6:18.

Hernán MA, Brumback B, Robins JM. Marginal structural models to estimate the causal effect of zidovudine on the survival of HIV-positive men. Epidemiology 2000; 11:561–570.

Hernán MA, Hernandez-Diaz S, Robins JM. A structural approach to selection bias. Epidemiology 2004; 15:615–625.

Hernán MA, Hernandez-Diaz S, Werler MM, Mitchell AA. Causal knowledge as a prerequisite for confounding evaluation: an application to birth defects epidemiology. Am J Epidemiol 2002; 155:176–184.

Hernán MA, Robins JM. Estimating causal effects from epidemiological data. J Epidemiol Community Health 2006a; 60:578–586.

Hernán MA, Robins JM. Instruments for causal inference: an epidemiologist's dream? Epidemiology 2006b; 17:360–372.

Höfler M. Causal inference based on counterfactuals. BMC Med Res Methodol 2005; 5:28.

Hosmer DW, Lemeshow S. Applied survival analysis: regression modeling of time-to-event data (2nd ed.). Hoboken, NJ: Wiley-Interscience, 2008.

Hosmer DW, Lemeshow S, Sturdivant RX. Applied logistic regression (3rd ed.). New York: Wiley and Sons, 2013.

Howard G, Cushman M, Howard VJ, Kissela BM, Kleindorfer DO, Moy CS, *et al.* Risk factors for intracerebral hemorrhage: the REasons for Geographic And Racial Differences in Stroke (REGARDS) study. Stroke 2013; 44:1282–1287.

Jewell NP. Statistics for epidemiology. New York: Chapman & Hall, 2004.

Joffe M, Gambhir M, Chadeau-Hyam M, Vineis P. Causal diagrams in systems epidemiology. Emerg Themes Epidemiol 2012; 9:1.

Kalbfleisch JD, Prentice RL. The statistical analysis of failure time data (2nd ed.). New York: Wiley and Sons, 2002.

Kent DM, Hayward RA. Limitations of applying summary results of clinical trials to individual patients: the need for risk stratification. JAMA 2007; 298:1209–1212.

Kleinbaum DG, Klein M. Logistic regression: a self-learning text (3rd ed.). New York: Springer, 2010.

Kleinbaum DG, Klein M. Survival analysis : a self-learning text (3rd ed.). New York: Springer, 2012.

Krieger N. Epidemiology and the web of causation: has anyone seen the spider? Soc Sci Med 1994; 39:887–903.

Lindsey JK, Jones B. Choosing among generalized linear models applied to medical data. Stat Med 1998; 17:59–68.

Little RJA, Rubin DB. Statistical analysis with missing data (2nd ed.). New York: Wiley, 2002.

Liu W, Brookhart MA, Schneeweiss S, Mi X, Setoguchi S. Implications of M bias in epidemiologic studies: a simulation study. Am J Epidemiol 2012; 176:938–948.

Lunceford JK, Davidian M. Stratification and weighting via the propensity score in estimation of causal treatment effects: a comparative study. Stat Med 2004; 23:2937–2960.

Luo Z, Gardiner JC, Bradley CJ. Applying propensity score methods in medical research: pitfalls and prospects. Med Care Res Rev 2010; 67:528–554.

Maldonado G, Greenland S. Simulation study of confounder-selection strategies. Am J Epidemiol 1993; 138:923–936.

Maldonado G, Greenland S. Estimating causal effects. Int J Epidemiol 2002; 31:422–429.

Martens EP, Pestman WR, de Boer A, Belitser SV, Klungel OH. Instrumental variables: application and limitations. Epidemiology 2006; 17:260–267.

McNutt LA, Wu C, Xue X, Hafner JP. Estimating the relative risk in cohort studies and clinical trials of common outcomes. Am J Epidemiol 2003; 157:940–943.

Miettinen OS. Stratification by a multivariate confounder score. Am J Epidemiol 1976; 104: 609–620.

Newhouse JP, McClellan M. Econometrics in outcomes research: the use of instrumental variables. Annu Rev Public Health 1998; 19:17–34.

Newman SC. Biostatistical methods in epidemiology. New York: Wiley and Sons, 2001.

Newman SC. Commonalities in the classical, collapsibility and counterfactual concepts of confounding. J Clin Epidemiol 2004; 57:325–329.

Pearl J. Causal diagrams for empirical research. Biometrika 1995; 82:669–688.

Pearl J. Causality: models, reasoning, and inference. Cambridge, UK: Cambridge University Press, 2000.

Peduzzi P, Concato J, Feinstein AR, Holford TR. Importance of events per independent variable in proportional hazards regression analysis. II. Accuracy and precision of regression estimates. J Clin Epidemiol 1995; 48:1503–1510.

Peduzzi P, Concato J, Kemper E, Holford TR, Feinstein AR. A simulation study of the number of events per variable in logistic regression analysis. J Clin Epidemiol 1996; 49:1373–1379.

Raghunathan TE. What do we do with missing data? Some options for analysis of incomplete data. Annu Rev Public Health 2004; 25:99–117.

Rassen JA, Brookhart MA, Glynn RJ, Mittleman MA, Schneeweiss S. Instrumental variables I: instrumental variables exploit natural variation in nonexperimental data to estimate causal relationships. J Clin Epidemiol 2009a; 62:1226–1232.

Rassen JA, Schneeweiss S, Glynn RJ, Mittleman MA, Brookhart MA. Instrumental variable analysis for estimation of treatment effects with dichotomous outcomes. Am J Epidemiol 2009b; 169:273–284.

Robins JM. Data, design, and background knowledge in etiologic inference. Epidemiology 2001; 12:313–320.

Robins JM, Hernán MA, Brumback B. Marginal structural models and causal inference in epidemiology. Epidemiology 2000; 11:550–560.

Robins JM, Mark SD, Newey WK. Estimating exposure effects by modelling the expectation of exposure conditional on confounders. Biometrics 1992; 48:479–495.

Rosenbaum PR. Model-based direct adjustment. J Am Stat Assoc 1987; 82:387–394.

Rosenbaum PR, Rubin DB. The central role of the propensity score in observational studies for causal effects. Biometrika 1983; 70:41–55.

Rosenbaum PR, Rubin DB. Reducing bias in observational studies using subclassification on the propensity scorects. J Amer Statist Assoc 1984; 79: 516–524.

Rosner B. Fundamentals of biostatistics (6th edition). Belmont, CA: Duxbury Press, 2006.

Royston P, Ambler G, Sauerbrei W. The use of fractional polynomials to model continuous risk variables in epidemiology. Int J Epidemiol 1999; 28:964–974.

Royston P, Sauerbrei W. Multivariable model-building: a pragmatic approach to regression analysis based on fractional polynomials for modelling continuous variables. Hoboken, NJ: Wiley, 2008.

Rubin DB, Thomas N. Matching using estimated propensity scores: relating theory to practice. Biometrics 1996; 52:249–264.

Sato T, Matsuyama Y. Marginal structural models as a tool for standardization. Epidemiology 2003; 14:680–686.

Schisterman EF, Cole SR, Platt RW. Overadjustment bias and unnecessary adjustment in epidemiologic studies. Epidemiology 2009; 20:488–495.

Schmoor C, Gall C, Stampf S, Graf E. Correction of confounding bias in non-randomized studies by appropriate weighting. Biom J 2011; 53:369–387.

Schneeweiss S, Rassen JA, Glynn RJ, Avorn J, Mogun H, Brookhart MA. High-dimensional propensity score adjustment in studies of treatment effects using health care claims data. Epidemiology 2009; 20:512–522.

Selvin S. Statistical tools for epidemiologic research. New York: Oxford University Press, 2011.

Shah BR, Laupacis A, Hux JE, Austin PC. Propensity score methods gave similar results to traditional regression modeling in observational studies: a systematic review. J Clin Epidemiol 2005; 58:550–559.

Shahar E. Causal diagrams for encoding and evaluation of information bias. J Eval Clin Pract 2009; 15:436–440.

Shpitser I, VanderWeele TJ. A complete graphical criterion for the adjustment formula in mediation analysis. Int J Biostat 2011; 7:16.

Stürmer T, Schneeweiss S, Brookhart MA, Rothman KJ, Avorn J, Glynn RJ. Analytic strategies to adjust confounding using exposure propensity scores and disease risk scores: nonsteroidal antiinflammatory drugs and short-term mortality in the elderly. Am J Epidemiol 2005; 161: 891–898.

Suarez D, Borràs R, Basagaña X. Differences between marginal structural models and conventional models in their exposure effect estimates: a systematic review. Epidemiology 2011; 22: 586–588.

Thompson RS, Rivara FP, Thompson DC. A case-control study of the effectiveness of bicycle safety helmets. N Engl J Med 1989; 320:1361–1367.

Trompet S, Jukema JW, Katan MB, Blauw GJ, Sattar N, Buckley B, et al. Apolipoprotein E genotype, plasma cholesterol, and cancer: a Mendelian randomization study. Am J Epidemiol 2009; 170:1415–1421.

VanderWeele TJ, Hernán MA, Robins JM. Causal directed acyclic graphs and the direction of unmeasured confounding bias. Epidemiology 2008; 19:720–728.

VanderWeele TJ, Robins JM. Directed acyclic graphs, sufficient causes, and the properties of conditioning on a common effect. Am J Epidemiol 2007a; 166:1096–1104.

VanderWeele TJ, Robins JM. Four types of effect modification: a classification based on directed acyclic graphs. Epidemiology 2007b; 18:561–568.

VanderWeele TJ, Shpitser I. A new criterion for confounder selection. Biometrics 2011; 67:1406–1413.

Vittinghoff E, Glidden DV, Shiboski SC, McCulloch CE. Regression methods in biostatistics: linear, logistic, survival, and repeated measures models (2nd ed.). New York: Springer, 2012.

Vittinghoff E, McCulloch CE. Relaxing the rule of ten events per variable in logistic and Cox regression. Am J Epidemiol 2007; 165:710–718.

Weinberg CR. Can DAGs clarify effect modification? Epidemiology 2007; 18:569–572.

Westreich D. Berkson's bias, selection bias, and missing data. Epidemiology 2012; 23:159–164.

Whitcomb BW, Schisterman EF, Perkins NJ, Platt RW. Quantification of collider-stratification bias and the birthweight paradox. Paediatr Perinat Epidemiol 2009; 23:394–402.

White IR, Royston P, Wood AM. Multiple imputation using chained equations: issues and guidance for practice. Stat Med 2011; 30:377–399.

Whittemore AS. Collapsibility of multidimensional contingency tables. J R Stat Soc B 1978; 40:328–340.

Wikipedia, 2012. Garrison Keillor. http://en.wikipedia.org/wiki/Garrison_Keillor.

Xiao Y, Abrahamowicz M, Moodie EEM. Accuracy of conventional and marginal structural Cox model estimators: a simulation study. Int J Biostat 2010; 6:Article 13.

Zhu SH, Anderson CM, Tedeschi GJ, Rosbrook B, Johnson CE, Byrd M, et al. Evidence of real-world effectiveness of a telephone quitline for smokers. N Engl J Med 2002; 347:1087–1093.

EXERCISES

1. Agriculture is a high-risk industry for fatal work-related injury in the United States, and tractor-related injuries are a major contributing factor. In a telephone survey of farm families in five Midwestern states (Carlson *et al.*, 2005), about 16,100 household members were asked whether they had experienced a tractor-related injury during the preceding year. Information about possible demographic and work-related risk factors at the beginning of that year was also obtained in these interviews.

   Data analysis employed multiple logistic regression, guided by the causal diagram shown in figure 12.23 (adapted from Carlson *et al.*, 2005). A statistical technique called "generalized estimating equations" was used to account for the non-independence of data on individuals within the same household, which affects the confidence limits but not the basic interpretation of the results. Selected findings are shown in Table 12.26 below the causal diagram.

   (a) Adjusted *odds ratios* were calculated. Can they be safely interpreted as adjusted *risk ratios* in this instance? Why or why not?

   (b) Suppose that the amount of time at risk and the timing of any tractor-related injuries had been available for each individual. What statistical technique would the investigators have probably used for multivariable analysis instead of logistic regression?

   (c) In the results table, the adjusted odds ratios for hours worked/week on the respondent's own farm were adjusted for age, gender, education, marital status, and prior injury status. Why were they not also adjusted for state of residence?

2. When comparing the conditions for collapsibility of the *RR* and *RD* with conditions for collapsibility of the *OR* in a $2 \times 2 \times k$ table, the text focused on the importance of differences in the weights in equations (12.1) and (12.2). It was noted that $w_{ei} = w_{ui}$ can be true while $w'_{ei} = w'_{ui}$ is not, or vice versa. In words, it is possible that there is no *C-E* association in the full study population while there *is* a *C-E* association among the controls (i.e., those with $Y = 0$), or vice versa.

   Another difference between the two sets of conditions for collapsibility is that Equation (12.1) involves r_{ui}, the *proportion* with $Y = 1$ among unexposed subjects in stratum i, while Equation (12.2) involves ψ_{ui}, the *odds* of $Y = 1$ among unexposed subjects in stratum i. In particular, if r_{ui} is constant across all strata, then Equation (12.1) will be satisfied and the *RR* or *RD* will be collapsible. If ψ_{ui} is constant across all strata, then Equation (12.2) will be satisfied and the *OR* will be collapsible.

   Are there tables in which r_{ui} is constant across all strata but ψ_{ui} is *not* constant across all strata, or vice versa?

3. Suppose that a case-control study is being conducted to investigate whether taking folate supplements during pregnancy reduces the risk of having a baby with a neural-tube defect (NTD), a relatively rare congenital malformation. Based on the best available background information, the researchers have developed the causal model shown in Figure 12.24.

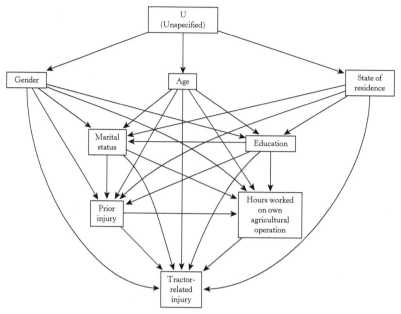

FIGURE 12.23

TABLE 12.26.

Exposure	No. of respondents	No. of events	Adjusted odds ratio Estimate	(95% CI)
Prior injury[a]				
No	13,039	66	1.00	(Reference)
Yes	3,081	69	2.02	(1.39 – 2.94)
Hours worked/week on own farm[b]				
0	2,759	3	0.63	(0.18 – 2.27)
1–20	7,699	24	1.00	(Reference)
21–40	2,282	17	1.20	(0.64, 2.26)
41–60	1,441	32	1.67	(0.88 – 3.15)
61–80	1,284	38	1.88	(1.00 – 3.53)
81+	475	14	1.85	(0.85 – 4.04)

[a] Adjusted for age, gender, state, education, and marital status
[b] Adjusted for age, gender, education, marital status, and prior injury status
(Based on data from Carlson *et al.* [2005])

According to the model, neural-tube defects (D) are thought to result from the interplay of genetic risk factors (H) and maternal serum folate during pregnancy (F). Both dietary intake of folate (C) and taking folate supplements (E) affect serum folate levels (F). Mother's education (A) affects dietary folate intake (C) as well as affecting whether a pregnant mother takes folate supplements (E). Mother's education also affects how many prior children the mother has had—i.e., her parity (B). Parity (B) and the mother's genetic predisposition (H) affect whether she has borne a prior child with a neural-tube defect (G). Having had a prior child with a neural-tube defect (G) affects whether a pregnant woman takes folate supplements (E). Assume for present purposes that this model correctly portrays the causal relationships among the variables shown.

(a) Of the variables shown, genetic predisposition would almost certainly be the hardest one to measure adequately, in part because of uncertainty about which specific genetic traits predispose to NTD occurrence. But suppose that all of the other variables shown can be measured satisfactorily. Would it be possible to control for some set of them to obtain an unconfounded estimate of the effect of taking folate supplements (E) on NTD occurrence (D) *without* controlling for genetic predisposition (H)?

(b) Suppose that the study used a matched case-control design in which each mother who bore a baby with an NTD was matched to a mother of similar age who bore a baby at the same hospital but without an NTD. What multivariable analysis method would be appropriate to obtain an adjusted estimate of the relative risk of NTD in relation to folate supplementation, controlling for other confounding factors on which cases and control were *not* matched?

4. Intracerebral hemorrhage is a subtype of stroke. Data on several potential risk factors for intracerebral hemorrhage were collected in a cohort study of 27,760 community-dwelling white and African-American adults recruited throughout the United States (Howard *et al.*, 2013). One potential risk factor of interest was systolic blood pressure (SBP), inasmuch as high SBP had been found to be associated with stroke incidence in several previous studies. In the study cohort, the mean SBP was 127.3 mmHg, with a standard deviation of 16.5.

In a proportional-hazards regression model that included age, sex, and race as other covariates, the estimated β-coefficient for SBP was found to be approximately 0.0166, which translates to an estimated hazard ratio of about 1.0167 (95% CI: 1.0039–1.0305). Similar results for SBP were obtained from other models that included several additional risk factors.

It has sometimes been argued that relative risks or hazard ratios less than about 2.0 should be discounted as evidence of a causal association. Do you feel that rule of thumb should be applied here? Why, or why not?

5. A research team is interested in the potential effects of neighborhood environment on cardiovascular disease (CVD). They have obtained data from a large cohort study that recruited people from multiple neighborhoods in several cities and identified new CVD cases among the participants over time. The researchers hypothesize that violent crime in a neighborhood may affect CVD risk. For one thing, neighborhood violence may affect whether people have safe opportunities to get regular exercise. Data from the cohort study (including race, family income, and physical activity level, among other variables) will be linked to additional data on the number of violent crimes in each neighborhood (defined operationally as a census tract) just before the cohort study began.

In planning their analysis, the investigators have constructed the causal diagram shown in Figure 12.25 involving some key variables (based on Fleischer and Diez Roux (2008)).

Assuming the diagram is correctly drawn, which of the variables shown need to be controlled in the analysis in order to prevent confounding when evaluating the main study hypothesis?

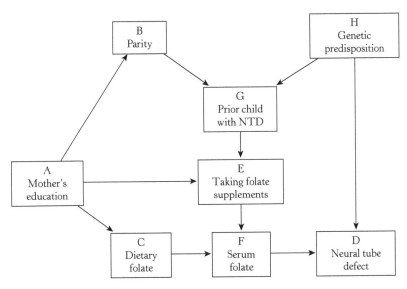

FIGURE 12.24

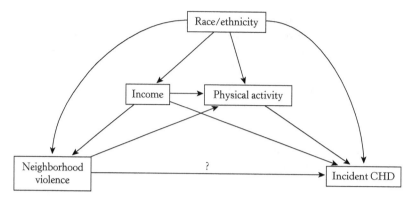

FIGURE 12.25

6. The California state health department set up a telephone "quit line" to help cigarette smokers in that state give up smoking (Zhu *et al.*, 2002). Normally, an interested smoker called the toll-free telephone number and received (1) a set of self-help smoking cessation materials in the mail, and (2) immediate linkage to a personal telephone counselor. Beginning with that initial call, the counselor provided personalized advice and encouragement on how to stop smoking. The counselor also followed the smoker over time to give ongoing support, initiating subsequent telephone contacts with the client if necessary.

During certain busy time periods, incoming call volume exceeded the program's capacity to provide a personalized counselor right away for every caller. Under those conditions, a randomly selected 60% of smokers who called in were handled in the usual way—sent self-help materials and connected on the same call to a personal counselor. The remaining 40% were sent the self-help materials and were told to call back after they had received those materials, to start work with a personal counselor who would be assigned at that time. All smokers in both groups agreed to permit follow-up assessments of their smoking status for program evaluation purposes.

Table 12.27 shows smoking status at three months after their initial call among participants in the randomized comparison described above.

(a) From the data given, what is your best estimate of the effect of being linked immediately to a personal counselor, as opposed to being told to call back later for counseling, on the probability of quitting smoking 3 months later?

(b) From the data given, can you estimate the impact of actually being linked to a personal counselor (versus not being linked to a counselor) on the quit proportion at 3 months? If so, what is it?

TABLE 12.27.

Group	n	Percent no longer smoking 3 months later
Linked to a counselor right away	1973	23.7%
Told to call back later for counseling;		
Did call back and were linked to a counselor	463	29.2%
Did not call back	846	9.6%

7. Angina pectoris is chest pain of cardiac origin, often brought on by exertion or stress. A randomized, double-blind, placebo-controlled trial has been conducted to evaluate a new drug, Anginex, which is intended to reduce the frequency of angina attacks by increasing coronary blood flow. Contrary to expectation, the results showed no overall association between being randomized to Anginex and the frequency of angina attacks as reported by patients. Compliance with the randomly assigned treatment was almost perfect, so non-compliance cannot be blamed for the negative result.

At the end of the trial, the investigators evaluated the success of blinding by asking patients in both treatment arms whether they thought they were on Anginex or on placebo. Of those actually on Anginex, 60% guessed correctly that they were taking Anginex, while only 40% of patients actually on placebo guessed that they were taking Anginex. These results were not altogether surprising, because Anginex is known to cause gastrointestinal discomfort in some patients as a side effect, and presence or absence of such side effects may have been a clue to patients as to what they

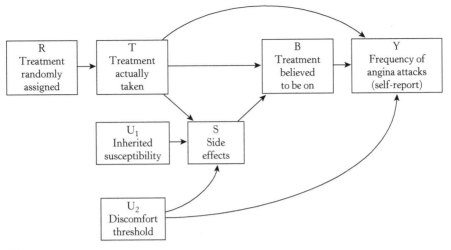

FIGURE 12.26

were taking. These side effects are thought to be more common among people with an inherited susceptibility to them and among those with low tolerance for discomfort.

Given the trial's negative result, the apparent partial failure of blinding was of concern to the investigators. They speculated that patients who thought they were on Anginex may have felt freer to engage in more vigorous physical activities or to expose themselves to stressful situations, thinking that being on Anginex would protect them from angina. Their increased exercise and exposure to stress may, in turn, have led to more angina attacks, thus "canceling out" any true pharmacological benefit of the drug on coronary blood flow.

After considerable discussion, the investigators distilled their theory about the circumstances into the causal model shown in Figure 12.26. All variables shown were measured except U_1 and U_2.

(a) One option under discussion is to re-analyze the trial data, stratifying on which drug each patient *believed* he/she was taking (B). Among patients who believed they were on Anginex, for example, angina frequency would be compared between those who actually were taking Anginex vs. those who were not. Such an analysis would aim to control for any psychological or behavioral effects of a belief that one was or was not on Anginex, thus focusing on the actual biological effects of being on Anginex vs. placebo.

Would this strategy yield a valid estimate of the biological effects of Anginex on angina frequency?

(b) Suppose the investigators stratified by both B and S. Would the B- and S-adjusted association between T and Y be a valid estimate of the biological effects of Anginex on angina frequency?

ANSWERS

1. (a) Yes. The one-year cumulative incidence of tractor-related injuries was under 5% overall and in all subgroups. Thus the rare-disease assumption would be easily satisfied here, and adjusted odds ratios should be good estimates of adjusted risk ratios.

(b) If detailed data on time at risk and injury occurrence had been available for each household member, proportional-hazards regression analysis could have been used.

(c) In that particular analysis, hours worked/week was the exposure, and tractor-related injury was the outcome. According to the causal diagram, state of residence was a direct cause of tractor-related injury, but state of residence was believed to affect hours worked only indirectly through its effects on marital status, education, and prior injury occurrence. These factors had already been included in the multivariable model, which blocks those backdoor paths.

Additional backdoor paths involving state of residence could go through U. However, from U, any such path would have to go through either age or gender, which had also been included in the multivariable model.

Thus, all backdoor paths between hours worked and tractor-related injuries that involved state of residence had already been blocked by controlling for the other five variables. Assuming that the causal diagram is correctly drawn, it was not necessary to adjust additionally for state of residence.

2. No, there are no such tables. If ψ_{ui} is constant across all strata, then r_{ui} must also be constant across all strata, and vice versa. Consider just two strata:

$$\psi_{u1} = \psi_{u2}$$

$$\frac{r_{u1}}{1 - r_{u1}} = \frac{r_{u2}}{1 - r_{u2}}$$

$$r_{u1}(1 - r_{u2}) = r_{u2}(1 - r_{u1})$$

$$r_{u1} - r_{u1}r_{u2} = r_{u2} - r_{u1}r_{u2}$$

$$r_{u1} = r_{u2}$$

which can be generalized to any number of strata. In short, any table in which ψ_{ui} is constant across strata will also have r_{ui} constant across strata, and vice versa. Therefore if there is no C-Y association among the unexposed, this will be reflected in both proportions and odds, and the RR, RD, and OR will all be collapsible.

3. (a) Yes. Starting from E, any backdoor path to D must go through either A or G. Therefore, controlling for both A and G would be sufficient to block all such paths, yielding an unconfounded estimate of the effect of E on D.

   Another, more elaborate, way to attack the problem is to identify all of the backdoor paths from E to D and then consider how to block each of them. There are four such paths: E-G-H-D, E-G-B-A-C-F-D, E-A-B-G-H-D, and E-A-C-F-D. Of these, the E-A-B-G-H-D path is special, because G is a collider on that path. Unless G is controlled, that path is already blocked without controlling for anything. However, the only way to block the E-G-H-D path is to control for G, because we cannot measure and control for H. Controlling for G is good because it blocks not only the E-G-H-D path but also the E-G-B-A-C-F-D path. However, controlling for G has the side effect of unblocking the E-A-B-G-H-D path because it induces an association between B and H. Fortunately, controlling additionally for A blocks both the newly reopened E-A-B-G-H-D path as well as the E-A-C-F-D path.

   Several other larger sets of covariates would also be sufficient to control confounding of the E-D association, but the two-element set {A, G} is the smallest set that would achieve the desired goal.

   One would never control for serum folate (F) as part of an effort to minimize confounding, because it is a descendant of the exposure, taking folate supplements (E). The causal diagram portrays serum folate as a mediating variable through which taking folate supplements would influence NTD risk.

   (b) The best choice would be conditional logistic regression. NTDs are said to be rare, so an adjusted odds ratio could be interpreted as an adjusted relative risk. Logistic regression yields adjusted odds ratios. *Conditional* logistic regression would be preferred over ordinary (unconditional) logistic regression for this kind of study because it would properly account for the matching of cases to controls.

4. The adjusted hazard ratio in question, calculated from a β-coefficient in a proportional-hazards regression model, estimates the factor by which the hazard rate would increase or decrease in relation to a *1-unit* change in the corresponding predictor variable, after controlling for other covariates in the model. But a 1-mmHg difference in SBP is quite small. A small increase in exposure will often produce only a small change in risk even if the underlying exposure, measured as a continuous variable, is a strong and important risk factor. The same interpretation problem would arise regardless of the presence or absence of other covariates in the regression model.

5. The main exposure is neighborhood violence, and the outcome is incident CVD. To control confounding, all backdoor paths from exposure to outcome must be blocked. Here, the exposure has two parents—income and race/ethnicity—each of which is also shown as a direct cause of incident CVD. Hence both income and race/ethnicity must be controlled. Since they are the only two parents of neighborhood violence, controlling them automatically blocks all backdoor paths involving the variables being considered here.

6. (a) This comparison (referred to as an *intent-to-treat* analysis), involves the two groups formed by randomization. The total number who successfully quit smoking in the call-back-later group was $(463 \times 0.292) + (846 \times 0.096) =$ 216, for an overall quit proportion of $216/(463 + 846) = 0.165 = 16.5\%$. The effect of immediate linkage to a counselor was to increase this quit proportion to $0.237 = 23.7\%$, an increase of 7.2 percentage points.

   (b) One might be tempted to compare quit proportions between those in the call-back-later arm who were linked to a counselor versus those in the same arm who did not call back to be linked to a counselor. However, this is not a randomized comparison and could be heavily influenced by self-selection. Those who called back to receive counseling might have been more motivated to quit than those who did not

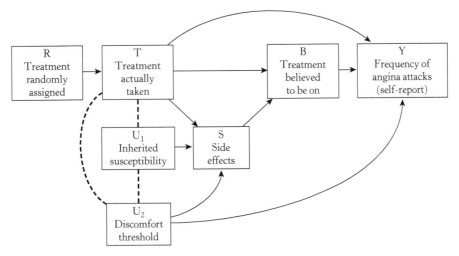

FIGURE 12.27

call back. Likewise, comparing the entire immediate-referral arm to the did-not-call-back subgroup of the opposite arm would be subject to the same self-selection bias.

However, it *is* possible to estimate indirectly the impact of being linked to a personal counselor by regarding randomized treatment assignment as an instrumental variable. Clients were much more likely to be linked to a counselor if they were connected right away than if they were told to call back. It is also unlikely that random assignment affected the likelihood of quitting in any other way, and randomization should have prevented confounding by other factors.

As calculated above, the overall proportion who quit successfully in the call-back-later group was 0.165. The estimated difference in quit proportions in relation to being linked to a counselor would be

$$\frac{(0.237 - 0.165)}{\left(\dfrac{1973}{1973} - \dfrac{463}{463 + 846}\right)} = 0.111$$

or 11.1 percentage points.

An alternative approach to a this kind of problem is described in Chapter 13, based on counterfactuals—see example 13-10.

7. (a) No. In causal-diagram terms, the investigators sought to evaluate the strength of the direct T-Y path (curved arrow) while blocking the "nuisance" path T-B-Y by stratifying on B. However, B has several ancestors. It is a shared descendant of T, U_1, and U_2, so controlling for B would induce associations among all pairs of these variables, as shown in Figure 12.27.

These induced associations would create two new backdoor paths from T to Y (namely, T-U_1-U_2-Y and T-U_2-Y), which would confound the direct T-Y causal path of interest. Unfortunately, neither backdoor path can be blocked, because U_1 and U_2 were not measured.

(b) No again. Like B, S is also a shared descendant of T, U_1, and U_2, so stratifying on it would induce the same associations as stratifying on B. Uncontrollable confounding of the T-Y causal path of interest by the T-U_1-U_2-Y and T-U_2-Y backdoor paths would remain a problem.

13

Randomized Trials

A lady declares that by tasting a cup of tea made with milk she can discriminate whether the milk or the tea infusion was first added to the cup. ... Our experiment consists in mixing eight cups of tea, four in one way and four in the other, and presenting them to the subject for judgment in a random order. ... Her task is to divide the eight cups into two sets of four, agreeing, if possible, with the treatments received.

—SIR RONALD FISHER

INTRODUCTION
Can *Ginkgo Biloba* Prevent Dementia?

Dementia, a chronic condition that includes Alzheimer's disease and related disorders, afflicts millions of Americans. Few modifiable risk factors have been identified. However, use of the herbal drug *Ginkgo biloba* has been popular in many areas of the world in an attempt to preserve memory. It contains antioxidants and other ingredients that may retard aggregation of amyloid protein into the neurotoxic brain deposits characteristic of Alzheimer's disease. In the United States, sales of *Ginkgo biloba* in 2006 were estimated to have exceeded $249 million, although evidence on the drug's effectiveness for preventing memory decline remained limited (DeKosky *et al.*, 2008).

To determine whether *Ginkgo biloba* actually prevents dementia, the Ginkgo Evaluation of Memory (GEM) study enrolled 3,069 older adult volunteers over an eight-year period at five study centers across the United States. Among the participants, 84% had normal cognition on entry, while the rest had mild cognitive impairment but not dementia. Subjects were then randomized to take either a twice-daily dose of *Ginkgo biloba* extract or twice-daily placebo. Participants were re-evaluated every 6 months using a standardized set of neuropsychological tests and were interviewed about possible side effects. The results were interpreted by an expert panel of clinicians to determine whether criteria for dementia were met. Neither the subjects themselves nor study staff responsible for follow-up or

outcome assessment knew which drug each subject was taking. An independent Data Safety and Monitoring Board reviewed the results periodically during the trial to determine whether the study should be stopped early, due either to proof of efficacy or to safety concerns.

After a median follow-up of 6.1 years, the incidence of dementia among *Ginkgo biloba* recipients was 3.3 cases per 100 person-years, compared to 2.9 among placebo recipients (hazard ratio = 1.12, 95% CI: 0.94–1.33). *Ginkgo biloba* also had no evident effect on the incidence of dementia in the subset of participants with mild cognitive impairment at baseline (hazard ratio = 1.13, 95% CI: 0.85–1.50). The investigators concluded that *Ginkgo biloba* could not be recommended for prevention of dementia.

The GEM study is an example of a *randomized trial*—a comparative study in which study subjects are assigned by a formal chance mechanism to two or more intervention strategies. Randomized trials occupy a special place among epidemiologic study designs because they can provide particularly strong evidence to support a hypothesis of a causal link between an exposure and an outcome. Randomized-trial results can sometimes reverse inferences drawn from non-randomized studies (Anderson *et al.*, 2004; Omenn *et al.*, 1996; Odgaard-Jensen *et al.*, 2011).

Why Randomize?

First, randomization generally offers excellent protection against confounding. As we saw in Chapter 12, a necessary condition for confounding is that there be an association between exposure and the potential confounder. Randomization tends to distribute potential confounders similarly among exposure groups, which removes this necessary precondition. In causal diagram form:

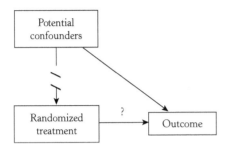

FIGURE 13.1

Randomization thus tends to break the links between exposure (here, the randomized treatment assignment) and all potential confounders, removing all backdoor paths from exposure to outcome. That said, while randomization balances potential confounders between exposure groups on average, some degree of imbalance may still occur by chance. With sufficiently large samples, any such imbalances are likely to be modest in size and can, if necessary, be addressed using the same kinds of analytic techniques that are routinely used to deal with confounding in non-randomized studies. Moreover, as discussed later, randomization can sometimes be implemented in such a way as to guarantee balance between exposure groups on a key potential confounder.

For example, in the GEM study, presence of the APOE $\epsilon4$ allele is known to be strongly associated with the risk of Alzheimer's disease and was thus an important potential confounding factor. Each of the 578 subjects who carried this genetic marker had an equal chance of being assigned to *Ginkgo biloba* or to placebo. It turned out that 297 subjects with the allele were assigned by chance to *Ginkgo biloba*, and 281 were assigned to placebo. The resulting prevalence of APOE ϵ 4 was 24.1% in the active treatment group and 23.0% in the placebo group—not identical, but very close indeed. The two groups also proved to be similar on a variety of other health-related characteristics that were assessed in the trial. Moreover, randomization works to prevent confounding even by factors that have not been measured or that may be unknown to the investigator.

Second, if potential study subjects or those who refer subjects into a trial can anticipate which treatment arm a subject would be assigned to, self-selection or selective referral can lead to a biased comparison. A desperately ill patient might prefer an experimental treatment to placebo and might choose to enroll only if likely to receive the experimental treatment. Such self-selection could skew the experimental-treatment arm toward sicker patients with worse prognosis. The specific characteristics that influence such choices in a particular context can be very difficult to identify, measure, and control adequately. The unpredictability of assignments that results from randomization helps prevent imbalances in those characteristics across treatment groups. In some trials, unpredictability due to randomization also makes it possible to keep participants unaware of which treatment group they are in ("blinded"), which helps avoid bias in self-reported outcomes and differential subject attrition.

Third, randomization supports statistical inference. It allows the probability of any given set of trial results under the null hypothesis to be calculated from statistical theory. This provides a solid basis for obtaining *p*-values and confidence limits: the assumptions behind standard statistical tests are satisfied by design.

When Can a Randomized Trial Design Be Used?

Some exposure–outcome relationships are more amenable than others to study in a randomized trial. Conditions that favor use of the randomized-trial design include the following:

1. *The exposure is potentially modifiable.* Factors such as genotype, family history, and race/ethnicity cannot be altered, so their influence on disease occurrence must be studied with non-randomized designs.
2. *The exposure is potentially modifiable by the investigator.* Certain exposures such as occupation, marital status, and smoking habits are, in principle, modifiable, but it is often impossible or impractical to assign people at random among the possible categories for research purposes. However, even this limitation does not always preclude use of a randomized trial in some form, as in the following example:

> **Example 13-1.** Many observational studies have found cigarette smoking during pregnancy to be associated with increased risk of having a low birth-weight baby. However, part of this association could represent confounding by maternal risk factors associated with smoking. Sexton and Hebel (1984) randomly assigned 935 pregnant smokers to either a smoking-cessation intervention or a

usual-care control group. By the eighth month of pregnancy, 57% of mothers in the intervention group still smoked, versus 80% of mothers in the control group. The average birth weight of babies born to all intervention-group mothers was 92 grams higher than that in the control group ($p < 0.05$). These results suggested not only that the intervention was effective at helping pregnant mothers to stop smoking, but also that maternal smoking was truly a cause of low birth weight.

Here, the exposure of main interest (smoking during pregnancy) was not the same as the randomized intervention actually studied (participation in a smoking-cessation program). But if it is safe to assume that the narrowly focused smoking cessation program did not influence birth weight in any other way than by changing mothers' smoking behavior, then the observed difference in birth weight represented a "diluted" effect of maternal smoking, biased away from finding a difference. When an association was found nonetheless, the case for a causal effect of smoking gained strong support.

3. *There is genuine uncertainty about which intervention strategy is superior.* Sometimes other available evidence indicates beyond a reasonable doubt that one intervention strategy is superior to another. If so, it may be unethical to offer people the inferior method in lieu of the superior one. For example, a tongue-in-cheek article in the *British Medical Journal* pointed out that parachutes are thought to "reduce the risk of injury after gravitational challenge, but their effectiveness has not been proved with randomised controlled trials" (Smith and Pell, 2003).

4. *The primary outcomes are relatively common and occur relatively soon.* Randomized trials almost always involve measuring outcomes prospectively in two or more comparison groups. As will be shown later, the power of a trial to detect an intervention effect on incidence depends on occurrence of a sufficient number of outcome events. For this reason, randomized trials are less well suited to studying rare or long-delayed outcomes, because large samples or prolonged follow-up would be needed to get the necessary number of outcome events.

Randomized trials can be expensive, especially when large numbers of participants are required, the period of follow-up is long, and/or the process of intervening and collecting data on each subject is costly. Still, it is important to keep in mind that the key distinguishing feature of a randomized trial is simply that the comparison groups be formed by a formal chance mechanism—a process that is technically quite easy to carry out and is neither costly nor time-consuming. Indeed, many randomized trials have been conducted speedily and at low cost when they concerned common, easily measured outcomes that occurred soon after the intervention was applied—e.g., Rosa *et al.* (1998); Klein *et al.* (1995). As recounted in the headnote to this chapter, Sir Ronald Fisher, inventor of the randomized trial, proved this point in a classic experiment about whether a lady could truly tell whether tea or milk was first added to the cup. (She did!)

Historical Milestones

Randomized trials are a relatively modern innovation in research design (Chalmers, 2001). Although a few comparative treatment experiments had been carried out before 1900, none used formal randomization to form the comparison groups. Fisher first developed randomized-trial methodology for use in agriculture (Fisher, 1935), and some terminology for experimental designs (e.g., "split plot") still reflects this legacy. A groundbreaking early randomized *clinical* trial showed that the antibiotic streptomycin was effective treatment for pulmonary tuberculosis (Medical Research Council, 1948). Growing appreciation of the design's unique benefits led to rapid development and acceptance of its use throughout the 1950s, including a large trial of the Salk vaccine for prevention of polio that involved 1.8 million schoolchildren (Dawson, 2004). In 1962, the United States Food and Drug Administration began requiring evidence of efficacy from properly controlled randomized trials before a new drug could be approved for general use in the United States (Junod, 2012). The 1970s–1980s saw mounting of many large multi-site trials, including the University Group Diabetes Program (University Group Diabetes Program, 1970a,b), the Multiple Risk Factor Intervention Trial for prevention of cardiovascular disease (Multiple Risk Factor Intervention Trial Research Group, 1982), and cooperative cancer chemotherapy groups (DeVita and Chu, 2008). In the 1990s, the Cochrane Collaboration—named for Archibald Cochrane, a tireless and influential advocate of randomized trials (Cochrane, 1972; Winkelstein, 2009)—was formed to provide critical systematic reviews of evidence from randomized trials relevant to medical practice and health policy (Friedrich, 2013). In 1996, the first CONSORT guidelines (discussed below) for reporting of trial results were published (Begg *et al.*, 1996) and were soon widely endorsed by medical journals. In 2004, the International Committee of Medical Journal Editors mandated that all clinical trials be registered in a publicly accessible trial registry (e.g., www.ClinicalTrials.gov), prior to patient enrollment, as condition of consideration for publication (DeAngelis *et al.*, 2004).

CONSORT

In an attempt to improve the completeness and quality of clinical trial reports in medical journals, an international committee of trialists, biostatisticians, epidemiologists, and journal editors developed the Consolidated Standards of Reporting Trials (CONSORT) in 1996 (Begg *et al.*, 1996). The CONSORT statement has since been revised periodically (Moher *et al.*, 2001; Schulz *et al.*, 2010), and expansions of it have been published for several specialized types of randomized trials (CONSORT, 2013).

The CONSORT statement has been endorsed by more than 600 medical journals. Accordingly, investigators who plan to conduct a randomized trial would be wise know what information journals will be likely to require in a trial report. The scientific basis for the CONSORT guidelines is presented in an extensively referenced companion publication (Moher *et al.*, 2010), which explains not only why each element should be addressed in a trial report, but also why the corresponding aspect of trial design and conduct is important scientifically. The CONSORT guidelines will be referenced repeatedly in this chapter.

TRIAL OBJECTIVES
Explanatory vs. Pragmatic Aims

Randomized trials are undertaken to determine whether one intervention strategy is better than another in some way. But why would the answer matter? Sometimes a potentially useful theory predicts a certain result, and the proposed trial would provide a rigorous test of the theory. Trials designed for this reason are often called *explanatory* trials (Schwartz and Lellouch, 1967; Thorpe *et al.*, 2009). They are akin to basic research. Their focus is on understanding causal mechanisms, and the main product is improved knowledge about how the world works.

Example 13-2. To follow up on earlier research that had found an inverse association between dietary calcium intake and body weight, Bendsen *et al.* (2008) sought to test the hypothesis that high calcium intake causes increased fecal excretion of dietary fat. Eleven adult volunteers were identified through advertisements in shops and campus websites. The investigators then provided subjects with two tightly controlled diets, one containing 2,300 mg. of daily calcium and the other containing 700 mg. of daily calcium. Randomization determined which of the two diets a given subject followed first, and after following that initial diet for seven days, the participant was switched to the other diet for seven more days. Total fat excretion was found to be 11.5 grams/day on the high-calcium diet and 5.4 grams/day on the low calcium diet ($p < 0.001$), supporting the theory that a high-calcium diet can promote weight loss.

In other situations, knowing which intervention strategy is better matters because a practical decision must be made between two or more possible courses of action. Time, money, lives, comfort, or other valued outcomes are at stake. Trials that are undertaken to guide decision-making in the "real world" are often called *pragmatic* trials. They are akin to applied research. The focus is on choosing between feasible alternatives that are potentially widely applicable (Tunis *et al.*, 2003). Whatever value the trial has as a test of a theory is a happy by-product.

Example 13-3. Women with breast cancer that has spread to a nearby lymph node are normally treated by surgical removal of the tumor, radiation therapy to the breast, and possibly chemotherapy. But there has been debate about whether the surgeon should do additional, more extensive dissection of axillary lymph nodes at the time of surgery in an attempt to find and remove other nodes that may contain cancer. Doing so may limit cancer spread, but it also prolongs surgery and poses risk of infection, lymphedema, and other complications.

Giuliano *et al.* (2011) conducted a collaborative randomized trial at 115 clinical centers, at which 891 eligible and consenting women with breast cancer and evidence of one or two affected local lymph nodes were randomized to receive either: (A) further dissection of at least ten axillary lymph nodes, or (B) no further axillary surgery. At follow-up, five-year survival was 91.8% for group A and 92.5% for group B. Disease-free survival was 82.2% for group A and 83.9% for group B. The investigators concluded that more-extensive axillary dissection offered little or no advantage in terms of survival or disease recurrence among such patients.

TABLE 13.1. INFLUENCE OF EXPLANATORY VS. PRAGMATIC ORIENTATIONS ON TRIAL DESIGN

Feature	Explanatory	Pragmatic
Experimental intervention	What theory predicts should work best, whether practical for wider application or not	Strategy practical for use in real-world settings
Comparison intervention	Sharply defined, often maximizing contrast between experimental and control conditions	Realistic practical alternative to experimental intervention, sometimes just "usual care"
Study subjects	Those in whom an effect of intervention is expected to be greatest, including highly compliant people	Relatively broad sample from the potential target population
Outcome variables	Variables most sensitive to effects predicted by theory	Outcomes most relevant to subjects and care providers

Explanatory and pragmatic aims are both perfectly good reasons for carrying out a trial. Sometimes the same study can satisfy both kinds of aims well. But choices about specific features of trial design must often be made between mutually exclusive alternatives. These choices can involve trade-offs between testing a theory rigorously and maximizing relevance to practical decision-making. Table 13.1 lists aspects of trial design that can be influenced by which kind of goal takes precedence. A clear view of whether a trial's primary purpose is explanatory or pragmatic provides a consistent philosophy to guide these choices.

A closely related distinction is between the *efficacy* and the *effectiveness* of an intervention (Porta, 2008; Koepsell *et al.*, 2011). *Efficacy* refers to how well an intervention *can* work under ideal circumstances—e.g., when administered by well-trained experts and aimed at perfectly compliant recipients—even if those conditions are artificial and hard to mimic outside the research setting. *Effectiveness* refers to how well an intervention *does* work under "field conditions"—e.g., when administered by ordinary practitioners and offered to a relatively unselected target population.

Clinical Trial Phases

The United States Food and Drug Administration (FDA) has set forth a typology of *phases* of clinical trials. The typology was originally developed to describe and classify trials of drugs, but terminology based on it is now widely used for trials of other kinds of experimental interventions as well. Note that the FDA typology uses the term "trial" to refer to an intervention study in humans, not necessarily a *randomized* intervention study.

- *Phase 1* trials aim to determine a safe dosage range and to identify side effects, usually by administering the drug or other intervention to 20–80 healthy volunteers. No control group is studied.
- *Phase 2* trials seek preliminary data about effectiveness by giving the experimental intervention to about 30–300 persons with the target health condition. Safety is also monitored. Some phase 2 studies lack a control group and base inferences only on changes over time in the treated individuals. Other phase 2 studies involve randomization between two arms, one of which is treated with a placebo or an alternative treatment.
- *Phase 3* trials are nearly always randomized, seeking to evaluate the intervention's effectiveness and assess its side effects and safety compared to placebo or an alternative. Phase 3 studies typically involve about 1,000–3,000 patients.
- *Phase 4* studies are conducted after a new drug or other treatment is on the market, to obtain additional data about its benefits and risks in regular use. Phase 4 studies are typically observational studies that can involve thousands of patients, but without a control group. Due to their larger size, they can often identify rare but important side effects.

This chapter relates most closely to phase 3 studies and to phase 2 studies that include a randomized control group.

TREATMENT ARMS

The alternative conditions to which trial participants are assigned are often termed *arms* or *treatment arms* of the trial. (The term "treatment" in this context should be interpreted broadly to mean an intervention of any kind, not necessarily a therapeutic one.) A simple and common trial design involves just two arms, commonly called the *experimental* and *control* arms. Other design variations are considered later.

Experimental

Interest in a particular new intervention (or an older one in which there is renewed interest) is usually what motivates a trial in the first place, and the trial is built around it. The form taken by this *experimental* intervention may be tailored to meet explanatory or pragmatic goals, as noted above.

Control

The extent to which an experimental intervention is found to affect outcomes can depend heavily on what it is compared to. Several common options for the control arm follow.

Nothing

If there is no widely accepted competitor for the experimental intervention, one option is simply to compare it to nothing at all. For example, a randomized trial of low-dose aspirin for prevention of coronary heart disease was conducted among male British physicians, in which participants agreed to take either 500 mg. of aspirin daily or to avoid aspirin and aspirin-containing products (Peto *et al.*, 1988). As one consequence of this design feature, the trial became an "open label" study, in which each participant knew full well whether he had been assigned to take aspirin or not. Such knowledge can influence self-reporting of outcomes, as discussed below.

Placebo

In drug trials, a *placebo* is a preparation that resembles the experimental drug to the senses but that omits the active ingredient and thus is believed to have no true biological effect (Vickers and de Craen, 2000). Placebos have long been credited with having the potential to make patients feel better by inducing expectations of benefit, although evidence in support of this claim is mixed (Hróbjartsson and Gøtzsche,

2001; Walsh *et al.*, 2002). In a randomized trial, the main function of a placebo is to help keep subjects unaware of which treatment they are receiving—i.e., to preserve *blinding*—which in turn helps prevent bias in ascertainment of outcomes or from differential attrition in the two arms. The GEM study of *Ginkgo biloba* used identical-appearing placebo tablets for just this purpose.

In trials of non-pharmacological interventions, the same function can be served by a "placebo-like" control intervention that appears similar to the experimental intervention but that lacks its presumably active component.

Example 13-4. Arthroscopic debridement and lavage has been a common orthopedic procedure to relieve knee pain due to osteoarthritis and resistant to drug therapy. The procedure involves cutting away damaged knee cartilage and rinsing out the joint space to remove fragments of debris, all done through an arthroscope to minimize the size of the surgical incision and to speed post-operative healing. Although about 650,000 such procedures were performed annually in the United States in the late 1990s, there was little firm evidence that the procedure improved outcomes. Moseley *et al.* (2002) conducted a randomized trial that compared arthroscopic surgery with sham surgery. They described what happened in the operating room and afterward for control-group subjects as follows:

> After the knee was prepped and draped, three 1-cm incisions were made in the skin. The surgeon asked for all instruments and manipulated the knee as if arthroscopy were being performed. Saline was splashed to simulate the sounds of lavage. No instrument entered the portals for arthroscopy. The patient was kept in the operating room for the amount of time required for a debridement. Patients spent the night after the procedure in the hospital and were cared for by nurses who were unaware of the treatment-group assignment.

It may seem alarming that half the participants in this trial underwent an invasive surgical procedure in which, deliberately, no action was taken to treat their underlying disease. However, it should be kept in mind that all the study subjects knew in advance that there was a 50% chance that they would receive arthroscopic surgery and an equal chance that they would receive sham surgery, and they willingly gave their informed consent to participate. The study protocol was also approved by an institutional review board. In the end, knee pain and functional outcomes up to two years later differed very little between patients in the two arms. In retrospect, then, subjects in the sham surgery arm did not necessarily receive inferior treatment, and they contributed to important new knowledge about the (in)effectiveness of a costly and invasive treatment for their condition.

Other novel examples of non-drug "placebos" include sham foot orthotics in a treatment trial for plantar fasciitis (Landorf *et al.*, 2006), sham hemodialysis in a trial of treatment for schizophrenia (Carpenter *et al.*, 1983), placebo steam in a trial of moist air for relief of upper respiratory infections (Macknin *et al.*, 1990), and sham electroconvulsive therapy in trials of treatment for depression (Johnstone *et al.*, 1980).

Delayed Intervention

In some instances, the only feasible comparison option may be to assign participants at random to receive the experimental intervention either right away or at a later time. Outcomes in both groups are monitored concurrently during the period when the early-intervention group has received the experimental intervention but the control group has not.

Example 13-5.   Gray *et al.* (2007) investigated the extent to which circumcision could reduce a man's risk of becoming infected with HIV in a high-prevalence area. Some 4,996 Ugandan men agreed to be randomized to receive circumcision either immediately or after a 24-month delay. Over the ensuing 24 months, the incidence of HIV infection was found to be 0.66 cases per 100 person-years in the early-circumcision group, compared to 1.33 cases per 100 person-years in the control group.

A delayed-intervention control strategy can be attractive when it is not practically or politically feasible to deny the experimental intervention entirely to control participants, and/or when resources are too scarce to provide that intervention to everyone immediately. A disadvantage is that once the control group receives the intervention, a concurrent randomized comparison of intervention vs. no intervention is no longer possible, which sacrifices the ability to gauge effects on longer-term outcomes.

Active Alternative

An older, established intervention may already be accepted as beneficial in comparison to nothing at all. If a new competitor then comes along, it is likely to be both more ethical and more relevant to compare the new intervention to the older one, rather than to compare the new one with placebo or with nothing. For example, randomized trials done in the 1960s showed that treatment of high blood pressure with certain antihypertensive drugs could reduce the risk of cardiovascular complications, compared to the risk among those who received no such treatment (Veterans Administration Cooperative Study Group on Antihypertensive Agents, 1967). Nowadays, a new antihypertensive drug would need to be shown to be at least as good as older drugs of proven benefit if the new drug is to merit a role in clinical practice (ALLHAT Collaborative Research Group, 2000).

Usual Care

A new treatment can be compared to what study subjects would otherwise receive. This option can be attractive when the trial is chiefly pragmatic in orientation. However, the researcher often has little control over what happens to participants who are assigned to usual care, and what they actually receive can prove to be an important determinant of trial results.

Example 13-6.   The Multiple Risk Factor Intervention Trial (MRFIT) sought to determine whether a multi-component intervention would reduce mortality from coronary heart disease (Multiple Risk Factor Intervention Trial Research Group, 1982). Some 12,866 high-risk men aged 35–57 years were randomized to either (1) a special intervention that included hypertension control, smoking cessation, and/or dietary reduction of blood cholesterol; or (2) usual care. When a subject entered the trial, risk-factor levels were evaluated through extensive testing during three baseline visits prior to randomization and annually thereafter. For men in the special-intervention group, data from these visits were used to tailor the intervention to their individual needs. For men in the usual-care group, reports from the baseline visits were sent to the participant's regular physician without specific recommendations about what should be done.

During follow-up averaging seven years, coronary heart disease mortality was slightly but not significantly lower in the special-intervention group than in the usual-care group (–7%, 95% confidence interval: –25% to +15%), while mortality from all causes was actually slightly higher in the special-intervention group. Blood-pressure levels, cholesterol, and smoking prevalence had all declined in special-intervention group men, but declines were also observed in the usual-care group. Coronary heart disease mortality in both groups proved to be much lower than had been expected when planning the trial. Possible explanations suggested for the trial's unexpected negative result included (1) the special intervention did not work; or (2) risk-factor changes in the usual-care group led to the trial's being unable to detect a modest relative benefit of the special intervention. A later report after ten years of follow-up found more convincing evidence of mortality reduction in special-intervention men (Multiple Risk Factor Intervention Trial Research Group, 1990).

ENROLLMENT OF STUDY SUBJECTS
Eligibility Criteria

The CONSORT guidelines mandate reporting the specific eligibility criteria for trial participants, and the settings and locations where the data were collected. Several factors come into play in setting eligibility criteria (Van Spall *et al.*, 2007):

Internal Validity

A trial's ability to reach a correct conclusion for subjects who actually take part is termed its *internal validity*. Examples of eligibility criteria motivated by a desire to protect internal validity include the following:

- *Subject retention.* People who expect to move away or who have an illness that may cut short their participation are often excluded.
- *Data quality.* People who do not share the native language of study personnel are often excluded because of the difficulty and expense of translating data instruments satisfactorily into other languages and concern about increases in measurement error.
- *Compliance.* In trials that seek to determine efficacy, potential subjects may be excluded if they would be unable or unwilling to comply with the intervention to which they are assigned. One strategy for enhancing compliance is to screen potential subjects during a *run-in* phase (Lang, 1990;

Pablos-Mendez *et al.*, 1998). Before being accepted and randomized, screenees are asked to do on a test basis what they would be expected to do during the main trial, such as taking a drug and/or providing certain data. Only those who show that they are willing and able to do so are accepted into the main phase of the trial. For example, in a trial of β-carotene and retinol for cancer prevention, only potential participants who took at least half of a supply of assigned placebo capsules during a three-month run-in phase were accepted into the trial (Thornquist *et al.*, 1993).

External Validity

Generalizability of a trial's findings to non-participants is termed its *external validity*. A pragmatic trial can be most useful if it includes a broadly representative sample of persons for whom the practical decision addressed by the trial would arise. The kinds of exclusions listed above, which seek to protect the trial's internal validity, may involve sacrificing generalizability.

The right balance between these competing goals depends in part on how much is already known about the experimental intervention. If there is uncertainty about whether it works even under highly favorable conditions, then establishing its efficacy may need to take priority—without it, there is little reason to consider wide dissemination. But if previous studies have shown that the intervention can work, at least in certain settings, the emphasis may properly shift to evaluating whether and how well it works in a broader target population (Rothwell, 2005; Weiss *et al.*, 2008; Koepsell *et al.*, 2011).

Risks and Benefits to Subjects

Finally, the experimental intervention, or the control condition, may pose unusual risks to certain kinds of people. A vaccine that is prepared in eggs could be dangerous to someone with a known allergy to eggs, so he or she would probably be excluded from a trial evaluating the vaccine. An experimental treatment may be known to be highly toxic or risky, but the disease itself may be almost uniformly fatal. Eligibility for a trial of such a treatment may thus be open only to persons for whom other therapeutic options have been exhausted.

Any exclusion rule that stems from special risks or benefits posed by *one* of the trial arms must nonetheless apply to *all* potential subjects. Bias could be introduced if such an exclusion were applied selectively after the outcome of randomization became known, because doing so would upset the similarity of the groups formed by random assignment, thus potentially losing the key benefit of randomization.

Number of Subjects

The CONSORT guidelines also mandate that a trial report specify how the trial's sample-size requirements were determined. The statistical methodology for estimating sample size for cohort studies, as described in Appendix 5B of Chapter 5, also applies to two-arm parallel-groups trials and is not repeated here. *Exposed* is replaced with *experimental arm* and *unexposed* with *control arm*. Chapter 5 also provides guidance on choosing input values for sample-size formulas and references to biostatistical sources for specialized designs.

When estimating a trial's sample-size requirements, specifying the size of the intervention effect—for example, the difference in incidence of outcome events between trial arms—often poses a challenge. Uncertainty about the size of this effect is, after all, the motivation for the trial in the first place, and it may seem circular to have to assume a value in order to plan the trial itself. This paradox can be resolved by thinking of the value specified for the intervention effect not as a prediction about what *will* happen, but as a judgment about the smallest effect that the trial needs to be able to detect. Ideally, that threshold value would be motivated by theory in an explanatory trial (How big an effect would it take to confirm or refute the theory?), or by practical considerations in a pragmatic trial (How big a difference in outcomes would justify opting for one strategy over the other, given the other factors affecting that decision?).

Perhaps because of the difficulty in making such judgments, investigators are sometimes tempted to specify the target intervention effect based on what was observed in a pilot study. That strategy can be hazardous, not only because it ignores the theoretical issue just discussed, but also because the small size of most pilot studies usually implies that the resulting estimate of intervention effect is quite imprecise. The pilot-study result may thus be far from the truth in either direction just by chance. A large effect that happens to be found in a small pilot study may spur enthusiasm for the intervention but could cause the main trial to be badly underpowered. A spuriously small effect size in a pilot study may cause a perfectly good intervention to be abandoned prematurely. Instead, a pilot study is best regarded as a small-scale evaluation of the feasibility of various aspects of study methodology, not as a preliminary test of the main hypothesis itself (Kraemer *et al.*, 2006; Gore, 1981b; Wittes and Brittain, 1990).

In some instances, the available number of subjects is limited by external factors, so that sample size is not under the investigator's sole control. To help determine whether a trial is worth doing under those circumstances, the formulas that are used to estimate sample size can often be rearranged to solve for β, the maximum tolerable probability of a Type II error under a specified alternative hypothesis. A decision on whether to proceed would be based on whether study power ($= 1 - \beta$) is judged to be high enough. One can also solve for the smallest detectable difference in outcome frequency, given specified values of the sample size, α, β, and possibly other design parameters.

In practice, setting a target sample size can be far easier than achieving it. Recruitment into trials is a frequent problem (Lovato *et al.*, 1997; Taylor *et al.*, 1984), particularly for minorities, older adults, and certain other subpopulations (Ford *et al.*, 2008; Swanson and Ward, 1995). Campbell *et al.* (2007) have evaluated and summarized evidence behind various ways to enhance enrollment into trials, and Lai *et al.* (2006) did so for minorities. A pilot study can be valuable for identifying recruitment problems that may arise and for verifying that the target number of subjects is realistic.

An important determinant of sample-size requirements is the expected frequency of the outcome events of main interest: other things being equal, rarer outcomes require larger sample sizes. This statistical fact is one reason why randomized trials are considered relatively inefficient for the detection of rare but serious adverse events. One proposed way to help overcome this limitation is to design and conduct *large, simple trials*—typically two-arm trials with uncomplicated eligibility criteria and bare-bones data collection requirements that focus on essential outcomes (Yusuf *et al.*, 1984). By minimizing the cost per participant, more subjects can be enrolled for a given overall trial cost. Moreover, recruiting a large number of subjects can be facilitated by keeping eligibility criteria simple. As one example, the Rotavirus Efficacy and Safety Trial (Vesikari *et al.*, 2006) studied 68,038 healthy infants in 11 countries to test whether a new vaccine against rotavirus increased the risk of intussusception, an important adverse outcome that had been associated with earlier anti-rotavirus vaccines and whose estimated incidence was about 50 cases per 100,000 infant-years (Heyse *et al.*, 2008). Within one year after receiving either the new vaccine or a placebo, 12 vaccine recipients and 15 placebo recipients developed intussusception (RR = 0.8, 95% CI: 0.3 – 1.8). The trial's large size yielded sufficiently narrow confidence limits around the final relative-risk estimate to provide reassurance that the new vaccine led to little or no increase in risk of intussusception.

Informed Consent

Randomized trials funded by any United States government agency must meet ethical standards concerning involvement of human subjects (U.S. Department of Health and Human Services, 1991). Many research organizations apply these policies regardless of their funding source. With rare exceptions, participants must give their informed consent to serve as research subjects. Required elements of informed consent involve informing potential subjects about:

- The fact that they would be participating in research
- Procedures involved
- The nature of risks and discomfort they might face
- Potential benefits to those who take part and to other people as a result of subjects' trial participation
- Alternative treatments or procedures that might be to subjects' advantage
- The extent to which information gathered would remain confidential
- Compensation available in the event of injury, if more than minimal risk is involved
- Whom subjects may contact with questions about the research
- The fact that participation is voluntary and that subjects may withdraw without penalty or loss of benefits to which they might otherwise be entitled.

Ethical aspects of the conduct of randomized trials are discussed more fully by Sugarman (2002), Kahn *et al.* (1998), and Kodish *et al.* (1990).

RANDOMIZATION

Random assignment of participants to treatment groups is the defining feature of a randomized trial. In this context, *random* does not mean simply "haphazard" or "with no apparent pattern"; rather, it means resulting from a formal chance mechanism by which each subject has a known probability of being assigned to a given treatment group, such that the outcome of that assignment is not predictable in advance.

Because randomization is so important, the CONSORT guidelines mandate reporting on three aspects of randomization, each of which is discussed further below:

- *Sequence generation*: The specific method that was used to generate the random-allocation sequence, including the type of randomization employed and details of any restrictions, such as blocking and block size.
- *Allocation concealment*: How the random-allocation sequence was kept concealed prior to subjects' assignments to treatment groups.
- *Implementation*: Who generated the random allocation sequence, who enrolled participants, and who assigned participants to treatments.

Generating the Sequence of Random Assignments

Several types of randomization can be used to generate a sequence of treatment-group assignments (Schulz and Grimes, 2002b). The choice among them involves two goals that can compete with each another:

- *Balance.* To prevent confounding, randomization should ideally form intervention groups that are similar on both measured and unmeasured characteristics that may influence outcomes. In a particular instance, the risk and extent of imbalance can depend on the specific type of randomization employed, as well as sample size.
- *Unpredictability.* To prevent bias due to self-selection or selective referral, neither potential subjects themselves nor others who refer potential subjects into a trial should be able to anticipate the intervention arm to which a subject would be assigned if he/she joined the trial. Maintaining unpredictability

depends in part on keeping the random-allocation sequence adequately concealed, as discussed later. But it also depends on the extent to which someone who looks closely at past treatment-group assignments could use that information to predict the next assignment.

The main types of randomization are described below. For simplicity, we assume here that the design calls for forming two treatment groups of approximately equal size; with minor changes, all of the methods can also be applied when the goal is a ratio of group sizes other than 1:1. Appendix 13A provides more technical details about how each can be implemented by computer and examples.

Simple Randomization

Simple (or unrestricted) randomization is tantamount to flipping a coin. Every subject has an equal chance of being assigned to either group, and all assignments are independent of one another. Simple randomization thus maximizes unpredictability: the sequence of past assignments provides no clue about the group to which the next patient is likely to be assigned.

The main disadvantage of simple randomization is the possibility of chance imbalances, particularly with small sample sizes. To illustrate: if 10 subjects with a certain characteristic are randomized between two groups, the probability that seven or more of them will end up in one group while the remaining three or fewer end up in the other group is about 0.34. With 30 subjects randomized, the probability of a split as lopsided as 70%:30% or worse is about 0.04; with 100 subjects randomized, it is about 0.00008; and with 1,000 subjects randomized, it is about 2×10^{-35}. In short, simple randomization balances the size and composition of the intervention groups better and better as the number of units randomized increases.

Restricted randomization refers to the use of another procedure along with random assignment in order to promote balance in the sizes or composition of study groups.

Block Randomization

Block randomization, the most common form of restricted randomization, involves first grouping study subjects into sets, or *blocks*. Within each block, an equal number of subjects is then randomly assigned to each treatment group.

The block size is usually a small integer multiple of the number of treatment groups. For example, if there are two treatment groups, block sizes of 2, 4, or another even number could be used. Often the basis for grouping subjects into blocks is their order of entry into the trial: for block size = 2, the first two subjects entering the trial belong to the first block, the next two subjects to the second block, etc. Doing so assures that the sizes of the treatment groups will be exactly equal at the end of each block during subject enrollment, even if recruitment ends early.

Block randomization gives priority to keeping the sizes of treatment groups balanced. However, it does so at the expense of unpredictability. For example, suppose that the recent sequence of treatment-group assignments (E = Experimental, C = Control) has been: E C E C C E E C C. It is not hard to detect a pattern: within each consecutive pair of subjects, there is one E and one C. The last subject was assigned to C, so the next will probably go to E in order to complete the pair. A care provider who really prefers that his patient, Mr. Jones, receive the experimental treatment may delay referral of Mr. Jones into the trial until it looks likely that he would be assigned to E. Even if the provider lacks complete information about recent assignments or does not detect the pattern, simply waiting to refer Mr. Jones until the previous trial participant went to C has a 3/4 chance of steering Mr. Jones toward receiving the experimental treatment. Needless to say, any such subversion of randomization in forming the treatment groups can create skewed trial results. Unfortunately, experience suggests that subversion of randomization does occur (Schulz, 1995), and it can be very difficult to "repair" a trial that is tainted by it.

One way to help prevent corruption of block randomization is to use larger block sizes. With a block size of four, as many as four participants in a row could be assigned to the same treatment group (the first two at the end of one block, the second two at the start of the next block), making it more difficult to detect a pattern and to subvert true random allocation. Block size can also be varied randomly to interject even greater unpredictability.

A special case of block randomization can be used to create two equal-sized treatment groups when the exact number of study subjects is known in advance. For example, if k subjects will be studied in a two-arm trial, exactly $k/2$ of them can be assigned to each of the two treatment groups. Having equal-sized treatment groups maximizes the statistical power of a trial, although there is generally only slight loss of power with modest departures from equal group sizes (Hewitt and Torgerson, 2006; Hedden *et al.*, 2006).

Stratified Randomization

Sometimes trial designers deem it important to *guarantee* that a strong potential confounding factor will be balanced between treatment groups. Stratified randomization can serve this purpose (Kernan *et al.*, 1999). Each level on the confounding factor becomes a stratum, and randomization is carried out separately within each stratum. Block randomization (or some other form of restricted randomization) must be used within each stratum to assure that the ratio of experimental to control subjects is equal across strata.

Because there may be many potential confounders, it can be tempting to try to "micromanage" randomization by stratifying simultaneously on several possible confounders. Unfortunately, this strategy soon becomes self-defeating. Within each stratum, block randomization assures equal allocation of subjects to treatment arms only at the completion of a block. If there are numerous small strata, many of them can contain uncompleted blocks when recruitment ends, and the desired balance may not be achieved, especially if larger block sizes are used to preserve unpredictability. Hence if stratified randomization is used, the number of strata is best kept small (Kernan *et al.*, 1999). As consolation, *post-hoc* stratification can always be used in the analysis to correct for imbalances, even if stratified randomization was not used to assign treatments.

Adaptive Allocation and Related Methods

A variety of other allocation methods have been described, mostly seeking to improve on the balancing property of randomization, including minimization (Scott *et al.*, 2002), biased-coin allocation (Efron, 1971), and urn randomization (Wei and Lachin, 1988). These methods are called *adaptive* because the probability of the next subject's assignment to a given study group is allowed to vary depending on the outcome of previous assignments. The strongest case for their use can be made for small trials, when the risk of imbalance with simple randomization is greatest, and for sequential trials (described below) that may end early with modest sample sizes (Hedden *et al.*, 2006). However, standard statistical tests that rely on an assumption of simple randomization may no longer apply, requiring that special analysis methods be used for proper statistical inference.

Remarks on Sequence Generation

While there are no universally accepted rules for which randomization method is best under which circumstances, some general guidance can be offered, based largely on Schulz and Grimes (2002b). For trials with about 100 or more subjects per group and no interim analyses planned, simple randomization can be expected to produce good balance, and it maximizes unpredictability. If total sample size is known in advance, single-block randomization equalizes group sizes, thus maximizing power. Otherwise, block randomization with many small blocks based on order of entry can keep group sizes balanced throughout recruitment, which facilitates interim analyses and possible early termination. Randomly varying block sizes promotes unpredictability. Stratified randomization is needed most in trials with fewer than about 50 subjects per treatment group when perhaps one or two strong prognostic factors are known *a priori*. Within strata, block randomization (possibly single-block, if stratum sample sizes are known in advance) is needed to keep treatment group sizes balanced. Adaptive allocation can be worth considering in special situations when there are good reasons to doubt the adequacy of conventional randomization methods and if resources are available to apply the non-standard analysis methods that may be required.

Regardless of the method chosen, randomization is not technically difficult or costly to carry out. In order to reap its major theoretical benefits, and in view of the CONSORT guidelines that call for detail in reporting, careful efforts should be made to randomize properly. Appendix 13A describes straightforward algorithms that use computer-generated random numbers produced by standard statistical software and that can be implemented so as to leave an audit trail.

Once the study design and type of randomization have been decided upon, the sequence of random assignments can almost always be generated at the beginning of the trial, before any subjects are enrolled. Doing so allows the sequence to be checked for technical correctness when there is still time to fix any programming errors gracefully. Early preparation of the allocation list can also simplify the process of assigning subjects to treatment groups when enrollment gets underway. Once a subject has been found eligible and has given consent, authorized study staff need only look up the subject's assignment on a list that has already been prepared.

Allocation Concealment

While there are good reasons to generate the allocation list for a trial early, access to the list must be carefully controlled in order to preserve unpredictability and prevent selection bias. Inadequate allocation concealment has been found in several studies to be associated with differences in trial results (Odgaard-Jensen et al., 2011), suggesting that bias is not just a theoretical possibility.

Fortunately, this kind of bias is almost always preventable. Probably the most effective method of allocation concealment is centralized randomization. When a potential new trial participant has been identified, the central study office is contacted by telephone or other means. A trained staff member whose primary responsibility is to protect study integrity receives the call, verifies the subject's eligibility, registers his/her identifying information, finds the subject's treatment assignment on a master allocation list that is kept secure at study headquarters, and then provides appropriate instructions to the caller about action to be taken for the newly enrolled subject. Alternatively, for placebo-controlled drug trials, trained pharmacy staff can register the subject and dispense sequentially numbered containers that have been pre-filled with the appropriately randomized experimental drug or placebo. Other systems include using sequentially numbered, sealed, opaque envelopes that contain treatment-group assignments and that can be opened in the field only after a new subject has been duly enrolled. However, it is difficult to make such a system completely tamper-proof without oversight by an independent third party responsible to the trial (Hewitt et al., 2005; Schulz and Grimes, 2002a).

Implementation

The CONSORT guidelines also call for reporting how key procedures related to randomization were actually carried out: in particular, who was responsible for which tasks. CONSORT recommends complete separation between (a) the persons who generate the random assignment sequence and who keep it concealed; and (b) those who enroll participants and carry out trial procedures once a subject has been assigned to a treatment group (Moher et al.,

2010). The aim is to maintain an information "firewall" that prevents premature disclosure of treatment assignments.

DATA COLLECTION
Baseline Characteristics

Information on study subjects at entry into a trial serves several purposes:

- *Verify eligibility*. Some data must be gathered to confirm that a subject qualifies for entry according to the trial's eligibility criteria.
- *Describe the study population*. Baseline data also serve to describe the study population and thus help consumers of the results to judge the scope of generalizability. Often the first table in a published trial report shows demographic and clinical characteristics of the groups formed by randomization, as called for by the CONSORT guidelines (Schulz et al., 2010; Altman and Dore, 1990; Assmann et al., 2000).
- *Assess potential confounding*. While randomization works well on average to create balanced treatment groups, "accidents of randomization" do occur. The initial table describing the study population in a trial report usually also permits a check on the degree to which randomization balanced the groups. Characteristics that are known determinants of the trial's main outcomes are especially important, because imbalance between treatment arms would make these factors confounders. Information on such factors may also be needed for use in stratified or blocked randomization.
- *Identify planned subgroups*. Some trials have *a priori* hypotheses about variation in the size of treatment effects across different subgroups (effect modification). Hence baseline information is needed to place study subjects in the relevant subgroup for later analysis. For example, in the Multiple Risk Factor Intervention Trial, the investigators hypothesized in advance that men with a normal baseline electrocardiogram would benefit most from intervention (Multiple Risk Factor Intervention Trial Research Group, 1982).
- *Enhance study power*. If a study outcome is also a characteristic that can be measured at baseline—e.g., blood pressure, body weight,

or bone density—then a trial's statistical power can often be enhanced by using each subject's baseline value in the analysis of later outcomes. To the extent that baseline and follow-up values are correlated within subjects, including the baseline value in the analysis can remove a source of between-subject variation that would otherwise be treated as part of random variation in outcomes (Fleiss, 1986, Chapter 7).

Outcomes

A trial's outcome measures usually follow naturally from its objectives. But like cohort studies, randomized trials lend themselves to studying multiple outcomes of a given exposure or intervention, and these outcomes can be distinguished from one another in several ways.

Primary and Secondary Outcomes

The CONSORT guidelines mandate that a trial's *primary* and *secondary* outcomes be clearly specified in trial reports. Primary outcomes are those deemed most important to users of trial results and are those used in sample-size or power calculations. Whether the trial has chiefly explanatory or pragmatic aims can affect the choice of measures: outcomes that matter for testing theory may matter less for guiding practice, and vice versa (Table 13.1). But it is often easy to add secondary outcome measures to the data collection plan without complicating the basic study design. The GEM study, for example, provided a convenient setting in which to examine the effects of *Ginkgo biloba* on endpoints other than dementia, including serious bleeding episodes, coronary heart disease, and stroke (DeKosky *et al.*, 2008).

Intermediate Outcomes

Investigators often have in mind a causal model under which an intervention should produce certain effects in a certain order. For example, in a trial of sodium fluoride to prevent bone fractures in postmenopausal women with osteoporosis, sodium fluoride was expected to increase cancellous bone formation and thus to increase bone density, leading to reduced incidence of fractures (Riggs *et al.*, 1990). Both bone density and fracture incidence were measured as outcomes. Bone density would be termed an *intermediate* outcome, while fracture occurrence would be a later *clinically important* outcome. Often,

as here, an intermediate outcome is a biomarker measuring some physiological variable or physical sign that the experimental treatment is expected to affect early but that may be imperceptible to participants. A later, clinically important outcome reflects a subject's symptoms, functioning, or survival (Lassere, 2008; Bucher *et al.*, 1999).

One function of an intermediate outcome is to permit testing assumptions about an intervention's mechanism of action. In the randomized trial described earlier (Example 13-1) of smoking cessation counseling to prevent low birth weight in infants of smoking mothers, two outcomes were measured: (1) whether pregnant smokers stopped smoking, and (2) infant birth weight. More than twice as many pregnant smokers in the intervention group as in the control group quit smoking (43% vs. 20%), and babies born to intervention-group mothers averaged 92 grams heavier. Together, these findings suggested that the intervention did indeed work as intended. But had there been no difference in mean birth weight between groups, one might wonder whether: (1) the intervention had been ineffective in getting pregnant mothers to stop smoking, or (2) the causal link between smoking in pregnancy and low infant birth weight was not as strong as had been supposed. Knowing whether maternal smoking behavior differed between groups would have provided a useful clue about where the hypothesized causal chain was broken.

The situation is different, however, if *only* an intermediate outcome is measured while the clinically important outcome is not. In that context, the intermediate outcome is often termed a *surrogate* outcome: it is used as a substitute for the clinically important outcome. An association between the surrogate outcome and the later clinically important endpoint may be considered to be already well established, so measurement of the surrogate outcome alone is proposed as sufficient for evaluating efficacy of an intervention. A major attraction of this approach is that the trial can almost certainly be completed earlier and may require many fewer subjects than if the clinically important outcome were the primary target. However, the following example illustrates a pitfall of this strategy:

Example 13-7. The Cardiac Arrhythmia Suppression Trial (CAST) (Echt *et al.*, 1991) was motivated by two observations: (1) myocardial infarction survivors whose electrocardiogram showed frequent premature ventricular contractions (PVCs) had an increased risk of sudden cardiac death, and (2) anti-arrhythmic drugs could reduce the frequency of PVCs in these patients. In early testing, two drugs—encainide and flecainide—were found to be particularly effective in suppressing PVCs (Cardiac Arrhythmia Pilot Study Investigators, 1988). The main CAST trial was then mounted to assess the ability of these drugs to save lives. After 10 months, the results shown in Table 13.2 were obtained, and the trial was stopped. Unexpectedly, both arrhythmic and non-arrhythmic cardiac deaths were *more* common among patients who received encainide or flecainide than among those who received placebo. Although the precise mechanisms for the observed excess deaths were unclear, these drugs evidently had important cardiac side effects beyond their ability to suppress PVCs. Encainide was subsequently taken off the market, and the clinical indications for flecainide were curtailed. Note that using PVC suppression alone as an intermediate endpoint to measure effectiveness would have been dangerously misleading.

The sodium fluoride trial to prevent bone fractures, described earlier, is a second example. Bone density was indeed 10–35% higher in sodium fluoride recipients than in placebo recipients, depending on anatomical location, but the incidence of non-vertebral fractures proved to be about three times *greater* in the sodium fluoride group. Although treatment with sodium fluoride made skeletal bones denser, it evidently also made them more fragile (Riggs et al., 1990).

These and other studies using intermediate outcomes (Lassere, 2008; Grimes and Schulz, 2005; Bucher et al., 1999; Psaty et al., 1999; Avorn, 2013)

TABLE 13.2. MORTALITY EXPERIENCE IN THE CARDIAC ARRHYTHMIA SUPPRESSION TRIAL

	Encainide or flecainide	Placebo
Patients randomized	755	743
Number of deaths due to:		
Arrhythmia	43	16
Other cardiac cause	17	5
Non-cardiac cause	3	5
All causes	63	26

(Based on data from Echt et al. [1991])

have taught sobering lessons about the potential danger of relying on surrogate outcomes as evidence of clinical effectiveness. The key problem is that an intervention can affect clinical outcomes through mechanisms other than those involving the intermediate outcome. These other mechanisms may not be known in advance but can turn out to be very important, even predominant.

Prentice (1989) set forth the following principle: a valid surrogate outcome is "a response variable for which a test of the null hypothesis of no relationship to the treatment groups under comparison is also a valid test of the corresponding null hypothesis based on the true endpoint." That is, the intermediate outcome measure must *fully* capture the effects of treatment on the clinical endpoint. Unfortunately, is difficult to verify that this requirement is met without having data on both the intermediate and the clinically important endpoints—a situation that, ironically, eliminates the need to rely exclusively on the intermediate outcome. Lassere (2008) and Weir and Walley (2006) review statistical approaches aimed at this problem.

Composite Endpoints

Some trials define their primary outcome as a *composite* endpoint: a subject is counted as having had an outcome event if he/she experiences any one of several possible clinical occurrences, some of which may be fatal and others nonfatal (Freemantle et al., 2003).

Example 13-8. The Trial to Assess Chelation Therapy (TACT) aimed to determine whether sodium EDTA infusions, a controversial treatment used mainly by alternative and complementary medicine practitioners, would improve outcomes after myocardial infarction (Lamas et al., 2013). A total of 1,708 participants from 134 clinical sites were randomized to either 40 EDTA infusions or 40 placebo infusions administered over several months. The primary endpoint was any occurrence of: death from any cause, reinfarction, stroke, undergoing coronary revascularization, or hospitalization for cardiac chest pain. The incidence of this composite outcome proved to be 18% lower (95% CI: 1%–31%) in EDTA recipients than in placebo recipients—a difference that barely crossed the threshold for statistical significance. Analyses that focused on individual components of the composite outcome showed roughly similar proportionate reductions in each of the individual components, but none were statistically significant at $p < 0.05$.

A major motivation for using a composite endpoint is to reduce the trial's sample-size requirements: incidence of the composite endpoint will be greater than the incidence of any of its components, leading to lower sample-size requirements to detect a certain proportionate reduction in incidence. Using a single composite outcome can also help circumvent a multiple-testing problem that might otherwise occur if statistical tests are conducted on each of several outcome types. A limitation of composite endpoints, however, is that they implicitly treat their different components as equally important—a view that may not be shared by consumers of trial results. In addition, reporting a single treatment effect may be taken to imply a similar effect on all components of the composite (Freemantle *et al.*, 2003). The trial results themselves may even suggest different effects on different components, but with insufficient precision to confirm or refute this inference conclusively. The TACT trial was criticized on those grounds (Nissen, 2013).

Blinding

Blinding (or *masking*, especially in trials of eye diseases) refers to keeping persons involved in a trial unaware of which study subjects are in which treatment arm during the trial. (Allocation concealment, discussed earlier, involves hiding information about the treatment group to which a subject will be assigned until after the assignment is made; blinding involves continuing to keep that information hidden throughout the trial.) The main reasons for this deliberate withholding of information are to prevent bias in ascertainment of outcomes and to minimize differential attrition of subjects.

A trial is *double-blind* if both the study subjects and the research staff members responsible for measuring outcomes are kept unaware of treatment-group assignments. A trial is *single-blind* if only one of these parties (usually study subjects) is kept unaware. However, blinding can also be extended to people who play other roles. In clinical trials, a patient's caregiver may not be the person who measures outcomes, but the caregiver's actions can nonetheless influence outcomes and be influenced by knowing which intervention the patient is receiving. The study protocol may therefore keep caregivers blinded while providing an escape mechanism to break the blinding if knowing to which arm of

the study the patient has been assigned becomes critical for care delivery. Even the statistician(s) responsible for day-to-day data analysis may be kept blinded to the identity of the intervention being received by each of the study groups, because it may be hard for a statistician who is in regular contact with other members of a research team to remain completely neutral as to the expected outcome. Most large trials create an independent Data Safety and Monitoring Board, whose members have exclusive access to information about which group is which. These people are charged with deciding whether any differences in outcomes across study groups justify breaking the blinding and halting the trial.

Blinding is not always possible. In community trials, for example, the intervention may involve a mass-media campaign to influence health behavior (Bauman and Koepsell, 2006), which is clearly at odds with keeping people unaware of which treatment arm they are in. Even when blinding is attempted, it may be only partly successful because it is difficult to design a perfect placebo. Certain characteristic side effects, for example, may be hard to mimic.

The success of blinding can often be evaluated at trial's end simply by asking people to guess which treatment they received (Colagiuri, 2010). In the GEM study, for example, 61% of all participants who completed an exit interview believed they had been taking placebo, and 39% believed they had been taking *Ginkgo biloba*, but those percentages were nearly identical in both treatment groups. However, attempts at blinding can also fall well short of their goal (Fergusson *et al.*, 2004; Byington *et al.*, 1985; Howard *et al.*, 1982). Sometimes differential attrition from the trial can also provide indirect evidence that suggests unblinding of at least some participants. For example, in the TACT trial of chelation therapy after myocardial infarction (Example 13-8), a larger proportion of patients in the placebo group dropped out during the trial, suggesting that some of them may have detected that they had been randomized to ineffective therapy (Lamas *et al.*, 2013; Nissen, 2013). Nonetheless, even if some trial participants correctly judge the nature of the intervention arm to which they have been assigned, removing part of the potential bias is arguably better than removing none at all.

ANALYSIS

Initial analyses describe the study sample and compare the treatment groups, especially with regard to known determinants of study outcomes, as a check on randomization. Occasional statistically significant differences can occur by chance, but an unexpectedly large number of them may raise suspicion about whether sequence generation or allocation concealment went awry.

Intent-to-Treat Principle

An important potential pitfall in the analysis and interpretation of randomized trials is illustrated by a now-famous example:

Example 13-9.   The Coronary Drug Project was a multicenter, randomized, double-blind, placebo-controlled trial, one aim of which was to test whether treatment with the lipid-altering agent clofibrate could reduce mortality from coronary heart disease (Coronary Drug Project Research Group, 1980). Compliance with the intended drug regimen was checked by pill counts at study visits. Among trial participants assigned to the clofibrate arm who actually took 80% or more of the clofibrate dispensed, five-year cumulative mortality was 15.0%, compared to 24.6% among patients who were less compliant ($p = 0.00011$). It is tempting to infer that clofibrate worked well among those who took it, but that it could not benefit patients who failed to take it. However, among patients in the control arm who were 80%+ compliant *with placebo*, five-year cumulative mortality was 15.1%, compared with 28.3% among those who were less compliant *with placebo* ($p < 5 \times 10^{-16}$). Multivariable adjustment for 40 baseline characteristics had little effect on these findings. Five-year cumulative mortality among all patients *randomized* to clofibrate was 20.0%, compared to 20.9% among those randomized to placebo ($p = 0.55$), suggesting that use of clofibrate itself had little effect.

Under the intent-to-treat principle, the primary analysis in a randomized trial should compare outcomes *between the groups formed by randomization*. In other words, each participant is categorized according to what intervention he or she was intended to receive. Recall that the main reason for using the randomized-trial design in the first place is to form groups that can be assumed to be similar, even with regard to unmeasured factors that may affect outcomes. If the composition of one or more of those groups is altered, this balancing property of randomization is lost. A study that began as a randomized trial would, in effect, be converted into a non-randomized study in which confounding may be present.

Several circumstances can tempt investigators to depart from the intent-to-treat principle:

- *Non-compliance* with the intended treatment can occur, as in the Coronary Drug Project.
- *Crossing over* can occur if persons who were originally randomized to one treatment end up receiving the other. For example, in a comparison of watchful waiting versus early surgical repair for men with a minimally symptomatic inguinal hernia, 23% of those randomized to watchful waiting ended up receiving surgical repair, while 17% of those randomized to early surgical repair ended up opting for watchful waiting (Fitzgibbons *et al.*, 2006).
- *Selective exclusions* can occur if participants are deliberately dropped from analysis after randomization. For example, in the Joint Study of Extracranial Arterial Occlusion (Sackett and Gent, 1979), the risk of recurrent transient ischemic attack, stroke, or death was reportedly reduced by 27% ($p = 0.02$) in patients who had surgery to bypass an arterial occlusion when the analysis was based on those "available for follow-up." However, this analysis excluded 15 patients who had been randomized to surgery but who died early or had perioperative strokes, while only one patient who had been randomized to medical treatment was excluded after randomization. In an intent-to-treat analysis, patients who were assigned to undergo surgery had only a 16% reduction in risk ($p = 0.09$).

Late exclusions can often be reduced by delaying randomization until as late as possible, so that some persons who are destined to drop out early do so before randomization.

The price paid for keeping the benefits of randomization in an intent-to-treat analysis is typically a diluted treatment effect. (Exclusions after randomization can shift the results in either direction depending on the reasons for exclusion.) In an *effectiveness* trial, this dilution may be an accurate reflection of what to expect under real-world conditions and thus may be consistent with trial goals. In an *efficacy* trial, a diluted treatment effect is unwanted, but at least the direction of bias is generally predictable, toward finding no difference. Any treatment effect found in an intent-to-treat analysis is thus likely to be a conservative estimate of efficacy.

Estimating Efficacy Indirectly

In some trials, efficacy of an intervention can be estimated from study data even in the face of non-compliance with the intended treatment, under certain assumptions. One method was described in Chapter 12, which involved using the randomized treatment-group assignment as an instrumental variable. Another method, based on counterfactuals, is illustrated in the following example:

Example 13-10. A randomized trial was conducted in Indonesia to determine whether vitamin A supplementation would reduce mortality among preschool children (Sommer and Zeger, 1991; Sommer et al., 1986). Of 450 study villages, 229 were randomly selected to have their age-eligible children receive two doses of oral vitamin A. Children in the control villages received no supplements. However, for various reasons, including logistical problems and parental non-compliance, about 20% of children in the vitamin-A villages did not receive vitamin A supplements as intended. During follow-up, child deaths were distributed as follows:

TABLE 13.3.

	n	No. of deaths	Cumulative mortality[a]
Intervention	12,094	46	3.8
Received vitamin A	9,675	12	1.2
Did not receive vitamin A	2,419	34	14.1
Control	11,588	74	6.4

[a] Deaths per 1,000 children

The effect of the overall intervention program can be estimated from an intent-to-treat analysis. The risk difference was $3.8 - 6.4 = -2.6$ deaths per 1,000 children, or a $(6.4 - 3.8)/6.4 \times 100\% = 41\%$ reduction in cumulative mortality.

However, the investigators also wanted to estimate the efficacy of vitamin A supplements *in children who actually received them*. A naïve estimate of $1.2 - 14.1 = -12.9$ deaths per 1,000 (a 91% reduction) would be confounded by whatever factors influenced receipt or non-receipt of vitamin A in

the study group, and these factors would be difficult to identify and control.

A better estimate that avoids this problem can come from envisioning the results if the treatment assignments had been reversed. Had the control group been assigned to receive vitamin A, some children in that group would have received the supplements and some would not. The two treatment groups and their subgroups can thus be organized and labelled as follows:

TABLE 13.4.

	n	No. of deaths	Cumulative mortality[a]
Intervention	12,094	46	3.8
A: Received vitamin A	9,675	12	1.2
B: Did not receive vitamin A	2,419	34	14.1
Control	11,588	74	6.4
C: Would have received vitamin A			
D: Would not have received vitamin A			

[a] Deaths per 1,000 children

Because randomization produces two exchangeable groups, whatever factors influence a child's receipt of vitamin A should be equally common in the control group and the intervention group. Therefore, given that $2,419/12,094 = 20\%$ of the intervention group did not receive vitamin A, we would expect that 20% of the control group would not have received vitamin A either, if it had been their assigned treatment. Subgroup D should thus contain about $11,588 \times 20\% \approx 2,318$ children. Moreover, it is reasonable to expect that the cumulative mortality in subgroup D should be the same as the cumulative mortality actually observed in subgroup B. This is because they are equivalent subgroups, and neither received vitamin A supplements (albeit for different reasons). Thus, there should be about $2,318 \times 14.1/1,000 \approx 33$ deaths among children in subgroup D. Now, given that the size and number of deaths in subgroup D have been estimated, the size and number of deaths in subgroup C can be obtained by subtraction from the entire control group, yielding:

TABLE 13.5.

	n	No. of deaths	Cumulative mortality[a]
Intervention	12,094	46	3.8
A: Received vitamin A	9,675	12	1.2
B: Did not receive vitamin A	2,419	34	14.1
Control	11,588	74	6.4
C: Would have received vitamin A	9,270	41	4.4
D: Would not have received vitamin A	2,318	33	14.1

[a] Deaths per 1,000 children

The effect of receiving vitamin A supplements can now be estimated as $1.2 - 4.4 = -3.2$ per 1,000 children, or about a 73% reduction in cumulative mortality. This result can be interpreted as the estimated efficacy of vitamin A supplements among children who received them, or who would have received them if assigned to do so.

Subgroup Analyses

The primary aim of most trials is to determine whether one strategy is better overall than another. Still, it is usually reasonable to assume that different subjects may respond differently to an intervention and that it may therefore be more effective in some subjects than in others. Often particular subgroups are identified in advance in whom an intervention effect is expected to be larger or smaller than in other subgroups. For example, in the study of β-carotene for prevention of lung cancer, the investigators hypothesized that participants who had a low serum β-carotene level at baseline would benefit more from active treatment than those who had a high baseline β-carotene level (Omenn et al., 1996). Even when there are few or no such a priori subgroup hypotheses, investigators often conduct exploratory analyses to search for larger or smaller intervention effects in multiple subgroups defined according to a variety of factors. The temptation to do so is especially great when trial results suggest little or no overall effect, which may represent a disappointing failure of what was thought to be a promising intervention. A "positive" effect in a subgroup can be viewed as rescuing an otherwise "negative" study. Pocock et al. (2002) found that in a sample of 50 trial reports in several major medical journals, 70% presented results of subgroup analyses.

Subgroup analyses are subject to several important pitfalls, however (Rothwell, 2005; Barraclough and Govindan, 2010; Oxman and Guyatt, 1992; Head et al., 2013; Yusuf et al., 1991):

1. *Increased risk of Type II errors.* The target number of subjects for most trials is driven by a main hypothesis that posits an *overall* treatment effect of a certain size. Because a subgroup is inevitably smaller than the full study population, statistical tests for a similar treatment effect within subgroups have less statistical power. In principle, if an a priori subgroup hypothesis is of sufficient scientific importance, trial size can be increased accordingly during the planning phase, but this is unusual.

2. *Increased risk of Type I errors.* Because a study population can be divided up in many ways, subgroup analyses can quickly present a multiple-comparisons problem (Schulz and Grimes, 2005). The more ways one looks for subgroup differences, the more likely it is that some "statistically significant" ones will be found, even if they reflect only the play of chance. This possibility is especially likely in a *post-hoc* exploratory search for an intervention effect in each of many subgroups.

To illustrate this point, investigators on a trial of early aspirin versus placebo in patients with suspected myocardial infarction found that, overall, early aspirin reduced 5-week mortality by about 23% (95% CI: 15%, 31%) (ISIS-2 Collaborative Group, 1988). However, after a search for subgroup differences, they found that whether early aspirin was beneficial or not appeared to depend on the presence or absence of a certain marker. Among subjects with this marker, mortality in the aspirin group was actually 9% *higher* than in the placebo group (95% CI: –15%, 37%), while among those without the marker, mortality in the aspirin group was 28% *lower* (95% CI: 18%, 38%). So what was this magic marker? Having an astrological sign of Gemini or Libra!

One way to help combat the multiple-comparisons problem is to apply interaction tests. For a factor C with two or more categories, one first conducts a single omnibus test of whether adding *all* (treatment group) $\times (C)$ interaction terms at once significantly improves the fit of a statistical model predicting outcomes, compared to a model that includes only treatment group and C (without their interactions) as predictors. Only if this omnibus interaction test is statistically significant does one proceed to examine treatment effects within the individual subgroups defined by different categories of C (Pocock et al., 2002). Methods also exist to "correct" subgroup-specific p-values for the number of different statistical tests done, but their use remains controversial (Savitz and Olshan, 1995; Bender and Lange, 2001). Methodologists generally advise limiting the severity of the multiple-comparisons problem by specifying only a few well-justified, planned subgroup comparisons in advance, and by interpreting *post-hoc* subgroup comparisons with great caution (Schulz and Grimes, 2005; Brookes *et al.*, 2004; Yusuf *et al.*, 1991).

3. *Formation of subgroups on characteristics that may be influenced by treatment assignment.* Bias can arise if subgroups are formed according to characteristics influenced by events after randomization. Whether a trial participant ends up in a certain subgroup may then depend on the treatment group to which he or she was assigned. In the Coronary Drug Project example, one might be tempted to try to circumvent the "dilution" of treatment effects that would occur in an intent-to-treat analysis by comparing outcomes only among patients who were compliant with their assigned treatment. But compliance was determined only after randomization and may well have depended on the particular treatment received. A patient who was compliant with placebo might not have complied with clofibrate, and vice versa. Hence this analysis cannot be considered a true randomized comparison.

Issues surrounding the interpretation of associations whose presence or size varies among subgroups of the study population are not confined to randomized trials and will be further discussed in Chapter 18.

DESIGN VARIATIONS

So far, we have mainly considered randomized trials in which individual study subjects are randomized to one of two arms and are then followed concurrently to assess and compare outcomes. But while random assignment to exposure groups is the defining characteristic of a randomized trial, a number of other design features can be used in conjunction with randomization to address different kinds of scientific questions. A few are discussed below. These features are not necessarily mutually exclusive and can be used in combination.

Noninferiority Trials

Most trials seek to determine whether one intervention strategy is superior to another. But suppose that one of two treatments has already been well studied, is deemed effective, and has become an accepted standard. The other treatment, of unknown effectiveness, is a new alternative that offers some other advantage(s) over the standard treatment: for example, it may be less costly, have fewer side effects, be more widely available, or be easier to use. If the new treatment is nearly as effective as the standard treatment, the new one would probably be preferred on the basis of its other advantages. The main goal of a trial comparing the two treatments is then to test whether the new treatment is no less effective than the standard: in other words, whether the new treatment is *noninferior*.

More formally, it is assumed that users would actually prefer the new treatment even if it were slightly less effective than the standard, in view of its other advantages. The difference-in-effectiveness value at which users would be indifferent between the new and old treatment is termed the *noninferiority threshold*, Δ. A value for Δ must be specified in order to plan a noninferiority trial. Δ can be specified in terms of the true difference in cumulative incidence of the primary outcome between treatments, or on a ratio scale (e.g., relative risk or hazard ratio). Considerations in setting a value for Δ are discussed by Mulla *et al.* (2012) and Fleming *et al.* (2011).

Once the trial has been completed, it produces an *observed* risk difference D for the primary outcome, and confidence limits for D that specify an interval within which the true difference probably lies. The trial's results are then interpreted according to where the confidence interval for D falls in relation to Δ.

Example 13-11. In an influenza pandemic, health care workers would be likely to be at high risk for infection. If no specific vaccine were available, other protective measures might be needed, such as face masks. Type N95 respirators are designed to filter out 95% of airborne particulate matter, but they are bulkier, costlier, and less widely available than standard surgical masks. Surgical masks offer some protection against airborne respiratory droplets, but they do not filter out smaller particles, and they allow more leakage around the mask edges.

Loeb *et al.* (2009) conducted a randomized noninferiority trial of surgical masks vs. fit-tested N95 respirators among 426 nurses at eight Ontario hospitals during the 2008–2009 influenza season. The investigators decided in advance on clinical grounds that surgical masks would be judged noninferior if the upper 95% confidence limit for the difference in cumulative incidence of laboratory-confirmed influenza infection (surgical mask minus respirator) was below 9 per 100.

At trial's end, the cumulative incidence of influenza infection in the surgical mask group was

TABLE 13.6. DIFFERENCES IN THE MEANING OF CONCEPTS INVOLVED IN STATISTICAL HYPOTHESIS TESTING BETWEEN SUPERIORITY AND NONINFERIORITY TRIALS

Notation:

Symbol	Denotes		
R_s	True cumulative incidence of adverse outcome with standard treatment		
R_n	True cumulative incidence of adverse outcome with new treatment		
Δ	Smallest clinically important difference in cumulative incidence, expressed as a positive quantity		
		Superiority trial	Noninferiority trial
Null hypothesis		$R_s - R_n = 0$	$R_n - R_s \geq \Delta$
Alternative hypothesis		$\lvert R_s - R_n \rvert \geq \Delta$ [a]	$R_n - R_s < \Delta$
Type I error		Conclude that one treatment is superior when in fact they are equally effective	Conclude that new treatment is noninferior when in fact it is inferior
Type II error		Conclude that treatments are equally effective when in fact one of them is superior	Conclude that new treatment is inferior when in fact it is not

[a] 2-sided

23.6 per 100, compared to 22.9 in the N95 respirator group, for a risk difference of +0.7 (95% CI: −7.3, +8.8) per 100. The upper 95% confidence limit for the risk difference was less than the pre-specified threshold of 9 per 100, so surgical masks were judged to be noninferior to N95 respirators for this purpose.

Although a value for Δ is needed to plan a noninferiority trial, the results are arguably best reported in terms of an estimate of effect (e.g., the risk difference D) and confidence limits for that estimate, rather than simply as a binary verdict about noninferiority. Doing so allows users to interpret the results in relation to their own noninferiority threshold, which may differ from that of the trial planners (Mulla et al., 2012).

Noninferiority trials differ from superiority trials in other ways as well. Concepts in the standard statistical-hypothesis testing framework have different meanings for noninferiority trials then for superiority trials, as summarized in Table 13.6. These differences call for different methods to estimate the required sample size (Julious and Owen, 2011). Also, non-compliance or crossovers, which usually attenuate treatment-group differences in an intent-to-treat analysis, will tend to bias results toward finding the new treatment to be noninferior. Accordingly, proposed extensions to the CONSORT guidelines for noninferiority trials recommend that results of both intent-to-treat and as-treated analyses be presented (Piaggio et al., 2006).

Equivalence trials are related to noninferiority trials but seek to test the hypothesis that the risk difference (or other effect measure) falls between $-\Delta$ and $+\Delta$: in other words, that neither treatment is superior to the other by more than a prespecified Δ (Christensen, 2007).

Sequential Trials

For both ethical and economic reasons, it can be desirable to end a trial early if the accumulated evidence shows that one treatment strategy is clearly superior. The CAST study was stopped early when it became clear that encainide and flecainide had unexpectedly increased cardiovascular mortality. Alternatively, the accumulated evidence may make it very unlikely that continuing the trial could reveal any meaningful difference in outcomes between treatment arms. Trials that involve continuous or periodic comparisons of outcomes as the study proceeds are termed *sequential* trials.

Example 13-12. Atherosclerotic narrowing of a major intracranial artery is a known strong risk factor for stroke. Angioplasty with stent placement became widely used in an attempt to remove stenosis and maintain blood flow, despite limited evidence on effectiveness of this procedure compared to medical therapy. Chimowitz *et al.* (2011) conducted a randomized trial of aggressive drug therapy, with or without angioplasty and stenting, in patients who had 70–99% occlusion of a major intracranial artery. As subject recruitment continued over a period of several years, the trial's Data Safety and Monitoring Board reviewed interim results every six months. The initial target sample size had been 764 patients, but after 451 patients were randomized, enrollment was stopped because the 30-day cumulative incidence of stroke or death was 14.7% in the stented group vs. 5.8% in the non-stented group ($p = 0.002$). Medication therapy alone remained superior in continued follow-up to one year after randomization.

The design and analysis of sequential trials must account for multiple "looks" at the results, which pose another kind of multiple-comparisons problem. Without special measures, repeated statistical testing would inflate the overall probability of a Type I error beyond the desired level. Fortunately, biostatistical methods are available to deal with this problem (Whitehead, 1999; Todd, 2007). It is possible technically to reanalyze the data each time a new outcome event has occurred. But in practice it is usually more feasible to plan a few interim analyses at regular intervals for review by a data monitoring committee (Ellenberg *et al.*, 2002; Slutsky and Lavery, 2004).

Factorial Trials

A *factorial* randomized trial involves one treatment group for every possible combination of two or more interventions.

Example 13-13. Adenomas of the colon are benign growths that can evolve over time into malignancy. When adenomas are detected by colonoscopy or X-ray, they are normally removed, but persons who have had an initial adenoma are at high risk for later recurrence. Results from observational studies suggested that people who take aspirin may be less likely to develop adenomas, and likewise for people with relatively high dietary intake of folate.

To determine whether aspirin use and/or folate supplements could prevent recurrent adenomas, Logan *et al.* (2008) conducted a trial in which consenting patients who had just had an adenoma removed were randomized to one of four possible combinations of aspirin (300 mg. daily) and/or folate (0.5 mg. daily):

TABLE 13.7.

Group	Drug(s) assigned
A	Aspirin + folate
B	Aspirin only
C	Folate only
D	Neither

To permit blinding, two kinds of placebos were used, one resembling aspirin and the other resembling folate. Depending on his/her treatment group assignment, each participant was thus instructed to take two pills daily: (1) either aspirin or an aspirin-like placebo, and (2) either folate or a folate-like placebo.

Over the subsequent three years, recurrent adenomas were detected as shown in Table 13.8. Based on these results, several comparisons of interest are possible:

The first three comparisons suggest that aspirin with folate, and aspirin alone, may have modestly reduced the risk of recurrent adenoma, while folate alone may have slightly increased the risk. However, confidence limits around all three *RR* estimates are fairly wide and include 1.00, so the results based on these comparisons are inconclusive.

The next two comparisons suggest that aspirin, when added to folate, may have reduced the risk by about 24%. Folate, when added to aspirin, had virtually no effect. But again, the confidence limits for both *RR* estimates are wide enough to include 1.00, so again these results are inconclusive.

These first five comparisons all involved pairwise contrasts between just two of the four groups, so each comparison used data on only half of all trial participants. The last two comparisons use data on *all* trial participants and take advantage of the fact that the factorial design prevents confounding of one drug's effect by that of the other drug. Among aspirin users (groups A + B), half took folate (group A) while the rest did not (group B). Likewise, among aspirin *non*-users (groups C + D), half took folate (group C), while the rest did not (group D). (The exact percentages of folate users differ slightly from 50% because the percentage of participants who underwent follow-up colonoscopy varied slightly among

TABLE 13.8.

Group	Active drug(s) assigned	No. of patients examined	No. with recurrent adenoma	Cumulative incidence
A	Aspirin + folate	217	50	23.0%
B	Aspirin only	217	49	22.6%
C	Folate only	215	65	30.2%
D	Neither	204	56	27.5%

TABLE 13.9.

Comparison	Groups compared	RR	(95% CI)
(Aspirin + folate) vs. nothing	A vs. D	0.84	(0.60–1.17)
Aspirin alone vs. nothing	B vs. D	0.82	(0.59–1.15)
Folate alone vs. nothing	C vs. D	1.10	(0.81–1.49)
(Aspirin + folate) vs. folate alone	A vs. C	0.76	(0.56–1.05)
(Aspirin + folate) vs. aspirin alone	A vs. B	1.02	(0.72–1.44)
Aspirin vs. no aspirin	(A + B) vs. (C + D)	0.79	(0.63–0.99)
Folate vs. no folate	(A + C) vs. (B + D)	1.07	(0.85–1.34)

the treatment groups.) Thus, the comparison of aspirin users vs. aspirin non-users cannot be confounded by folate use. By similar logic, the comparison of folate users vs. folate non-users cannot be confounded by aspirin use.

These last two comparisons estimate the overall effects of aspirin and of folate. The confidence limits for the RR comparing aspirin vs. no aspirin exclude 1.00, reflecting the added precision gained from being able to use data on the full study population. These comparisons presuppose negligible effect modification: that is, aspirin and folate are assumed to be neither synergistic nor antagonistic. Statistically, this assumption can be checked with a significance test for an aspirin × folate interaction effect. Here, that interaction test yields a p-value of 0.745, which is compatible with no true interaction and justifies estimating a single overall effect for each drug.

The factorial trial design offers two main advantages (McAlister et al., 2003; Green, 2002; Stampfer et al., 1985):

- If the effect of each intervention is independent of the other(s)—i.e., there is no synergy or antagonism—then the entire study population can be used to estimate and test the main effect of each intervention. This proved to be the case in the adenoma study, which was thus able to evaluate two interventions for little more than the cost of evaluating one.

- If the effect of each intervention is *not* independent of the other(s), the factorial design can detect and quantify the synergy or antagonism between them. This would not be possible if a separate study were done for each intervention, or if a three-arm trial (intervention #1 vs. intervention #2 vs. nothing) were conducted instead. The added information thus gained may be helpful in choosing a particularly effective combination of intervention approaches, or in raising cautions that one intervention's effectiveness may be compromised among persons exposed to another.

The factorial design strategy can be extended to simultaneous study of three or more interventions. Cook et al. (2007) describe a 2 × 2 × 2 factorial trial of three chemopreventive agents against cardiovascular disease in women, and Day et al. (2002)

evaluated three intervention approaches to prevention of falls in older adults using a $2 \times 2 \times 2$ factorial design.

Randomizing Within an Individual

In all of the trials considered so far, individual people were randomized to different treatments. But entities smaller in scale than a person can be randomized as well. Being able to make comparisons within the same people offers two main advantages. First, patient-level characteristics that may influence outcomes, such as overall disease severity and symptom perceptions, apply in common to both intervention and control conditions. Hence the potential for confounding by these characteristics is largely eliminated. Second, statistical power is usually enhanced because the variability in responses *within* the same individual tends to be smaller than the variability in responses *between* different individuals (Gore, 1981a). Accordingly, when these designs can be used, they often require fewer participants than a parallel-groups design in which each person receives only one treatment (Louis *et al.*, 1984).

Randomizing Body Parts

When a treatment is expected to affect only a localized part of the body, other similar parts of the same person's body can receive a different treatment and thus provide a matched control. One such trial sought to determine whether laser photocoagulation treatments could slow the progression of retinal complications of diabetes (Blankenship, 1979). For each eligible diabetic patient, one eye was chosen at random to be treated with laser photocoagulation, while the other eye served as a matched control.

Crossover Trials

In a crossover trial, each subject receives each of the alternative treatments at a different time. The *order* of exposure is randomized (Mills *et al.*, 2009).

Example 13-14. A crossover trial was conducted to test whether taking the drug candesartan, an angiotensin II receptor blocker, could prevent migraine attacks in people prone to such headaches (Tronvik *et al.*, 2003). Sixty patients who typically had two to six migraine attacks per month were randomized into two groups. One group took candesartan for 12 weeks, followed by a four-week "washout" period with no treatment, then took placebo for 12 more weeks. The other group took placebo for 12 weeks, then had a four-week "washout" period,

then took candesartan for 12 weeks. The mean number of days with headache proved to be 18.5 during placebo periods vs. 13.6 during candesartan periods ($p < 0.001$), implying that the drug was effective for migraine prevention.

A crossover design is most suitable when the expected effects of treatment occur promptly after treatment is begun and taper off within a reasonable time period after it is stopped.

N-of-1 Trials

The so-called *n-of-1* trial design extends the concept behind crossover trials even further, conducting a randomized trial on only a single individual (Guyatt *et al.*, 1986, 1988; Gabler *et al.*, 2011).

Example 13-15. The stimulant drug methylphenidate has been tried as empirical treatment for geriatric patients with severe depression or apathy. But uncertainty persists about the drug's effectiveness, and patients have been observed to respond differently to it. Jansen *et al.* (2001) conducted five separate *n-of-1* trials on five different older adults with depression or apathy. Each trial involved five one-week periods. Each period involved giving either methylphenidate or placebo on Monday and Tuesday, giving no drug on Wednesday, and then giving the opposite drug on Thursday and Friday. Randomization applied to each one-week period determined whether methylphenidate was given first or second during that period. A geriatrician who was blinded to each patient's treatment status evaluated outcomes using standardized measures of depression, apathy, and possible drug side effects. Upon trial completion, three patients were judged to be significantly improved when taking methylphenidate; one was significantly worse when taking methylphenidate; and one patient was unable to complete the trial due to loss of speech, which made it impossible to assess key outcomes.

N-of-1 trials thus use randomization to guide choice of the best treatment approach for an individual patient. As with crossover studies, *n-of-1* trials are most suitable when the therapy under investigation produces its effects promptly and when those effects wane fairly soon after the treatment is stopped.

Randomizing Groups of Individuals

The design variations just discussed involved randomizing something within an individual. Another

TABLE 13.10. SELECTED RESULTS OF A GROUP-RANDOMIZED TRIAL OF INFLUENZA VACCINATION IN CANADIAN HUTTERITE COLONIES

Group	Influenza cases	Person-days	Incidence rate[a]	Vaccine effectiveness[b] Est.	(95% CI)
Vaccine recipients				55%	(−21%, 84%)
Influenza vaccine arm	41	70,377	5.8		
Control arm	79	58,954	13.4		
Vaccine non-recipients				61%	(8%, 83%)
Influenza vaccine arm	39	182,866	2.1		
Control arm	80	151,902	5.3		
Everyone				59%	(5%, 82%)
Influenza vaccine arm	80	253,243	3.2		
Control arm	159	210,856	7.5		

[a] Influenza cases per 10,000 person-days
[b] From proportional-hazards regression, accounting for clustering within colonies
(Based on data from Loeb *et al.* [2010])

variation involves randomizing aggregates of individuals. As discussed in Chapter 16, a group-randomized trial can also be considered as a type of ecological study.

Example 13-16. The overall public health impact of vaccination against many infectious diseases is believed to depend in part on *herd immunity*: people who have not been vaccinated themselves may benefit nonetheless by being surrounded by other vaccinated people who cannot serve as a source of infection. One strategy for prioritizing influenza vaccination has been to target schoolchildren and adolescents. Young people spend much of their time in schools where the virus can spread easily, and they can then infect adults at home and elsewhere. To test this vaccination strategy, 49 Hutterite colonies in three Canadian provinces agreed to be randomized to have their children receive either influenza vaccine or hepatitis A vaccine, which served as a control (Loeb *et al.*, 2010). Each Hutterite colony was a close-knit, relatively isolated community of Anabaptist families, typically with a population of 60–120 people. All eligible children within a given colony received the same vaccine. Over a six-month follow-up period that included a flu season, the results summarized in Table 13.10 were obtained. The incidence of influenza was reduced by more than half among both influenza vaccine recipients and non-recipients living in the same communities, demonstrating herd immunity in action.

A *group-randomized* design is worth considering when:

- By its nature, the experimental intervention applies non-selectively to an entire group. For example, fluoridation of a community's water supply or broadcasting health promotion messages via the mass media would affect nearly everyone in a community, so randomizing individuals within those communities to receive or not to receive such interventions would be difficult or impossible.
- Intervention effects are thought to be transmissible from person to person. The Hutterite colony influenza vaccination trial provided one such example, but non-biological attributes such as attitudes, norms, or behaviors can also be viewed as contagious within a social group. For example, Peterson *et al.* (2000) randomized 40 school districts either to implement a smoking-prevention intervention or to serve as controls. The intervention sought to change norms about the desirability of smoking, so that schoolchildren would reinforce each other's decisions not to smoke. The intervention mechanism itself thus depended on interactions between individuals within a school. In other contexts, transmissibility of intervention effects may instead be a potential

source of unwanted contamination of controls if individuals were randomized (Torgerson, 2001). That contamination may be largely avoidable if groups that are not in close communication with each other are randomized instead.

Study planning and data analysis for a group-randomized trial are typically more complex than when individuals are randomized (Murray, 1998; Donner and Klar, 2000; Atienza and King, 2002; Bauman and Koepsell, 2006). Because outcome measurements on people within the same group are likely to be correlated, analyzing the data as if individuals had been randomized tends to exaggerate statistical significance (Eldridge *et al.*, 2004; Donner *et al.*, 1981; Koepsell *et al.*, 1991). Avoiding this non-conservative bias requires taking both individual-level and group-level random variation within treatment arm into account (Murray, 1998; Donner and Klar, 2000; Murray *et al.*, 2008). The total number of individuals studied to achieve a certain level of statistical power must usually be greater in a group-randomized study than in an individual-randomized study of the same topic.

CONCLUSION

Most of the time, epidemiologists must rely on non-randomized study designs. These methods provide us with many ways to detect and to quantify associations, and there is broad consensus (albeit not unanimity) about how evidence from observational studies can be interpreted to support or refute causal inferences. Nonetheless, a relationship observed in a randomized trial provides perhaps the sturdiest bridge we have from association to causation. Historically, results from a randomized trial have not uncommonly contradicted a theory that had been built on multiple prior observational studies. These surprises ought to keep us vigilant and humble when we seek to interpret the results of observational studies. They also show why randomized trials deserve a special place in our set of research tools and why well-trained epidemiologists need to know when and how to use them.

APPENDIX 13A: ALGORITHMS FOR RANDOMIZATION BY COMPUTER

Four methods of randomization are described and illustrated below. For each method, the starting point is a list of subject identifiers (ID). If all subjects are known in advance, each subject's ID may be his/her position on a master list of subjects (which can be in any order). If instead a randomized assignment list is to be created before any subjects are enrolled, the starting IDs may simply be a list of consecutive integers that will refer to subjects' order of entry into the trial. Here, each method is illustrated for the first eight subjects.

All methods involve pairing each subject ID with a random number drawn from a uniform distribution between 0 and 1. All widely used statistical packages and some spreadsheet programs provide a function to generate such random numbers. Below, the variable containing these random values is labelled *RN*.

For illustration, assume that the design involves two groups, Experimental and Control, of approximately equal size. With minor changes, these allocation methods could be used to create two groups of different sizes, or to allocate subjects among three or more groups.

Simple Randomization

A suitable way to carry out simple randomization is: if $RN > 0.5$, assign the subject to Experimental; otherwise, assign the subject to Control. For example:

TABLE 13.11.

ID	RN	Assignment
1	0.81422	Experimental
2	0.90634	Experimental
3	0.32979	Control
4	0.05449	Control
5	0.32959	Control
6	0.06776	Control
7	0.72420	Experimental
8	0.29415	Control

Block Randomization

For block size = 2, a suitable way to carry out block randomization is: whichever subject within a given block has the larger value of *RN* is assigned to Experimental, and the other block member is assigned to Control. For example:

TABLE 13.12.

ID	Block	RN	Assignment
1	1	0.81422	Control
2	1	0.90634	Experimental
3	2	0.32979	Experimental
4	2	0.05449	Control
5	3	0.32959	Experimental
6	3	0.06776	Control
7	4	0.72420	Experimental
8	4	0.29415	Control

TABLE 13.14.

Stratum	ID (within stratum)	Block (within stratum)	RN	Assignment
Males				
	1	1	0.81422	Control
	2	1	0.90634	Experimental
	3	2	0.32979	Experimental
	4	2	0.05449	Control
Females				
	1	1	0.32959	Experimental
	2	1	0.06776	Control
	3	2	0.72420	Experimental
	4	2	0.29415	Control

For larger block sizes of size k, say, this rule can be generalized to assign the $k/2$ subjects within each block who have the largest values of RN to Experimental, and assign the remaining block members to Control.

Single-Block Randomization

If it is known that there will be k subjects in all, the above block-randomization method can be applied to all k subjects treated as a single block. The $k/2$ subjects who have the largest values of RN are assigned to Experimental and the remaining subjects to Control. For example, if $k = 8$:

TABLE 13.13.

ID	RN	Assignment
1	0.81422	Experimental
2	0.90634	Experimental
3	0.32979	Experimental
4	0.05449	Control
5	0.32959	Control
6	0.06776	Control
7	0.72420	Experimental
8	0.29415	Control

Stratified Randomization

Randomization is carried out separately within each stratum, using block randomization (or some other form of restricted randomization) to achieve equal or nearly equal Experimental and Control group sizes within the stratum. For example, if gender is the stratification factor and block size = 2:

NOTE

1. Technically, they are *pseudo*-random numbers. Computers are deterministic machines and cannot generate truly random numbers. Instead, they apply well-studied numerical algorithms to carry out calculations that produce a stream of digits that behave as though they were random (Knuth, 1997). If the underlying algorithm is known, every digit in the sequence can be predicted with certainty; but otherwise, the sequence appears to be random and can pass various tests for randomness.

REFERENCES

ALLHAT Collaborative Research Group. Major cardiovascular events in hypertensive patients randomized to doxazosin vs chlorthalidone: the antihypertensive and lipid-lowering treatment to prevent heart attack trial (ALLHAT). JAMA 2000; 283:1967–1975.

Altman DG, Dore CJ. Randomisation and baseline comparisons in clinical trials. Lancet 1990; 335:149–153.

Anderson GL, Limacher M, Assaf AR, Bassford T, Beresford SAA, Black H, *et al.* Effects of conjugated equine estrogen in postmenopausal women with hysterectomy: the Women's Health Initiative randomized controlled trial. JAMA 2004; 291:1701–1712.

Assmann SF, Pocock SJ, Enos LE, Kasten LE. Subgroup analysis and other (mis)uses of baseline data in clinical trials. Lancet 2000; 355:1064–1069.

Atienza AA, King AC. Community-based health intervention trials: an overview of methodological issues. Epidemiol Rev 2002; 24:72–79.

Avorn J. Approval of a tuberculosis drug based on a paradoxical surrogate measure. JAMA 2013; 309:1349–1350.

Barraclough H, Govindan R. Biostatistics primer: what a clinician ought to know: subgroup analyses. J Thorac Oncol 2010; 5:741–746.

Bauman A, Koepsell TD. Epidemiologic issues in community interventions. Chapter 6 in Brownson RC, Petitti DB (eds.), Applied epidemiology (2nd ed.). New York: Oxford University Press, 2006.

Begg C, Cho M, Eastwood S, Horton R, Moher D, Olkin I, et al. Improving the quality of reporting of randomized controlled trials. The CONSORT statement. JAMA 1996; 276:637–639.

Bender R, Lange S. Adjusting for multiple testing—when and how? J Clin Epidemiol 2001; 54:343–349.

Bendsen NT, Hother AL, Jensen SK, Lorenzen JK, Astrup A. Effect of dairy calcium on fecal fat excretion: a randomized crossover trial. Int J Obes (Lond) 2008; 32:1816–1824.

Blankenship GW. Diabetic macular edema and argon laser photocoagulation: a prospective randomized study. Ophthalmology 1979; 86:69–78.

Brookes ST, Whitely E, Egger M, Smith GD, Mulheran PA, Peters TJ. Subgroup analyses in randomized trials: risks of subgroup-specific analyses; power and sample size for the interaction test. J Clin Epidemiol 2004; 57:229–236.

Bucher HC, Guyatt GH, Cook DJ, Holbrook A, McAlister FA. Users' guides to the medical literature: XIX. Applying clinical trial results. A. How to use an article measuring the effect of an intervention on surrogate end points. Evidence-Based Medicine Working Group. JAMA 1999; 282:771–778.

Byington RP, Curb JD, Mattson ME. Assessment of double-blindness at the conclusion of the β-Blocker Heart Attack Trial. JAMA 1985; 253:1733–1736.

Campbell MK, Snowdon C, Francis D, Elbourne D, McDonald AM, Knight R, et al. Recruitment to randomised trials: Strategies for Trial Enrollment and Participation Study. The STEPS study. Health Technol Assess 2007; 11:iii, ix–105.

Cardiac Arrhythmia Pilot Study Investigators. Effects of encainide, flecainide, imipramine and moricizine on ventricular arrhythmias during the year after acute myocardial infarction: the Cardiac Arrhythmia Pilot Study (CAPS). Am J Cardiol 1988; 61:501–509.

Carpenter WT, Sadler JH, Light PD, Hanlon TE, Kurland AA, Penna MW, et al. The therapeutic efficacy of hemodialysis in schizophrenia. N Engl J Med 1983; 308:669–675.

Chalmers I. Comparing like with like: some historical milestones in the evolution of methods to create unbiased comparison groups in therapeutic experiments. Int J Epidemiol 2001; 30:1156–1164.

Chimowitz MI, Lynn MJ, Derdeyn CP, Turan TN, Fiorella D, Lane BF, et al. Stenting versus aggressive medical therapy for intracranial arterial stenosis. N Engl J Med 2011; 365:993–1003.

Christensen E. Methodology of superiority vs. equivalence trials and non-inferiority trials. J Hepatol 2007; 46:947–954.

Cobb LA, Thomas GI, Dillard DH, Merendino KA, Bruce RA. An evaluation of internal-mammary-artery ligation by a double-blind technic. N Engl J Med 1959; 260:1115–1118.

Cochrane AL. Effectiveness and efficiency: random reflections on health services. London: Nuffield Provincial Hospitals Trust, 1972.

Colagiuri B. Participant expectancies in double-blind randomized placebo-controlled trials: potential limitations to trial validity. Clin Trials 2010; 7:246–255.

CONSORT, 2013. Extensions of the CONSORT statement. http://www.consort-statement.org/extensions/.

Cook NR, Albert CM, Gaziano JM, Zaharris E, MacFadyen J, Danielson E, et al. A randomized factorial trial of vitamins C and E and beta carotene in the secondary prevention of cardiovascular events in women: results from the Women's Antioxidant Cardiovascular Study. Arch Intern Med 2007; 167:1610–1618.

Coronary Drug Project Research Group. Influence of adherence to treatment and response of cholesterol on mortality in the Coronary Drug Project. N Engl J Med 1980; 303:1038–1041.

Dawson L. The Salk Polio Vaccine Trial of 1954: risks, randomization and public involvement in research. Clin Trials 2004; 1:122–130.

Day L, Fildes B, Gordon I, Fitzharris M, Flamer H, Lord S. Randomised factorial trial of falls prevention among older people living in their own homes. BMJ 2002; 325:128–133.

DeAngelis CD, Drazen JM, Frizelle FA, Haug C, Hoey J, Horton R, et al. Clinical trial registration: a statement from the International Committee of Medical Journal Editors. JAMA 2004; 292:1363–1364.

DeKosky ST, Williamson JD, Fitzpatrick AL, Kronmal RA, Ives DG, Saxton JA, et al. Ginkgo biloba for prevention of dementia: a randomized controlled trial. JAMA 2008; 300:2253–2262.

DeVita VT Jr, Chu E. A history of cancer chemotherapy. Cancer Res 2008; 68:8643–8653.

Donner A, Birkett N, Buck C. Randomisation by cluster: sample size requirements and analysis. Am J Epidemiol 1981; 114:906–914.

Donner A, Klar N. Design and analysis of cluster randomisation trials in health research. New York: Edward Arnold, 2000.

Echt DS, Liebson PR, Mitchell LB, Peters RW, Obias-Manno D, Barker AH, et al. Mortality and morbidity in patients receiving encainide, flecainide, or placebo. The Cardiac Arrhythmia Suppression Trial. N Engl J Med 1991; 324:781–788.

Efron B. Forcing a sequential experiment to be balanced. Biometrika 1971; 58:403–417.

Eldridge SM, Ashby D, Feder GS, Rudnicka AR, Ukoumunne OC. Lessons for cluster randomized trials in the twenty-first century:a systematic review of trials in primary care. Clin Trials 2004; 1:80–90.

Ellenberg SS, Fleming TR, DeMets DL. Data monitoring committees in clinical trials: a practical perspective. Hoboken, NJ: Wiley and Sons, 2002.

Fergusson D, Glass KC, Waring D, Shapiro S. Turning a blind eye: the success of blinding reported in a random sample of randomised, placebo controlled trials. BMJ 2004; 328:432.

Fisher RA. The design of experiments. London: Oliver and Boyd, 1935.

Fitzgibbons RJ Jr, Giobbie-Hurder A, Gibbs JO, Dunlop DD, Reda DJ, McCarthy M Jr, et al. Watchful waiting vs repair of inguinal hernia in minimally symptomatic men: a randomized clinical trial. JAMA 2006; 295:285–292.

Fleiss JL. The design and analysis of clinical experiments. New York: Wiley and Sons, 1986.

Fleming TR, Odem-Davis K, Rothmann MD, Li Shen Y. Some essential considerations in the design and conduct of non-inferiority trials. Clin Trials 2011; 8:432–439.

Ford JG, Howerton MW, Lai GY, Gary TL, Bolen S, Gibbons MC, et al. Barriers to recruiting underrepresented populations to cancer clinical trials: a systematic review. Cancer 2008; 112:228–242.

Freemantle N, Calvert M, Wood J, Eastaugh J, Griffin C. Composite outcomes in randomized trials: greater precision but with greater uncertainty? JAMA 2003; 289:2554–2559.

Friedrich MJ. The Cochrane Collaboration turns 20: assessing the evidence to inform clinical care. JAMA 2013; 309:1881–1882.

Gabler NB, Duan N, Vohra S, Kravitz RL. N-of-1 trials in the medical literature: a systematic review. Med Care 2011; 49:761–768.

Giuliano AE, Hunt KK, Ballman KV, Beitsch PD, Whitworth PW, Blumencranz PW, et al. Axillary dissection vs no axillary dissection in women with invasive breast cancer and sentinel node metastasis: a randomized clinical trial. JAMA 2011; 305:569–575.

Gore SM. Assessing clinical trials—design I. Br Med J 1981a; 282:1780–1781.

Gore SM. Assessing clinical trials—first steps. Br Med J 1981b; 282:1605–1607.

Gray RH, Kigozi G, Serwadda D, Makumbi F, Watya S, Nalugoda F, et al. Male circumcision for HIV prevention in men in Rakai, Uganda: a randomised trial. Lancet 2007; 369: 657–666.

Green S. Design of randomized trials. Epidemiol Rev 2002; 24:4–11.

Grimes DA, Schulz KF. Surrogate end points in clinical research: hazardous to your health. Obstet Gynecol 2005; 105:1114–1118.

Guyatt G, Sackett D, Adachi J, Roberts R, Chong J, Rosenbloom D, et al. A clinician's guide for conducting randomized trials in individual patients. CMAJ 1988; 139:497–503.

Guyatt G, Sackett D, Taylor DW, Chong J, Roberts R, Pugsley S. Determining optimal therapy—randomized trials in individual patients. N Engl J Med 1986; 314:889–892.

Head SJ, Kaul S, Tijssen JGP, Serruys PW, Kappetein AP. Subgroup analyses in trial reports comparing percutaneous coronary intervention with coronary artery bypass surgery. JAMA 2013; 310:2097–2098.

Hedden SL, Woolson RF, Malcolm RJ. Randomization in substance abuse clinical trials. Subst Abuse Treat Prev Policy 2006; 1:6.

Hewitt C, Hahn S, Torgerson DJ, Watson J, Bland JM. Adequacy and reporting of allocation concealment: review of recent trials published in four general medical journals. BMJ 2005; 330: 1057–1058.

Hewitt CE, Torgerson DJ. Is restricted randomisation necessary? BMJ 2006; 332:1506–1508.

Heyse JF, Kuter BJ, Dallas MJ, Heaton P, REST Study Team. Evaluating the safety of a rotavirus vaccine: the REST of the story. Clin Trials 2008; 5: 131–139.

Hooton TM, Roberts PL, Stapleton AE. Cefpo-doxime vs ciprofloxacin for short-course treatment of acute uncomplicated cystitis: a randomized trial. JAMA 2012; 307:583–589.

Howard J, Whittemore AS, Hoover JJ, Panos M. How blind was the patient blind in AMIS? Clin Pharmacol Ther 1982; 32:543–553.

Hróbjartsson A, Gøtzsche PC. Is the placebo powerless? An analysis of clinical trials comparing placebo with no treatment. N Engl J Med 2001; 344:1594–1602.

Hulley S, Grady D, Bush T, Furberg C, Herrington D, Riggs B, et al. Randomized trial of estrogen plus progestin for secondary prevention of coronary heart disease in postmenopausal women. Heart and Estrogen/progestin Replacement Study (HERS) Research Group. JAMA 1998; 280:605–613.

ISIS-2 Collaborative Group. Randomised trial of intravenous streptokinase, oral aspirin, both, or neither among 17,187 cases of suspected acute myocardial infarction: ISIS-2. ISIS-2 (Second International Study of Infarct Survival) Collaborative Group. Lancet 1988; 2:349–360.

Jansen IHM, Olde Rikkert MGM, Hulsbos HAJ, Hoefnagels WHL. Toward individualized evidence-based medicine: five "n-of-1" trials of methylphenidate in geriatric patients. J Am Geriatr Soc 2001; 49:474–476.

Johnstone EC, Drakin JFW, Lawler P, Frith CD, Stevens M, McPherson K, et al. The Northwick Park electroconvulsive therapy trial. Lancet 1980; 2:1317–1320.

Julious SA, Owen RJ. A comparison of methods for sample size estimation for non-inferiority studies with binary outcomes. Stat Methods Med Res 2011; 20:595–612.

Junod, 2012. FDA and clinical drug trials: a short history. At http://www.fda.gov/AboutFDA/What-WeDo/History/Overviews/.

Kahn JP, Mastroianni AC, Sugarman J. Beyond consent: seeking justice in research. New York: Oxford, 1998.

Kannus P, Parkkari J, Niemi S, Paganen M, Palvanen M, Jarvinen M, et al. Prevention of hip fracture in elderly people with use of a hip protector. N Engl J Med 2000; 343:1506–1513.

Kernan WN, Viscoli CM, Makuch RW, Brass LM, Horwitz RI. Stratified randomization for clinical trials. J Clin Epidemiol 1999; 52:19–26.

Klein EJ, Shugerman RP, Leigh-Taylor K, Schneider C, Portscheller D, Koepsell T. Buffered lidocaine: analgesia for intravenous line placement in children. Pediatrics 1995; 95:709–712.

Knuth DE. The art of computer programming. Volume 2: Seminumerical algorithms (3rd ed.). Reading, MA: Addison-Wesley, 1997.

Kodish E, Lantos JD, Siegler M. Ethical considerations in randomized controlled clinical trials. Cancer 1990; 65:2400–2404.

Koepsell TD, Martin DC, Diehr PH, Psaty BM, Wagner EH, Perrin EB, et al. Data analysis and sample size issues in evaluations of community-based health promotion and disease prevention programs: a mixed-model analysis of variance approach. J Clin Epidemiol 1991; 44:701–713.

Koepsell TD, Zatzick DF, Rivara FP. Estimating the population impact of preventive interventions from randomized trials. Am J Prev Med 2011; 40:191–198.

Kraemer HC, Mintz J, Noda A, Tinklenberg J, Yesavage JA. Caution regarding the use of pilot studies to guide power calculations for study proposals. Arch Gen Psychiatry 2006; 63:484–489.

Kramer MS, Barr RG, Dagenais S, Yang H, Jones P, Ciofani L, et al. Pacifier use, early weaning, and cry/fuss behavior: a randomized controlled trial. JAMA 2001; 286:322–326.

Lai GY, Gary TL, Tilburt J, Bolen S, Baffi C, Wilson RF, et al. Effectiveness of strategies to recruit underrepresented populations into cancer clinical trials. Clin Trials 2006; 3:133–141.

Lamas GA, Goertz C, Boineau R, Mark DB, Rozema T, Nahin RL, et al. Effect of disodium EDTA chelation regimen on cardiovascular events in patients with previous myocardial infarction: the TACT randomized trial. JAMA 2013; 309:1241–1250.

Landorf KB, Keenan AM, Herbert RD. Effectiveness of foot orthoses to treat plantar fasciitis: a randomized trial. Arch Intern Med 2006; 166:1305–1310.

Lang JM. The use of a run-in to enhance compliance. Stat Med 1990; 9:87–95.

Lassere MN. The Biomarker-Surrogacy Evaluation Schema: a review of the biomarker-surrogate literature and a proposal for a criterion-based, quantitative, multidimensional hierarchical levels of evidence schema for evaluating the status of biomarkers as surrogate endpoints. Stat Methods Med Res 2008; 17:303–340.

Loeb M, Dafoe N, Mahony J, John M, Sarabia A, Glavin V, et al. Surgical mask vs N95 respirator for preventing influenza among health care workers: a randomized trial. JAMA 2009; 302:1865–1871.

Loeb M, Russell ML, Moss L, Fonseca K, Fox J, Earn DJD, et al. Effect of influenza vaccination of children on infection rates in Hutterite communities: a randomized trial. JAMA 2010; 303:943–950.

Logan RFA, Grainge MJ, Shepherd VC, Armitage NC, Muir KR, ukCAP Trial Group. Aspirin and folic acid for the prevention of recurrent colorectal adenomas. Gastroenterology 2008; 134: 29–38.

Louis TA, Lavori PW, Bailar JC 3rd, Polansky M. Crossover and self-controlled designs in clinical research. N Engl J Med 1984; 310:24–31.

Lovato LC, Hill K, Hertert S, Hunninghake DB, Probstfield JL. Recruitment for controlled clinical trials: literature summary and annotated bibliography. Control Clin Trials 1997; 18:328–352.

Macknin ML, Mathew S, Medendorp SV. Effect of inhaling heated vapor on symptoms of the common cold. JAMA 1990; 264:989–991.

McAlister FA, Straus SE, Sackett DL, Altman DG. Analysis and reporting of factorial trials: a systematic review. JAMA 2003; 289:2545–2553.

Medical Research Council. Streptomycin treatment of pulmonary tuberculosis: a Medical Research Council investigation. Br Med J 1948; II:769–782.

Mills EJ, Chan AW, Wu P, Vail A, Guyatt GH, Altman DG. Design, analysis, and presentation of crossover trials. Trials 2009; 10:27.

Moher D, Hopewell S, Schulz KF, Montori V, Gøtzsche PC, Devereaux PJ, et al. CONSORT 2010 explanation and elaboration: updated guidelines for reporting parallel group randomised trials. BMJ 2010; 340:c869.

Moher D, Schulz KF, Altman D. The CONSORT statement: revised recommendations for improving the quality of reports of parallel-group randomized trials. JAMA 2001; 285:1987–1991.

Moseley JB, O'Malley K, Petersen NJ, Menke TJ, Brody BA, Kuykendall DH, et al. A controlled trial of arthroscopic surgery for osteoarthritis of the knee. N Engl J Med 2002; 347:81–88.

Mulla SM, Scott IA, Jackevicius CA, You JJ, Guyatt GH. How to use a noninferiority trial: users' guides to the medical literature. JAMA 2012; 308:2605–2611.

Multiple Risk Factor Intervention Trial Research Group. Multiple risk factor intervention trial. Risk factor changes and mortality results. JAMA 1982; 248:1465–1477.

Multiple Risk Factor Intervention Trial Research Group. Mortality rates after 10.5 years for participants in the Multiple Risk Factor Intervention Trial. Findings related to a priori hypotheses of the trial. JAMA 1990; 263:1795–1801.

Murray DM. Design and analysis of group-randomized trials. New York: Oxford, 1998.

Murray DM, Pals SL, Blitstein JL, Alfano CM, Lehman J. Design and analysis of group-randomized

trials in cancer: a review of current practices. J Natl Cancer Inst 2008; 100:483–491.

Nissen SE. Concerns about reliability in the Trial to Assess Chelation Therapy (TACT). JAMA 2013; 309:1293–1294.

Odgaard-Jensen J, Vist GE, Timmer A, Kunz R, Akl EA, Schünemann H, et al. Randomisation to protect against selection bias in healthcare trials. Cochrane Database Syst Rev 2011; :MR000012.

Omenn GS, Goodman GE, Thornquist MD, Balmes J, Cullen MR, Glass A, et al. Effects of a combination of beta carotene and vitamin A on lung cancer and cardiovascular disease. N Engl J Med 1996; 334:1150–1155.

Oxman AD, Guyatt GH. A consumer's guide to subgroup analyses. Ann Intern Med 1992; 116: 78–84.

Pablos-Mendez A, Barr RG, Shea S. Run-in periods in randomized trials. Implications for the application of results in clinical practice. JAMA 1998; 279:222–225.

Peterson AV Jr, Kealey KA, Mann SL, Marek PM, Sarason IG. Hutchinson Smoking Prevention Project: long-term randomized trial in school-based tobacco use prevention—results on smoking. J Natl Cancer Inst 2000; 92: 1979–1991.

Peto R, Gray R, Collins R, Wheatley K, Hennekens C, Jamrozik K, et al. Randomised trial of prophylactic daily aspirin in British male doctors. Br Med J 1988; 296:313–316.

Piaggio G, Elbourne DR, Altman DG, Pocock SJ, Evans SJW, CONSORT Group. Reporting of noninferiority and equivalence randomized trials: an extension of the CONSORT statement. JAMA 2006; 295:1152–1160.

Pocock SJ, Assmann SE, Enos LE, Kasten LE. Subgroup analysis, covariate adjustment and baseline comparisons in clinical trial reporting: current practice and problems. Stat Med 2002; 21:2917–2930.

Porta M (ed.). A dictionary of epidemiology (5th edition). New York: Oxford, 2008.

Prentice RL. Surrogate endpoints in clinical trials: definition and operational criteria. Stat Med 1989; 8:431–440.

Psaty BM, Weiss NS, Furberg CD, Koepsell TD, Siscovick DS, Rosendaal FR, et al. Surrogate end points, health outcomes, and the drug-approval process for the treatment of risk factors for cardiovascular disease. JAMA 1999; 282:786–790.

Riggs BL, Hodgson SF, O'Fallon WM, Chao EY, Wahner HW, Muhs JM, et al. Effect of fluoride treatment on the fracture rate in postmenopausal women with osteoporosis. N Engl J Med 1990; 322:802–809.

Rosa L, Rosa E, Sarner L, Barrett S. A close look at therapeutic touch. JAMA 1998; 279:1005–1010.

Rothwell PM. External validity of randomised controlled trials: "To whom do the results of this trial apply?" Lancet 2005; 365:82–93.

Sackett DL, Gent M. Controversy in counting and attributing events in clinical trials. N Engl J Med 1979; 301:1410–1412.

Savitz DA, Olshan AF. Multiple comparisons and related issues in the interpretation of epidemiologic data. Am J Epidemiol 1995; 142:904–908.

Schulz KF. Subverting randomization in controlled trials. JAMA 1995; 274:1456–1458.

Schulz KF, Altman DG, Moher D, CONSORT Group. CONSORT 2010 statement: updated guidelines for reporting parallel group randomized trials. Ann Intern Med 2010; 152:726–732.

Schulz KF, Grimes DA. Allocation concealment in randomised trials: defending against deciphering. Lancet 2002a; 359:614–618.

Schulz KF, Grimes DA. Generation of allocation sequences in randomised trials: chance, not choice. Lancet 2002b; 359:515–519.

Schulz KF, Grimes DA. Multiplicity in randomised trials II: subgroup and interim analyses. Lancet 2005; 365:1657–1661.

Schwartz D, Lellouch J. Explanatory and pragmatic attitudes in therapeutical trials. J Chron Dis 1967; 20:637–648.

Scott NW, McPherson GC, Ramsay CR, Campbell MK. The method of minimization for allocation to clinical trials: a review. Control Clin Trials 2002; 23:662–674.

Sexton M, Hebel JR. A clinical trial of change in maternal smoking and its effect on birth weight. JAMA 1984; 251:911–915.

Slutsky AS, Lavery JV. Data safety and monitoring boards. N Engl J Med 2004; 350:1143–1147.

Smith GC, Pell JP. Parachute use to prevent death and major trauma related to gravitational challenge: systematic review of randomised controlled trials. BMJ 2003; 327:1459–1461.

Sommer A, Tarwotjo I, Djunaedi E, West KP Jr, Loeden AA, Tilden R, et al. Impact of vitamin A supplementation on childhood mortality. A randomised controlled community trial. Lancet 1986; 1:1169–1173.

Sommer A, Zeger SL. On estimating efficacy from clinical trials. Stat Med 1991; 10:45–52.

Stampfer MJ, Buring JE, Willett W, Rosner B, Eberlein K, Hennekens CH. The 2 × 2 factorial design: its application to a randomized trial of aspirin and carotene in U.S. physicians. Stat Med 1985; 4:111–116.

Sugarman J. Ethics in the design and conduct of clinical trials. Epidemiol Rev 2002; 24:54–58.

Swanson GM, Ward AJ. Recruiting minorities into clinical trials: toward a participant-friendly system. J Natl Cancer Inst 1995; 87:1747–1759.

Taylor KM, Margolese RG, Soskolne CL. Physicians' reasons for not entering eligible patients in a randomized clinical trial of surgery for breast cancer. N Engl J Med 1984; 310:1363–1367.

Thornquist MD, Omenn GS, Goodman GE, Grizzle JE, Rosenstock L, Barnhart S, et al. Statistical design and monitoring of the Carotene and Retinol Efficacy Trial (CARET). Controlled Clin Trials 1993; 14:308–324.

Thorpe KE, Zwarenstein M, Oxman AD, Treweek S, Furberg CD, Altman DG, et al. A Pragmatic-Explanatory Continuum Indicator Summary (PRECIS): a tool to help trial designers. CMAJ 2009; 180:E47–E57.

Todd S. A 25-year review of sequential methodology in clinical studies. Stat Med 2007; 26:237–252.

Torgerson DJ. Contamination in trials: is cluster randomisation the answer? BMJ 2001; 322:355–357.

Tronvik E, Stovner LJ, Helde G, Sand T, Bovim G. Prophylactic treatment of migraine with an angiotensin II receptor blocker. JAMA 2003; 289:65–69.

Tunis SR, Stryer DB, Clancy CM. Practical clinical trials: increasing the value of clinical research for decision making in clinical and health policy. JAMA 2003; 290:1624–1632.

University Group Diabetes Program. A study of the effects of hypoglycemic agents on vascular complications in patients with adult-onset diabetes: I. Design, methods and baseline results. Diabetes 1970a; 19 (Suppl. 2):747–783.

University Group Diabetes Program. A study of the effects of hypoglycemic agents on vascular complications in patients with adult-onset diabetes: II. Mortality results. Diabetes 1970b; 19 (Suppl. 2):787–830.

US Department of Health and Human Services. 45 Code of Federal Regulations 46. Fed Reg 1991; 56:28012.

Van Spall HGC, Toren A, Kiss A, Fowler RA. Eligibility criteria of randomized controlled trials published in high-impact general medical journals: a systematic sampling review. JAMA 2007; 297:1233–1240.

Vesikari T, Matson DO, Dennehy P, Van Damme P, Santosham M, Rodriguez Z, *et al.* Safety and efficacy of a pentavalent human-bovine (WC3) reassortant rotavirus vaccine. N Engl J Med 2006; 354:23–33.

Veterans Administration Cooperative Study Group on Antihypertensive Agents. Effects of treatment on morbidity in hypertension. Results in patients with diastolic blood pressures averaging 115 through 129 mmHg. JAMA 1967; 202:116–122.

Vickers AJ, de Craen AJ. Why use placebos in clinical trials? A narrative review of the methodological literature. J Clin Epidemiol 2000; 53:157–161.

Walsh BT, Seidman SN, Sysko R, Gould M. Placebo response in studies of major depression: variable, substantial, and growing. JAMA 2002; 287:1840–1847.

Wei LJ, Lachin JM. Properties of the urn randomization in clinical trials. Control Clin Trials 1988; 9:345–364.

Weir CJ, Walley RJ. Statistical evaluation of biomarkers as surrogate endpoints: a literature review. Stat Med 2006; 25:183–203.

Weiss NS, Koepsell TD, Psaty BM. Generalizability of the results of randomized trials. Arch Intern Med 2008; 168:133–135.

Whitehead J. A unified theory for sequential clinical trials. Stat Med 1999; 18:2271–2286.

Winkelstein W Jr. The remarkable Archie: origins of the Cochrane Collaboration. Epidemiology 2009; 20:779.

Wittes J, Brittain E. The role of internal pilot studies in increasing the efficiency of clinical trials. Stat Med 1990; 9:65–72.

Yusuf S, Collins R, Peto R. Why do we need some large, simple randomized trials? Stat Med 1984; 3:409–422.

Yusuf S, Wittes J, Probstfield J, Tyroler HA. Analysis and interpretation of treatment effects in subgroups of patients in randomized clinical trials. JAMA 1991; 266:93–98.

EXERCISES

1. Internal mammary artery ligation enjoyed brief popularity in the 1950s for treatment of coronary artery disease until randomized trials showed the procedure to be of little or no benefit. A key trial by Cobb *et al.* (1959) involved randomizing twelve men and five women to either internal mammary artery ligation or sham surgery.

   (a) According to the published report, all five of the women were randomly assigned to the ligated group. But the probability that all of the women would be assigned to the new procedure by chance alone is only about 0.03. Does this imply that the randomization scheme had been improperly carried out or subsequently subverted?

   (b) Under what circumstances would the resulting imbalance in the sex composition of the two treatment groups bias the outcome of the study?

   (c) Is there any way by which the investigators could have prevented the gender imbalance, yet still allocate subjects at random to the two groups? If so, how?

   (d) During follow-up of 3–15 months, patients who received sham surgery tended to report marked improvement in their symptoms and reduced need for nitroglycerin tablets to control their angina attacks. Does this indicate that sham surgery was effective for relieving angina? Why or why not?

   (e) Suppose you were a devoted advocate of the internal mammary artery ligation technique. Other than possible confounding due to sex or other factors, are there any arguments you would invoke as to why this study should not be considered proof that the technique is valueless?

2. Use of infant pacifiers has been found in several observational studies to be associated with early termination of breastfeeding. Partly on that basis, many pediatricians and some professional organizations have discouraged the use of pacifiers, even though many parents find them a convenient way to respond to a baby's crying or fussing.

   Kramer *et al.* (2001) sought to test whether pacifier use is actually a *cause* of early weaning. They randomized 281 mothers who planned to breastfeed their newborn baby to one of two types of counseling sessions. For intervention-group mothers, counseling included a recommendation that they avoid use of pacifiers, and education about other ways to comfort a crying or fussing baby. Control-group mothers received no such advice or education about pacifiers. Follow-up interviews were conducted by research staff who were kept unaware of each mother's treatment group assignment.

   Among intervention-group mothers, 38.6% reported that they totally avoided pacifier use, compared with 16.0% of control-group mothers (ratio 2.4, 95% CI: 1.5–3.8). Other interview data also showed less-frequent pacifier use among intervention-group mothers. But at three months postpartum, the percentage of mothers who had weaned their infant was nearly equal: 18.9% in the intervention group vs. 18.3% in the control group. The reported frequency of crying or fussing was also similar. The researchers concluded that there was no causal link between pacifier use and early weaning, and they recommended that organizations promoting breastfeeding re-examine their opposition to pacifiers.

(a) What features of the research problem made it amenable to study with a randomized trial design?

(b) The trial report describes the study as "double-blind." Do you agree? Why or why not? Does it matter in this case?

(c) The trial report states: "we estimated that a reduction in daily pacifier use from 60% to 40% would reduce the risk of weaning before the age of 3 months from 40% to 35%. With an α level of .05 and a β of .10, approximately 140 infants were required per group." It is not clear from this statement whether the target sample size was based on the hypothesized difference in daily pacifier use or on the hypothesized difference in early weaning. Can you determine which difference was used in the sample-size calculations?

(d) When the investigators analyzed outcome data from the trial according to actual *use* of pacifiers (without regard to randomized treatment-group assignments), they found that pacifier use was indeed associated with early weaning, just as previous observational studies had observed. But they argued that the lack of association between pacifier use and early weaning in the randomized-trial analysis "trumped" the positive association seen in the observational-study analysis. What key confounding factor(s) do you think could be controlled in the randomized-trial analysis but not in the observational-study analysis?

3. Cystic fibrosis is a chronic inherited disease that involves abnormally viscous respiratory secretions, which put affected persons at increased risk for lung infections and long-term decline in pulmonary function. Imagine that you are a co-investigator on a proposed trial of a newly developed drug that is supposed to liquefy respiratory secretions in cystic fibrosis patients, making the secretions easier to clear. The trial will be a two-arm, parallel-groups trial comparing the new drug with placebo.

Four cystic fibrosis specialty centers in different cities have contacted the patients for whom they currently provide ongoing care, in order to determine each patient's eligibility and willingness to participate. Other clinical practices and outcomes vary among the centers, so the investigators want to allocate trial participants in such a way that care-center affiliation is guaranteed not to confound the main treatment comparison.

A total of 100 potential participants have been identified—10 at Center A, 20 at Center B, 30 at Center C, and 40 at Center D—which has been determined to be an adequate total sample size to test the main study hypothesis. Select an appropriate method of randomization, and generate the sequence of treatment group assignments using the method you have chosen.

4. The Heart and Estrogen/progestin Replacement Study (HERS) was a randomized trial that sought to confirm many prior observational studies showing lower risk of coronary heart disease (CHD) associated with use of estrogen supplements during menopause (Hulley *et al.*, 1998). The investigators described it as a "secondary prevention trial" because participating women already had CHD, as evidenced by prior myocardial infarction (MI), past coronary artery bypass graft surgery or percutaneous coronary revascularization, or angiographic evidence of at least a 50% occlusion of one or more major coronary arteries. The main study hypothesis was that hormone supplements would prevent future CHD events, including MI and sudden cardiac death, in this high-risk cohort. However, the results appeared to be at odds with the observational evidence. The abstract from the main published report appears below:

Context. Observational studies have found lower rates of coronary heart disease (CHD) in postmenopausal women who take estrogen than in women who do not, but this potential benefit has not been confirmed in clinical trials.

Objective. To determine if estrogen plus progestin therapy alters the risk for CHD events in postmenopausal women with established coronary disease.

Design. Randomized, blinded, placebo-controlled secondary prevention trial.

Setting. Outpatient and community settings at 20 United State clinical centers.

Participants. A total of 2,763 women with coronary disease, younger than 80 years, and postmenopausal with an intact uterus. Mean age was 66.7 years.

Intervention. Either 0.625 mg. of conjugated equine estrogens plus 2.5 mg. of medroxyprogesterone acetate in 1 tablet daily (n = 1,380) or a placebo of identical appearance (n = 1,383). Follow-up averaged 4.1 years; 82% of those assigned to hormone treatment were taking it at the end of 1 year, and 75% at the end of 3 years.

Main Outcome Measures. The primary outcome was the occurrence of nonfatal myocardial infarction (MI) or CHD death. Secondary cardiovascular outcomes included coronary revascularization, unstable angina, congestive heart failure, resuscitated cardiac arrest, stroke or transient ischemic attack, and peripheral arterial disease. All-cause mortality was also considered.

Results. Overall, there were no significant differences between groups in the primary outcome or in any of the secondary cardiovascular outcomes: 172 women in the hormone group and 176 women in the placebo group had MI or CHD death (relative hazard [RH], 0.99; 95% confidence interval [CI], 0.80–1.22). The lack of an overall effect occurred despite a net 11% lower low-density lipoprotein cholesterol level and 10% higher high-density lipoprotein cholesterol level in the hormone group compared with the placebo group (each $p < 0.001$). Within the overall null effect, there was a statistically significant time trend, with more CHD events in the hormone group than in the placebo group in year 1 and fewer in years 4 and 5. More women in the hormone group than in the placebo group experienced venous thromboembolic events (34 vs. 12; RH, 2.89; 95% CI, 1.50–5.58) and gallbladder disease (84 vs. 62; RH, 1.38; 95% CI, 1.00–1.92). There were no significant differences in several other end points for which power was limited, including fracture, cancer, and total mortality (131 vs. 123 deaths; RH, 1.08; 95% CI, 0.84–1.38).

Conclusions. During an average follow-up of 4.1 years, treatment with oral conjugated equine estrogen plus medroxyprogesterone acetate did not reduce the overall rate of CHD events in postmenopausal women with established coronary disease. The treatment did increase the rate of thromboembolic events and gallbladder disease. Based on the finding of no overall cardiovascular benefit and a pattern of early increase in risk of CHD events, we do not recommend starting this treatment for the purpose of secondary prevention of CHD. However, given the favorable pattern of CHD events after several years of therapy, it could be appropriate for women already receiving this treatment to continue.

(a) The HERS trial's primary aim was to test the efficacy of postmenopausal hormone therapy for preventing future CHD events in a high-risk cohort of women. But it also sought to evaluate the safety of this regimen in terms of the incidence of other non-cardiovascular health conditions, including several forms of cancer. In what way might a randomized trial of this sort be limited in its ability to establish safety in comparison to other epidemiologic study designs?

(b) The study's criteria for eligibility included a long list of exclusions:

> Women were excluded for the following reasons: CHD event within 6 months of randomization; serum triglyceride level higher than 3.39 mmol/L (300 mg/ dL); use of oral, parenteral, vaginal, or transdermal sex hormones within 3 months of the screening visit; history of deep vein thrombosis or pulmonary embolism; history of breast cancer or breast examination or mammogram suggestive of breast cancer; history of endometrial cancer; abnormal uterine bleeding, endometrial hyperplasia, or endometrium thickness greater than 5 mm on baseline evaluation; abnormal or unobtainable Papanicolaou test result; serum aspartate aminotransferase level [a liver-function test] more than 1.2 times normal; unlikely to remain geographically accessible for study visits for at least 4 years; disease (other than CHD) judged likely to be fatal within 4 years; New York Heart Association class IV or severe class III congestive heart failure; alcoholism or other drug abuse; uncontrolled hypertension (diastolic blood pressure ≥ 105 mm Hg or systolic blood pressure ≥ 200 mm Hg); uncontrolled diabetes (fasting blood glucose level ≥ 16.7 mmol/L [300 mg/dL]); participation in another investigational drug or device study; less than 80% compliance with a placebo run-in prior to randomization; or history of intolerance to hormone therapy.

Identify at least two exclusions that were included chiefly to protect the safety of participants. Identify two others that were included chiefly to protect the internal validity of the trial.

(c) After the study was published, a critic contended that the results may have been biased because diagnostic tests were not performed on all women at the outset of the trial to ascertain the extent of coronary and other vascular disease in participants, in order to prove that the two treatment groups were similar on these factors. Would you agree that this was a serious flaw?

(d) Lipid-lowering drugs are often prescribed in order to reduce low-density lipoprotein ("bad") cholesterol and to raise high-density lipoprotein ("good") cholesterol. These drugs turned out to be prescribed more often during the course of the trial for placebo recipients than for estrogen/progestin recipients. Should this differential use of lipid-lowering drugs be considered a potential confounding factor in evaluating the effectiveness of these hormones for preventing future CHD events?

5. Hooton *et al.* (2012) conducted a randomized trial that compared two antibiotics from different drug classes for uncomplicated urinary tract infection in women. Drug A was ciprofloxacin, a fluroquinolone; Drug B was cefpodoxime, a new, third-generation cephalosporin. At the time of the study, Drug A was widely used, but bacterial resistance to it was becoming more frequent, leading to concerns about overuse and possible treatment failures. Drug B was thought not to have these shortcomings and was equally easy to take. The trial was designed as a noninferiority trial, with a noninferiority threshold of 10 percentage points in the percent clinically cured after 30 days.

In an intent-to-treat analysis, 139/150 (93%) of women treated with drug A were clinically cured after 30 days, compared with 123/150 (82%) of women treated with drug B, for a difference of 11% (95% CI: 3%–18%).

(a) Was Drug A superior to Drug B?

(b) Was Drug B noninferior to Drug A?

(c) How can you reconcile these two conclusions?

6. Falls are common in older adults. Kannus *et al.* (2000) conducted a randomized trial of thin, inexpensive pads that can be positioned over the greater femoral trochanter and worn under clothing. If the wearer falls, the hip pad is intended to cushion the blow and keep the upper femur from breaking.

The trial involved 1,801 ambulatory adults who resided in 20 Finnish geriatric treatment units. The treatment units were randomly allocated in a 1:2 ratio to be either a hip-pad unit or a control unit.

(a) In principle, each individual adult could have been randomized either to wear hip pads or to serve as a control. Why do you suppose the investigators chose to randomize treatment units instead?

(b) The published trial report contains a table comparing the baseline characteristics of residents of units assigned to the hip-pad and control groups, from which the results shown in Table 13.15 are excerpted.

We normally expect only about 5% of baseline comparisons to be statistically significant at the 0.05 level. Why do you think so many of the differences shown in this table resulted in such small *p*-values?

(c) After the treatment units had been randomized, older adults on each unit were asked whether they would be willing to take part in the study. Some 31% of patients on hip-pad units declined, vs. 9% of patients on control units. Could this difference have led to bias? If so, how might it have been avoidable by designing the trial differently?

(d) Suppose that you are thinking about conducting a confirmatory trial in which older adults in assisted-living settings would be individually randomized with equal probability to hip-pad or control conditions and then followed for 18 months. Drawing on the Finnish study results, you consider it reasonable to assume that the 18-month cumulative incidence of hip fracture among controls should be about 7.5%. You would like the study to have 80% power to detect a 50% reduction in hip-fracture incidence in the hip-pad group. You plan to test the results for statistical significance with a two-tailed test at the 0.05 level. Assume that dropouts will be negligible. How many subjects would be needed in each arm?

ANSWERS

1. (a) *Imply* is too strong a word. Even under a properly implemented random allocation process, all five women could be assigned to the ligated group with probability $(1/2)^5 = 1/32 \approx 0.03$— an unusual but not impossible outcome of random allocation. After all, people do win the lottery.

(b) Because of the apparent "accident of randomization," gender was strongly associated with exposure (whether the internal mammary artery was ligated). If gender itself were associated with any of the outcomes under study, then it could become a confounding factor for those outcomes. The results were not reported separately by gender, however, so we cannot actually compare outcomes between men and women within the ligated group.

(c) They could have used randomly permuted blocks within each gender stratum. For example, if blocks of size two were used, the first two women recruited for study would be considered

TABLE 13.15. BASELINE CHARACTERISTICS OF
RESIDENTS IN THE INTERVENTION AND CONTROL
GROUPS IN A RANDOMIZED TRIAL OF HIP PADS

| | Percent or mean ± s.d. | | |
Characteristic	Hip-pad group ($n = 653$)	Control group ($n = 1,148$)	p-value
Sex			0.41
Female	77%	79%	
Male	23%	21%	
Age (years)	81 ± 6	82 ± 6	0.006
Weight (kg.)	63.1 ± 11.8	65.5 ± 13.1	< 0.001
Medical conditions			
Heart disease	52%	51%	0.46
Dementia	33%	26%	0.001
Hypertension	20%	23%	0.13
Past stroke	21%	15%	0.002
Mental status			< 0.001
Normal	39%	42%	
Mild impairment	19%	25%	
Moderate impairment	22%	22%	
Severe impairment	21%	12%	
Walking ability			0.001
Independently	39%	35%	
With cane or walker	49%	57%	
With help	12%	8%	

(Based on data from kANNUS *et al.* [2000])

to belong to the same block. A random number would then be chosen to decide which of the two women would be assigned to the ligated group, with the other woman automatically going to the non-ligated group.

(d) No. This was only a before–after comparison. Symptoms of coronary heart disease tend to vary over time within an individual, waxing and waning in severity. Patients would be unlikely to consider surgery at a time when their symptoms were relatively mild or improving; instead, they would be looking for new therapeutic options when their symptoms were relatively severe or were getting worse. Even in the absence of any therapeutic benefit, we might expect such patients' symptom severity to improve over time as they regress toward their respective mean severity levels. More convincing evidence of the effectiveness of sham surgery would come from a randomized comparison group that did not undergo sham surgery.

(e) A clinically important effect of mammary-artery ligation would be very difficult to detect with only 17 study subjects due to low statistical power. Also, the follow-up period was relatively short and may have missed any longer-term differences in outcomes between the ligated and non-ligated groups.

2. (a) • Parents largely controlled whether and how often a pacifier was used to calm their baby. As the results showed, this form of parenting behavior could, in turn, be modified by the investigators through an educational intervention.

• The key outcome, early weaning, was relatively common. It also occurred relatively soon after birth, so that prolonged follow-up was not required.

• Besides early weaning, cry/fuss behavior was also of interest as a secondary outcome. A randomized-trial design lends itself to studying multiple outcomes.

- There was uncertainty about the balance of good and bad effects of pacifiers.

(b) Use of the term "double-blind" is questionable in this case. Although the research staff who interviewed participants about study outcomes were unaware of which mother was in which treatment group, the educational intervention itself should have made mothers well aware of whether they had been discouraged from using pacifiers. This educational message could have influenced their perceptions and/or reporting of the frequency of pacifier use and cry/fuss behavior.

(c) The target sample size of 140 per group appears to have been based on the hypothesized difference in pacifier use. Applying the sample-size estimation method in Appendix 5B:

p_0 = estimated frequency of daily pacifier use in

control group

$= 0.6$

p_1 = hypothesized frequency of daily pacifier

use in experimental group

$= 0.4$

$Z_\alpha \approx 1.96$ for $\alpha = 0.05$, two-sided

$Z_\beta \approx 1.28$ for $\beta = 0.10$

$k = 1$ for two equal-sized treatment groups

$$\bar{p} = \frac{p_1 + 1 \cdot p_0}{1 + 1} = .5$$

$$n_1 = \frac{\left[\begin{array}{c} \sqrt{\bar{p}(1-\bar{p})(1+1/k)} \cdot Z_\alpha \\ + \sqrt{p_1(1-p_1) + p_0(1-p_0)/k} \cdot Z_\beta \end{array} \right]^2}{(p_1 - p_0)^2}$$

≈ 130 (rounded up to next integer)

The investigators may have used a slightly different sample-size formula, some of which incorporate a continuity correction, or they may have boosted the target sample size slightly to allow for dropouts. In any event, repeating the above calculations with $p_0 = 0.4$ and $p_1 = 0.35$ yields $n \approx 1,968$, so it is clear that the study was too small to detect a 5-percentage-point difference in early weaning with the specified power.

(d) While we cannot know for sure, mothers who used pacifiers more often may have been less committed to longer-term breastfeeding to begin with, or they may have experienced more discomfort or inconvenience from it once they started. In the randomized-trial analysis, we can expect those possibly subtle factors to be fairly well balanced between groups, even though they were not directly measured.

3. Confounding by center can be prevented by assuring that equal numbers of patients are assigned to the new drug and to placebo within each center. The number of willing and eligible patients at each center is already known, so each center's patients can be randomized as a single block. A simple algorithm for achieving the desired result is:

(a) Construct a data set with 100 observations (rows). Call its first column (variable) **Center**, and assign the value "A" for the first 10 observations, "B" for the next 20, "C" for the next 30, and "D" for the last 40.

(b) Add another column called **Assignment**, and give half of the observations within each center the value "New drug" and the other half "Placebo" in any order. A convenient way to do this is simply to assign "New drug" and "Placebo" in alternating order from the first observation to the last.

(c) Add another column called **RN**, and fill it in with random numbers from a uniform distribution in the range 0–1. Statistical packages and spreadsheet programs typically have a built-in function for this purpose.

(d) Sort the rows by **RN** within **Center**. This "shuffles" (randomly permutes) the rows within each center without changing the number of patients assigned to each treatment group.

(e) For convenience, another column called **Seq** can be added, which will contain the sequence number of each row (which corresponds to patient) within a center. That is, rows for center A will be numbered 1...10, those for center B will be numbered 1...20, etc.

Standard statistical packages, such as Stata, SAS, R, or SPSS, can all implement the above method. It is also possible to coax a spreadsheet program such as Excel into doing the same job, or to do the whole task "by hand" using a table of random numbers. But for production work, it is preferable to write a computer file that contains the actual input commands for a statistical package to do the job, so that there is an audit trail that allows the method to be checked.

It is also possible, but unnecessary, to make treatment-group assignments in smaller blocks of, say, 2 within each center. In this case, the number of patients at each center is known in advance, so all patients at a center can be allocated within a single block to maximize unpredictability.

4. (a) Randomized trials are not statistically efficient for detecting rare or delayed, but nonetheless serious, unintended effects of a therapy. For example, the investigators noted that the HERS trial had insufficient power to determine whether long-term use of hormones would affect the risk of breast cancer, given that "only" 2,763 women were included and that the total length of the study was only 4.1 years.

(b) Some exclusions intended chiefly to protect participants' safety were:

- History of intolerance to hormone therapy
- History of endometrial cancer
- History of deep vein thrombosis or pulmonary embolism
- History of breast cancer or abnormal mammogram
- Abnormal liver function tests

Some exclusions intended chiefly to protect the trial's internal validity were:

- Unlikely to remain geographically accessible for study visits for 4+ years
- Alcoholism or drug abuse
- Disease (other than CHD) judged likely to be fatal within 4 years

(c) Given the large sample size, it is reasonable to assume that randomization balanced the groups well on unknown or unmeasured potential confounders, including the nature and extent of preexisting coronary heart disease.

(d) No. The less-frequent use of lipid-lowering drugs among estrogen recipients was probably because estrogens had a similar effect on lipid levels, as reported in the study abstract. Placebo had no such effect. But because lipid-lowering drug use would thus be causally downstream from the treatment that was assigned at random, it cannot be considered a confounding factor. Part of the overall effect of hormone replacement on heart disease risk may include making it less likely that the recipient would receive other lipid-lowering drugs.

5. (a) A verdict on *superiority* is generally based on whether there is a statistically significant difference in outcomes. In this case, the 95% confidence interval for the difference in percentage clinically cured excluded 0, so Drug A would be considered superior to Drug B by this criterion.

(b) A verdict on *noninferiority* is based on whether we can confidently infer from the trial's results that the true difference in outcomes lies below the prespecified noninferiority threshold. In this case, the confidence interval for the difference in percentage clinically cured extended from 3% to 18%, which straddles the threshold of 10%. This result implies that the true difference in percentage clinically cured could plausibly be either above or below the noninferiority threshold. The trial thus did not show that Drug B is noninferior to Drug A by this criterion.

(c) The terms *superiority* and *noninferiority*, while well entrenched, can occasionally lead to some apparently paradoxical combinations. The difficulty is that each involves a binary verdict, but these verdicts are based on two different thresholds. Superiority depends on whether the confidence interval for the difference in outcomes excludes zero. Noninferiority depends on whether that confidence limit excludes Δ, a prespecified non-zero value at which somewhat worse outcomes for a new treatment would be balanced by its other advantages over a standard treatment. In this case, the confidence limits excluded zero but included Δ. The results suggest that Drug A probably does cure a larger percentage of afflicted women than Drug B, but its margin of effectiveness may or may not be large enough to sway the choice between drugs.

(Another theoretically possible result would be a confidence interval for the differences in percentage clinically cured extending from, say, 3% to 8%, which would exclude both zero and Δ. By the superiority/noninferiority terminology, such a result would imply that Drug A was superior to Drug B, but that Drug B was noninferior to Drug A!)

Confusion of this sort can be largely avoided by focusing instead on the observed difference in outcomes and its confidence interval once the trial is completed. This information conveys the degree of uncertainty about comparative effectiveness once evidence from the trial is available, and it allows users to apply their own decision threshold in choosing between the alternatives. See Mulla *et al.* (2012) and Piaggio *et al.* (2006) for more discussion of these issues.

6. (a) They feared that randomizing individual patients within a unit would pose too great a risk of "contamination" if those who were randomized to the control group felt short-changed, got access to hip pads on their own, and started wearing them.

(b) Randomization was conducted at the treatment-unit level, but the statistical testing for this table was apparently done as if individual patients had been randomized. (Note that the n's atop the columns total to 1,801, not 20.) The mix of patients was evidently quite variable among treatment units, with some units catering to older adults, some to adults with dementia, etc. When entire treatment units were randomized, all adults in a unit that served generally older people or people with dementia were assigned *en bloc* to one of the treatment groups.

Randomizing clusters generally does not balance the treatment arms as evenly as randomizing individuals, because fewer units are randomly allocated. Proper statistical significance testing must account for the cluster randomization and would no doubt have shown many fewer baseline comparisons to be statistically significant in this instance.

(c) Yes, it could have led to bias. Many control-group participants probably would have declined participation had they been assigned to the hip-pad group, but they remained in the study. No comparable subjects remained in the hip-pad group—they declined to take part. Hence selection bias occurring after randomization may have rendered two groups of participants dissimilar.

This bias might have been avoided if potential participants had been asked *first* if they would be willing to be randomized to either a hip-pad group or a control group. Only those who consented would then have been randomized and taken part in the rest of the study.

(d) For power = 80%, $\beta = 0.2$, which corresponds to $Z_\beta \approx 0.84$. For a two-tailed test at $\alpha = 0.05$, $Z_\alpha \approx 1.96$.

$p_0 =$ cumulative incidence in controls

$\quad = 0.075$

$p_1 =$ cumulative incidence in hip-pad group

$\quad = 0.075 \times 0.5 = 0.0375$

$\bar{p} = \dfrac{p_0 + p_1}{2}$

$\quad = 0.05625$

$Z_\alpha \approx 1.96$ for $\alpha = 0.05$, two-sided

$Z_\beta \approx 0.84$ for $\beta = 0.20$

$k = 1$ for two equal-sized treatment groups

$$n_1 = \frac{\left[\begin{array}{c} \sqrt{\bar{p}(1-\bar{p})(1+1/k)} \cdot Z_\alpha \\ + \sqrt{p_1(1-p_1) + p_0(1-p_0)/k} \cdot Z_\beta \end{array} \right]^2}{(p_1 - p_0)^2}$$

$$\approx 591$$

14

Cohort Studies

Cohort studies, sometimes called follow-up studies, compare the subsequent occurrence of illness, injury, or death among groups of persons whose exposure status differs "naturally," i.e., not as the result of random assignment. Sometimes the "exposure" to be studied is an exogenous one, such as infection with hepatitis B virus or consumption of dietary fiber. Other times it is a characteristic of persons, such as ABO blood type or their height and weight. The exposure or characteristics under study can be present as discrete categories, such as blood type O, A, B, or AB, or as a gradient on a continuous scale (such as fiber intake) when no natural categories exist.

The follow-up of study subjects for the occurrence of illness, injury, or death may already have occurred prior to the time of the initiation of the study. For example, many studies of the possible relationship of occupational exposures to health identify persons employed in earlier years and monitor the mortality rates of these workers up until the time the study is initiated. These are often called "retrospective" cohort studies. Alternatively, a cohort study may ascertain exposure status at the outset, with follow-up to occur in the future. Studies of this type are "prospective" cohort studies. In either case, the studies are able to determine cumulative incidence or incidence rates directly from the experience of the study subjects, which sets them apart from most case-control studies. What sets cohort studies apart from randomized controlled trials, of course, is that, in them, something other than chance alone led an individual study subject to receive a particular exposure or to possess a particular characteristic. Therefore, in contrast to the interpretation of randomized controlled trials, the interpretation of the results of cohort studies must consider the reason for the person's being exposed or not (or the reason underlying their level of exposure) as a possible explanation for the results seen.

COHORT IDENTIFICATION

Some cohort studies seek to enlist as participants a sample of persons who reside in a defined geographic area. From those who agree to take part in the study, exposure information and health outcomes are ascertained. During the second half of the 20th century in the United States, studies of this type have taken place in such locations as Framingham, Massachusetts; Tecumseh, Michigan; Evans County, Georgia; and Washington County, Maryland. More commonly, however, cohort studies are fashioned around persons who have distinctive and measurable exposures, or among groups of persons for which there are special resources that allow for either cohort identification and/or cohort follow-up.

Cohort Studies Initiated Because of the Presence of a Distinctive Exposure

Assessments of the potential impact of ionizing radiation on the incidence of cancer have exploited the presence of identifiable groups of persons who had been exposed to such radiation in various contexts. As examples, epidemiologists have conducted studies of cancer occurrence among survivors of the atomic detonations in Hiroshima and Nagasaki (Shimizu et al., 1990); Israeli children who received scalp irradiation for tinea capitis (Ron et al., 1988); British patients with ankylosing spondylitis who underwent radiation therapy (Court-Brown and Doll, 1957); persons exposed to radiation on the job (such as radiologic technologists (Linet et al., 2005), Chernobyl cleanup workers (Rahu et al., 2006), and uranium miners (Darby et al., 1995)); and children who, while in utero, had been exposed to diagnostic

X-rays given to their mothers (Harvey *et al.*, 1985). Most of what we know of the health effects of irradiation on human beings comes from studies such as these.

Special Resources for Cohort Identification and/or Follow-up

Some cohort studies have been mounted among persons enrolled in life insurance plans, since follow-up for mortality in such persons can be achieved with nearly complete success by monitoring claims submitted by beneficiaries of cohort members. For example, one of the early cohort studies of smoking and mortality involved the mailing of brief questionnaires to former World War II servicemen who held government life insurance policies (Kahn, 1966). Subsequent mortality rates from lung cancer and other conditions could then be compared between men who had and had not reported being a cigarette smoker.

Similarly, the strong incentive for members of prepaid health care plans to receive medical care from within the plan enables cohort studies to be conducted in such individuals at relatively low cost. Studies done in these settings can determine if the incidence of various illnesses that generally require medical treatment among health plan members differs according to the presence of various antecedent medical conditions or to the use of prescription drugs, since these can be ascertained through the records of many prepaid health care plans as well.

Finally, it is also relatively easy to do cohort studies among women seeking prenatal care, since the large majority of them will continue to seek care from the same provider through the time of the delivery of their child. This allows for relatively complete access to information on pregnancy outcomes that occur among patients of a given provider of prenatal care.

Occasionally, investigators have at their disposal an unusual ability to collect follow-up information on potential cohort members, allowing a cohort study to take place that would not otherwise be feasible. For example, prior to the advent of the National Death Index in the United States, the American Cancer Society conducted a large cohort study (Hammond, 1966) that utilized the very large number of Cancer Society volunteers to both identify potential cohort members and to help monitor their whereabouts and vital status. Also, several studies of college alumni have been conducted (Lee and Paffenbarger, 1998; Sesso *et al.*, 1998) because of the existence of alumni association records that maintain a listing of their

members' addresses. In each of these instances, the cohort study was done prospectively, with a questionnaire being sent out to potential cohort members at the outset and the follow-up for mortality occurring subsequently.

Increasingly, with the advent of population-based disease registries, it has been possible to follow cohort members for the occurrence for diseases that are ascertained by these registries. Thus, the follow-up of cancer incidence among Israeli children treated with scalp irradiation was done simply by linking the identity of the irradiated children with those who later appeared in the records of the Israel Tumor Registry (Ron *et al.*, 1988).

METHODS OF ASCERTAINMENT OF EXPOSURE STATUS
Records

Records, of one sort or another, serve as the means of characterizing the exposure status of study participants in many cohort studies. *Occupational* records, available from employers or unions, can identify the fact of employment in a job or industry in which a particular exposure is known to be (or to have been) present. Often, additional relevant information is available from this source as well, such as the duration and recency of employment, as well as the type of job held and the location(s) of that job within the work environment. A discussion of the ascertainment of occupational exposures, along with other aspects of occupational cohort studies, can be found in Checkoway and Eisen (1998).

The availability of *medical* and *pharmacy* records over a period of years on members of prepaid health care plans, or enrollees in government health insurance programs, has allowed many cohort studies to be conducted. Examples include the evaluation of the possible influence of vasectomy on the incidence of coronary heart disease (Walker *et al.*, 1981; Petitti *et al.*, 1983; Nienhuis *et al.*, 1992), the use of appetite-suppressant drugs on the incidence of valvular heart disease (Jick *et al.*, 1998), and the prescription of antidepressant medications in relation to a woman's subsequent risk of breast cancer (Fulton-Kehoe *et al.*, 2006).

Some cohort studies have been made feasible because of "exposure" information contained in *vital* records. For example, women who underwent elective induction of labor were identified from birth certificates of the state of Washington during 1989–1993, and the occurrence of Cesarean section and selected unfavorable pregnancy outcomes was compared between them and otherwise comparable women delivering a child whose labor had not been induced (Dublin *et al.*, 2000). In some countries *census* records can be used to characterize employment status. This has permitted an examination of the possible influence of occupation on those health outcomes (e.g., cancer incidence) that are routinely ascertained on residents of those countries (Lynge and Thygesen, 1990).

Interviews or Questionnaires

The principal advantage of most prospective cohort studies, relative to retrospective cohort studies, is the ability to obtain information on current and past exposures from the study participants who are to be enrolled for follow-up, and to do so in a way that directly fits the aim(s) of the study. For example, in one cohort study, a questionnaire was returned by 51,529 male dentists, veterinarians, and other health professionals, which provided information on a number of prior and present health conditions and exposures. Health outcomes were monitored in this group by means of follow-up questionnaires, sent every two years, with medical records obtained pertinent to illnesses that were reported. The information contained in these questionnaires permitted the investigators to characterize exposures in some detail (e.g., a history of vasectomy *and* the age at which that operation occurred). For an outcome of particular interest, such as prostate cancer, it also allowed them to assess other factors (such as race) that could confound the examination of a possible association with vasectomy (Giovanucci *et al.*, 1993).

Some cohort studies seek interviews or questionnaires from participants only at the outset of follow-up, whereas others seek to update some or all of that information periodically. If it is believed that the action of the exposure in causing or preventing an illness could be relatively short-term, clearly it is desirable to have updated information.

Example 14-1. The Nurses' Health Study enrolled female registered nurses in 11 states of the United States in a prospective cohort study in 1976. Detailed information on a number of characteristics of these women was first collected at the time, and then updated every two years as part of a questionnaire sent to participants that inquired about health outcomes (and also about changes in these characteristics). Analyses of the incidence of pulmonary embolism among members of this cohort

(Goldhaber *et al.*, 1997) compared women with and without various attributes (e.g., obesity, cigarette smoking, a diagnosis of hypertension) only as of the time of the most recent questionnaire, given the rapidity with which known risk factors for pulmonary embolism (e.g., surgery, immobility) exert their harmful effect.

Direct Measurements Made on Cohort Members

For individual subjects, many exposures of interest cannot be determined with any accuracy, or perhaps at all, from either records or interviews, but can be determined by direct measurement. For example, blood samples were obtained from civil servants in Taiwan and tested for the presence of the hepatitis B surface antigen (an indicator of chronic active hepatitis B infection). During the next several years, the death rate from primary liver cancer among persons who tested positive was some 200 times that of those who tested negative (Beasley *et al.*, 1981). As other examples:

- In a number of cohort studies, the incidence of vascular disease has been compared among persons who differ in terms of their levels of serum cholesterol and other lipids (Dawber *et al.*, 1963; Tyroler *et al.*, 1971; Klag *et al.*, 1993).
- Investigators at the Portsmouth Naval Shipyard mounted a retrospective cohort study in which each participant's exposure to occupational radiation was assessed by reading the dose recorded on that person's radiation film badge (Rinsky *et al.*, 1981).
- The results of psychiatric evaluations of Swedish military recruits during 1969–1970 were examined as possible predictors of the incidence of suicide among these men during the subsequent 13 years (Allebeck *et al.*, 1988).

If the characteristic being measured exhibits short-term variability (e.g., serum cholesterol or systolic blood pressure, which can vary hour-to-hour), the value obtained will not necessarily reflect the study participant's long-term mean level. The impact of this misclassification will be to dull the study's ability to assess the degree of association between the characteristic and a given health outcome, resulting in what has been termed "regression dilution" bias (Clarke *et al.*, 1999). For characteristics that do vary, it is desirable (although not always practical) to obtain repeated measurements as a way of minimizing this bias. Thus, most cohort studies that obtain a blood-pressure reading do so several times on each participant during his/her study examination. If the cohort is to be followed for health outcomes over an extended period and the characteristic exhibits long-term changes (e.g., weight, blood pressure), then remeasurement of that characteristic during the course of follow-up may be important as well. Additional discussion of the issue of remeasurement of exposure status, as well as other exposure measurement questions that arise in the conduct of prospective cohort studies, can be found in White *et al.* (1998).

BASES FOR ESTIMATING THE EXPECTED OCCURRENCE OF DISEASE AMONG ''EXPOSED'' COHORT MEMBERS

In cohort studies in which there is heterogeneity of exposure status among study participants, the occurrence of disease can be contrasted between persons who have or who have not been exposed, or across levels of exposure. For example, in a group of 715 monozygotic twins, all of whom had served in the United States armed forces during 1965–1975, the prevalence of post-traumatic stress disorder in 1987 was compared between those who had and those who had not served in Southeast Asia (Goldberg *et al.*, 1990). In the Framingham study, the incidence of heart attack was calculated for persons in each fourth of the distribution of serum cholesterol (Kannel *et al.*, 1971). In the Women's Health study, women in the lowest seventh of the distribution of body mass index (BMI)—weight in kilograms divided by the square of the height in meters, a measure of obesity—served as the reference category for women in each of the other sevenths of the distribution in terms of the incidence of coronary heart disease (Kurth *et al.*, 2005).

The selection of subjects to be used as a basis for comparison to "exposed" individuals should not be conditioned in any way on events that occur during follow-up for health outcomes. Failure to adhere to this admonition can lead to a distorted estimate of the risk associated with an exposure. For example, in a study of the occurrence of Cesarean section following elective induction of labor at a given gestational age, at first glance it might seem appropriate to choose as comparison subjects women who

delivered a child of the same gestational age, without induction. However, this choice would omit women from the non-exposed group who went on to deliver later in the pregnancy, in whom the occurrence of Cesarean section tends to be particularly high (Caughey *et al.*, 2006). Failure to appropriately include them in the comparison group would be expected to give rise to a spuriously high estimate of risk of Cesarean section associated with elective induction of labor.

When every member of the cohort under study has sustained the exposure of interest, then some external basis for the expected rate must be found. One possibility is the rate of the health outcome(s) of interest in members of cohorts who sustained other exposures, ones that are believed not to influence the occurrence of the health outcome. For example, the mortality rate from lung cancer in asbestos textile workers was compared in one of several analyses to that of cotton textile workers (Gardner, 1986). Cancer mortality among American radiologists was compared to that of a sample of physicians in other specialties (Seltser and Sartwell, 1965).

Another basis for comparison is the rate of the health outcome present in the geographic population in which cohort members reside. This approach commonly is used when mortality is the outcome of concern, given the availability of mortality statistics for most geographic populations. For other health outcomes, such as cancer incidence and birth defects, data may be available for the relevant geographic area, or, if not, rates may be "borrowed" from another area if it is felt that they are likely to reflect the rates that would have prevailed in the appropriate population.

Each approach for generating the "expected" mortality or morbidity among exposed cohort members has potential strengths and weaknesses. The rates among non-exposed persons within the cohort itself, when available, are generally to be preferred, since for both exposed and non-exposed persons the means of cohort identification and follow-up for illness outcomes should then be comparable. Also, the distribution of demographic and other potentially confounding factors often is similar between these two groups. However, when the size of the non-exposed group is relatively small, and the outcome of interest is relatively uncommon, then this choice might provide but a statistically flimsy basis for estimating the expected rate among exposed persons.

Example 14-2. Blair *et al.* (1998) sought to assess the possibility that occupational exposure to trichloroethylene (TCE), a carcinogen in some animal experiments, was associated with an increased incidence of one or more forms of cancer in humans. They identified a cohort of persons who had been employed in an aircraft maintenance facility in Utah during 1952–1956, and monitored their mortality experience through 1990. Based on a review of each individual's job title(s), about 7,000 persons were characterized as having been exposed to TCE, about 3,300 as having exposure to one or more other industrial chemicals but not TCE, and about 3,700 as not having exposure to chemicals in the workplace.

The primary comparison was site-specific mortality from cancer between TCE-exposed persons and persons not exposed to chemicals. For relatively common cancers, this comparison probably was a valid one, more so than a comparison of the TCE-exposed cohort to an external population. However, for relatively uncommon cancers, this strategy led to problems. For example, 10 deaths from esophageal cancer occurred in TCE-exposed persons, corresponding to a rate 5.6 times that of persons with no known chemical exposure. However, the rate in non-exposed persons was based on but a single death from esophageal cancer, so the 95% confidence interval around the relative risk of 5.6 was very wide (0.7–44.5), severely restricting the interpretation of this association. Since the mortality rate from esophageal cancer among the entire cohort of 14,000 was actually slightly below that of the population as a whole, it is highly unlikely that esophageal cancer mortality in persons with TCE exposures similar to the 7,000 TCE-exposed persons in this study is truly elevated by a factor of 5.6; most or all of the apparent excess must be attributable to an atypically *low* rate in non-exposed persons, which, given the low frequency of esophageal cancer, could easily have occurred by chance.

When a comparison internal to the study is not available, there may be advantages in selecting the experience of a group of individuals who have sustained different sorts of exposures than the one of interest. Comparing the mortality of radiologists in the United States to that of other physicians (Seltser and Sartwell, 1965) was likely to provide a more valid contrast than a comparison with mortality rates for the population in general. By choosing the experience of non-radiologist physicians, it was possible to achieve a greater degree of comparability with

respect to a number of social and economic factors that bear on the risk of developing and dying from a variety of causes (and that might bear on the likelihood that the cause of death was correctly classified). Nonetheless, the success of the above strategy is contingent on the comparison cohort's not having their own exposure(s) that have an impact on the health outcomes of interest. If, for example, the mortality from a given cancer among TCE-exposed workers were compared only to that of workers with other chemical exposures, and no differences were found, it could mean either that:

- there is no association between exposure to TCE and the occurrence of that cancer; or that
- exposure to TCE as well as to one or more other chemicals used in aircraft maintenance is associated with an altered cancer risk to a similar degree.

Example 14-3. In a cohort of American asbestos textile workers, 24 deaths from lung cancer occurred (Gardner, 1986). This was exactly twice the number expected based on United States mortality rates (95% confidence interval = 1.3–3.0), but was 7.4 times the number predicted when the death rates among cotton textile workers served as a basis for comparison (95% confidence interval = 3.1–20.3). Which of these estimates of the relative risk is likely to be closer to the truth? While the use of population rates as a source for the expected number of deaths is likely to produce a figure that is spuriously high (and therefore a relative risk that is too low—see below)—the magnitude of that bias is generally modest. Alternatively, the relative risk of 7.4 could be spuriously high if the occupational exposures sustained by cotton textile workers provided them some protection against the development of lung cancer. Given that the mortality rate from lung cancer in cotton textile workers was but 27 percent of the United States population rate, this appears to be a credible hypothesis. The true relative risk of lung cancer in the American asbestos textile workers probably was considerably closer to 2.0 than to 7.4.

In summary, there may be instances in which the experience of a comparison group of persons exposed to something other than the agent of interest will reflect that of non-exposed persons who are otherwise comparable to the exposed cohort, and thus provide a valid result. However, the use of such a comparison group can also lead to a potentially large bias in either direction. If possible, rates of illness in parallel cohorts should be supplemented by rates available for the broader defined population in which the cohort is situated.

Many cohort studies employ population rates as a basis for comparison to the illness or mortality experience of a particular cohort of exposed individuals. These rates generally are based on a sizeable number of events and so are, statistically speaking, quite precise. Nonetheless, some care must be used when interpreting the results of such a comparison. Specifically, it is necessary to address the following questions:

1. *Have the outcome events under study been ascertained comparably between the exposed cohort and the general population?* For events that are identified by means of linkage with death or other registries, under-ascertainment in the cohort can occur more readily than in the general population, since only in the former group do specific persons have to be followed over time and the occurrence of illness or death linked to their identity. For example, a cohort study of possible adverse effects of cosmetic breast implants compared the incidence of breast cancer among women in Alberta, Canada, who had received these implants (and who had no prior history of breast cancer) with that of all adult female Alberta residents (Berkel *et al.*, 1992). The study observed a modest deficit of breast cancer among cohort members, but one possible explanation lay in the fact that follow-up for the occurrence of breast cancer relied on linkage of the identities of these women to the records of the population-based cancer registry serving Alberta. The investigators did not monitor individual cohort members for migration outside the province, or for changes in surname, and so a number of breast cancers diagnosed in these women could have been missed.

The criteria for defining outcome events need to be comparable between the exposed cohort and general population as well. When for both groups the same source of information is used to characterize the events, such as a statement of cause of death on a death certificate, or a report in a cancer or a congenital malformations registry, this comparability is easily achieved. But problems can arise when the information available differs between the groups.

Example 14-4. In a cohort mortality study of United States insulation workers, Selikoff *et al.*

(1980) were particularly interested in deaths from mesothelioma. However, during the period of follow-up in that study, 1967–1976, this malignancy was only beginning to be recognized as such, and it was suspected that some mesothelioma deaths were being attributed to other causes. To address this concern, the investigators sought to obtain medical and pathology records of cohort members who died of cancer, so that they might identify possibly undiagnosed cases of mesothelioma. This strategy did, in fact, uncover nearly one additional mesothelioma death for every one actually listed as such on the death certificate. Nonetheless, since the assessment of excess mortality from mesothelioma was obliged to rely on a comparison of the rates in the cohort with rates in the population as a whole, and since the deaths that composed the numerator of the latter rates did not undergo the same intensive reevaluation, the authors' primary analysis used death certificate information only. The goal of comparability of outcome ascertainment in exposed and unexposed groups was given priority, properly so, over the goal of accuracy of classification of outcome status in just one of the two groups. Use of the revised assignment of cause of death in the insulation workers would be appropriate only for estimating their *absolute* mortality rate from mesothelioma.

2. *To what extent has the rate of illness in the exposed cohort influenced the size of the rate for the population as a whole?* Cohort studies seek to contrast the incidence of illness and/or death in exposed and non-exposed individuals. In most cohort studies that use population rates as a basis for comparison, the contribution of events in exposed persons to the total number in the general population is so small that the population's rate is very similar to that of non-exposed persons. However, if more than a small proportion of the population has been exposed, and if the relative risk associated with exposure is very high, then an appreciable degree of bias can be produced by the use of general population rates as a basis for comparison. Figure 14.1 (taken from Jones and Swerdlow, 1998) illustrates this bias and the circumstances that produce it. If the observed standardized mortality ratio (i.e., relative risk) is below 1.5, little relative bias is present, no matter how common the exposure. If the prevalence of the exposure in the population is less than five percent, only for observed standardized mortality ratios of more than five does the bias exceed 25%.

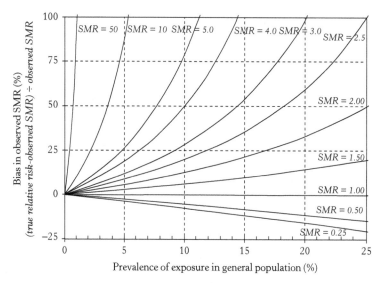

FIGURE 14.1 Bias in observed standardized mortality ratio (SMR) in relation to population prevalence of exposure. (*Source:* Jones and Swerdlow [1998])

3. *On average, are cohort members different from the general population in ways that bear on disease incidence or mortality, beyond differences in those demographic characteristics that are measured in both groups and for which statistical adjustment can be performed?* This question was of concern to William Farr of the British General Register Office, who in the mid-19th century wished to determine if, during peacetime, British soldiers suffered an atypically high mortality rate (Farr, 1979). During 1839–1853, the annual mortality among soldiers averaged 33.0 per 1,000, whereas men of corresponding ages in England and Wales it was but 9.2 per 1,000. Farr pointed out that this difference of nearly 24 per 1,000 actually had to be an *under*estimate of the adverse impact on mortality of being a soldier in peacetime Britain, since

> the mortality of the troops in peacetime ought to be lower than that of civilians. First of all, there was a process of selection involved. Soldiers were "picked lives." They had passed a medical examination at the time of recruitment, while those who failed remained in the general population. Furthermore, men who developed chronic diseases in the army were discharged and reappeared in the civilian ranks.

This incomparability between British soldiers and British men as a whole with regard to their underlying risk of death would nowadays be viewed as an example of confounding. It arises to at least

some degree in most occupational cohort mortality studies that use population death rates for comparison, and has been termed "healthy worker" bias (McMichael, 1976). The two components of this bias that Farr noted—selective recruitment and selective retention—have been given their own designations as well; i.e., "healthy hire effect" and "healthy worker survivor effect" (Arrighi and Hertz-Picciotto, 1996). In the absence of a workplace exposure that has an influence on mortality, persons who are employed would be expected to have a lower death rate than the population in general because, in order to obtain and retain a job, a certain level of good health generally is required. The magnitude of this bias differs among the various causes of death, being greatest for the illnesses for which there is a long interval between the onset of disability and death (such as might be true for chronic obstructive lung disease or multiple sclerosis), and smallest for those that typically produce death rapidly (such as pulmonary embolism). While it is possible for healthy worker bias to be present in cohort studies of disease incidence, in general its magnitude will be considerably smaller than in mortality studies, since hiring and retention are not often strongly influenced by the presence of risk factors for disease incidence. So, for example, while persons disabled by lung cancer or chronic lung disease may be preferentially excluded from many types of employment, generally persons with only a predisposition to these conditions, by virtue of their being cigarette smokers, would not.

If studies of mortality in relation to occupation are based on a comparison of death rates between retirees and the population at large, a bias akin to the healthy worker bias can emerge, though in the opposite direction. This results from the fact that some persons retire because they have developed a condition that can prove fatal, so members of the retired cohort below the typical retirement age will have an over-representation of that condition relative to the demographically comparable population as a whole. In the absence of any negative impact of a particular occupation on mortality, death rates among persons who have retired from that occupation will tend to be higher than those of the population in which they reside.

Example 14-5. In a cohort mortality study intended to estimate potential hazards from asbestos exposure, Enterline *et al.* (1987) ascertained deaths among white men who had retired during 1941–1967 after having been production or maintenance employees of a United States asbestos products company. Cause-specific mortality rates were compared to those of American white men as a whole. In order to minimize bias that likely would arise from an over-representation in the exposed group of men who had retired due to ill health, the investigators restricted their analysis to the person-time that accrued in each of the men after he had turned 65 years of age. This was the age that retirement would have been anticipated for all men in this industry, healthy or not.

When rates of illness or death are compared between patients who have received a specific medical intervention and the population as a whole—perhaps to assess the presence of adverse effects associated with that intervention—two particular sources of potential bias commonly must be considered:

1. *Could the condition that necessitated the treatment itself have an impact on the incidence of the disease(s) being studied?* Solely from a comparison of treated patients and the population in general, it would not be possible to disentangle the impact of the treatment from that of the illness that necessitated the treatment. So, for example, when mortality from a variety of causes was observed to be higher in British patients prescribed an H2 blocker, cimetidine, during the first year after the drug had been prescribed, relative to mortality rates in demographically comparable persons in England and Wales (Colin-Jones *et al.*, 1983), the interpretation was ambiguous: Either the drug, or the conditions that led to the drug being prescribed, or both, could have been responsible. If confounding of this sort (known as "confounding by indication") is likely to be present, it is necessary for the comparison group to comprise persons who have the same condition(s) as the treated cohort, but who are treated in a different way or not treated at all (Weiss, 2006).

2. *At the time treatment was being considered, were members of the treated group evaluated for the presence of a condition, with only those* not *having the condition allowed to receive the treatment?* A comparison of the subsequent incidence of this condition between the treated patients and the population at large—most of whom would probably not have received such an evaluation—would give rise to "healthy screenee bias"; i.e., a spuriously low rate in the patient group (Weiss and Rossing, 1996). For example, women who receive cosmetic breast implants would be expected to have a lower incidence of breast cancer following implantation than women in general, even if this treatment had no anti-carcinogenic effect at all. This would result from the fact that all the treated women, but only some in the comparison group, would have had a thorough breast evaluation around the time the implant was being considered, and only those believed not to have breast cancer could go on to have (by definition) a "cosmetic" implant.

Because population rates as a basis for comparison have some attractive features—and, often, because there is no better alternative available!—epidemiologists have developed strategies to minimize the healthy worker and healthy screenee biases. The primary one involves omitting from the analysis the part of the follow-up experience of exposed individuals that is most susceptible to these biases; i.e., that which accrues relatively soon after exposure status is defined. The actual length of time chosen will differ from study to study, depending on the suspected duration of the incomparability between the exposed cohort and the comparison population. For example, most screen-detectable breast cancers (which are likely to be more prevalent among women in general than in women who have just received a cosmetic breast implant) are expected to progress to clinically evident disease within 2–3 years. Thus, a comparison with population rates that is more likely to be valid (assuming no other forms of bias are present) would tabulate rates of breast cancer among cosmetic implant recipients starting about three years after their surgery. In an occupational cohort mortality study, outcome events and person-time that accrue during the period immediately following the point in time that the criteria for exposure have been met could be deleted from the analysis. The duration of this period would depend on the investigators' perception of the typical duration of disability prior to death from the causes of death of particular interest.

FOLLOW-UP OF COHORT MEMBERS

Ideally, a cohort study will be able to completely enumerate all relevant health outcomes that occur among study participants, and also determine for all participants whether follow-up has been truncated (due to death, or to migration beyond the reach of the follow-up mechanisms). If the duration of follow-up is quite short—e.g., a few hours, perhaps during an assessment of rapidly developing adverse effects of various anesthetic agents—then it might be possible to meet this ideal. In most cohort studies, however, when the period of follow-up extends from months to decades, ascertainment of both the numerator and the denominator of the rate of illness or death will be incomplete to at least some extent, allowing for the possibility of bias. If the degree of under-ascertainment is relatively modest, and is present to a comparable extent for exposed and non-exposed persons, the bias will be small or absent. But as the degree of under-ascertainment grows—especially if it is present for only the exposed individuals, as in a study that compares the morbidity or mortality of these persons to that of the population as a whole—then the validity of the results will be increasingly threatened.

The means by which outcome events are enumerated in cohort members depends upon the specific outcome(s) of interest and the resources available in the setting in which the study is done. In the United States, deaths in 1979 and later among study subjects can be identified by means of linkage with the National Death Index (Bilgrad, 1990), whereas in some parts of the world, death certificates are not made available for health research. In Scandinavia, cohort studies of cancer incidence routinely rely on population-based registries to determine the development of cancer in specified individuals. In contrast, the *absence* of cancer registries that serve the entire population in which cohort members reside for most or all of the period of follow-up

has obliged cohort studies done in many other parts of the world to rely on cancer mortality as an outcome, rather than cancer incidence. The occurrence of a number of outcomes of potential interest (e.g., urinary tract infections, rheumatic diseases, smoking cessation) are not ascertained routinely by any sort of registry. Their identification would require conducting a review of medical records, or an interview with or measurement upon individual cohort members. Studies that utilize records, interviews, and/or measurements as a means of assessing illness occurrence need to take particular care to develop standardized criteria for the presence of outcome events, and need to apply these criteria without knowledge of each subject's exposure status.

Example 14-6.   As part of a prospective cohort study of 115,886 American nurses, Manson *et al.* (1990) examined the possible influence of obesity on the incidence of coronary heart disease. After enrollment in 1976, participants were queried every two years regarding the development of a myocardial infarction or angina pectoris. (The occurrence of fatal cases was ascertained by means of the National Death Index.) Medical records were sought for each woman who responded affirmatively regarding one or both conditions. Using these records, physicians (who were blinded to the presence or absence of a women's weight and other possible risk factors) applied a standard set of criteria to judge whether a woman had sustained a myocardial infarction or had developed angina pectoris.

In order to determine for each cohort member the amount of person-time that he/she is contributing to the denominator of the incidence rate, in many studies it is necessary to monitor periodically that person's whereabouts. In the Nurses' Health Study, the return of the biennial questionnaire serves to ascertain not only the development of relevant outcomes, but also that the woman is still reachable to report such outcomes if they were to occur. (As mentioned earlier, this questionnaire also elicits updated information on exposure status.) There are instances in which it is likely that all outcomes that occur in cohort members will be ascertained through a reliable linkage procedure with a database that covers a geographic area outside of which migration is expected to be minimal; e.g., the United States National Death Index or a cancer registry in a Nordic country. In such an instance, no additional follow-up is needed beyond the linkage procedure. However, there are other circumstances in which considerable resources need to be devoted to tracking study participants (Bender *et al.*, 2006).

Example 14-7. Hagan *et al.* (2001) sought to assess determinants of the acquisition of hepatitis C virus (HCV) infection among intravenous drug users (IDUs). They obtained information on patterns of drug use and other potential risk factors from a group of HCV-seronegative IDUs. Cohort members then were followed for a period of one year, at which time a blood sample and additional interview information was to be obtained. To arrange for the blood-drawing, and re-interview, letters were mailed to the address given at the outset, but if there was no response, the investigators tried calling the participant and (if necessary) persons whose phone numbers had been provided by the participant at the beginning of the study. In addition, censuses of the county jail and of drug treatment facilities were checked for the presence of any cohort members, as were state prison and death records.

On occasion, criteria for eligibility of persons to serve as cohort members are tailored to maximize the likelihood of successful follow-up. For example, in the cohort study of aircraft maintenance workers in Utah (see Example 14-2), persons who had been employed at the facility for less than one year were not included. Such persons would be expected to be relatively mobile, residentially, and thus the most likely to have left the state during the follow-up period. Since one of the means of identifying health outcomes in this study was the Utah Cancer Registry, including the short-term workers would have led, for cancer incidence, to a relatively lower level of follow-up. Restriction of the cohort to aircraft maintenance workers of one year or longer also had the desirable feature of excluding workers whose cumulative exposures to TCE would very likely have been quite low.

NATURE OF THE ILLNESS OUTCOME: PREVALENCE VERSUS INCIDENCE

Some studies compare, not the occurrence of an illness between persons who have and have not had a given exposure, but rather the presence of that condition at a specified point in time. Such studies (termed "cross-sectional" because they have no longitudinal component) often are done to investigate possible harmful effects of the work environment, by examining employed persons with different levels or types of exposure on the job. Examples are studies of lung function in pipe coverers in 1940s shipyards who had been exposed to asbestos to varying degrees (Fleischer *et al.*, 1946), or studies of musculoskeletal disorders in persons whose work requires repetitive and/or forceful movements of the hand and wrist (Silverstein *et al.*, 1987). However, a cross-sectional study will not give a valid result if persons whose health has been impaired by their occupational exposure(s) are no longer employed when the study is done. For example, the investigation conducted in the shipyard (Fleischer *et al.*, 1946) observed the prevalence of asbestosis not to be elevated among pipe coverers who had sustained a substantial exposure to asbestos. It is highly likely that selective retirement of men whose health already had been compromised by their asbestos exposure led to a result that falsely minimized the occurrence of asbestosis associated with this occupation.

FREQUENCY OF THE OUTCOME EVENT: IS A GIVEN COHORT LARGE ENOUGH TO CONTRIBUTE USEFUL ETIOLOGICAL INFORMATION FOR A RARE ILLNESS?

In the wake of the development of the hypothesis that *in utero* exposure to diethylstilbestrol (DES) could predispose to the occurrence of clear cell adenocarcinoma of the vagina 15–20 years later, Lanier *et al.* (1973) conducted a cohort study. They identified 804 female infants whose mother had been prescribed an estrogen (primarily DES) while pregnant with them.

Telephone interviews, mailed questionnaires, and/or review of medical records obtained 11–30 years later on these girls and women failed to identify a single case of vaginal adenocarcinoma. This negative finding should not be interpreted as indicating the true absence of an association, but rather as an instance in which the occurrence of the disease, even among exposed individuals, was too low to allow identification of an association in an "undersized" cohort. (The cumulative incidence of clear cell adenocarcinoma of the vagina subsequently has been estimated to be about one per 1,000 girls exposed *in utero* to DES.)

As illustrated by the above example, one potential limitation of cohort studies can relate to the relatively small number of outcome events that may occur during follow-up of a particular study population, and to the resulting statistical imprecision of the results. However, with the increasing availability over the years of automated data systems on large, defined populations, cohort studies increasingly are able to address the etiologies of even quite-rare conditions.

Example 14-8. Using data from the Danish Civil Registration System, Madsen *et al.* (2002) enumerated the 537,303 children born in Denmark during 1991–1998. Among these children, Danish National Board of Health Records revealed that 82% had subsequently received the measles, mumps, and rubella (MMR) vaccine. The occurrence of autism in these children was ascertained using records of the Danish Psychiatric Central Register. A total 316 cases of autistic disorder were identified, the incidence being nearly identical in children who did and those who did not receive vaccination against MMR (relative risk = 0.92, 95% confidence interval = 0.68–1.24).

Clearly, being able to address (by means of a cohort study) the important question of the safety of MMR was greatly facilitated by the existence of national data files that identify the cohort, as well as the receipt of MMR and the occurrence of autism among cohort members.

Similar to some randomized trials of uncommon outcomes, cohort studies of relatively rare events may assess strong predictors of these events ("surrogate" outcomes) among their study participants. For example, Agot *et al.* (2007) wished to learn if the favorable results of randomized trials of adult circumcision in relation to HIV acquisition generalized to men outside the settings of these trials. Specifically, they were concerned that in the community at large, receipt of circumcision might be followed by "behavioral disinhibition" with higher risk activities in circumcised men negating the suspected lower biological susceptibility to HIV afforded by circumcision. In their cohort study in Kenya, the relatively small number of young adult men undergoing circumcision ($n = 324$) and relatively short follow-up period (one year) meant that it was unlikely that the study would be able to reliably document a lower incidence of new HIV infection compared to that among participants who chose to remain uncircumcised. Thus, the study of Agot *et al.* assessed (by means of periodic interviews during follow-up) a history of unprotected sexual intercourse, number of sexual partners, etc. To the extent that the interview information was accurate, their observation of a similar frequency of "high risk" activities between men who had previously chosen, or not chosen, to be circumcised argues that, in Kenya, the biological resistance to HIV infection that circumcision confers is not likely to be overridden by changes in the behavior of circumcised men.

ISSUES IN THE ANALYSIS AND INTERPRETATION OF COHORT STUDIES

1. *For purposes of analysis, how soon after exposure should outcome events that occur in cohort members begin to be counted?*

Generally, the answer to this question is "immediately," in order to capture the full range of consequences of the exposure. An exception would be made if "healthy worker" bias or "healthy screenee" bias were anticipated (see pp. 326–327). Another exception would be made if there were reasons to believe that persons in whom the diagnosis was made very early in the following period had that disease present in an occult form before exposure commenced. While the presence of the disease in those persons could not have been affected by the exposure, it could possibly have influenced the likelihood of receipt of exposure, or the presence or level of a characteristic under study. In this situation, a more valid analysis would exclude cases (and the associated person-time) for a long enough period of time after the beginning of follow-up to allow for most or all of these prevalent-but-undetected cases to have been diagnosed.

Example 14-9. A number of studies have observed the incidence of colon cancer to be relatively high among persons with relatively low levels of serum cholesterol. However, in an analysis of the combined results of these studies (Law and Thompson, 1991), the increased risk was confined to the first two years of follow-up: No association was present once cases diagnosed in the first two years after the serum sample had been drawn were excluded. Since it is unlikely that an elevated serum cholesterol value could influence the development of a colon tumor so rapidly, and then not over the longer term, it seems more probable that the presence of the tumor or its antecedent pathology led to metabolic changes that resulted in, on average, a reduction in serum cholesterol. Figure 14.2 depicts the patterns of results that would, and would not, tend to support the hypothesis that a low serum cholesterol (or another metabolic characteristic with which it is correlated) is

(A) Pattern of results in support of an etiological role for serum
    cholesterol:

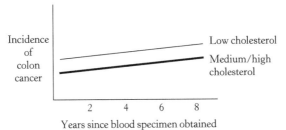

(B) Pattern of results in support of the hypothesis that colon cancer
    depresses serum cholesterol:

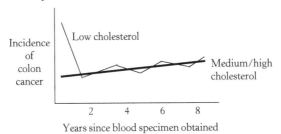

FIGURE 14.2 Does a low serum cholesterol predispose to colon cancer, or does the presence of cancer cause a lowering of serum cholesterol?

a cause of colon cancer. To avoid being influenced by "reverse causality," an analysis would simply ignore diagnoses and person-time that accrued during the early part of the period of follow-up.

Example 14-10. Because administration of phenobarbital was known to lead to tumor development in mice, Clemmesen and Hjalgrim-Jensen (1981) sought to determine the impact of long-term use of this drug in humans. They identified 8,077 Danes who had been hospitalized for treatment with an anticonvulsive agent during 1933–1963, most of whom would have received phenobarbital while hospitalized and for a long period of time thereafter. With the help of records from the Danish tumor registry, they sought to identify brain tumors that arose in cohort members through 1976. Table 14.1 describes the results of the study.

While the observed association was very strong during the first 10–15 years of follow-up, it is unlikely that much of it reflects a causal role of phenobarbital in the development of brain tumors: 1) It would be an unusual carcinogen that predisposed to a brain tumor in the first 10–15 years after exposure but scarcely at all after that time; and 2) An alternative noncausal hypothesis is highly plausible—that the presence of an undiagnosed brain tumor led to a seizure disorder, which in turn led to treatment with anticonvulsants. In the era before intracranial imaging techniques became available, often seizure patients would have a brain tumor identified as the likely basis for their disorder some years after the onset of the seizures. Of course, there will be uncertainty regarding precisely what period of time after initiating anticonvulsant medication should be excluded when interpreting these data. Nonetheless, it seems likely that the relative risks observed 15–19 and > 20 years (1.8 and 1.9, respectively) are a better indication of the possible capacity of phenobarbital use to cause brain tumors in humans than the relative risk of 11.6 observed during the first decade of follow-up.

2. How are changes in the exposure status of cohort members handled?

Persons with a history of occupational exposure to asbestos are at an increased risk of mesothelioma. It has been observed in cohort studies that several decades are required for the inhalation of asbestos fibers (and the body's response to them) to lead to the development of mesothelioma. Additional asbestos inhalation by persons whose occupational exposure had begun several decades earlier does not appear to contribute to risk in any substantial way during his/her maximum lifespan (Peto *et al.*, 1982). In retrospect, if no attempt had been made to characterize more recent asbestos exposures once the criteria for the presence of the initial exposures had been met, the validity of studies of the incidence of mesothelioma among these persons would not have been compromised to any appreciable degree. In contrast, if in this same cohort one had been studying the impact of the combination of cigarette smoking and asbestos exposure on the risk of lung cancer, it would have been important to obtain updated information on smoking status during the entire period of follow-up. This is because of the beneficial influence that smoking cessation exerts on lung cancer incidence among cigarette smokers without a history of occupational exposure to asbestos (Hammond, 1966).

Some cohort studies ascertain exposure status only when subjects are first enrolled, so they are not able to consider the issue of changes in the presence or level of exposure. For example, some 1.2 million persons were enrolled in a cohort study conducted by the American Cancer Society, in which mortality rates during a 14-year follow-up period were related to characteristics and exposures reported on a questionnaire at the start of the study. Using these data, Calle *et al.* (1999) examined the association of body mass index with mortality from all causes combined. Other cohort studies of BMI and disease have obtained updated information on exposure status during the follow-up period, and conducted analyses that took account of this additional information. For example, in the Nurses' Health Study, participants were asked about their weight and height every two years, and in their analysis of the relationship of BMI to the incidence of coronary heart disease, Manson *et al.* (1990) recategorized women after each additional questionnaire was returned. Thus, the person-time contribution of a woman to the denominator

of the incidence rate (and to the numerator, if coronary disease occurred) could be made to more than one BMI category as the follow-up continued. For characteristics such as BMI that do change over time, and for outcome events whose occurrence is sensitive to relatively recent exposure status, being able to take into account the updated data can serve to reduce exposure misclassification. (If there is a suspected "lag" between the presence of an exposure and its impact on disease occurrence, analyses also can be done in which the suspected induction time is ignored—see Rothman *et al.*, (2008, pp. 102–106), for details.)

Among exposed cohort members, duration of exposure often increases with continuing follow-up. For example, among a group of persons with a given occupational exposure whose death rates are being monitored, those who continue on the job generally will increase their duration of exposure to one or more agents present in that workplace, while those who quit or retire will not. Duration of exposure is a central feature of the analysis of many cohort studies, but some care must be taken in order not to bias that analysis. Specifically, cohort members can not be permitted to contribute events to the numerator of a rate, nor person-time to the denominator, until they meet the criteria for a particular category of duration. If, for example, one wished to determine the mortality rate from a particular disease in employees of at least 10 years' duration, only illnesses and person-time that took place beginning at 10 years from first employment would enter the calculation. Person-time in these individuals would not begin at the time of first employment, since, by definition, none of these persons could have died during the ensuing 10 years! In a comparison of mortality in workers with an occupational exposure of <10 and ≥10 years duration, only data gathered beginning 10 years after the date of first employment of *any* study subject would enter into the analysis. A similar

TABLE 14.1.

Time since first hospitalization (yrs.)	Malignant brain tumors		
	Observed	Expected	Relative risk
<10	45	3.87	11.6
10–14	13	2.42	5.4
15–19	4	2.28	1.8
>20	9	4.79	1.9

sort of "immortal time bias" is encountered occasionally in pharmacoepidemiologic studies as well (Suissa, 2008).

CONCLUSION

To the extent that they can ascertain exposure status prior to disease occurrence, cohort studies have been and will remain indispensable for evaluating the impact of exposures whose presence or magnitude cannot be retrospectively ascertained in a valid way. Despite the complexities that sometimes arise in the design and conduct of cohort studies, their longitudinal nature—begining with exposure status, then documenting disease occurrence—makes them relatively easy to understand.

Because this longitudinal character is shared with randomized controlled trials, epidemiologists reporting the results of those studies have an obligation to remind their audience (and themselves!) of the limitations of their studies that are imposed by the absence of randomization. They must not lose sight of the fact that associations between exposure and disease that are observed in cohort studies, even when it is clear that the exposure has preceded the presence of disease, are not necessarily causal associations.

Example 14-11. Greenberg *et al.* (1996) conducted a randomized controlled trial in which 1,720 patients with non-melanotic skin cancer were assigned to receive either 50 mg. per day of beta-carotene or a placebo. During the follow-up period (median of 4.3 years), total mortality was identical in the two groups (relative risk = 1.0, 95% confidence interval = 0.8–1.3), as was mortality from the two major cause-of-death categories, cardiovascular disease and cancer. However, plasma beta-carotene measured at entry into the study was inversely related to mortality: Relative to the death rate of subjects in the lowest fourth of the distribution of plasma beta-carotene, mortality among persons in the second, third, and upper fourth was 0.7, 0.6, and 0.6, respectively, adjusted for age, sex, BMI, and history of cigarette smoking. These estimates were reasonably statistically precise; for example, the 95% confidence interval of the relative risk for persons in the highest fourth of the distribution was 0.4–0.9. Since the dose of beta-carotene use in the study produced approximately a 10-fold increase in the beta-carotene levels compared to those prior to treatment, and since the administration of beta-carotene clearly had

no impact on mortality rates, it seems almost certain that the association observed between low levels of beta-carotene and mortality does not reflect a cause–effect relationship, at least in the short term. After seeing the results of their study, Greenberg, *et al.* concluded as follows: "Although the possibility exists that beta-carotene supplementation produces benefits that are too small or too delayed to have been detected in this study, non-causal explanations should be sought for the association between plasma concentrations of beta-carotene and diminished death."

REFERENCES

Agot KE, Kiarie JN, Nguyen HQ, Odhiambo JO, Onyango TM, Weiss NS. Male circumcision in Siaya and Bondo Districts, Kenya: prospective cohort study to assess behavioral disinhibition following circumcision. J Acquir Immune Defic Syndr 2007; 44:66–70.

Allebeck P, Allgulander C, Fisher LD. Predictors of completed suicide in a cohort of 50,465 young men: role of personality and deviant behavior. Br Med J 1988; 297:76–78.

Arrighi HM, Hertz-Picciotto IH. Controlling the healthy worker survivor effect: an example of arsenic exposure and respiratory cancer. Occup Environ Med 1996; 53:455–462.

Beasley RP, Lin CC, Hwang LY, Chen CS. Hepatocellular carcinoma and hepatitis B virus. Lancet 1981; 2:1129–1133.

Bender R, Jockel KH, Trautner C, Spraul M, Berger M. Effect of age on excess mortality in obesity. JAMA 1999; 281:1498–1504.

Bender TJ, Beall C, Cheng H, Herrick RF, Kahn AR, Matthews R, *et al.* Methodologic issues in follow-up studies of cancer incidence among occupational groups in the United States. Ann Epidemiol 2006; 16:170–179.

Berkel H, Birdsell DC, Jenkins H. Breast augmentation: a risk factor for breast cancer? N Engl J Med 1992; 326:1649–1653.

Bilgrad R. National Death Index User's Manual. DHHS Pub. No. (PHS) 90-1148. Washington, D.C.: U.S. Department of Health and Human Services, 1990.

Blair A, Hartge P, Stewart PA, McAdams M, Lubin J. Mortality and cancer incidence of aircraft maintenance workers exposed to trichloroethylene and other organic solvents and chemicals: extended follow up. Occup Environ Med 1998; 55:161–171.

Calle EE, Thun MJ, Petrelli JM, Rodriguez C, Heath CW Jr. Body-mass index and mortality in a prospective cohort of U.S. adults. N Engl J Med 1999; 341:1097–1105.

Caughey AB, Nicholson JM, Cheng YW, Lyell DJ, Washington AE. Induction of labor and cesarean delivery by gestational age. Am J Obstet Gynecol 2006; 195:700–705.

Checkoway H, Eisen EA. Developments in occupational cohort studies. Epidemiol Rev 1998; 20:100–111.

Clarke R, Shipley M, Lewington S, Youngman L, Collins R, Marmot M, et al. Underestimation of risk associations due to regression dilution in long-term follow-up of prospective studies. Am J Epidemiol 1999; 150:341–353.

Clemmesen J, Hjalgrim-Jensen S. Does phenobarbital cause intracranial tumors? A follow-up through 35 years. Ecotoxicol Environ Saf 1981; 5:255–260.

Colin-Jones DG, Langman MJ, Lawson DH, Vessey MP. Postmarketing surveillance of the safety of cimetidine: 12 month mortality report. Br Med J (Clin Res Ed) 1983; 286:1713–1716.

Court-Brown WM, Doll R. Leukemia and aplastic anaemia in patients irradiated for ankylosing spondylitis. Medical Research Council Special Report Series No. 295. London: Her Majesty's Stationery Office, 1957.

Darby SC, Whitley E, Howe GR, Hutchins SJ, Kuisiak RA, Lubin JH, et al. Radon and cancers other than lung cancer in underground miners: a collaborative analysis of 11 studies. J Natl Cancer Inst 1995; 87:378–384.

Dawber TR, Kannel WB, Lyell LP. An approach to longitudinal studies in a community: The Framingham Study. Ann NY Acad Sci 1963; 107:539–556.

Dublin S, Lydon-Rochelle M, Kaplan RC, Watts DH, Critchlow CW. Maternal and neonatal outcomes after induction of labor without an identified indication. Am J Obstet Gynecol 2000; 183: 986–994.

Enterline PE, Hartley J, Henderson V. Asbestos and cancer: a cohort followed up to death. Br J Ind Med 1987; 44:396–401.

Farr W. Quoted in: Eyler EM. Victorian social medicine. Baltimore: Johns Hopkins University Press, 1979. p. 163

Fleischer WE, Viles FJ, Gode RL. A health survey of pipe covering occupations in construction naval vessels. J Ind Hyg Toxicol 1946; 28:9–16.

Fulton-Kehoe D, Rossing MA, Rutter C, Mandelson MT, Weiss NS. Use of antidepressant medications in relation to the incidence of breast cancer. Br J Cancer 2006; 94:1071–1078.

Gardner MJ. Considerations in the choice of expected numbers for appropriate comparisons in occupational cohort studies. Med Lav 1986; 77:23–47.

Giovanucci E, Ascherio A, Rimm EB, Colditz GA, Stampfer MJ, Willett WC. A prospective cohort study of vasectomy and prostate cancer in U.S. men. JAMA 1993; 269:873–877.

Goldberg J, True WR, Eisen SA, Henderson WG. A twin study of the effects of the Vietnam War on posttraumatic stress disorder. JAMA 1990; 263:1227–1232.

Goldhaber SZ, Grodstein F, Stampfer MJ, Manson JE, Colditz GA, Speizer FE, et al. A prospective study of risk factors for pulmonary embolism in women. JAMA 1997; 277:642–645.

Greenberg ER, Baron JA, Karagas MR, Stukel TA, Nierenberg DW, Stevens MM, et al. Mortality associated with low plasma concentration of beta carotene and the effect of oral supplementation. JAMA 1996; 275:699–703.

Hagan H, Thiede H, Weiss NS, Hopkins SG, Duchin JS, Alexander ER. Sharing of drug preparation equipment as a risk factor for hepatitis C virus incidence. Am J Public Health 2001; 91:23–27.

Hammond EC. Smoking in relation to the death rates of one million men and women. J Natl Cancer Inst 1966; Monograph #19:127–204.

Harvey EB, Boice JD, Honeyman M, Flannery JT. Prenatal x-ray exposure and childhood cancer in twins. N Engl J Med 1985; 312:541–545.

Jick H, Vasilakis C, Weinrauchand LA, Meier CR, Jick SS, Derby LE. A population-based study of appetite-suppressant drugs and the risk of cardiac-valve regurgitation. N Engl J Med 1998; 339:719–727.

Jones ME, Swerdlow AJ. Bias in the standardized mortality ratio when using general population rates to estimate expected number of deaths. Am J Epidemiol 1998; 148:1012–1017.

Kahn HA. The Dorn study of smoking and mortality among US veterans: Report on eight and one-half years of observation. NCI Monograph 1966; 19:1–125.

Kannel WB, Castelli WP, Gordon T, McNamara PM. Serum cholesterol, lipoproteins, and the risk of coronary heart disease. The Framingham Study. Ann Intern Med 1971; 74:1–12.

Kelman CW, Kortt MA, Becker NG, Li Z, Mathews JD, Guest CS, et al. Deep vein thrombosis and air travel: record linkage study. BMJ 2003; 327:1072.

Klag MJ, Ford DE, Mead LA, He J, Whelton PK, Liang KY, et al. Serum cholesterol in young men and subsequent cardiovascular disease. N Engl J Med 1993; 328:313–318.

Kurth T, Gaziano JM, Rexrode KM, Kase CS, Cook NR, Manson JE, et al. Prospective study of body mass index and risk of stroke in apparently healthy women. Circulation 2005; 111:1992–1998.

Lanier AP, Noller KL, Decker DG, Elveback LR, Kurland LT. Cancer and stilbestrol. A follow-up of 1,719 persons exposed to estrogens in utero and born 1943–1959. Mayo Clin Proc 1973; 48:793–799.

Law MR, Thompson SG. Low serum cholesterol and the risk of cancer: an analysis of the published prospective studies. Cancer Causes Control 1991; 2:253–261.

Lee IM, Paffenbarger RS Jr. Physical activity and stroke incidence: the Harvard Alumni Health Study. Stroke 1998; 29:2049–2054.

Linet MS, Freedman DM, Mohan AK, Doody MM, Ron E, Mabuchi K, *et al.* Incidence of haematopoietic malignancies in US radiologic technologists. Occup Environ Med 2005; 62:861–867.

Lynge E, Thygesen L. Primary liver cancer among women in laundry and dry cleaning work in Denmark. Scand J Work Environ Health 1990; 16:108–112.

Madsen KM, Hviid A, Vestergaard M, Schendel D, Wohlfahrt J, Thorsen P, *et al.* A population-based study of measles, mumps, and rubella vaccination and autism. N Engl J Med 2002; 347: 1477–1482.

Manson JE, Colditz GA, Stampfer MJ, Willett WC, Rosner B, Monson R, *et al.* A prospective study of obesity and risk of coronary heart disease. N Engl J Med 1990; 322:882–889.

McMichael AJ. Standardized mortality ratios and the "healthy worker effect": scratching below the surface. J Occup Med 1976; 18:165–168.

Nienhuis H, Goldacre M, Seagroatt V, Gill L, Veseey M. Incidence of disease after vasectomy: a record linkage retrospective cohort study. Br Med J 1992; 304:743–746.

Persson I, Yuen J, Bergkvist L, Schairer C. Cancer incidence and mortality in women receiving estrogen and estrogen-progestin replacement therapy. Int J Cancer 1996; 67:327–332.

Petitti DB, Klein R, Kipp H, Friedman GD. Vasectomy and the incidence of hospitalized illness. J Urology 1983; 129:760–762.

Peto J, Seidman H, Selikoff IJ. Mesothelioma mortality in asbestos workers: Implications for models of carcinogenesis and risk assessment. Br J Cancer 1982; 45:124–135.

Rahu M, Rahu K, Auvinen A, Tekkel M, Stengrevics A, Hakulinen T, *et al.* Cancer risk among Chernobyl cleanup workers in Estonia and Latvia, 1986–1998. Int J Cancer 2006; 119:162–168.

Rinsky RA, Zumwalder RD, Waxweiler RJ, Murray WE, Bierman PJ, Landrigan PJ, *et al.* Cancer mortality at a naval nuclear shipyard. Lancet 1981; 1:231–235.

Ron E, Modan B, Boice JD Jr. Mortality from cancer and other causes following radiotherapy for ringworm of the scalp. Am J Epidemiol 1988; 127:713–725.

Roscoe RJ, Deddens JA, Salvan A, Schnorr TM. Mortality among Navajo uranium miners. Am J Public Health 1995; 85:535–540.

Rothman KJ, Greenland S, Lash TL. Modern epidemiology (3rd ed.). Philadelphia: Lippincott Williams & Wilkins, 2008.

Selikoff IJ, Hammond EC, Seidman H. Latency of asbestos disease among insulation workers in the United States and Canada. Cancer 1980; 46:2736–2740.

Seltser R, Sartwell PE. The influence of occupational exposure to radiation on the mortality of American radiologists and other medical specialists. Am J Epidemiol 1965; 81:2–22.

Sesso HD, Paffenbarger RS Jr, Lee IM. Physical activity and breast cancer risk in the College Alumni Health Study (United States). Cancer Causes Control 1998; 9:433–439.

Shimizu Y, Kato H, Schull WJ. Studies of the mortality of A-bomb survivors. 1950–1985. Part 2. Cancer mortality based on the recently revised doses. Radiation Res 1990; 121:120–141.

Silverstein BA, Fine LJ, Armstrong TJ. Occupational factors and carpal tunnel syndrome. Am J Ind Med 1987; 11:343–358.

Suissa S. Immortal time bias in pharmaco-epidemiology. Am J Epidemiol 2008; 167:492–499.

Tyroler HA, Heyden S, Bartel A, Cassel J, Cornoni JC, Hames CG, *et al.* Blood pressure and cholesterol as coronary heart disease risk factors. Arch Intern Med 1971; 128:907–914.

Velentgas P, Daling JR, Malone KE, Weiss NS, Williams MA, Self SG, *et al.* Pregnancy after breast carcinoma: outcomes and influence on mortality. Cancer 1999; 85:2424–2432.

Walker AM, Jick H, Hunter JR, Danford A, Rothman KJ. Hospitalization rates in vasectomized men. JAMA 1981; 245:2315–2317.

Weiss NS. Clinical epidemiology: the study of the outcome of illness (3rd ed.). New York: Oxford, 2006.

Weiss NS, Rossing MA. Healthy screenee bias in epidemiologic studies of cancer incidence. Epidemiology 1996; 7:319–322.

White E, Hunt JR, Casso D. Exposure measurement in cohort studies: the challenges of prospective data collection. Epidemiol Rev 1998; 20:43–56.

EXERCISES

1. Roscoe *et al.* (1995) enumerated deaths from 1960–1990 among 757 Navajo uranium miners in the south-

TABLE 14.2. SURVIVAL FROM BREAST CANCER* BY NUMBER OF SUBSEQUENT PREGNANCIES

No. of pregnancies following diagnosis	No. of patients	%	Survival (%)		
			3 years	5 years	10 years
0	83	76.2	86.7	72.8	58.5
1+	26	23.8	96.2	96.2	84.1
Total	109	100.0	89.0	78.5	64.7

* Survival from date of diagnosis of breast cancer

TABLE 14.3. STANDARDIZED MORTALITY RATIO IN PATIENTS HOSPITALIZED FOR OBESITY

Gender	Age range	Person-years	No. of deaths	SMR	95% CI	p-value
Men	18–29	5,109	36	2.46	1.72–3.41	<.001
	30–39	3,425	63	2.30	1.77–2.95	<.001
	40–49	3,297	105	1.99	1.62–2.40	<.001
	50–74	7,483	161	1.31	1.11–1.52	.001
	TOTAL	19,314	365	1.67	1.51–1.85	<.001
Women	18–29	13,661	31	1.81	1.23–2.57	.003
	30–39	10,139	85	2.10	1.68–2.60	<.001
	40–49	10,916	176	1.70	1.46–1.97	<.001
	50–74	25,305	371	1.26	1.13–1.39	<.001
	TOTAL	60,021	663	1.45	1.34–1.57	<.001

Source: Bender *et al.* (1999)

western United States. They estimated standardized mortality ratios, using the combined New Mexico and Arizona non-white mortality rates as a basis for comparison. In this study, there was a low standardized mortality ratio, not only for cirrhosis of the liver (0.5, 95% confidence interval = 0.2–0.7), usually an alcohol-related disease, but for "alcoholism" (SMR = 0.4, 95% confidence interval = 0.1–1.1) as well. What do you believe to be the most likely explanation for the reduced mortality from these two causes among the Navajo uranium miners?

2. Among 22,597 Swedish women to whom non-contraceptive hormone therapy had been prescribed during 1977–80 and who had not previously been diagnosed with cancer, Persson *et al.* (1996) found that 102 died from breast cancer through 1991. Based on the mortality rate from breast cancer among the Swedish female population of the same ages during the same period of time, 195.9 breast cancer deaths would have been expected (relative risk = 0.5, 95% confidence interval = 0.4–0.6).

It is likely that this study underestimated the size of the true relative risk relating hormone use to mortality from breast cancer. Why?

3. Most epidemiologists seeking to assess the impact of the cessation of cigarette smoking on a person's risk of death have excluded from consideration both deaths and person-time during the first year after a study participant stops smoking. What do you believe to be the rationale behind this?

4. The following is excerpted from an investigation of the possible influence of pregnancy following breast cancer in young women on the likelihood of survival:

One or more pregnancies occurred in approximately one-quarter of our patients. The age distributions of women who did and did not have a subsequent pregnancy were similar. Patients with subsequent pregnancies had an excellent prognosis [see Table 14.2].

Beyond the possible beneficial influence of pregnancy itself on survival, what are the two most likely explanations for the observed association?

5. The following is a portion of an abstract of an article (Bender *et al.*, 1999), along with Table 14.3, derived from that article.

TABLE 14.4. OBSERVED AND EXPECTED NUMBERS OF FIRST VENOUS THROMBOEMBOLISM EVENTS BY TIME IN DAYS SINCE MOST RECENT FLIGHT ARRIVAL

Traveler category	Days since most recent flight arrival				
	0–14	15–30	31–60	61–100	Total
Observed	46.0	23.0	32.0	52.0	153.0
Expected (A)	102.6	113.2	212.3	283.0	711.1
Expected (B)	22.1	24.4	45.7	60.9	153.0

Context: The effect of age on excess mortality from all causes associated with obesity is controversial. Few studies have investigated the association between body mass index (BMI), age, and mortality, with sufficient numbers of subjects at all levels of obesity.

Objective: To assess the effect of age on the excess mortality associated with all degrees of obesity.

Design: Prospective cohort study.

Setting and Participants: A total of 6,193 obese patients with mean (SD) BMI of 36.6 (6.1) kg/m^2 and mean ($\pm$SD) age of 40.4 (12.9) years who had been referred to the obesity clinic of Heinrich-Heine University, Dusseldorf, Germany, between 1961 and 1994. Median follow-up time was 14.8 years.

Main Outcome Measure: All-cause mortality through 1994 among 6,053 patients for whom follow-up data were available (1,028 deaths) analyzed as standardized mortality ratios (SMRs) using the male-female population of the geographic region (North Rhine Westphalia) as reference.

Results: The cohort was grouped into approximate quartiles according to age (18–29, 30–39, 40–49, and 50–74 years) and BMI (25 to <32, 32 to <36, 36 to <40, and >40 kg/m^2) at baseline. The SMRs showed a significant excess mortality with an SMR for men of 1.67 (95% confidence interval, 1.51–1.85; $p < .001$) and an SMR for women of 1.45 (95% confidence interval, 1.34–1.57; $p < .001$). The excess mortality associated with obesity declined with age. For men, the SMRs of the four age groups were 2.46, 2.30, 1.99, and 1.31, respectively; for women, they were 1.81, 2.10, 1.70, and 1.26, respectively (Poisson trend test, $p < .001$).

(a) There are features of the choice of exposed and comparison cohorts that could lead to bias. Among persons of all ages (combined), how is it possible that this study could have overestimated the association between obesity and mortality? How is it possible that the association could have been underestimated? (Assume that the SMRs that were calculated have eliminated potential confounding by age and other demographic characteristics.)

(b) The authors concluded the paper by stating that "the excess mortality associated with obesity declined considerably with age." Assuming for the moment that the results of this study are valid, is the mortality burden associated with obesity greater in 18–29-year-olds than 50–74-year-olds? Provide your answer in quantitative terms.

6. Kelman *et al.* (2003) identified 5,408 residents of Western Australia who had been hospitalized for deep vein thrombosis or pulmonary embolism during 1981–1999. Using airline records covering the same period of time, they found that 153 of these persons had taken an international flight during the 100 days prior to hospitalization. The distribution of the dates of hospitalization of these 153 cases, in terms of the time since the most recent flight, is shown in Table 14.4. Included in the table are two rows providing the expected number of cases, in each of the time periods, based on either:

(a) Rates of hospitalization for deep vein thrombosis/pulmonary embolism among Western Australians in general, adjusted to the age and sex distribution of the international travelers hospitalized for these conditions; or

(b) The 153 cases distributed in proportion to the fraction of the 100 days present in each time period. For example, for the first 14 days, the expected number of cases was $153 \times (14.5/100.5) = 22.1$.

Compared to the rate of deep vein thrombosis/pulmonary embolism in the general population, persons who completed international air travel in the prior two weeks had a low risk ($46/102.6 = 0.45$).

However, these persons' risk was more than twice that predicted based on the expectation of an evenly distributed incidence over the first 100 days following arrival ($46/22.1 = 2.1$). What do you believe accounts for the disparity between the two relative risk estimates?

7. The following question pertains to a news item that appeared in *The Lancet*, Oct. 25, 2003:

People screened for lung cancer by spiral CT have accelerated and prolonged quit rates of smoking, regardless of whether the screening shows disease. Researchers found that 1 year after scanning, 14% of smokers had stopped smoking; by contrast, the rate among the general smoking population was 5–7%. The findings suggest that screening is an ideal place to provide cessation messages, say the researchers.

Assume that the difference between the figures of 14% and 5–7% is not due to chance and is not due to differences in demographic characteristics between persons who do and do not receive spiral CT screening. What is an explanation for this difference apart from a genuine impact of attending the screening program on the likelihood of smoking cessation?

ANSWERS

1. Alcoholism and cirrhosis almost certainly are less prevalent in Navajos who initiate or maintain employment in uranium mines than in Navajos who do not. The presence of this "healthy worker" bias is the most plausible explanation for the observed reduced mortality among these miners, certainly more so than a beneficial effect of underground exposure to uranium.

Nonetheless, being employed in any manner probably reduces one's risk of becoming or staying an alcoholic, and it is possible that this accounts for a portion of the low SMRs for cirrhosis and alcoholism as well.

2. Women diagnosed with breast cancer prior to 1977–1980 are absent from the cohort of hormone users. In contrast, the breast cancer mortality rates in the women against whom the hormone users are being compared—Swedish women in general—are based on deaths that occurred during 1977–1991, irrespective of when a given woman's diagnosis took place. Therefore, even if hormone use had no bearing on mortality from breast cancer, an apparent deficit would be seen among the hormone users due to this lack of comparability.

3. Many people with smoking-related conditions stop smoking once that condition is diagnosed. Because of this, in the short term, persons who stop smoking actually have a higher mortality rate than continuing smokers. In studies in which the reason for smoking cessation is not ascertained (or is not ascertained reliably), the potential beneficial impact of stopping smoking is most validly measured by excluding that period of time during which the diseases that caused the smoking cessation in study participants led to death. While some of these fatal diseases last longer than one year, excluding the first year after cessation probably removes much of the bias.

4. (a) Women with high probability of survival—that is, those with no recurrence of their tumor—may be those most likely to seek to become pregnant, and also able to become pregnant. This would be an example of confounding.

(b) The way this analysis has been constructed guarantees that, even in the absence of a true benefit of pregnancy on survival, one will be observed.

TABLE 14.5. MORTALITY DIFFERENCE BETWEEN OBESITY CLINIC PATIENTS AND GENERAL POPULATION, BY GENDER AND AGE

| Sex | Age | Mortality per 1,000 person-years | | Mortality difference |
		Clinic patients	Population	
Male	18–29	36/5,109 = 7.05	7.05 ÷ 2.46 = 2.86	7.05 − 2.86 = 4.19
Male	50–74	161/7,483 = 21.52	21.52 ÷ 1.31 = 16.42	21.5 − 16.4 = 5.10
Female	18–29	31/13,661 = 2.27	2.27 ÷ 1.81 = 1.25	2.27 − 1.25 = 1.02
Female	50–74	371/25,305 = 14.66	14.66 ÷ 1.26 = 11.64	14.66 − 11.64 = 3.02

Having a pregnancy assures that a woman has survived until that time—no such "advantage" is conferred to nonpregnant cases of breast cancer. In other words, the calculated mortality rate is spuriously low among women who had a pregnancy, and thus the estimated survival is spuriously high, because these women were allowed to accrue person-time prior to the pregnancy without the possibility of a death occurring.

In order to overcome these sources of bias it is necessary to select, as a basis for comparison to each of those who become pregnant, one or more other women with breast cancer who are similar to them with regard to predictors of survival (e.g., time since breast cancer diagnosis, history of a recurrence) at the time of the pregnancy. Deaths and person-years would be tabulated for women in both groups only from the date the pregnancy begins (Velentgas *et al.*, 1999).

5. (a) The observed association between obesity and mortality could have been overestimated if there had been selective referral to the clinic of obese persons in ill health. However, it also could be underestimated due to inclusion of persons with obesity in the comparison cohort.

(b) Table 14.5 can be constructed from the data. In both men and women, the mortality burden associated with obesity—when viewed as a difference rather than as a ratio—is, if anything, greater at older ages, not smaller.

6. A "healthy traveler" bias almost certainly is the basis for the much greater number of cases of deep vein thrombosis/pulmonary embolism expected from population incidence rates than the number actually observed among the travelers. Persons at greatest risk of venous thrombosis and embolism—those who are bedridden, recovering from surgery, or who suffer from one of a number of serious illnesses—are substantially under-represented among international travelers.

The proportional-incidence analysis that generated the second set of expected numbers of cases no doubt gives a more valid estimate of the influence of international air travel on the incidence of deep vein thrombosis/pulmonary embolism during the two weeks following international travel. This analysis assumes only that air travel has little or no impact on the occurrence of these conditions beyond the first two weeks after travel has been completed.

7. There could be confounding present: Those persons concerned about their smoking-related risk of lung cancer could preferentially be present among screenees and be more inclined to stop smoking during the following year.

15

Case-Control Studies

In 1971, Herbst *et al.* (1971) reported that the mothers of seven of eight teenage girls diagnosed with clear cell adenocarcinoma of the vagina in Boston during 1966–1969 reported having taken a synthetic hormone, diethylstilbestrol (DES), while that child was *in utero*. None of the mothers of 32 girls without vaginal adenocarcinoma, matched to the mothers of cases with regard to hospital and date of birth, had taken DES during the corresponding pregnancy. Within a year, a New York study of five cases and eight girls without vaginal cancer obtained similar results (Greenwald *et al.*, 1971). The introduction of prenatal DES use into obstetrical practice in the United States during the 1940s–1950s, followed by the appearance of this hitherto unseen form of cancer some 20 years later, supported a causal connection between *in utero* exposure to DES and vaginal adenocarcinoma. The means by which *in utero* DES exposure might predispose to the occurrence of clear cell vaginal adenocarcinoma was unknown in 1971. Nonetheless, a causal inference was made at that time by the Food and Drug Administration, which specified pregnancy as a contraindication for DES use. (At present, it is believed that DES acts by interfering with normal development of the female genital tract, resulting in the persistence into puberty of vaginal adenosis in which adenocarcinoma can arise (Ulfelder and Robboy, 1976)).

The investigation by Herbst *et al.* was a case-control study: a comparison of prior exposures or characteristics of ill persons (cases) with those of persons at risk of developing the illness. Generally, the prior experience of persons at risk is estimated from observations on a sample of them (controls). A difference in the frequency or levels of exposure between cases and controls—i.e., an association—may be a reflection of a causal link.

At first glance, the case-control approach appears to proceed backwards, from consequence to potential cause. Nonetheless, if a case-control study enrolls cases and controls from the same underlying population at risk of the outcome, and can measure exposure status validly in them, the results obtained will closely resemble those from a properly done cohort study. A case-control, cohort, or any other form of non-randomized study does have the potential to observe a spurious association because of the influence of some other factor associated with both exposure and outcome. Even so, the evidence that is provided by well-done case-control studies can carry great weight when evaluating the validity of a causal hypothesis. Indeed, a number of causal inferences have been based largely on the results of case-control studies. These include, in addition to the DES–vaginal adenocarcinoma relationship, the connection between aspirin use in children and the development of Reye's syndrome (Hurwitz *et al.*, 1985), and the use of super-absorbent tampons and the incidence of toxic shock syndrome (Stallones, 1982).

One of the criteria used to assess the validity of a causal hypothesis is the strength of the association between exposure and disease, usually as measured by the ratio of the incidence rate in exposed and non-exposed persons. In most case-control studies, it is not possible to measure incidence rates in either of these groups. Nonetheless, from the frequency of exposure observed in cases and controls, it is usually possible to estimate closely the ratio of the incidence rates. The way this is done—through the use of the odds ratio—as well as the underlying rationale were discussed in Chapter 9.

RETROSPECTIVE ASCERTAINMENT OF EXPOSURE STATUS IN CASES AND CONTROLS

Epidemiologic studies seek to obtain information on exposures present during an etiologically relevant period of time. That period varies across etiologic relationships. For example, excess consumption of alcohol predisposes to motor vehicle injuries within minutes to hours, but it predisposes to cirrhosis of the liver only after a number of years. Most case-control studies are required to consider explicitly how best to assess in retrospect subjects' exposure status during a period of time in which it might have been acting to influence disease risk. Possible sources of data on exposure status include interviews or questionnaires, available records, or physical or laboratory measurements.

Interviews/Questionnaires

For many exposures, a subject's memory is an excellent window to the past. A number of important etiologic relationships have been identified through interview-based case-control studies. As a general rule, study participants will report longer-term and more recent experiences with the greatest accuracy. Paying attention to the ways in which questions are asked (White *et al.*, 2008) will maximize the accuracy of the information received, along with using visual aids when appropriate (e.g., pictures of medicines, or of containers of household products; calendars for important life events to enhance recall of the timing of other exposures). This type of attention, together with using the same questions for cases and controls asked in the same way, will also minimize the potential for bias that could result from the subject's or interviewer's awareness of case or control status.

One virtue of exposure ascertainment via interview or questionnaire is that information can be sought for multiple points in time. It is possible that a given exposure plays an etiologic role only if present at a certain age, for a certain duration, or at a certain time in the past. Because there is often little guidance before a study starts to suggest the most relevant age, length, or recency, key exposures are often elicited throughout much of the subject's lifetime. Still, care must be taken not to include exposures that took place after the illness began.

Example 15-1. Victora *et al.* (1989) conducted a case-control study of infant death from diarrhea in relation to type of feeding. They asked mothers of cases whether their child was or was not being breastfed immediately prior to the onset of the fatal illness. Mothers of controls were queried about type of feeding prior to a comparable point in time. Mothers were also asked if subsequent to the onset of the illness there had been any changes in type of feeding: following the development of diarrhea, many breastfed children are supplemented with formula and cow's milk. Relative to infants who were solely breastfed, those who also drank powdered or cow's milk prior to their illness had about four times the risk of diarrheal death. However, the authors showed that if one inappropriately considered the feeding method that was present during the illness, about a 13-fold increase in risk associated with supplementation would have been estimated.

In most interview-based case-control studies, information is not sought from cases until days to months have elapsed following the diagnosis of their condition. These persons are queried regarding exposures that occurred during what is presumed to be the etiologically relevant period prior to diagnosis. For controls, in whom there is no "diagnosis" date, what is the appropriate time frame in which to focus the questions that are asked of them? If exposures that occurred some time in the past, or that occurred over an extended period, are the most likely to be relevant, controls generally are asked about events during the same calendar time as the cases. However, when studying exposures that potentially can act acutely to lead to illness, having the case recall events immediately prior to illness and the control do the same for the corresponding time in the past may lead to bias: Only the cases will have the onset of their illness to help in recalling events that took place shortly prior to that time. This difference could lead to relatively more complete ascertainment of exposure among cases.

In response to this concern, some case-control studies investigating potentially rapidly acting exposures query controls about the time period prior to the date of interview instead of the date of their case's diagnosis (or, in an unmatched study, the date of a typical case's diagnosis). So, in a study of risk factors for meningococcal disease in adolescents (Tully *et al.*, 2006), cases were asked about events during the two weeks prior to diagnosis (which occurred, on average, 53 days prior to interview); controls, about events during the two weeks just prior to the interview itself. The investigators felt that case-control comparability of recall of exposures plausibly involved in transmission (e.g., "intimate kissing with multiple partners") would be greater using this approach than one in which the controls were asked about the two-week period ending 53 days prior to interview. However, while a sound approach when trying to estimate the short-term influence of many exposures, this strategy can backfire if recall of an exposure diminishes over time to the same degree in cases and controls. For example, in the study of meningococcal disease, a far smaller proportion of cases than controls reported attending religious observances during their respective two-week intervals (odds ratio, adjusted for other risk factors = 0.1, 95% confidence interval = 0.02–0.6). Almost certainly this difference had more to do with relatively poorer recall of churchgoing among cases (who had to think back some two months) than to a genuine salutary effect of church attendance on the incidence of meningococcal disease!

Records

Case-control studies have exploited vital, registry, employment, medical, and pharmacy records, to name only some, as a means of obtaining information on exposures. However, because the information contained in the records will usually have been assembled for purposes other than epidemiologic research, it may not provide precisely that information desired by the epidemiologist. For example, a death certificate or an occupational record may state an individual's job, but often not his/her actual exposure to the substance(s) of interest to the study. Or, a pharmacy record will indicate a prescription's having been filled, but not whether the patient took the medication on a given day, or took it at all. This sort of imprecision will impair a study's ability to discern a true association between an exposure and a disease: the greater the imprecision, the greater the impairment. Nonetheless, some very strong associations have been identified through record-based case-control studies. For example (and as described more fully in Chapter 10), in a study based entirely on tumor registry records, Daling et al. (1982) observed that men with anal cancer were substantially less likely to be married than men with other types of cancer. This served as a stimulus to conduct interview-based studies that could elicit information regarding receptive anal intercourse, the exposure suspected to underlie the association with never having been married. The latter studies showed an exceedingly strong association with a history of receptive anal

intercourse among men (odds ratio of 50) (Daling et al., 1987).

In case-control studies in which medical records are used to characterize exposure status, care must be taken to restrict the information obtained to that which preceded the case's diagnosis and the presence of symptoms, if any, that led to the diagnosis. The records of controls must be truncated at similar points in time. Without this safeguard, it is possible that bias will arise from there being systematically more complete information available to review on cases than controls: the case's illness may have stimulated an inquiry by medical personnel into his/her past, whereas no corresponding inquiry would necessarily have occurred for control subjects.

Example 15-2. Weinmann et al. (1994) conducted a case-control study of renal cell cancer in relation to antecedent use of anti-hypertensive medications within the membership of Kaiser-Permanente Northwest. For cases and their matched controls (demographically similar members of the health care plan without this disease), outpatient and inpatient medical records were reviewed for information regarding medication use up to a date three months prior to the case's diagnosis. By selectively not including the last three months in the data collection period, the investigators sought to minimize differences between cases and controls regarding the quantity of information contained in the records on prior medication use. Also, they felt it implausible that use of a drug during such a relatively short time as the three months prior to diagnosis would have an influence on the development of that patient's renal cell cancer.

Physical and Laboratory Measurements

The recognized limitations of interviews and records in characterizing a variety of potentially relevant exposures have stimulated the conduct of epidemiologic studies that use laboratory and other methods of measurement. A woman cannot tell an investigator the level of her reproductive hormones, the concentration of various micronutrients in her blood, or whether her cervix is infected with human papillomavirus, while laboratory tests can. Unfortunately, such tests tell us only what these things are at the time the specimens have been obtained. For some exposures, there will be a high correlation between the measured level following case and control identification and that present during the etiologically relevant time period. For example, lead enters and does not leave the dentine of teeth. Therefore, in young school-age children, lead dentine levels are an indicator of cumulative lead exposure, a good portion of which could be relevant to the development of intellectual impairment and other adverse neurological outcomes (Needleman *et al.*, 1990). Or, in a case-control study of vaccine efficacy against tuberculosis, the presence of a BCG vaccination scar is just as reliable an indicator of exposure status when measured after illness is present as it would be if it had been possible to assess the presence of a scar earlier in time (Rodrigues and Smith, 1999). In contrast, one would not rely on serum levels of reproductive hormones of postmenopausal women with breast cancer and controls to indicate what their premenopausal levels were, much less the hormonal status during their very early reproductive years (at which time it is plausible that hormones can exert the greatest impact on future risk of breast cancer).

Example 15-3. Green *et al.* (1999) compared 88 children who had been diagnosed with leukemia and 133 controls regarding exposure to magnetic fields. During a 2-day period that took place an average of 2.5 years after the diagnosis had been made, study participants wore a personal monitoring device that assessed these fields once each minute. (The study was restricted to children who continued to live in the same residence as the one they had in the 6–12 months prior to the time of diagnosis.) Earlier studies of the possible association between magnetic field exposure and leukemia typically had estimated exposures based on the electric wire configuration of the household, or on direct measures within the household itself, but had not used personal monitors. The study of Green *et al.* observed a substantially stronger association between exposure to magnetic fields and leukemia than nearly all prior studies of this question. While it is possible that this stronger association is genuine—a result of a relatively more accurate means of assessing exposure status—it is also possible that some bias has been introduced by having to rely on magnetic field measurements obtained several years after each child's leukemia had been diagnosed, or by behavioral changes produced by the leukemia.

Some case-control studies are nested within cohort studies in which specimens (e.g., blood, urine) have been obtained prior to diagnosis on all cohort members, but have not yet been analyzed for

the exposure(s) in question. At a later time, measurements are made upon the specimens from cohort members who developed a particular illness (cases) and on controls sampled from: (1) the cohort as a whole (case-cohort studies); or (2) cohort members who did not develop the illness as of the date of diagnosis of their respective cases (nested case-control studies) (Wacholder, 1991). The results obtained from studies of this type cannot be influenced by metabolic and other changes that occur following the diagnosis of the illness. However, the results can be influenced by such changes that take place between the time the illness first develops and the time it is diagnosed as such. So, in order to lessen the chance that occult illness in cases has influenced levels of a suspected etiologic factor, many studies of this type exclude from the analyses specimens obtained within the period prior to diagnosis that might correspond to the duration of the preclinical stage of disease.

Example 15-4. In a Finnish study (Woodson *et al.*, 2003), 29,133 male smokers were monitored for cancer incidence. Blood samples were obtained periodically and frozen on a random sample of 800 of these men. During follow-up, 21 of the 800 men were diagnosed with prostate cancer. On them and on 21 demographically matched controls, blood specimens obtained during the year prior to diagnosis (and the corresponding date in controls) and others obtained 2–3 years prior to diagnosis were thawed and assayed for two substances hypothesized to influence cancer development:

- Insulin-like growth factor–1 (IGF-1)
- Insulin-like growth factor binding protein–3 (IGFBP-3)

The table below compares the change over time in IGF-1 and IGFBP-3, separately in cases and controls:

While the results of this study are based on but 21 men with prostate cancer, they suggest that in the several years preceding cancer diagnosis there is a rise in serum levels of IGF-1. Because it is suspected that tumors are present for at least several years prior to diagnosis, the rise in IGF-1 probably has no etiologic significance and is instead a manifestation of the presence or growth of not-yet-diagnosed prostate cancer.

These results suggest that case-control studies of prostate cancer in relation to serum levels of IGF-1 that use specimens obtained at or after diagnosis are

TABLE 15.1.

	Cases	Controls	p*
Mean serum IGF-1 (ng/ml)			
Within 1 year of diagnosis	86.4	79.0	
2–3 years before diagnosis	73.1	82.1	
Difference	+18%	–4%	0.02
Mean serum IGFBP-3 (ng/ml)			
Within 1 year of diagnosis	2067.7	2144.3	
2–3 years before diagnosis	2033.2	2240.5	
Difference	+1.7%	–4.3%	0.29

*For the size of difference between cases and controls

likely to produce a spuriously positive association. In contrast, there is no suggestion of a change in serum levels of IGFBP-3 during the several years prior to diagnosis, so case-control comparisons of IGFBP-3 concentrations based on specimens obtained close to the time of diagnosis may well yield a valid result.

Among the large majority of case-control studies in which exposure status is not measured until the illness or injury has been diagnosed, some are concerned only with an exposure or characteristic that would have been the same at all times in a person's life. This is true for a genetically determined characteristic such as ABO blood type or the absence of glutathione transferase M1 activity (an enzyme that metabolizes several potentially carcinogenic constituents of cigarette smoke). Clearly, these studies are no less valid for having had to measure exposure in retrospect.

CASE DEFINITION

Ideally, the cases in a case-control study would comprise all (or a representative sample of) members of a defined population who develop a given health outcome during a given period of time. For studies of disease etiology, that outcome is disease occurrence. For studies that seek to determine the efficacy of early disease detection or treatment, the outcome generally is mortality or the onset of complications of the disease; such studies have been described in detail elsewhere (Selby, 1994; Weiss, 1994) and will not be covered any further here.

The population from which cases are to be drawn may be defined geographically, or it may be defined on the basis of other characteristics, such as membership in a prepaid health care plan or an occupational group. The identification of all newly ill persons in a defined population can be facilitated by the presence of a reporting system, such as a cancer or malformation registry, that seeks to accomplish this identification for other purposes. On occasion, care for the condition being studied may be centralized, so that it would be necessary to review the records of only one or a few institutions to identify all cases in the population in which those institutions are located. However, in many instances it is not feasible to identify all cases that occur in a given population, so case-control studies are often based on but a portion of them, perhaps cases identified from hospital records or from the records of selected providers from whom patients had sought health care. The study of Herbst et al. (1971) of vaginal adenocarcinoma was of this type. Whether or not the cases are derived from a defined population, it is necessary that they be drawn in an unselected manner with regard to exposure status; that is, by including in the study all eligible cases diagnosed or receiving care during a defined time period.

While the goal of a case-control study of etiology is to enroll incident cases, in some circumstances it may be necessary to enroll prevalent cases at a particular point in time, irrespective of when each one's illness had begun. For some conditions, the date of occurrence may simply not be known. For example, in the absence of very close sero-monitoring, one generally cannot determine when a person acquired an HIV infection. Second, for uncommon diseases of long duration, an incidence series may yield too few cases for meaningful analysis. The disadvantages of using prevalent cases in a case-control study relate in part to the added problems of accurate exposure ascertainment. For prevalent conditions whose date of diagnosis is known, pre-illness exposure information on study subjects must be obtained for more distant points in the past, on average, than would be necessary for an incident series. For prevalent conditions whose date of occurrence is unknown (e.g., HIV infection), there will be uncertainty as to the best point in time before which one should elicit exposure information. Also, by studying persons remaining alive with a given condition, one is studying at the same time not only etiologic factors, but also factors that influence the duration of the condition, including those associated with survival.

Example 15-5. Ponsonby et al. (2005) interviewed prevalent cases of multiple sclerosis in Tasmania, as well as community controls, during

1999–2001. By comparing the proportion of cases and controls who had, during their first 6 years of life, resided with a younger sibling 0–2 years of age, they sought to test the hypothesis that childhood infection patterns and related immune responses bear on the occurrence of multiple sclerosis. Even though cases were not interviewed on average until nearly 10 years after diagnosis (at a mean age of 43.5 years), it seems likely that information obtained from them and from controls on exposure to a younger sibling during their childhood years would be accurate. Nonetheless, because a number of persons with rapidly progressive multiple sclerosis who had been diagnosed in Tasmania during the 1990s probably had already succumbed to their illness prior to the initiation of the interviewing, the results of this study may apply only to those forms of multiple sclerosis with a lengthy natural history.

Ideally, the criteria used to identify and select individual cases for study should be objective ones of high sensitivity and specificity for the disease. Specificity is of particular concern, since the inadvertent inclusion of persons without disease in the case group will generally obscure any true association with exposure (see Chapter 10). With this in mind, in the case-control study of Reye's syndrome in relation to antecedent analgesic use conducted by the Centers for Disease Control (Hurwitz *et al.*, 1985), only cases with a substantial degree of neurological impairment (stage 2 or higher) were included. The use of this criterion minimized the chances that children with diseases other than Reye's syndrome, diseases that generally would have a lesser degree of severity, would be included in the case group. It also was intended to serve as protection against selective misclassification of Reye's syndrome based on knowledge of exposure status, since the hypothesis that aspirin was associated with Reye's syndrome was well known by the time the study took place. Conceivably, the knowledge that the child had consumed aspirin could have led some physicians to diagnose Reye's syndrome in cases with an atypical illness.

CONTROL DEFINITION

Occasionally, the proportion of ill persons who have had a specific exposure is so high, unequivocally more than would be expected in the population from which they were derived, that the presence of an association (though not its magnitude) can be surmised from a case series alone (Cummings and Weiss, 1998). For example, an investigation revealed that all persons with a form of pneumonia that was epidemic in Spain in 1981 had ingested adulterated rapeseed oil. Consumption of such oil was known not to be universal in this population. Thus, a causal inference was drawn, leading to efforts to eliminate further use of that oil. This action was taken before any formal comparison of cases with controls was made (Tabuenca, 1981).

However, in the vast majority of instances, an explicit control group is needed to estimate the frequency and degree of exposure that would have taken place among cases in the absence of an exposure–disease association. An ideal control group would be one that consists of individuals:

1. Selected from a population whose distribution of exposure is that of the population from which the cases arose;
2. Who are identical to the cases with respect to their distribution of all characteristics:

   (a) that influence the likelihood and/or degree of exposure, and
   (b) that, independent of their relation this to exposure, are also related to the occurrence of the illness under study or to its recognition; and

3. In whom the presence of the exposure can be measured accurately and in a manner that is identical to that used for cases.

If the criteria above are not met in a particular study, then selection bias, confounding, or information bias, respectively, may be present.

Minimizing Selection Bias

If the cases identified in the study are all, or a representative sample, of those that occurred in a defined population, one can seek to achieve comparability by choosing as controls persons sampled from that same population. For geographically defined populations, a number of different methods of sampling have been used, including random digit dialing of telephone numbers, area sampling, neighborhood sampling, voters' lists, population registers, motor vehicle licenses, and birth certificates, among others. When cases are members of a prepaid health care plan who develop an illness or injury, a sample of persons who were members of the health plan when the illness or injury occurred can serve as controls. When cases are ill or injured members of an employed population, controls can be selected from that same group of employees.

Example 15-6. Enumeration of the defined population from which the cases arose may require an innovative approach. Smith *et al.* (2001) identified recreational boating fatalities in Maryland and North Carolina among persons 18 years and above during 1990–1998, seeking to determine the presence and magnitude of an association with alcohol consumption. Of 221 fatal cases on whom blood alcohol levels were measured, 55% tested positive. To provide a basis for comparison, the investigators devised a plan to randomly sample recreational boats on the waterways of the two states, then to obtain a breath sample for alcohol testing from the boat operator and a random sample of any passengers aboard ($n = 3,943$). Only 17% of the persons chosen as controls had a positive result, and the disparity between cases and controls grew with increasing alcohol levels.

In some studies, cases have not been selected from a definable population at risk for the disease, but rather from persons treated for a particular illness at one or a few hospitals or clinics. Selection bias may be present in such studies if: (a) controls are not chosen from persons who, had they developed the illness under study, would have received care at these hospitals or clinics; and (b) persons who do and do not receive care from these sources differ with regard to their frequency or level of exposure.

Therefore, when cases are chosen from a narrow range of providers of health care, often controls are chosen from other ill persons treated by these providers. Such ill controls may also be used if, irrespective of the source of cases, there is no feasible way to sample from the population at large, or if sampling from the population at large would be likely to result in a substantial level of non-response or information bias (see below). For these reasons, in some studies of fatal illness, exposures in persons with a given cause of death are compared to exposures in a sample of persons who died for other reasons (Gordis, 1982).

However, the choice of ill or deceased controls can itself give rise to selection bias if the illnesses (or causes of death) represented in the control group are in some way associated with the exposure of interest. For example, ill or recently deceased persons tend to have been smokers of cigarettes more often than other persons (McLaughlin *et al.*, 1985), since smoking is associated with a variety of causes of illness and death. Because smoking histories of ill persons overstate the cigarette consumption of the population

from which the cases arose (even if that population cannot be defined), the odds ratio associated with smoking based on the use of ill persons as controls will be spuriously low.

To minimize selection bias related to having chosen ill or deceased controls, an attempt can be made to omit potential controls with conditions known to be related (positively or negatively) to the exposure. For example, in the analysis of a hospital-based case-control study of bladder cancer in relation to prior use of artificial sweeteners, the investigators excluded from their control group persons who were hospitalized for obesity-related diseases (Silverman *et al.*, 1983). They showed that, without this restriction, the control group would have a spuriously high proportion of users of artificial sweeteners relative to the population from which their cases actually had come. This approach will succeed to the extent that one judges correctly which conditions truly are exposure-related, and how accurately the presence of those conditions can be determined. For many exposures, this may pose little problem, and judicious exclusion will yield a control group capable of providing an unbiased result. For others, such as cigarette smoking or alcohol drinking, it has been shown that admitting diagnoses or statements of cause of death are incapable of identifying all persons with illnesses related to these exposures (McLaughlin *et al.*, 1985).

Occasionally, controls are chosen from individuals who are tested for the presence of the disease under study and are found not to have it. For example, persons demonstrated to have coronary artery occlusion on coronary angiography have been compared to angiography patients without occlusion with regard to potential risk factors (Thom *et al.*, 1992). As another example, the prior use of oral contraceptives was compared between women diagnosed with venous thromboembolism and women seen at the same institution for suspected venous thromboembolism who turned out not to have this condition (Bloemenkamp *et al.*, 1999). It may be relatively inexpensive to select controls from persons who receive the same diagnostic evaluation as do cases, and it is also possible to achieve case-control comparability with regard to the choice of a health care provider (and the correlates of that choice). This approach can have an impact on the study's validity when the frequency or degree of exposure differs between otherwise-comparable members of a population who do and do not receive the test:

1. It will increase the validity if the disease being investigated is generally asymptomatic, and therefore would not be detected in the absence of testing. Thus, the relationship of the use of oral contraceptives to the incidence of *in situ* cancer of the cervix is best studied in women who have received cervical screening, by comparing oral contraceptive use between cases of *in situ* cancer and women with a negative screen. This is because:

   (a) In most societies, screening is more commonly administered to women who use oral contraceptives than to women who do not; and
   (b) *In situ* cancers are asymptomatic and will not be identified in the absence of cervical screening.

   Therefore, if controls are chosen from women in general, who may or may not have received cervical screening, an apparent excess of oral contraceptive users would be present among cases of *in situ* cancer even if no true association were present.

2. The choice of test-negative controls, however, will detract from a study's validity if the large majority of persons who develop the disease soon would get diagnosed whether or not the test was administered. There was a controversy in the late 1970s regarding the suitability, in case-control studies of postmenopausal estrogen use and endometrial cancer, of a control group restricted to women with no evidence of cancer on endometrial biopsy. Among women without endometrial cancer, estrogen use differs greatly between those who have undergone biopsy and those who have not, because estrogen use predisposes to uterine bleeding of a nonmalignant nature that often leads to endometrial biopsy. The investigators who believed that there was a great prevalence of occult endometrial cancer in the population suggested that the optimal control group ought to be women undergoing endometrial biopsy and found not to have cancer (Horwitz and Feinstein, 1978). However, the majority of investigators believed that no such large pool of prevalent, occult disease existed, and that choosing biopsy-negative controls would lead to a spuriously high estimate of estrogen use in the population at risk, and thus a spuriously low odds ratio (Shapiro *et al.*, 1985).

No matter how controls are defined in a case-control study, selection bias may be introduced to the extent that exposure information is not obtained on all who have been selected to take part. The magnitude of the bias will increase in relation to the frequency of missing data and the degree to which exposure frequencies or levels differ between study subjects on whom exposure status is and is not known. The problem of incomplete ascertainment of exposure on study subjects is particularly common in interview- or questionnaire-based case-control studies. Strategies for minimizing the degree of non-response in case-control studies are discussed in detail elsewhere (White *et al.*, 2008).

Minimizing Information Bias

In case-control studies in which information on exposure status is sought by means of an interview or questionnaire, the chief safeguards against information bias entail asking questions (a) about events that are salient to the respondent; (b) that are framed in an unambiguous way; and (c) that are presented identically to both cases and controls. Employment of these safeguards, however, will not prevent differential accuracy of reporting between cases and controls in all circumstances. Some past exposures/events will simply be more salient to persons with an illness, who might have dwelt on possible reasons that it occurred, than to persons without that illness. Other exposures may be viewed as socially undesirable, and there may be a difference between cases and healthy controls in their willingness to admit to them. If the anticipated difference in the quality of information between cases and otherwise-appropriate controls is too great, a control group that is less than ideal in other respects may be selected instead so as to minimize the potential for information bias. For example, some studies of prenatal risk factors for a particular congenital malformation that utilize maternal interviews as the source of exposure data have selected as controls infants with other malformations (Rosenberg *et al.*, 1983). This control group will provide a more valid result than a control group that consists of infants in general if: (a) mothers of malformed and mothers of normal infants report prenatal exposures to a different degree even in the absence of an association, and (b) the exposure in question is not associated with the occurrence of the malformations present in control infants. (For some exposures, such as use of multivitamin supplements during pregnancy, there is an association with a broad range of malformation types (Werler *et al.*, 1999), making it difficult or impossible to define a subgroup of malformed infants as controls that would yield an unbiased result.)

Daling *et al.* (1987) had the foregoing in mind when conducting their case-control study of anal cancer in relation to a history of anal intercourse, and this led them to eschew the geographic population from which their cases had arisen as a sampling frame for controls. They feared that interviews that sought information about prior anal intercourse might be more complete among men with cancer than men in the population at large. Thus, they chose as controls men with a cancer of a different site (colon). They had reason to believe that colon cancer was unlikely to have been etiologically related to prior anal intercourse, and suspected that in terms of their willingness to answer sensitive questions reliably, men with colon cancer would be more similar to men with anal cancer than would be men selected at random.

When the measurement of the exposure under consideration is inherently imprecise, or when there is a large subjective component involved, it may be difficult or impossible to identify a control group that will provide information comparable to that provided by cases. An instructive example comes from a case-control study of Down's syndrome (Stott, 1958) conducted shortly before the chromosomal basis for the etiology of this condition had been learned. The study sought to determine whether emotional "shocks" during pregnancy might be a risk factor. The author interviewed mothers of children with Down's syndrome with regard to the occurrence of a "situation or event [that would be] stress- or shock-producing ... in an emotionally stable woman." Identical interviews were administered to mothers of normal children, and also to mothers of retarded children who did not have Down's syndrome. Even though it is not possible that an emotional shock in pregnancy could play any etiologic role in a condition already determined at conception, a far higher proportion of mothers of cases of Down's syndrome reported an emotional shock than did mothers of normal controls (odds ratio estimated from the data = 17.0). The use of other retarded children as controls only partially reduced the spuriously high odds ratio, to a value of 4.3.

When conducting an interview-based study of a rapidly fatal disease, or a disease that impairs a person's ability to provide valid interview data, it is necessary to obtain information from at least some surrogate respondents. Typically, these respondents are close relatives of the cases. For purposes of comparability, similar information generally ought to be obtained from surrogates of controls, even though the control him/herself would be expected to provide more accurate data.

Example 15-7. In their case-control study of vigorous exercise as a possible precipitant of primary

cardiac arrest, Siscovick et al. (1984) compared information obtained from the wives of men in whom an arrest had occurred with that obtained from wives of men identified at random (controls) in the same community. (Though it would have been feasible to interview the control men themselves, the large majority of the cases had died.) The investigators were willing to accept the likely greater degree of exposure misclassification arising from the use of interviews with spouses of controls as the price for achieving a higher degree of case-control comparability of exposure data.

Results of case-control studies based on exposure information provided by surrogate respondents need to be interpreted with particular caution. Though by no means present in every instance (Nelson et al., 1990; Campbell et al., 2007), there can be a large difference in the validity of the responses given by case and control surrogates. For example, Greenberg et al. (1985) investigated the basis for an apparent strong association between cancer mortality and "nuclear" work among employees of a naval shipyard that had been found in a comparison of work histories provided by surrogates of men who died from cancer and of those who died of other conditions. They observed that, regarding work in the nuclear part of the industry, surrogates of the cases generally provided information similar to that contained in employment records of the shipyard. In contrast, the surrogates of controls substantially misclassified the nature of their relatives' jobs as not involving radiation. Using the more accurate data provided by employment records, which included individual radiation dosimetry (Rinsky et al., 1981), little or no association was present between cancer mortality and radiation exposure received at the shipyard.

What was undoubtedly a spuriously negative association was found in a case-control study of lung cancer and passive cigarette smoking that used, for one analysis, information obtained from surrogate respondents (Janerich et al., 1990). In this analysis, the relative risk of lung cancer among nonsmokers associated with a spouse's having smoked—0.33 (i.e., a 67% reduction in risk)—would seem almost certainly due to a spurious minimization or denial of smoking by spouses of cases, who may have feared their habit caused their spouse to develop lung cancer.

Differentially accurate assessment of exposure status between cases and controls is not confined to interview or questionnaire-based studies. Most laboratory-based studies seek to prevent this by testing samples blind to case/control status. If feasible, it is desirable to do this blinding as well in studies in which exposure is to be determined from medical or other records. However, there are instances in which the nature of the information available in records has already been influenced by whether the subject is a case or a control. For example, it was found that among 100 infertile women who underwent laparoscopy (Strathy *et al.*, 1982), 21 had endometriosis. Only 2% of 200 women undergoing laparoscopy for another indication, tubal ligation, were noted in the records of their procedure to have endometriosis. Taken at face value, these data would suggest that the presence of endometriosis predisposes to infertility. However, the interpretation of this association is not straightforward, since the means of identification and/or recording of endometriosis in cases and controls (women undergoing tubal ligation) may well have not been comparable—only in the infertile women was the laparoscopy expressly done as a diagnostic tool to investigate the possible presence of conditions such as endometriosis.

Additional delineation of the rationale underlying control definition and selection can be found in Wacholder *et al.* (1992a,b,c).

CONTROL OF CONFOUNDING IN CASE-CONTROL STUDIES
Characteristics of Confounding Variables in Case-Control Studies

Confounding is present when the estimate of the relationship between an exposure and disease is distorted by the influence of another factor. In any study design, confounding generally will occur to the extent that the other factor is associated both with exposure (though not as a result of the exposure) and with the occurrence of the disease or its recognition. In case-control studies alone, a factor may confound even if it is not associated with an altered risk of disease, if the proportions of cases and controls vary across levels or categories of the factor. For example, in a collaborative study of ovarian cancer in relation to use of oral contraceptives (Weiss *et al.*, 1981), an attempt was made to identify and interview all incident cases during a several-year period in two United States populations. In one of the populations (western Washington State), several controls per case were interviewed, whereas the control/case ratio in the other (Utah) was 1.0. Thus, the design created an association between study population and

disease status among persons actually studied. Since oral contraceptive use was more common in Washington women than in Utah women, failure to take into account the state of residence in the analysis (e.g., by adjustment) would have led to a spuriously high estimate of the frequency of oral contraceptive use in controls relative to that in cases.

Means of Controlling for Confounding

One straightforward way of preventing confounding is to restrict cases and controls to a single category or level of the potentially confounding variable. For example, in their study of physical activity in relation to primary cardiac arrest, Siscovick *et al.* (1982) excluded persons with conditions, such as clinically recognized heart disease, that could both predispose to cardiac arrest and might be expected to alter the persons level of activity. A second way is to obtain information on exposures or characteristics that may differ between cases and controls, and then make statistical adjustments for those that also are found to be related to the exposure or characteristic under investigation (see Chapter 11).

Alternatively, it is possible to match controls to cases (either to individual cases, or to groups of cases with a shared characteristic) on the category or level of a potentially confounding factor. However, it should be kept in mind that in case-control studies, matching alone is not sufficient to eliminate a variable's confounding influence, and that failure to consider a matching variable in the analysis of the study can lead to a biased result (Rothman *et al.*, 2008). It is appropriate to match if:

- The variable is expected to be strongly related to both exposure and to disease. Thus, in a case-control study of breast cancer in relation to use of hair dye, it would make sense to match on gender (if the study had not already been restricted to women) since: (a) in most cultures, use of hair dye is more common in women than in men; and (b) in the absence of matching, the case-to-control ratio would be very uneven between women and men. While confounding by gender could be prevented even without matching by adjustment in the analysis, the statistical precision of the unmatched study would be substantially reduced relative to that of a case-control study having a more similar proportion of female cases and controls.

- Information on possible matching variables can be obtained inexpensively. There are some means of control selection in which information regarding some confounders can be obtained at no cost. For example, from voters' lists or prepaid health plan membership records, it would generally be possible to directly choose one or more controls who were nearly identical to a given case's age. On the other hand, if a population-sampling scheme such as random digit dialing were being employed, the age of the respondent would not be known in advance of approaching him/her. Rather than omitting already contacted controls who did not match a particular case's age, the matching can be done much more broadly. Additional control for finer categories of age can be accomplished in the data analysis.

- Information on exposure status cannot be obtained inexpensively. The higher the cost of exposure ascertainment, the greater the incentive to limit the number of control subjects to the number of cases. Differences between cases and controls regarding confounding factors particularly will reduce the statistical power of a study that does not have a surplus of controls. Enriching the group of controls selected with persons more similar to the cases with regard to confounding factors (i.e., matching) can prevent this loss of statistical power.

In case-control studies of genetic characteristics as possible etiologic factors, some investigators have used a matched design in which a specified type of relative (e.g., parent, sibling, cousin) is chosen as a control for each case (Yang and Khoury, 1997; Witte et al., 1999; Ahsan et al., 2002). This approach has the advantage of minimizing potential confounding by other genetic characteristics with which the one of interest is associated. It has a disadvantage, though: the exclusion of a possibly-large fraction of cases for whom there is no relative available of the type needed to provide a sample for genetic analysis.

Analyses of studies that have matched controls to cases on a given characteristic can adjust for that characteristic as if no matching had taken place. Alternatively, these analyses can explicitly consider cases and controls as matched sets. In the instance of matched case-control pairs and a dichotomous

exposure variable, the following table could be constructed:

TABLE 15.2.

Case	Control	
	Exposed	Non-exposed
Exposed	a	b
Non-exposed	c	d

Only the b pairs in which the case was exposed but not the matched control, and the c pairs in which the reverse was true, would enter the analysis. The odds ratio would be calculated as b/c. When there is more than one control per case, or an uneven number of controls per case, an odds ratio that accounts for the matching can be calculated as well (Breslow and Day, 1980; Hosmer and Lemeshow, 2000).

CASE-CONTROL STUDIES THAT DIRECTLY COMPARE DISEASE OR EXPOSURE SUBGROUPS

Imagine that an ordinary case-control study has been conducted in which ill and well persons are to be compared in terms of the proportion who have received a given exposure. If the ill individuals can be subdivided on the basis of a manifestation of their illness (e.g., histologic type of cancer, or hemorrhagic versus thrombotic stroke), it is straightforward to compare separately each of the subgroups of cases to the controls. Similarly, when comparing a single case group to controls for the presence of an exposure with multiple categories (e.g., type of oral contraceptive, brand of cellular phone), odds ratios can be calculated for each type of exposure subcategory, using nonexposed persons as a common referent category.

For a variety of reasons, primarily relating to feasibility, some case-control studies do not include a group of non-diseased individuals, but instead compare exposure status among subgroups of cases. In such studies, if there are reasons to believe that one of the subgroups is typical of the underlying population at risk in terms of the likelihood or levels of exposure, a valid estimate of the effect of the exposure on the incidence of the other disease subgroups can be obtained.

Example 15-8.   In 10,748 drivers involved in fatal road crashes in France during 2001–2003, Laumon *et al.* (2005) obtained postmortem blood samples and analyzed them for levels of a metabolite of cannabis. Among the 6,766 drivers judged to have been at fault in the crash, 8.8% tested positive, in contrast to 2.8% of the other 3,006 drivers (odds ratio = 3.3, 95% confidence interval = 2.6–4.2). This difference persisted to roughly the same degree after control for blood alcohol levels and other confounding variables.

The results of the study of Laumon *et al.* (2005) will provide an accurate assessment of the impact of cannabis consumption on fatal road crashes if each of these crashes has a single driver at fault, and that for a given crash the authors could perfectly identify which driver that was. To the extent that these conditions do not hold, the misclassification that ensues will tend to make the size of the observed association smaller than the true one. Trying to estimate through any other means the prevalence of cannabis use in drivers otherwise comparable to those killed in road crashes would present considerable logistical difficulties. Thus, a comparison of at-fault and other fatally injured drivers is probably necessary to assess this particular hazard of cannabis use, even if that assessment provides but a conservative estimate of the increase in risk.

Some epidemiologic studies include, among both cases and controls, only persons who sustained a broadly defined exposure, within which a particular exposure subcategory is of interest. Under certain circumstances these studies also can provide useful information.

Example 15-9.   In a study of oropharyngeal cancer, Gillison *et al.* (2000) compared the smoking and drinking habits of persons whose tumors were positive for human papillomavirus type 16 (HPV16) and those whose tumors were negative. All but one of the 25 persons with a tumor that was HPV16-negative had smoked cigarettes, as opposed to 27 of 34 of those with an HPV16-positive tumor. Similarly, half of the HPV16-negative patients consumed 100 grams or more of alcohol per week prior to diagnosis, in contrast to but 5 of 34 of the persons whose tumor was HPV16-positive.

Because the study did not include men and women without cancer as a basis for comparison,

from these data alone it is impossible to distinguish the two possible interpretations of these results (we will also assume that neither chance nor bias is an explanation): (a) Smoking and drinking particularly predispose to the occurrence of HPV16-negative oropharyngeal tumors; or (b) Smoking and drinking protect against the occurrence of HPV16-positive tumors. However, there are ample data from other studies (Mayne *et al.*, 2006) that did include controls without cancer to indicate that smoking and drinking are strongly positively associated with the incidence of oropharyngeal cancer in general. (These studies were conducted before it was possible to assess a tumor's HPV status.) Thus, the most plausible explanation is (a) above: smoking and drinking predispose to the incidence of oropharyngeal cancer through a causal pathway that does not require the presence of an infection with HPV16. The hypothesis that smoking and drinking also predispose to oropharyngeal cancer when HPV infection is present, but simply to a relatively smaller degree, could be tested in a case-control study only by including controls without oropharyngeal cancer.

Example 15-10.   *Helicobacter pylori (H. pylori)* is a heterogeneous bacterial species. A number of studies (summarized by Spechler *et al.* (2000)) have examined the possibility that those *H. pylori* strains that express cytoxin-associated gene A (cagA) are particularly virulent in terms of their ability to produce gastric pathology. These studies have compared the presence of serum antibodies to the cagA protein among patients with gastric disease (e.g., ulcer or carcinoma) and healthy individuals (e.g., blood donors), with both cases and controls being serologically positive for *H. pylori* infection. Most (though not all) such studies observed a higher proportion of *H. pylori* infections to be cagA-positive in cases than in controls.

The exclusion of *H. pylori*-negative persons in the analysis of data from these studies, strictly speaking, limits the interpretation of the results: Examined in isolation, the data are equally compatible with the hypothesis that *H. pylori* strains that express cagA predispose to gastric pathology as with the hypothesis that cagA-negative strains lead to a reduced risk (relative to the absence of *H. pylori* infection).

Here is an older example in which the restriction of the study population to "exposed" individuals alone prevented an appreciation of the impact of each of the exposure subgroups on disease risk.

Example 15-11. In 1975, a study was conducted on 20 women under 40 years of age in the United States who developed endometrial cancer and who had a history of oral contraceptive use (Silverberg and Makowski, 1975). Thirteen (65%) of these women had taken a sequential preparation (almost all of which was the brand Oracon), substantially more than the eight percent expected based on United States national sales of oral contraceptives. This observation is compatible with the hypothesis that use of Oracon predisposes to endometrial cancer, but is equally compatible with the hypothesis that use of other types of oral contraceptives protects against this disease. In fact, both hypotheses turned out to be correct: When a case-control study was done that was not restricted to users of oral contraceptives (Weiss and Sayvetz, 1980), Oracon users were observed to have about a seven-fold increased risk of endometrial cancer, and users of non-sequential oral contraceptives ("combination" pills) a 50% lower risk, relative to women who had not taken oral contraceptives.

WHEN SHOULD WE LOOK TO RESULTS OF CASE-CONTROL STUDIES FOR ANSWERS TO QUESTIONS OF DISEASE ETIOLOGY?

Randomized trials will not be able to answer all of our questions regarding the reasons diseases occur. Many potential disease-causing or disease-preventing exposures cannot be manipulated, either at all—e.g., most genetic characteristics—or in any practical way for the purposes of a study. For many exposure–disease relationships, either the disease is too uncommon or the induction period is too long to conduct a randomized trial that is not infeasibly large in size or long in duration. Finally, it generally will not be possible to conduct separate randomized trials to measure the impact of all potential types, amounts, and durations of a class of exposure.

Also, for many of the same reasons, it is not possible to rely solely on cohort studies for answers. Just as with randomized trials, the disease outcome being studied may be too rare to allow a cohort approach to be useful. This explains why the etiologies of vaginal adenocarcinoma and Reye's syndrome, for example, have been evaluated exclusively by case-control studies—these diseases are simply too uncommon

for most cohort studies to generate any cases, even in "exposed" individuals. Prospective cohort studies are also of limited use when the induction period for the exposure-disease relationship is either very short or very long. If the induction period is very short, and the exposure status of an individual varies over time, a cohort study would need to assess exposure status repeatedly among cohort members. For this reason, studies of alcohol consumption in relation to the occurrence of injuries typically are case-control in nature (Holcomb, 1938). Similarly, unless information on exposure status can be ascertained retrospectively at the time the cohort is formed, it would rarely be feasible to initiate a cohort study of a suspected etiologic relation that requires several decades to manifest itself.

While case-control studies may be of particular value in the evaluation of the etiology of uncommon diseases, they may have difficulty obtaining statistically precise results if the frequency of the exposure in the population under study is either extremely common or extremely uncommon (Crombie, 1981). Thus, only an association as strong as the one between cigarette smoking and lung cancer could have emerged reliably from case-control studies of several hundred British men conducted in the late 1940s (Doll and Hill, 1950), given that well over 90% of that population were cigarette smokers. For very uncommon exposures—e.g., occupational exposure to a specific substance suspected of posing a risk to health, or an infrequently prescribed drug—unless there truly is a strong association and there are a large number of subjects available, even the best-designed case-control study can offer no more than a suggestion of an association with the occurrence of a given illness.

REFERENCES

Abenhaim L, Moride Y, Brenot F, Rich S, Benichou J, Kurz X, et al. Appetite-suppressant drugs and the risk of primary pulmonary hypertension. International Primary Pulmonary Hypertension Study Group. N Engl J Med 1996; 335:609–616.

Ahsan H, Hodge SE, Heiman GA, Begg MD, Susser ES. Relative risk for genetic associations: the case-parent triad as a variant of case-cohort design. Int J Epidemiol 2002; 31:669–678.

Anton-Culver H, Lee-Feldstein A, Taylor TH. Occupation and bladder cancer risk. Am J Epidemiol 1992; 136:89–94.

Bloemenkamp KW, Rosendaal FR, Buller HR, Helmerhorst FM, Colly LP, Vandenbroucke JP. Risk of venous thrombosis with use of current low-dose oral contraceptives is not explained by diagnostic suspicion and referral bias. Arch Intern Med 1999; 159:65–70.

Breslow NE, Day NE. Statistical methods in cancer research. Volume I: The analysis of case-control studies. Lyon, France: International Agency for Research on Cancer, 1980.

Campbell PT, Sloan M, Kreiger N. Utility of proxy versus index respondent information in a population-based case-control study of rapidly fatal cancers. Ann Epidemiol 2007; 17:253–257.

Crombie IK. The limitations of case-control studies in the detection of environmental carcinogens. J Epidemiol Community Health 1981; 35:281–287.

Cummings P, Weiss NS. Case series and exposure series: the role of studies without controls in providing information about the etiology of injury or disease. Inj Prev 1998; 4:34–57.

Daling JR, Weiss NS, Hislop TG, Maden C, Coates RJ, Sherman KJ, et al. Sexual practices, sexually transmitted diseases, and the incidence of anal cancer. N Engl J Med 1987; 317:973–977.

Daling JR, Weiss NS, Klopfenstein LL, Cochran LE, Chow WH, Daifuku R. Correlates of homosexual behavior and the incidence of anal cancer. JAMA 1982; 247:1988–1990.

Doll R, Hill AB. Smoking and carcinoma of the lung. Br Med J 1950; 2:739–748.

Gillison ML, Koch WM, Capone RB, Spafford M, Westra WH, Wu L, et al. Evidence for a causal association between human papillomavirus and a subset of head and neck cancers. J Natl Cancer Inst 2000; 92:709–720.

Gordis L. Should dead cases be matched to dead controls? Am J Epidemiol 1982; 115:1–5.

Green LM, Miller AB, Agnew DA, Greenberg ML, Li J, Villeneuve PJ, et al. Childhood leukemia and personal monitoring of residential exposures to electric and magnetic fields in Ontario, Canada. Cancer Causes Control 1999; 10:233–243.

Greenberg ER, Rosner B, Hennekens C, Rinsky R, Colton T. An investigation of bias in a study of nuclear shipyard workers. Am J Epidemiol 1985; 121:301–308.

Greenwald P, Barlow JJ, Nasca PC, Burnett WS. Vaginal cancer after maternal treatment with synthetic estrogens. N Engl J Med 1971; 285:390–392.

Herbst AL, Ulfelder H, Poskanzer DC. Adenocarcinoma of the vagina: association of maternal stilbestrol therapy with tumor appearance in young women. N Engl J Med 1971; 284:878–881.

Holcomb RL. Alcohol in relation to traffic accidents. JAMA 1938; 111:1076–1085.

Horwitz RI, Feinstein AR. Alternative analytic methods for case-control studies of estrogens and endometrial cancer. N Engl J Med 1978; 299:1089–1094.

Hosmer DW, Lemeshow S. Applied logistic regression (2nd ed.). New York: John Wiley & Sons, 2000.

Hurwitz ES, Barrett MJ, Bregman D, Gunn WJ, Schonberger LB, Fairweather WR, et al. Public Health Service study on Reye's syndrome and medications. Report of the pilot phase. N Engl J Med 1985; 313:849–857.

Janerich DT, Thompson WD, Varela LR, Greenwald P, Chorost S, Tucci C, et al. Lung cancer and exposure to tobacco smoke in the household. N Engl J Med 1990; 323:632–636.

Laumon B, Gadegbeku B, Martin JL, Biecheler MB. Cannabis intoxication and fatal road crashes in France: population based case-control study. BMJ 2005; 331:1371.

Mayne ST, Morse DE, Winn DM. Cancers of the oral cavity and pharynx. In: Schottenfeld D, Fraumeni JF (eds.). Cancer epidemiology and prevention (3rd ed.). New York: Oxford, 2006 pp.674–696.

McLaughlin JK, Blot WJ, Mehl ES, Mandel JS. Problems in the use of dead controls in case-control studies. II. Effect of excluding certain causes of death. Am J Epidemiol 1985; 122:485–494.

Meier CR, Jick SS, Derby LE, Vasilakis C, Jick H. Acute respiratory-tract infections and risk of first-time acute myocardial infarction. Lancet 1998; 351:1467–1471.

Nam RK, Zhang WW, Trachtenberg J, Jewett MA, Emami M, Vesprini D, et al. Comprehensive assessment of candidate genes and serological markers for the detection of prostate cancer. Cancer Epidemiol Biomarkers Prev 2003; 12:1429–1437.

Needleman HL, Schell A, Bellinger D, Leviton A, Allred EN. The long-term effects of exposure to low doses of lead in childhood. An 11-year follow-up report. N Engl J Med 1990; 322:83–88.

Nelson LM, Longstreth WT Jr, Koepsell TD, van Belle G. Proxy respondents in epidemiologic research. Epidemiol Rev 1990; 12:71–86.

Ponsonby AL, van der Mei I, Dwyer T, Blizzard L, Taylor B, Kemp A, et al. Exposure to infant siblings during early life and risk of multiple sclerosis. JAMA 2005; 293:463–469.

Rinsky RA, Zumwalde RD, Waxweiler RJ, Murray WE Jr, Bierbaum PJ, Landrigan PJ, et al. Cancer mortality at a naval nuclear shipyard. Lancet 1981; 1:231–235.

Rodrigues LC, Smith PG. Use of the case-control approach in vaccine evaluation: Efficacy and adverse effects. Epidemiol Rev 1999; 21:56–72.

Rosenberg L, Mitchell AA, Parsells JL, Pashayan H, Louik C, Shapiro S. Lack of relation of oral clefts to diazepam use during pregnancy. N Engl J Med 1983; 309:1282–1285.

Rothman KJ, Greenland S, Lash TL. Modern epidemiology (3rd ed.). Philadelphia: Lippincott Williams & Wilkins, 2008.

Rowe B, Milner R, Johnson C, Bota G. The association of alcohol and night driving with fatal snowmobile trauma: a case-control study. Ann Emerg Med 1994; 24:842–848.

Selby JV. Case-control evaluations of treatment and program efficacy. Epidemiol Rev 1994; 46:91–101.

Shapiro S, Kelly JP, Rosenberg L, Kaufman DW, Helmrich SP, Rosenshein NB, et al. Risk of localized and widespread endometrial cancer in relation to recent and discontinued use of conjugated estrogens. N Engl J Med 1985; 313:969–972.

Silverberg SG, Makowski MD. Endometrial carcinoma in young women taking oral contraceptive agents. J Obstet Gynecol 1975; 46:503–506.

Silverman DT, Hoover RN, Swanson GM. Artificial sweeteners and lower urinary tract cancer: hospital vs. population controls. Am J Epidemiol 1983; 117:326–334.

Siscovick DS, Weiss NS, Fletcher RH, Lasky T. The incidence of primary cardiac arrest during vigorous exercise. N Engl J Med 1984; 311:874–877.

Siscovick DS, Weiss NS, Hallstrom AP, Inui TS, Peterson DR. Physical activity and primary cardiac arrest. JAMA 1982; 248:3113–3117.

Smith GS, Keyl PM, Hadley JA, Bartley CL, Foss RD, Tolbert WG, et al. Drinking and recreational boating fatalities: a population-based case-control study. JAMA 2001; 286:2974–2980.

Spechler SJ, Fischbach L, Feldman M. Clinical aspects of genetic variability in Helicobacter pylori. JAMA 2000; 283:1264–1266.

Stallones RA. A review of the epidemiologic studies of toxic shock syndrome. Ann Intern Med 1982; 96:917–920.

Stott DH. Some psychosomatic aspects of casualty in reproduction. J Psychosomatic Res 1958; 3:42–55.

Strathy JH, Molgaard CA, Coulam CB, Melton LJ 3d. Endometriosis and infertility: a laparoscopic study of endometriosis among fertile and infertile women. Fertil Steril 1982; 38:667–672.

Tabuenca JM. Toxic-allergic syndrome caused by ingestion of rapeseed oil denatured with aniline. Lancet 1981; 2:567–568.

Thom DH, Grayston JT, Siscovick DS, Wang SP, Weiss NS, Daling JR. Association of prior infection with Chlamydia pneumoniae and angiographically demonstrated coronary artery disease. JAMA 1992; 268:68–72.

Tully J, Viner RM, Coen PG, Stuart JM, Zambon M, Peckham C, et al. Risk and protective factors for meningococcal disease in adolescents: matched cohort study. BMJ 2006; 332:445–450.

Ulfelder H, Robboy SJ. The embryologic development of the human vagina. Am J Obstet Gynecol 1976; 126:769–776.

Victora CG, Smith PG, Vaughan JP, Nobre LC, Lombardi C, Teixeira AM, et al. Infant feeding and deaths due to diarrhea. A case-control study. Am J Epidemiol 1989; 129:1032–1041.

Wacholder S. Practical considerations in choosing between the case-cohort and nested case-control designs. Epidemiology 1991; 2:155–158.

Wacholder S, McLaughlin JK, Silverman DT, Mandel JS. Selection of controls in case-control studies. I. Principles. Am J Epidemiol 1992a; 135:1019–1028.

Wacholder S, Silverman DT, McLaughlin JK, Mandel JS. Selection of controls in case-control studies. II. Types of controls. Am J Epidemiol 1992b; 135:1029–1041.

Wacholder S, Silverman DT, McLaughlin JK, Mandel JS. Selection of controls in case-control studies. III. Design options. Am J Epidemiol 1992c; 135:1042–1050.

Weinmann S, Glass AG, Weiss NS, Psaty BM, Siscovick DS, White E. Use of diuretics and other antihypertensive medications in relation to the risk of renal cell cancer. Am J Epidemiol 1994; 140:792–804.

Weiss NS. Application of the case-control method in the evaluation of screening. Epidemiol Rev 1994; 16:102–108.

Weiss NS, Lyon JL, Liff JM, Vollmer WM, Daling JR. Incidence of ovarian cancer in relation to the use of oral contraceptives. Int J Cancer 1981; 28:669–671.

Weiss NS, Sayvetz TA. Incidence of endometrial cancer in relation to the use of oral contraceptives. N Engl J Med 1980; 302:551–554.

Werler MM, Hayes C, Louik C, Shapiro S, Mitchell AA. Multivitamin supplementation and risk of birth defects. Am J Epidemiol 1999; 150:675–682.

White E, Armstrong BK, Saracci R. Principles of exposure measurement in epidemiology: collecting, evaluating, and improving measures of disease risk factors (2nd ed.). New York: Oxford, 2008.

Witte JS, Gauderman WJ, Thomas DC. Asymptotic bias and efficiency in case-control studies of candidate genes and gene-environment interactions: Basic family designs. Am J Epidemiol 1999; 149:693–705.

Woodson K, Tangrea JA, Pollak M, Copeland TD, Taylor PR, Virtamo J, et al. Serum insulin-like growth factor I: tumor marker or etiologic factor? A prospective study of prostate cancer among Finnish men. Cancer Res 2003; 63:3991–3994.

Yang Q, Khoury MJ. Evolving methods in genetic epidemiology. III. Gene-environment interaction in epidemiologic research. Epidemiol Rev 1997; 19:33–42.

EXERCISES

1. A study of bladder cancer in relation to occupation among women was conducted in Southern California (Anton-Culver *et al.*, 1992). For women diagnosed with this condition during 1984–1988, current occupation was ascertained from medical records. As a basis for comparison, interviews were conducted with a random sample of similar-aged women who resided in the same counties as the cases. A far greater proportion of cases than controls were categorized as "home-makers": Relative to women who had a professional, technical, or managerial occupation, homemakers were estimated to have about a five-fold increase in the risk of bladder cancer (95% confidence interval of the relative risk = 2.4–12.0). The authors hypothesized that the hobbies and household tasks of the home-makers might expose them to carcinogenic agents to a greater extent than other women. What is a (possibly more plausible) noncausal explanation for the association?

2. The following data were obtained in an epidemiologic study of hip and forearm fracture. Female residents of King County, Washington, ages 50–74 years, who were treated for either of these conditions during a 2-year period by one of 59 orthopedists in the County ($n = 320$) were identified and interviewed regarding prior receipt of postmenopausal unopposed estrogen therapy. Similar information was obtained from a sample of King County women of the same ages ($n = 567$). The results are shown in Tab. 15.3.

   (a) Relative to the risk of hip or forearm fracture in estrogen non-users, what is the risk in women who

TABLE 15.3. HIP AND FOREARM FRACTURES IN RELATION TO DURATION OF UNOPPOSED ESTROGEN USE AMONG FEMALE RESIDENTS OF KING COUNTY, WASHINGTON

Duration of unop-posed estrogen use	Cases	Controls
None	210	272
1–5 years	60	108
6+ years	50	187
Total	320	567

used unopposed estrogens for 1–5 years? For 6+ years?

   (b) Assume that long-term unopposed estrogen use (e.g., 6+ years) truly protects against the occurrence of fracture of the hip and forearm. From the data provided, can you determine the amount by which the rate of hip or forearm fracture is reduced in women who have used unopposed estrogens for 6+ years? If yes, what is that amount? If no, why not?

3. During the mid-1980s, several epidemiologists conducted a case-control study of childhood cancer in relation to birth weight. Cases were all children under two years of age in King County, Washington, who developed cancer during 1974–1982. Controls were selected from this county's birth certificates, and were matched to the cases on the basis of year of birth and sex. The results of the study are summarized in Tab. 15.4.

   The study was criticized for having included in the analysis children with birth weights <2500 grams, because of the relatively high mortality of this group during the first days and weeks of life.

   (a) Does this criticism have some merit? If yes, why? If no, why not?

   (b) Should this criticism influence the conclusion that high birth weight (i.e. >4000 grams) was associated with cancer incidence in the first two years of life? If yes, why? If no, why not?

4. While primary pulmonary hypertension can be a fatal disease, it may be present in a relatively mild form, at least temporarily. Therefore, some persons may not seek medical attention for symptoms of primary pulmonary hypertension in its early stages, or their physician may fail to diagnose the condition.

   Some time ago, data became available to suggest strongly that a particular appetite suppressant agent, aminorex, could predispose to the development of primary pulmonary hypertension. Years later, a case-control study of primary pulmonary hypertension (Abenhaim *et al.*, 1996) observed an elevated odds ratio associated with use (before the onset of symptoms) of several newer appetite suppressant drugs. The odds ratio was particularly high in the analysis pertaining to patients with moderate and severe symptoms and signs, but was only slightly elevated when restricted to cases with less serious illness. Does this pattern of results suggest that the association between use of the newer appetite suppressant drugs and primary pulmonary hypertension is not genuine, but rather is due to differential recognition of pulmonary hypertension according to prior use of these drugs?

TABLE 15.4. BIRTH WEIGHT DISTRIBUTION OF CHILDREN
DIAGNOSED WITH CANCER PRIOR TO AGE 2 YEARS, AND OF
CONTROLS

| | Birth weight (grams) | | | | | |
	<2500	2501 –3500	3501 –4000	4001 –4500	>4500	All
Cases (%)	5.6	44.9	27.0	16.9	5.6	100.0
Controls (%)	6.1	53.2	29.6	9.1	1.9	100.0

5. One of the early studies of the possible association between the use of oral contraceptives and the risk of myocardial infarction (MI) was conducted in Great Britain. During 1973, investigators identified and obtained information on all cases of MI in women under the age of 40 years who resided in a portion of that country, and in 50% of the women ages 40–44. Controls were selected from patient rosters of general practitioners. The data from the study are shown in Tab. 15.5.

(a) Without adjusting for age, estimate the risk of myocardial infarction in current users of oral contraceptives relative to that in women who were not current users. Now estimate the corresponding relative risk adjusted for age. Why do the two estimates differ? Which one do you believe more accurately reflects the size of the association between oral contraceptive use and the incidence of myocardial infarction?

(b) On the basis of these and other data, you have concluded that the current use of the oral contraceptives available in 1973 was a cause of myocardial infarction, and to roughly the same relative degree across age groups. By what percentage do you estimate the incidence rate of this disease would have fallen in British women under 45 years of age if oral contraceptives had no longer been used?

6. The following is a hypothetical abstract from an article reporting results of a case-control study of testicular

cancer in relation to occupation: "The men with testicular cancer ($n = 18$) were much more likely to be plastics workers (33%) than controls (11% of 159 men). Occupational histories showing exposure to agent X for five out of six cases known to have been plastics workers further support a causal association between agent X and testicular cancer."

Do you agree that a causal association between exposure to agent X and testicular cancer is strengthened by the observation that exposure to agent X had occurred among five of six cases known to be plastics workers? If yes, why? If no, why not?

7. The following is excerpted from the abstract of an article that appeared in the *Lancet* (Meier *et al.*, 1998):

Background: There is growing interest in the role of infections in the etiology of acute myocardial infarction (MI). We undertook a large, population-based study to explore the association between risk of MI and recent acute respiratory-tract infection.

Methods: We used data from general practices in the UK (General Practice Research Database). Potential cases were people aged 75 years or younger, with no history of clinical risk factors, who had a first-time diagnosis of MI between January 1, 1994, and October 31, 1996. Four controls were matched to each case on age, sex, the practice attended, and the absence of clinical risk factors for MI. The date of the MI in the case was

TABLE 15.5. ORAL CONTRACEPTIVE USE IN MYOCARDIAL
INFARCTION CASES AND CONTROLS, BY AGE

Current oral contraceptive use	<40 years		40–44 years	
	Cases	Controls	Cases	Controls
Yes	21	17	8	2
No	26	59	44	50
	47	76	52	52

defined as the index date. For both cases and controls the date of the last respiratory-tract infection before the index date was identified.

Findings: In the case-control analysis of 1922 cases and 7649 matched controls, significantly more cases than controls had an acute respiratory-tract infection in the 10 days before the index date (54 [2.8%] vs. 72 [0.9%]). The odds ratios adjusted for smoking and body-mass index, for first-time MI in association with an acute respiratory-tract infection 1–5, 6–10, 11–15, or 16–30 days before the index date (compared with participants who had no such infection during the preceding year) were 3.6 [95% CI 2.2–5.7, 2.3 (1–4.2), 1.8 (1.0–3.3), and 1.0 (0.7–1.6)] (test for trend $p < 0.01$).

Interpretation: Our findings suggest that in people without a history of clinical risk factors for MI, acute respiratory tract infections are associated with an increased risk of MI for a period of about two weeks.

Because this study was conducted within the U.K. General Practice Research Database, controls could be readily selected from the defined population from which each case came; i.e., the patients of an individual general practitioner.

In the United States, where many physicians do not have such a well-defined group of patients who necessarily would seek primary care from them, a different case-control design might be considered. Imagine that in a United States study of this question, for each case that developed an MI, four controls (matched for age and sex) could be selected from among those who visited the case's primary care physician on the day of the case's MI. Would you expect this latter design to produce a biased estimate of the relationship of recent acute respiratory tract infections to the incidence of MI? If yes, why, and in which direction? If no, why not?

8. The following is excerpted from the abstract of an article that appeared in *Cancer Epidemiology, Biomarkers & Prevention* (Nam *et al.*, 2003):

We examined whether selected polymorphisms in 11 candidate genes help predict the presence of prostate cancer. We studied 1031 men who underwent one or more prostate biopsies because of an elevated PSA level or abnormal digital rectal exam. Of the 1031 men, 483 had cancer on any biopsy (cases) and 548 men had no cancer (controls).

The authors conducted this study to determine whether they could enhance their ability to predict which men suspected of having prostate cancer actually did have this condition. Under what circumstances might their results also provide a valid assessment of the potential role of the 11 genes in the *etiology* of prostate cancer?

9. A study of risk factors for snowmobile fatalities during 1985–1990 identified 108 deaths from this cause in a Canadian province (Rowe *et al.*, 1994). Based on blood alcohol determinations, a greater proportion of those persons had evidence of recent alcohol use than controls (demographically comparable drivers of automobiles and motorcycles who died in crashes during 1985–1990): odds ratio = 4.3, 95% confidence interval = 2.5–7.0.

Do you believe the control group chosen for this study led to bias in the estimate of the relative risk of fatal snowmobile trauma associated with alcohol use? If yes, why, and would an unbiased estimate be greater or smaller than that obtained by the authors? If not, why not?

10. Scleroderma is an uncommon connective tissue disorder that has been postulated to be related to the presence of a silicone breast implant. To address this question, a case-control study was conducted in a large metropolitan area in Australia. Implants were performed in Australia as early as the 1960s, and the frequency of this operation rose steadily through 1990. The investigators sought to identify all cases of scleroderma that had occurred among residents of that area between 1980 and 1990. They did so by reviewing the records of medical laboratories for the presence of tests done to diagnose scleroderma, the records of dermatologists and rheumatologists practicing in the area, the records of all hospitals in the area, and death certificates. Strict criteria for the presence of scleroderma were developed prior to the start of the study, and each potential case was evaluated for the presence of these criteria without regard to her history of a breast implant. Controls of the same ages as the cases (as of the time of their diagnosis) were selected by means of a random sample of residents of this area in 1990. Cases and controls were asked detailed questions regarding a history of silicone brest implants and other implants elsewhere in the body prior to the onset of symptoms (for cases) or to the date of interview (for controls). Four of 251 cases had had a breast implant, versus five of 289 control women.

    (a) Estimate the risk of scleroderma in women who have had a breast implant relative to that in women who had not.

    (b) Assume the identification of cases of scleroderma was complete, and that the information provided by study subjects was accurate, including that provided by next of kin of the scleroderma cases who died prior to the start of the study. What do you believe to be the major threat to the validity of this study? Why? In what direction do you think the observed estimate of relative risk would be biased in relation to the true relative risk?

ANSWERS

1. Given the very different means by which current occupation was assessed in cases and controls—medical records and interviews, respectively—it seems that a large degree of information bias could have been present in this study. In their "Discussion", the authors acknowledge that "traditionally, one would use similar methodology to interview both cases and controls, to determine with the same degree of accuracy and completeness the risk factor of occupation. Alternatively, this study, which used previously collected data from two different sources, required no additional resources for data collection." Earlier (Chapter 6) we commented that epidemiologists often are data scavengers, and that the analysis of previously collected data can often yield valid and useful information. Nonetheless, there are situations in which this is not so. We recommend that the "tradition" of case-control comparability regarding exposure ascertainment be respected!

2. (a) The two relative risks can be estimated by means of the respective odds ratios. For 1–5 year's use relative to never used, $OR = 60/210 \div 108/272 = 0.72$. For ≥ 6 year's use relative to never used, $OR = 50/210 \div 187/272 = 0.35$.

   (b) The amount by which estrogen use reduces risk of fracture cannot be estimated from these data alone. What would be required in addition is the *rate* of fracture in one of the three categories of women or in the 50–74 year old female population as a whole.

3. The study was criticized for having included in the analysis children with birth weights <2500 grams, because of the relatively high mortality of this group during the first days and weeks of life.

   (a) The criticism is valid. Proportionately fewer children who live to develop cancer will have low birth weights than those in a matched sample of newborns. Thus, even if there were no association between birth weight and cancer in early childhood, with this design the risk of cancer in high birth weight babies relative to that in low birth weight babies would be expected to slightly exceed 1.0.

   (b) Compared to infants of average birth weight (e.g., 2501–3500 g.), the cancer risk in those of

TABLE 15.6. ODDS RATIO FOR CANCER IN RELATION TO BIRTH WEIGHT

Birth weight	Case	Control	Odds ratio
>4000 g.	22.5	11.0	2.23
≤2500 g.	5.6	6.1	1
>4000 g.	22.5	11.0	2.42
2501–3500 g.	44.9	53.2	1

high birth weight was also elevated, as shown in Tab. 15.6.

Thus, assuming that among infants who weigh >2500 g. at birth there is no increase in infant mortality with decreasing birth weight, the authors' conclusion is valid.

4. Bias can arise in a non-randomized study when some persons with a disease go undiagnosed, and when there is reason to believe that exposed persons (e.g., to appetite suppressant drugs) are relatively less likely to go undiagnosed. In the present example, it might be true that some physicians, aware of the association between use of aminorex and the incidence of pulmonary hypertension: (1) were relatively more alert to the presence of this condition in patients taking appetite suppressant drugs, or (2) had a relatively lower threshold for making a diagnosis of pulmonary hypertension in users of these other appetite suppressant drugs.

   In such a situation it might be expected that, unlike persons with mild pulmonary hypertension, those with a more severe form of the disease would be recognized as having it, irrespective of their exposure status. If this were true, the most valid assessment of an association with the exposure of concern would be restricted to them. Since the association between primary pulmonary hypertension and use of appetite suppressant drugs was particularly great once the milder cases had been excluded from the analysis, this bias does not appear to be present here.

5. (a) Age is a confounder, in that: (1) current OC use was more common in younger than in older women; and (2) the ratio of cases/controls differed (by design) in the two age categories.

$$\text{Crude } OR(= RR) = \frac{29/70}{19/109} = 2.38$$

Adjusted $OR(= RR)$

$$= \frac{(21 \times 59 \div 123) + (8 \times 50 \div 104)}{(17 \times 26 \div 123) + (44 \times 2 \div 104)}$$

$$= 3.14$$

TABLE 15.7. TWO SETS OF HYPOTHETICAL RESULTS IN A CASE-CONTROL STUDY OF TESTICULAR CANCER

Plastics worker	Exposed to agent X	Cases	Controls	Odds ratio
No	—	12	141	1.0
Yes	—	6	18	3.9
	Yes	5	9	6.5
	No	1	9	1.3
No	—	12	141	1.0
Yes	—	6	18	3.9
	Yes	5	15	3.9
	No	1	3	3.9

(b)

$$PAR\% = \frac{RR-1}{RR}(P_c) \times 100\%$$

$$= \frac{3.14-1}{3.14}(P_c) \times 100\%$$

Since only half the deaths in women ages 40–44 were included, as opposed to all deaths in women under 40,

$$P_c = \frac{21+2(8)}{47+2(52)} = .245$$

$$PAR\% = \frac{RR-1}{RR}(P_c) \times 100\%$$

$$= \frac{3.14-1}{3.14}(.245) \times 100\%$$

$$= 16.7\%$$

6. The observation would only support an association if, among men *without* testicular cancer who had been workers, fewer than 5/6 had been exposed to agent X. Note the difference in the interpretation of the top and bottom panels in Tab. 15.7.

Only the data in the upper table, in which the proportion of plastics workers exposed to agent X differs between cases (83%) and controls (50%), support the hypothesis of there being a subgroup of plastics workers at particularly high risk of testicular cancer.

7. Yes, the results would be biased, because respiratory infections are a common reason for visiting a doctor.

An atypically high proportion of controls chosen in this manner would be expected to have a respiratory infection on the index date, leading to a falsely low estimate of the association between recent respiratory infection and the incidence of the MI.

8. The study could be expected to provide a valid result if each genotype had no relation to the occurrence of the conditions (in aggregate) that the men in the control group had. That is, a valid result would be obtained if the genotype distribution for a particular polymorphism among these controls reflected that of the underlying population from which the cases of prostate cancer were derived.

9. The control group for this study comprised persons with alcohol-related causes of death; i.e., those due to motor vehicle and motorcycle accidents. Therefore, the observed odds ratio is probably lower than the true one.

10. (a) $RR \approx OR = \frac{4}{247} \div \frac{5}{284} = 0.92$

(b) The greatest potential source of bias in this study is the difference in time periods during which implants could have been received by cases and controls. The relevant time period for cases was that prior to the onset of symptoms, the average date of which was almost certainly earlier than 1985 (the approximate mean year of diagnosis). The relevant time period for controls was prior to interview in 1990. Because breast implant procedures became more common in more recent years, the cases would have a spuriously low frequency relative to controls, leading to a spuriously low odds ratio.

16

Ecological and Multi-Level Studies

No man is an island, entire of itself; every man is a piece of the continent, a part of the main.

—JOHN DONNE

INTRODUCTION

Most United States citizens are legally entitled to own a gun for personal protection, but whether it is to a person's advantage to do so has long been a matter of debate (Hemenway and Azrael, 2000; Cummings and Koepsell, 1998; Kleck and Gertz, 1995). Some argue that keeping a gun in the home can deter criminals and allow potential victims to defend themselves. Others argue that brandishing a gun may provoke gunfire from an intruder, or that easy access to a gun in the home could escalate a domestic conflict into firearm violence.

Killias (1993) reported on a study that sought to clarify the relationship between gun ownership and the risk of homicide or suicide. A sample of households in 13 nations had participated in an international crime survey, which yielded country-specific estimates of the proportion of households with a gun. This information was then combined with death rates due to homicide in each country. Figure 16.1 shows the results for all homicides. The prevalence of gun ownership was found to have a significant positive correlation with the homicide rate. In other analyses, the prevalence of gun ownership

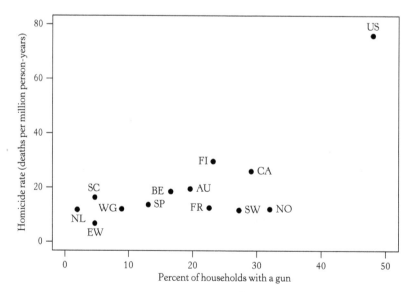

Key: AU = Australia, BE = Belgium, CA = Canada, EW = England and Wales, FI = Finland, FR = France, NL = Netherlands, NO = Norway, SC = Scotland, SP = Spain, SW = Sweden, US = United States, WG = West Germany

FIGURE 16.1 Ecological association between prevalence of guns in households and homicide rate in 13 countries, 1983–1989.

(Based on data from Killias [1993])

was also positively correlated with the death rates for gun-related homicides, for all suicides, and for gun-related suicides, and with the proportions of homicides and of suicides due to guns. The article concluded that "the correlations detected in this study suggest that the presence of a gun in the home increases the likelihood of homicide or suicide."

The Killias study is an example of an *ecological* study. Ecological studies investigate exposure–outcome associations among groups of people by examining how the frequency of exposure in each of several groups is related to the frequency of the outcome in that group.

Ecological studies are commonly undertaken for one of two reasons. First, only aggregate information on each group may be available to the investigator, even though both exposure and outcome status would surely vary among individuals within each group. For example, in the Killias study, only estimates of the overall prevalence of gun ownership were available for each country, not the gun-ownership status of each individual or household within each country. Hence there was no way to determine from the data available whether a particular homicide victim in one of the study countries was any more or less likely to own a gun than were other individuals in that country. Each of the 13 countries became a single unit of observation. In this situation, an exposure–outcome association at the population level is studied as a proxy for an exposure–outcome association at the individual level. As discussed below, there are a number of potential pitfalls involved in making this inference across levels.

Second, the exposure of interest may actually vary only at the group level, not among individuals within groups. For example, legal penalties for drinking and driving vary among states, but everyone within a state is subject to the same state law. In this situation, an exposure–outcome association must necessarily be examined at the aggregate level because there is no variation in exposure within a group.

In principle, the aggregate populations in ecological studies can be of any size, including households, classrooms, workplaces, institutions, communities, geographic regions, or entire nations. Often they are geopolitically defined populations for which the necessary data are routinely collected, inasmuch as most ecological studies use existing data (Dufault and Klar, 2011).

Ecological studies are best regarded as a class of study designs, not a single design (Morgenstern,

1995; Walter, 1991a). Whether aggregate populations or individuals are the units of study is one dimension on which study designs can be distinguished from each other. In other respects, ecological designs can be classified in much the same way as studies of individuals, as described in Chapter 5. For example:

- *Group-randomized trials.* Community intervention trials involve assigning entire communities at random to intervention or control conditions. They are the ecological counterparts to randomized trials of individuals. For example, Finkelstein *et al.* (2008) studied the effectiveness of a community program to reduce unnecessary antibiotic prescribing for children by randomizing 16 Massachusetts communities to either intervention or control status. All care providers in the same community thus belonged to the same treatment group. Computerized health records were then used to track antibiotic prescribing for children of different ages in relation to whether they lived in an intervention or a control community.

- *Ecological cohort studies.* The frequency of disease (or other outcome) can be compared between a set of exposed populations and a set of non-exposed control populations, even if the investigator had no control over which populations were exposed. For example, Boice *et al.* (2006) ascertained cancer mortality rates in four counties located near the Hanford nuclear facility in Washington State, from which radioactive iodine had been released into the air during 1944–1957. Cancer mortality in these exposed counties was compared with cancer mortality in five demographically similar counties elsewhere in the state that had little or no radioactive iodine exposure.

- *Cross-sectional ecological studies.* Two or more characteristics that pertain to the same point in time or time period can be compared among several study populations. Killias's international study of gun ownership and homicide rates exemplifies this type of study.

- *Longitudinal ecological studies.* Studies of changes in frequency of an outcome over time in entire populations correspond to longitudinal studies of individuals. For example, Héry *et al.* (2010) examined the incidence of cutaneous melanoma in Iceland over a 53-year period in relation to the growing use of tanning beds in that country and increasing travel abroad to sunny destinations. However, no individual-level data were available on melanoma status in relation to the use of tanning beds.

Several useful reviews of methodological issues that arise in ecological studies have been published: Wakefield (2008); Morgenstern (1995); Walter (1991a,b). Dufault and Klar (2011) have reviewed the quality of reporting of ecological studies in several epidemiology journals and offered recommendations for improvement.

GROUP-LEVEL AND INDIVIDUAL-LEVEL VARIABLES

Groups are made up of individuals—a statement that highlights two levels of aggregation at which characteristics relevant to disease occurrence can be ascertained. *Individual-level* variables include such familiar characteristics as a person's age, gender, gun-ownership status, and so on. However, individual-level measurements are often unavailable in an ecological study. *Group-level* variables can be divided into two kinds:

- An *aggregate* measure summarizes the distribution of an individual-level characteristic that may vary within a group—in other words, it is a summary statistic derived from individual-level data. For example, mean age, median age, and the proportion of persons aged 65 years or older are all aggregate measures that distill the age distribution of group members into a single, group-level number. Aggregate measures have also been termed *derived* variables (Susser, 1994a; Diez-Roux, 2002).

  An aggregate measure of an individual characteristic can take on new meaning at the group level as a descriptor of the environment within which people live. Returning to the issue of gun ownership and homicide, a person's risk of becoming a homicide victim may be influenced not only by whether he or she owns a gun, but also by the general availability of guns in the community as reflected by the population prevalence of gun ownership. Individual gun ownership and the population prevalence of gun ownership, which are the same characteristic measured at two different levels, could both affect a person's homicide risk by different mechanisms.

- An *intrinsically group-level* measure (termed an *integral* measure by some authors (Diez-Roux, 2002; Pickett and Pearl, 2001; Susser, 1994a; Selvin and Hagstrom, 1963) characterizes an entire group as a unit. For example, a city's size, its population density, and whether the city has a law requiring registration of handguns are all intrinsically city-level characteristics. Such a measure automatically applies to all members of a group, so there is no individual-level variation on that measure within the group. One important class of intrinsically group-level measures is the presence or absence of policies or programs that apply to all members of a population and that may affect disease frequency.

Group-level variables, whether aggregated summaries of individual-level variables or intrinsically group-level, are also sometimes termed *contextual* variables (Diez-Roux, 2002).

More generally, populations may be divided up at several possible levels of aggregation, and hence of measurement—census tract, city, state, and nation are examples—which may be nested within each other to form a hierarchy of levels. *Multi-level studies*, discussed later in this chapter, use data pertaining to two or more different levels of aggregation. For present purposes, however, two levels are enough to introduce the main methodological issues in ecological studies, including special problems that arise when only aggregate-level data are available. The two levels are sometimes termed the *macro* and *micro* levels.

STUDYING EFFECTS OF INDIVIDUAL-LEVEL EXPOSURES

One of the main uses of ecological studies in epidemiology has been to study the relationship between an individual-level exposure and individual-level disease risk, using the association between exposure prevalence and disease frequency at the population level as a proxy for the individual-level association of real interest. For example, Delong (2011) reported finding a positive state-level association between the proportion of children in a state who had received recommended vaccines by the age of two years and the state's prevalence of autism or a speech/language impairment. It was suggested that this macro-level association supported the possible existence of a micro-level association between a child's receipt of a battery of vaccinations and his/her risk of developing autism or a speech disorder. The Killias study of gun ownership and homicide provides another such example.

Other historically notable examples of ecological studies that sought to assess individual-level associations include:

- Smoking and lung cancer. Lung cancer mortality rates were found to be higher in countries where per capita tobacco sales were higher, which was used to support the inference that smoking causes lung cancer (Advisory Committee to the Surgeon General, 1964).
- Poverty and pellagra. As described in Chapter 7, Goldberger *et al.* (1920) found pellagra to be more common in South Carolina cotton mill villages where a higher proportion of men had per capita incomes below $6 or $8 per month. The investigators went on to show that this association held at the individual level and appeared to be explained by income-related differences in diet.
- Fluoride in drinking water and dental caries. Dean (1938) observed that the prevalence of dental caries was lower among children in several Midwestern communities that had relatively high fluoride content in their drinking water.

Advantages

One of the chief attractions of using ecological studies to examine individual-level associations is that preexisting population-level data may be readily available. If so, an ecological study can be completed relatively quickly and at low cost.

A second advantage can arise when exposure frequency varies substantially *between* populations but not very much *within* populations. This situation is sketched in Figure 16.2, in which the exposure and outcome variables are assumed continuous for illustration. By construction, the true relationship between exposure and outcome is positive and linear, with random error around a common regression line. Each rectangle encloses the individual-level observations from one of three hypothetical communities.

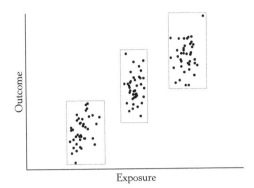

FIGURE 16.2 Example showing substantial between-population variation in exposure, but little within-population variation.

Exposure varies only over a fairly narrow range within each community, but the mean exposure level varies considerably among the communities. As a result, the underlying linear relationship between exposure and outcome is easier to detect if data from all three communities are considered (Pearson's $r = 0.90$), but it is less evident within each community ($r = 0.42, 0.04,$ and 0.20, respectively).

As an example, Rose noted that studying the relationship between water hardness and mortality from cardiovascular disease using traditional case-control studies of individuals *within* British regions would have been futile: nearly everyone obtained most of their water from public water supplies, resulting in relatively uniform exposure to hard or soft water within a region. Among regions, however, water hardness varied widely, and this permitted detection of an inverse association (Rose, 1985). Similarly, relatively large geographic and cultural differences in dietary fat intake may make it easier to detect associations between dietary fat and the incidence of breast cancer in ecological studies than in individual-level studies within geographic regions (Goodwin and Boyd, 1987).

A third advantage can become important if the exposure is subject to a high degree of measurement error or short-term biological variation at the individual level (Piantadosi *et al.*, 1988; Susser, 1994a,b). If so, then aggregation of individual measurements to the population level can reduce the effects of such errors, enabling the detection of associations that might otherwise be missed (Prentice and Sheppard, 1995).

Estimating Attributable Risk and Relative Risk

The results of ecological studies are sometimes reported simply in terms of correlation coefficients

TABLE 16.1. RESULTS FROM ECOLOGICAL REGRESSION ANALYSES OF DATA IN FIGURE 16.1

Analysis	R_0	R_1	Relative risk[a]	Attributable risk[a]
Linear least-squares				
Unweighted	1.4	100.1	71.5	98.7
Weighted	−8.0	159.9	?	168.9
Poisson	6.1	1135.0	186.1	1128.9
Negative binomial	9.0	317.1	35.2	308.1

Rates shown as deaths per million person-years
[a] Exposed = gun owner; non-exposed = gun non-owner

(Dufault and Klar, 2011), which at least convey the direction and approximate strength of the group-level association between exposure prevalence and disease frequency. For the Killias study data in Figure 16.1, the Pearson correlation between prevalence of gun ownership and homicide rate among countries is +0.73, and the Spearman rank correlation is +0.47, both suggesting moderately strong positive associations.

For epidemiologic purposes, however, relative risk and attributable risk are more informative measures of association and are easier to compare with results from other kinds of studies. Point estimates of relative risk and attributable risk can be obtained from ecological data using a generalization of a method described by Morgenstern (1982, 1995):

1. Apply regression analysis to the group-level data, modeling disease frequency as a function of exposure prevalence. Several forms of regression can be used for this purpose, as described below.
2. Use the fitted regression model to predict disease frequency for a population in which everyone is exposed, and call it R_1. Similarly, predict disease frequency for a population in which nobody is exposed, and call it R_0.
3. Estimate relative risk as R_1/R_0 and attributable risk as $R_1 - R_0$.

Although we will later note several pitfalls in inferring individual-level associations from ecological data, the data from the Killias study of the prevalence of guns in households in relation to homicide rates can be used to illustrate this method and some problems that can arise. Table 16.1 shows the results of applying four types of regression:

- Unweighted least-squares regression. Like the ordinary Pearson and Spearman correlation coefficients, this method gives equal weight to each of the 13 data points. It posits a linear

relationship between exposure prevalence and outcome frequency. However, one difficulty is that the *homoscedasticity* (equal-variance) assumption required under ordinary least-squares regression is almost surely violated, because a rate from a smaller country will be less precise than one from a larger country, due to smaller numbers.
- Weighted least-squares regression. This method also posits a linear relationship between exposure prevalence and outcome frequency, but it aims to satisfy the homoscedasticity assumption more nearly by weighting each country's data point by its estimated population. A remaining problem is that both unweighted and weighted least-squares regression permit negative predicted values of R_0 or R_1, which is impossible for a rate or a proportion.
- Poisson regression. This method assumes a linear relationship between log(rate) and exposure prevalence, gives more weight to data from larger countries, and guarantees that the predicted values of R_0 or R_1 will always be positive. However, the residuals often exhibit more variation than expected under the Poisson distribution.
- Negative binomial regression. This method posits a log-linear model form similar to that of Poisson regression, but it also allows for extra-Poisson variation in rates.

The results shown in Table 16.1 for all four regression models suggest a strong positive association between prevalence of gun ownership and homicide rate, but the estimates of relative and attributable risk vary greatly across models. One reason is that estimating R_0 and R_1 involves extrapolating the fitted regression relationships well beyond

TABLE 16.2. HYPOTHETICAL RESULTS OF AN ECOLOGICAL STUDY OF GUN OWNERSHIP AND HOMICIDE, ILLUSTRATING CROSS-LEVEL BIAS

| | Ecological data | | Individual-level data | | | | | | |
| | | | Gun owners | | | Gun non-owners | | | |
Country	Prevalence of gun ownership	Homicide rate[a]	Homicides	Pop. at risk[b]	Homicide rate[a]	Homicides	Pop. at risk[b]	Homicide rate[a]	Relative risk
A	.20	21.0	210	18	11.7	1,680	72	23.3	0.50
B	.22	22.0	408	33	12.4	2,892	117	24.7	0.50
C	.26	24.0	359	26	13.8	2,041	74	27.6	0.50
D	.34	28.0	1,147	68	16.9	4,453	132	33.7	0.50

[a] Homicides per million person-years
[b] In millions

the range of observed exposure prevalences to estimate what the homicide rates would be in hypothetical countries in which 0% or 100% of households own guns. Subtle differences in the shape of the regression relationships become greatly magnified when extrapolated that far, leading to very different predictions. In the case of weighted least-squares regression, the estimated value of R_0 is actually negative—an impossibility that precludes calculating RR at all under that model.

Because the number of population data points in an ecological study is often small, there may be very limited power to determine whether one model form fits significantly better than another (Greenland, 1992; Richardson *et al.*, 1987). In this example, a comparison of goodness-of-fit statistics across models indicates that the negative binomial regression model fits the data best, suggesting that the bottom row of Table 16.1 may contain the most credible estimates of relative and attributable risk. Still, estimates of attributable and relative risk obtained from ecological studies must usually be viewed only as rough approximations.

Pitfalls

Ecological studies of individual-level associations between exposure and disease are vulnerable to several potential sources of bias, some of which have no direct counterpart in studies of individuals.

To continue with the gun ownership and homicide example, so far several ways of viewing the data have led to the same general conclusion that a positive association exists between gun ownership and homicide risk. But now consider the hypothetical data in Table 16.2 from an imaginary study, similar in design to the Killias study, but for simplicity confined

to just four countries. As in the Killias study, at the country level, the homicide rate is positively associated with the prevalence of gun ownership. In fact, by construction, there is a perfect linear relationship between these two country-level variables.

But the key feature of Table 16.2 is that we are allowed to peek at the individual-level data behind the country-specific homicide rates and prevalences of gun ownership on which the ecological analysis was based. Surprisingly, within each country, the homicide rate among gun owners is actually only *half* the rate among gun non-owners. The individual-level association is not even in the same direction as the association seen in the population-level data.

Figure 16.3 illustrates this phenomenon graphically for continuous exposure and outcome variables. *Within* each of four populations, as exposure increases, outcome decreases. But *across* populations, as the mean exposure level increases, the mean level or rate of the outcome increases.

The hypothetical data in Table 16.2 and Figure 16.3 show that associations at the population level need not necessarily reflect associations of similar magnitude, or even of similar direction, at the individual level. The *ecological fallacy* occurs when a population-level association is erroneously taken to imply a similar individual-level association. It is an inferential pitfall long known to sociologists (Robinson, 1950). More generally, *cross-level bias* occurs when an association at one level of aggregation is assumed to represent the association at another level, when in fact the associations at the two levels are unequal.

Unfortunately, the kind of detailed individual-level data shown on the right side of Table 16.2 are seldom available in an ecological study. (If they

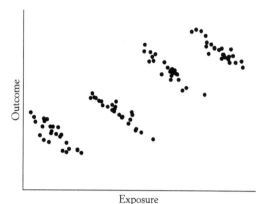

FIGURE 16.3 Example of different population-level and individual-level associations between continuous exposure and outcome variables.

were, the motivation for the ecological analysis might vanish altogether.) Hence there is usually no way to determine empirically whether cross-level bias is present, and, if so, how large it is. Perhaps the best available defense is to understand situations that can lead to this bias, including the following:

- *Group itself meets necessary conditions to be a confounder.* For example, in Table 16.2, the prevalence of gun ownership rises steadily from 0.20 to 0.34 as we scan down the rows, while the homicide rate in gun non-owners rises steadily from 23.3 to 33.7 per million person-years. Thus, country is associated both with exposure and with outcome in non-exposed persons. This is an epidemiologic version of conditions first described by Firebaugh (1978) as producing cross-level bias in sociological data. This pattern of associations can, in turn, arise in several ways:

  - The groups may differ on the distribution of one or more extraneous individual-level risk factors, such as age and gender. For example, if young males are more likely to own guns and are also at greater risk for homicide, then a country whose population is heavily weighted toward young males may have both a high prevalence of gun ownership and a high homicide rate among gun non-owners.
  - An intrinsically group-level factor may be a confounder. For example, lax law enforcement could be associated both with

widespread gun ownership and with high homicide rates in gun non-owners.
  - The exposure itself may have effects at the group level above and beyond its effects at the individual level. In other words, an individual's risk may depend not only on his/her own exposure status, but also on the exposure status of other individuals in the group. For example, homicide risk to a gun non-owner may be greater in a country where owning a gun is common than where it is rare.

  Herd immunity is a special case of this phenomenon. A person's risk of developing a certain disease can depend not only on his or her own immunity status but also on whether a large proportion of people with whom he/she comes in contact are immune. Herd immunity is important for many contagious diseases because it implies that eradication of the disease may be possible without vaccinating everyone in a population against it. But as noted in Chapter 13, a similar phenomenon can also occur for various non-infectious diseases whenever one person's exposure status can affect another person's disease risk. For example, whether a household has a working smoke detector may influence the risk to people in other nearby households of being injured by fire.

- *Unequal distribution of an effect modifier across groups.* Greenland and Morgenstern (1989) present a hypothetical example in which esophageal cancer incidence in non-smokers is the same across groups, but the incidence among smokers varies across groups because a characteristic that enhances smoking's harmful effect is more common in some groups than in others. In their example, an ecological analysis suggests a spurious inverse association between smoking and esophageal cancer, although more generally a bias in either direction could result. Piantadosi (1994) also discusses the statistical basis for this phenomenon.
- *Model misspecification.* For many graded exposures, the relationship between exposure and risk at the individual level is non-linear. In an ecological study, the only available data may be the mean exposure level for each group, which does not capture information

about the distribution of exposure among individuals. The same mean exposure level could result from most individuals falling near the mean, or from two subgroups at opposite ends of the exposure range. These two patterns could correspond to quite different expected overall disease rates. Moreover, in the ecological analysis, the number of groups available for study may be small. As a result, a simple linear or log-linear model between disease rate and mean exposure level may appear to fit the ecological data adequately, even though it is actually a poor reflection of the individual-level relationship of real interest (Greenland, 1992).

Measurement error and control of confounding factors also pose special challenges in ecological studies. As discussed in Chapter 10, in individual-level studies, non-differential misclassification of exposure normally biases estimates of excess risk toward the null value. In ecological studies, however, non-differential error in exposure measurement can have just the opposite effect, causing estimates of excess risk to be biased *away* from the null (Brenner *et al.*, 1992).

Control over confounding factors can also be hard to achieve with ecological data. Confounders can operate at either the individual level or the group level. Some may have non-linear associations with disease risk at the individual level, making it difficult to remove confounding by them if only group-level means are available (Greenland and Morgenstern, 1989; Greenland, 1992; Greenland and Robins, 1994). For many of the diseases considered in Chapter 7, for example, non-linear associations are seen between incidence or mortality and age. The possibility of non-linear associations motivates using more finely detailed information about distribution of the confounder in each group, if this information is available. For example, rather than including just mean age in a group-level regression analysis in an attempt to remove confounding by age, better control may be gained by including several age-related variables, each of which reflects the proportion of group members falling into a particular age group (Greenland and Robins, 1994).

Rate standardization (see Chapter 11) can also be used to control confounding in ecological studies—for example, by using the age-adjusted rate, rather than the crude rate, for each group. It then becomes important to standardize the prevalence of

exposure and of other covariates to the same reference population (Rosenbaum and Rubin, 1984).

Sometimes the researcher has choices in designing an ecological study, such as what kind of groups to study and on what basis the groups studied are selected. Ecological studies should theoretically be less prone to bias and have greater power when within-group variation in exposure is small but between-group variation in exposure prevalence is large (Wakefield, 2008; Greenland, 1992). On the other hand, to prevent confounding, it is preferable that groups be similar to each other on potential confounders—a condition that can be hard to satisfy while simultaneously seeking to maximize exposure heterogeneity between groups.

In view of the many ways in which ecological studies can go wrong as a method of estimating individual-level associations, one might wonder why any self-respecting epidemiologist would choose to venture into such a minefield of possible biases. Indeed, some have argued that ecological studies should be used only for hypothesis generation (Piantadosi, 1994). Even that limited role would be hard to justify if these studies were just as likely to mislead as to point toward the truth.

Piantadosi *et al.* (1988) conducted one of the few studies in which the magnitude of ecological bias could be examined empirically with real data. They carried out parallel ecological and individual-level analyses of the associations between several pairs of variables in the Second National Health and Nutrition Examination Survey. Figure 16.4 plots the state-level correlation against the corresponding individual-level correlation for each of 13 pairs of variables: that is, the figure shows the correlation between correlations. While anomalies did occur in which the state-level and individual-level correlations had different signs (e.g., for race and weight), it is reassuring to note a general correspondence between associations at the two levels as to direction and magnitude. How generally this correspondence holds is, of course, unknown. For the earlier example of gun ownership and homicide, at least, individual-level case-control studies have also found a positive association between owning a gun and homicide risk (e.g., Kellermann *et al.*, 1993), supporting one of the broad conclusions reached in the Killias study. On the other hand, a systematic review of individual-level studies of a possible association between autism and use of measles, mumps, and rubella vaccine found essentially no association (Demicheli *et al.*, 2012), contrary

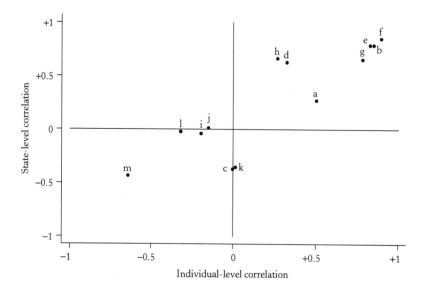

Key:

Point label	Variable #1	Variable #2
a	Height	weight
b	Weight	Body mass index
c	Height	Body mass index
d	Age	Body mass index
e	Calories	protein
f	Calories	Fat
g	Protein	Fat
h	Income	Education
i	Race	Income
j	Race	Education
k	Race	Weight
l	Sex	Weight
m	Sex	Height

FIGURE 16.4 Scatterplot of state-level vs. individual-level correlations for 13 pairs of variables in the Second National Health And Nutrition Examination Survey.

(Based on data from Piantadosi *et al.* [1998])

to the ecological study results mentioned earlier (Delong, 2011).

STUDYING EFFECTS OF GROUP-LEVEL EXPOSURES

A second application of ecological designs in epidemiology is studying the health effects of group-level characteristics. Several authors have argued that social and environmental context, as reflected in both intrinsically group-level characteristics and derived measures that summarize individual-level characteristics at the group level, can greatly influence health, but that such contextual factors have received comparatively little attention in epidemiologic research (Putnam and Galea, 2008; Schwartz, 1994; Susser and Susser, 1996; Diez-Roux, 1998; March and Susser, 2006; Gordon, 1966). Dismissing all ecological studies as being unacceptably vulnerable to bias risks ignoring this large, important class of factors that affect disease frequency.

A key type of group-level exposure that can affect health is programs and policies that apply to entire populations. Chapter 21 considers epidemiologic approaches to evaluating policies in more depth, but ecological studies provide one such approach.

Example 16-1. During the 1990s, several American states passed laws making gun owners criminally liable if a child gained unsupervised access to a gun and injured him- or herself or someone else. Cummings *et al.* (1997) sought to determine whether the presence of such a law was associated with lower rates of firearm death in children.

The number of child suicides, homicides, and unintentional deaths due to firearms and the number of children at risk were obtained over the Internet from the National Center for Health Statistics for all possible groups formed by simultaneous stratification on age category, gender, race, state, and calendar year from 1979–1994. During this period, 12 states had enacted such laws, which took effect at various times. Each group of children was considered exposed if a law was in effect in that state for six months or more of that calendar year; otherwise, the group was considered non-exposed. Negative binomial regression was used to model the number of firearm deaths as a function of number of children at risk, state, calendar year, and the presence or absence of a qualifying safe, firearm, storage law. Age, gender, and race were also examined as potential confounders but had little impact on the results once state and calendar year were included in the regression models.

When a safe-storage law was in effect, the incidence of unintentional firearm deaths among children under 15 years of age was 23% lower than without such a law ($RR = 0.77$, 95% C.I.: 0.63–0.94). Weaker negative associations were found with gun suicide ($RR = 0.81$, 95% C.I.: 0.66–1.01) and gun homicide ($RR = 0.89$, 95% C.I.: 0.76–1.05).

Here the exposure of interest was presence or absence of a firearm safe storage law—an intrinsically group-level characteristic that applied to all children in the states and years studied. In a sense, this situation is a limiting case in which all of the variation in exposure is between groups, and none is within groups. We saw earlier that when ecological studies are used to study individual-level exposures by proxy, the need to extrapolate well beyond the exposure prevalences actually observed can lead to large errors in estimating relative risk and attributable risk. In

happy contrast, when investigating group-level exposures, we see that the study populations actually *were* either fully exposed or fully unexposed, thus ameliorating this source of error. Cross-level bias is also of less concern, because the target level of inference is at the group level—the level at which such an exposure would be potentially modifiable. However, it is still possible for individual- or group-level confounding factors to bias the observed group-level association.

In this example, potential confounding was addressed by cross-classifying the study population by age, gender, race, state, and calendar time. Safe-storage laws were in effect for some of the resulting groups and not for others, but everyone in each group was either exposed or not exposed. Cross-classification permitted accounting for systematic variation in firearm mortality rates associated with the stratification factors, thus better isolating the remaining variation in rates associated with presence or absence of a law.

No doubt there were other unmeasured differences among groups that influenced firearm mortality rates, which contributed to extra-Poisson variation in rates (see Chapter 4). Negative binomial regression was used to account for this extra-Poisson variation, yielding wider but more defensible confidence limits around rate ratio estimates (McCullagh and Nelder, 1989; Gardner *et al.*, 1995).

Ecological designs have been used to study health effects of a variety of other macro-level exposures, such as population income inequality in relation to various measures of health (Lynch *et al.*, 2004); frequency of outpatient antibiotic use in relation to antibiotic resistance (Goossens *et al.*, 2005); geographic covariation in the frequency of inflammatory bowel disease and of multiple sclerosis, suggesting possible shared environmental causes for these seemingly disparate diseases (Green *et al.*, 2006); and alcoholic beverage prices in relation to mortality from cirrhosis of the liver (Seeley, 1960). Blakely and Woodward (2000) discuss several generic mechanisms by which ecological factors can affect individual health.

MULTI-LEVEL STUDIES

Most diseases can be regarded as resulting from a web of contributing causes that operate at different levels. For example, an individual's obesity status is almost certainly determined not only by his/her personal eating behavior but also by household income and food-purchase choices, which in turn are influenced by broader societal factors affecting food prices and availability. Even if an epidemiologic study focuses narrowly on a particular exposure, researchers may need to consider factors at different levels as potential confounders or effect modifiers. Ecological studies have only limited ability to do so, because most depend on preexisting group-level data. On the other hand, individual-level studies are often restricted to a single setting or may deliberately match study subjects on, say, area of residence. Those design features control for possible confounding by area, but they also prevent studying the possibility that the effects of an individual-level exposure of interest may also have contextual effects that can only be detected by studying multiple areas with different exposure prevalences. For example, the risk of motor vehicle collision injury may depend not only on an individual driver's blood alcohol level but also on the distribution of blood alcohol levels among other drivers on the road. Restricting or matching on area also precludes studying other area-level factors as exposures in their own right.

In some research situations, data are available or obtainable on *both* individual-level and group-level characteristics, and possibly on characteristics measured at additional levels of aggregation. *Multi-level* epidemiologic studies use both individuals and groups as units of analysis (Gelman and Hill, 2007; Diez-Roux, 2004, 2000; Von Korff *et al.*, 1992). One purpose of such studies is to allow concurrent investigation of a wider range of exposures and potential confounding factors, based on a broader conceptualization of determinants of a certain health outcome. Data analysis seeks to disentangle individual-level effects from group-level effects, thus avoiding the ecological fallacy and other forms of cross-level bias. Variation in the effect of an individual-level exposure across groups—that is, cross-level effect modification—can also be detected.

Another purpose of multi-level studies is to help explain why the frequency of an outcome varies among groups. Two broad possibilities are *compositional effects*, meaning that the distribution of individual-level risk factors varies among groups; and *contextual effects*, meaning that group-level determinants of outcome vary among groups.

Multi-level studies require special statistical methods for proper data analysis. Conventional multivariable analysis, as described in Chapter 12, assumes statistical independence of observations (or, more properly, of error terms). To the extent that

this independence assumption is violated, the resulting regression coefficient estimates (or quantities derived from them, such as odds ratio estimates) and their confidence limits can be biased. Fortunately, several other suitable statistical approaches are available. These techniques vary as to their assumptions and modeling capabilities, but all allow for the possibility that observations on individuals within the same group may be correlated.

The following example used a data analysis method that goes by several names: multi-level modeling, hierarchical modeling, mixed- or random-effects regression, and generalized linear mixed modeling (Gelman and Hill, 2007; Raudenbush and Bryk, 2002; Austin *et al.*, 2001; Diez-Roux, 2000). The example illustrates how individual-level predictors, group-level predictors, and cross-level interactions can be examined together.

Example 16-2. Considerable research effort in mental health epidemiology has sought to elucidate the relationship between immigration and psychiatric illness. Possible mechanisms for such an association include differential migration of persons with and without preexisting mental illness, stresses of acculturating to a new environment, family disruption, and cultural factors affecting recognition of and care-seeking for mental illness.

Menezes *et al.* (2011) used data from the large Canadian Community Health Survey to study how the likelihood of having certain psychiatric disorders varied in relation to both (1) whether the subject was an immigrant and (2) neighborhood immigrant concentration, while controlling for other sociodemographic characteristics of respondents and neighborhoods. A standardized and validated set of interview questions, which had been translated into several languages, was used to classify whether a respondent had had a given psychiatric disorder within the previous 12 months. The survey also captured information on respondents' sociodemographic characteristics. Survey data were later linked to Canadian national census data on immigrant concentration and socioeconomic factors in *dissemination areas*—predefined census geographic areas with a population of about 400–700 persons—which were used to define neighborhoods operationally.

Multi-level logistic regression (discussed below) was used for data analysis. Table 16.3 summarizes the results for substance dependence, which was one of

TABLE 16.3. INDIVIDUAL- AND NEIGHBORHOOD-LEVEL CHARACTERISTICS IN
RELATION TO SUBSTANCE DEPENDENCE IN THE CANADIAN COMMUNITY HEALTH
SURVEY, AS ESTIMATED BY MULTI-LEVEL LOGISTIC REGRESSION

Characteristic	OR	(95% CI)
Individual:		
Immigrant status	0.472	(0.338–0.660)
Age	0.950	(0.945–0.956)
Female gender	0.401	(0.351–0.458)
Annual income (per $1000)	1.188	(1.113–1.267)
Marital status		
Married	1.000	(Reference)
Common-law union	2.160	(1.680–2.776)
Widowed	1.190	(0.612–2.313)
Separated	4.011	(2.960–5.435)
Divorced	3.111	(2.332–4.150)
Single	3.086	(2.522–3.777)
Education		
Less than secondary	1.000	(Reference)
Secondary	1.174	(0.980–1.405)
Other post-secondary	1.388	(1.139–1.692)
Post-secondary	0.836	(0.702–0.995)
Neighborhood:		
Immigrant concentration (per 1%)	0.990	(0.941–1.042)
Mean annual income (per $1,000)	1.017	(0.917–1.128)
Socioeconomic disadvantage score (per 1 SD)	1.190	(1.116–1.270)
Cross-level interaction:		
Immigrant status × immigrant concentration	0.704	(0.587–0.845)

(Based on data from Menezes *et al.* [2011])

several disorders studied. Three exposures were of primary interest:

- *Immigrant status*, which referred to whether the individual survey respondent was foreign-born (coded as 1) or native-born (coded as 0).
- *Immigrant concentration*, which referred to the proportion of persons in the respondent's neighborhood who were foreign-born, as obtained from census data. In the analysis, this characteristic was represented as $\frac{P-\bar{P}}{SD}$, where P was the proportion foreign-born in the respondent's neighborhood, $\bar{P}$ was the average proportion foreign-born across all neighborhoods (here, 15.5%), and SD was the standard deviation in that proportion across all neighborhoods (here, 16.2%). The result of such a transformation is often termed a z-score.

- *Immigrant status × immigrant concentration* was the product of the preceding two variables—that is, a cross-level interaction term.

At first glance, if only the main effects of immigrant status and immigrant concentration are considered, it might appear that substance dependence was much less likely if the respondent was an immigrant ($OR = 0.472$, 95% CI = 0.338–0.660), while the immigrant concentration in the respondent's neighborhood made little difference ($OR = 0.990$, 95% CI = 0.941–1.042). However, results for the cross-level interaction term ($OR = 0.704$, 95% CI = 0.587–0.845) imply that the effect of each of these two exposures depended on the level of the other.

Figure 16.5, which was constructed from these regression results, shows how the odds of substance dependence varied in relation to both individual

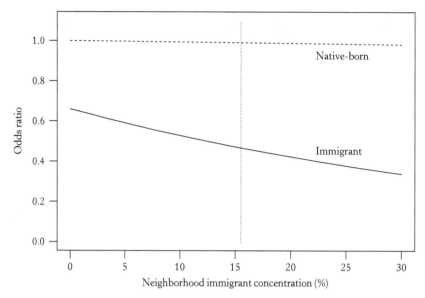

FIGURE 16.5 Individual immigrant status and neighborhood immigrant concentration in relation to odds of substance dependence.
(Based on data from Menezes *et al.,* [2011])

immigrant status and neighborhood immigrant concentration. For a native-born Canadian, the likelihood of substance dependence varied very little in relation to whether he/she lived in a neighborhood with few immigrants or many immigrants. For a foreign-born individual, the likelihood of having substance dependence was always lower than for a native-born Canadian, but more markedly so if the he/she lived in a neighborhood with a high immigrant concentration. The dotted vertical line marks the mean immigrant concentration across neighborhoods, which is the x-axis location at which the *OR* for immigrant status is exactly 0.472—the main-effect value shown in Table 16.3. Overall, these results are consistent with the notion that the social climate in an immigrant-dense neighborhood may exert relatively strong influence on the substance-using behavior of an immigrant, while native-born individuals remain relatively immune to such influence.

Example 16-2 also provides a context in which statistical models can offer further insight into the ecological fallacy and how multi-level studies avoid it. First, suppose that only individual-level survey data had been available, that covariates other than immigrant status can be ignored, and that a linear probability model is used for analysis. Let:

y_i = presence of substance dependence in person i
$\quad$ (1 = yes, 0 = no)

x_i = immigrant status of person i
$\quad$ (= 1 if immigrant, = 0 if not)

ϵ_i = error term for person i

Then a simple individual-level regression model relating substance dependence to individual immigrant status would be:

$$y_i = \alpha + \beta \cdot x_i + \epsilon_i \qquad (16.1)$$

The quantities α and β would be estimated from the data. The value of β would be interpretable as the difference in the probability of substance dependence between an immigrant and a native-born respondent.

Now suppose instead that only neighborhood-level information on the prevalence of substance dependence (from survey data) and immigrant concentration (from census data) had been available. Let:

$\bar{y}_g$ = prevalence of substance dependence in neighborhood g

$\bar{x}_g$ = immigrant concentration (proportion immigrants) in neighborhood g

ϵ_g = error term for neighborhood g

Note that $\bar{y}_g$ and $\bar{x}_g$ are just neighborhood-specific means of y_i and x_i, respectively. An ecological regression model would be:

$$\bar{y}_g = \alpha^* + \beta^* \cdot \bar{x}_g + \epsilon_g \qquad (16.2)$$

β^* in model (16.2) would be interpretable as the difference in prevalence of substance dependence between two hypothetical neighborhoods with 100% and 0% immigrant concentration. The ecologic fallacy involves conflating β^* in model (16.2) with β in model (16.1). Figure 16.3 is a graphical reminder that these two slopes can be completely different.

Now consider the multi-level logistic regression model that was actually used to obtain the results in Table 16.3. There are several differences from the simplified models just examined: use of a logistic model form, immigrant concentration represented not as a simple proportion but as a z-score, inclusion of a cross-level interaction term, and incorporation of additional covariates. But an especially important difference is that it includes both individual immigrant status and neighborhood immigrant concentration as predictors, allowing them to play possibly different roles. Building on the notation used above, let[1]:

$\hat{y}_i$ = estimated probability of substance
dependence in person i

$z_{g[i]}$ = immigrant concentration (as z-score) in
neighborhood g, to which person i belongs

$\alpha_{g[i]}$ = intercept for neighborhood g, to
which person i belongs

$\beta_1 \ldots \beta_3$ = fitted regression coefficients

The logistic regression model is:

$$\log\left(\frac{\hat{y}_i}{1 - \hat{y}_i}\right) = \alpha_{g[i]} + \beta_1 \cdot x_i + \beta_2 \cdot z_{g[i]}$$
$$+ \beta_3 \cdot x_i \cdot z_{g[i]} + (\text{other terms})$$

The "other terms" would be terms involving all other predictor variables shown in Table 16.3, each multiplied by a fitted β-coefficient.

A key statistical feature of this two-level model is that the α_g group-specific intercept terms are not constants to be estimated from the data, as intercept terms would be in conventional regression. Rather, the α_g are assumed to follow a normal distribution, whose mean and variance are estimated from the data. The variance of this distribution quantifies the amount of group-level variation in outcomes that is

unexplained by the predictor variables. Often this variance is of interest in its own right in multi-level studies. Among other purposes, it can be used to quantify the relative contributions of within- and between-group variation in outcomes.

More elaborate multi-level models can involve:

- Examining the degree to which the residual group-level variance (i.e., variance of the α_g terms) changes when other individual- or group-level predictors are included in the model. Doing so explores the degree to which compositional and contextual effects contribute to group-level variation.
- Allowing the β-coefficient(s) for one or more individual-level predictor(s) to vary by group, analogously to α_g above, in order to test for and quantify unexplained variation in the effects of those predictors from group to group.
- Estimating adjusted group-specific means, taking into account varying group sizes.

A different approach to data analysis in multi-level studies employs *generalized estimating equations (GEE)* (Liang and Zeger, 1986, 1993; Hanley *et al.*, 2003). This approach treats group-level variation—or, equivalently, the correlation of observations within groups—as a nuisance rather than as an object of study. This method avoids distributional assumptions about unexplained group-level variation, but it requires a sufficient number of groups for accurate estimates and proper confidence-limit coverage. For logistic regression models, GEE yields estimates of population-averaged (marginal) effects, while mixed-effects regression yields estimates of group-specific effects. GEE and mixed-effects regression approaches have been compared and contrasted by Hubbard *et al.* (2010); Gardiner *et al.* (2009); and Begg and Parides (2003). Johns *et al.* (2012) illustrate use of GEE in a multi-level study of neighborhood cohesion in relation to period prevalence of post-traumatic stress disorder.

Complex-survey analysis methods offer yet another approach to data analysis in multi-level studies when study subjects constitute a true probability sample from a larger defined population (Korn and Graubard, 1999; Graubard and Korn, 1999, 1996; Lumley, 2010). These methods seek to account properly for stratified and clustered sampling and for differential selection probabilities among study subjects. The goal of such *design-based* analysis methods is to estimate parameters in the larger defined population from which the sample has been drawn. In contrast, the *model-based* methods described earlier assume random sampling from an infinite hypothetical superpopulation or ongoing data-generating process. Lemeshow *et al.* (1998) discuss this distinction and compare the results of the two approaches to analysis for an epidemiologic study of dementia and wine intake. Diez-Roux *et al.* (2001) illustrate use of complex survey analysis methods in a study of neighborhood socioeconomic environment and the incidence of coronary heart disease.

Study Design Considerations

As shown above, incorporating individual-level data can transform a purely ecological study into a multi-level study. Doing so can avoid the ecological fallacy and other forms of cross-level bias, permit confounding to be better addressed, and allow the study of both individual- and group-level exposures. Having both individual- and group-level data also can yield gains in precision or statistical power (Glynn *et al.*, 2008).

These advantages notwithstanding, individual-level data can be costly to collect, while group-level data may be cheaply available from government or other existing sources. Several authors (Haneuse and Bartell, 2011; Wakefield and Haneuse, 2008; Glynn *et al.*, 2008; Jackson *et al.*, 2006) have shown how ecological data can be used to develop an efficient sampling plan for obtaining supplementary individual-level data. A two-level study is conducted in two phases: (1) ecological data are obtained first and used to characterize groups on some combination of outcome, exposure, and possibly other covariates; and (2) the phase-1 data are used to design an efficient sampling plan for individual-level data collection in some or all of the groups (Wakefield and Haneuse, 2008). Simulation studies have suggested that the sample of individuals at phase 2 need not be large to yield large benefits (Glynn *et al.*, 2008). The optimal sampling design at phase 2 depends on several factors, including outcome frequency, exposure prevalence, and their variability among groups. In general, more information is gained from sampling areas with relatively high or relatively low exposure prevalence, and individuals in relatively rare outcome or exposure categories (Glynn *et al.*, 2008). In that vein, Haneuse and Wakefield (2008) have proposed designs that combine ecological and case-control data.

CONCLUDING REMARKS

Ecological studies have sometimes been disparaged as a relatively weak source of evidence in epidemiology because of their vulnerability to bias when group-level associations are studied as proxies for individual-level associations. That application of ecological studies is indeed based on strong and usually untestable assumptions, and cautious interpretation is warranted when the design is used for that purpose.

However, many of those potential biases are greatly diminished or vanish altogether when ecological studies are used to study the effects of exposures that apply to an entire group. Accordingly, ecological studies can be a very useful tool for evaluating policies and programs—a theme to be explored further in Chapter 21.

Epidemiologic study designs that use data at both the group and individual levels are becoming increasingly common, with good reason. At the price of added complexity, these multi-level studies have the potential to combine the best features of ecological and individual-level studies.

In any case, our understanding of why certain people develop certain diseases can often be advanced by thinking about how people organize themselves into groups, and how they interact within those groups. Ecological and multi-level studies have a special role to play in translating those ideas into epidemiologic research.

NOTE

1. The notation used here is adapted from Gelman and Hill (2007). Another common notation for two-level models uses two subscripts to index individuals, one to identify the group and a second to identify an individual within that group (Diez-Roux, 2000).

REFERENCES

Advisory Committee to the Surgeon General. Smoking and health. Public Health Service Pub. No. 1103. Washington, D.C.: U.S. Department of Health, Education, and Welfare, 1964.

Austin PC, Goel V, van Walraven C. An introduction to multilevel regression models. Can J Public Health 2001; 92:150–154.

Barker DJP, Morris J, Nelson M. Vegetable consumption and acute appendicitis in 59 areas in England and Wales. BMJ 1986; 292:927–930.

Begg MD, Parides MK. Separation of individual-level and cluster-level covariate effects in regression analysis of correlated data. Stat Med 2003; 22:2591–2602.

Blakely TA, Woodward AJ. Ecological effects in multi-level studies. J Epidemiol Community Health 2000; 54:367–374.

Boice JD Jr, Mumma MT, Blot WJ. Cancer mortality among populations residing in counties near the Hanford site, 1950–2000. Health Phys 2006; 90:431–445.

Brenner H, Greenland S, Savitz DA. The effects of nondifferential exposure misclassification in ecologic studies. Am J Epidemiol 1992; 135:85–95.

Cummings P, Grossman DC, Rivara FP, Koepsell TD. State gun safe storage laws and child mortality due to firearms. JAMA 1997; 278:1084–1086.

Cummings P, Koepsell TD. Does owning a firearm increase or decrease the risk of death? JAMA 1998; 280:471–473.

Dean HT. Endemic fluorosis and its relation to dental caries. Public Health Rep 1938; 53:1443–1452.

Delong G. A positive association found between autism prevalence and childhood vaccination uptake across the U.S. population. J Toxicol Environ Health A 2011; 74:903–916.

Demicheli V, Rivetti A, Debalini MG, Di Pietrantonj C. Vaccines for measles, mumps and rubella in children. Cochrane Database Syst Rev 2012; 2:CD004407.

Diez-Roux AV. Bringing context back into epidemiology: variables and fallacies in multilevel analysis. Am J Public Health 1998; 88:216–222.

Diez-Roux AV. Multilevel analysis in public health research. Annu Rev Public Health 2000; 21:171–192.

Diez-Roux AV. A glossary for multilevel analysis. J Epidemiol Community Health 2002; 56:588–594.

Diez-Roux AV. The study of group-level factors in epidemiology: rethinking variables, study designs, and analytical approaches. Epidemiol Rev 2004; 26:104–111.

Diez-Roux AV, Merkin SS, Arnett D, Chambless L, Massing M, Nieto FJ, *et al.* Neighborhood of residence and incidence of coronary heart disease. N Engl J Med 2001; 345:99–106.

Donne J. Devotions upon emergent occasions, no. 17. In: Gardner H, Healy T (eds.). Donne's selected prose. Oxford, England: Clarendon Press, 1967.

Dufault B, Klar N. The quality of modern cross-sectional ecologic studies: a bibliometric review. Am J Epidemiol 2011; 174:1101–1107.

Finkelstein JA, Huang SS, Kleinman K, Rifas-Shiman SL, Stille CJ, Daniel J, *et al.* Impact of a 16-community trial to promote judicious antibiotic use in Massachusetts. Pediatrics 2008; 121: e15–e23.

Firebaugh G. A rule for inferring individual-level relationships from aggregate data. Am Sociol Rev 1978; 43:557–572.

Gardiner JC, Luo Z, Roman LA. Fixed effects, random effects and GEE: what are the differences? Stat Med 2009; 28:221–239.

Gardner W, Mulvey EP, Shaw EC. Regression analyses of counts and rates: Poisson, overdispersed Poisson, and negative binomial models. Psychol Bull 1995; 118:392–404.

Gelman A, Hill J. Data analysis using regression and multilevel/hierarchical models. New York: Cambridge University Press, 2007.

Glynn AN, Wakefield J, Handcock MS, Richardson TS. Alleviating linear ecological bias and optimal design with subsample data. J R Statist Soc A 2008; 171:179–202.

Goldberger J, Wheeler GA, Sydenstricker E. A study of the relation of family income and other economic factors to pellagra incidence in seven cotton-mill villages of South Carolina in 1916. Public Health Rep 1920; 35:2673–2714.

Goodwin PJ, Boyd NF. Critical appraisal of the evidence that dietary fat intake is related to breast cancer risk in humans. JNCI 1987; 79: 473–485.

Goossens H, Ferech M, Vander Stichele R, Elseviers M, ESAC Project Group. Outpatient antibiotic use in Europe and association with resistance: a cross-national database study. Lancet 2005; 365:579–587.

Gordon JE. Ecologic interplay of man, environment and health. Am J Med Sci 1966; 252:341–356.

Graubard BI, Korn EL. Modelling the sampling design in the analysis of health surveys. Stat Methods Med Res 1996; 5:263–281.

Graubard BI, Korn EL. Analyzing health surveys for cancer-related objectives. J Natl Cancer Inst 1999; 91:1005–1016.

Green C, Elliott L, Beaudoin C, Bernstein CN. A population-based ecologic study of inflammatory bowel disease: searching for etiologic clues. Am J Epidemiol 2006; 164:615–23; discussion 624–628.

Greenland S. Divergent biases in ecologic and individual-level studies. Stat Med 1992; 11:1209–1223.

Greenland S, Morgenstern H. Ecological bias, confounding, and effect modification. Int J Epidemiol 1989; 18:269–274.

Greenland S, Robins J. Invited commentary: ecological studies—biases, misconceptions, and counterexamples. Am J Epidemiol 1994; 139: 747–760.

Haneuse S, Bartell S. Designs for the combination of group- and individual-level data. Epidemiology 2011; 22:382–389.

Haneuse SJPA, Wakefield JC. The combination of ecological and case-control data. J R Stat Soc Series B Stat Methodol 2008; 70:73–93.

Hanley JA, Negassa A, Edwardes MDd, Forrester JE. Statistical analysis of correlated data using generalized estimating equations: an orientation. Am J Epidemiol 2003; 157:364–375.

Hemenway D, Azrael D. The relative frequency of offensive and defensive gun uses: results from a national survey. Violence Vict 2000; 15:257–272.

Héry C, Tryggvadóttir L, Sigurdsson T, Olafsdóttir E, Sigurgeirsson B, Jonasson JG, et al. A melanoma epidemic in Iceland: possible influence of sunbed use. Am J Epidemiol 2010; 172:762–767.

Hubbard AE, Ahern J, Fleischer NL, Van der Laan M, Lippman SA, Jewell N, et al. To GEE or not to GEE: comparing population average and mixed models for estimating the associations between neighborhood risk factors and health. Epidemiology 2010; 21:467–474.

Jackson C, Best N, Richardson S. Improving ecological inference using individual-level data. Stat Med 2006; 25:2136–2159.

Johns LE, Aiello AE, Cheng C, Galea S, Koenen KC, Uddin M. Neighborhood social cohesion and post-traumatic stress disorder in a community-based sample: findings from the Detroit Neighborhood Health Study. Soc Psychiatry Psychiatr Epidemiol 2012; 47:1899–1906.

Kellermann AL, Rivara FP, Rushforth NB, Banton JG, Reay DT, Francisco JT, et al. Gun ownership as a risk factor for homicide in the home. N Engl J Med 1993; 329:1084–1091.

Killias M. International correlations between gun ownership and rates of homicide and suicide. Can Med Assoc J 1993; 148:1721–1725.

Kleck G, Gertz M. Armed resistance to crime: the prevalence and nature of self-defense with a gun. J Criminal Law Criminol 1995; 86:150–187.

Korn EL, Graubard BI. Analysis of health surveys. New York: Wiley, 1999.

Lehrer S, Green S, Stock RG. Association between number of cell phone contracts and brain tumor incidence in nineteen U.S. States. J Neurooncol 2011; 101:505–507.

Lemeshow S, Letenneur L, Dartigues JF, Lafont S, Orgogozo JM, Commenges D. Illustration of analysis taking into account complex survey considerations: the association between wine consumption and dementia in the PAQUID study. Personnes Ages Quid. Am J Epidemiol 1998; 148:298–306.

Liang KY, Zeger SL. Longitudinal data analysis using generalized linear models. Biometrika 1986; 73:3–22.

Liang KY, Zeger SL. Regression analysis for correlated data. Annu Rev Public Health 1993; 14:43–68.

Lumley T. Complex surveys: a guide to analysis using R. New York: Wiley, 2010.

Lynch J, Smith GD, Harper S, Hillemeier M, Ross N, Kaplan GA, et al. Is income inequality a determinant of population health? Part 1. A systematic review. Milbank Q 2004; 82:5–99.

March D, Susser E. The eco- in eco-epidemiology. Int J Epidemiol 2006; 35:1379–1383.

McCullagh P, Nelder JA. Generalized linear models (2nd ed.). London: Chapman and Hall, 1989.

Menezes NM, Georgiades K, Boyle MH. The influence of immigrant status and concentration on psychiatric disorder in Canada: a multi-level analysis. Psychol Med 2011; 41:2221–2231.

Messias E, Eaton WW, Grooms AN. Economic grand rounds: Income inequality and depression prevalence across the United States: an ecological study. Psychiatr Serv 2011; 62:710–712.

Morgenstern H. Uses of ecologic analysis in epidemiologic research. Am J Public Health 1982; 72:1336–1344.

Morgenstern H. Ecologic studies in epidemiology: concepts, principles, and methods. Annu Rev Public Health 1995; 16:61–82.

Piantadosi S. Invited commentary: ecologic biases. Am J Epidemiol 1994; 139:761–764.

Piantadosi S, Byar DP, Green SB. The ecological fallacy. Am J Epidemiol 1988; 127:893–904.

Pickett KE, Pearl M. Multilevel analyses of neighbourhood socioeconomic context and health outcomes: a critical review. J Epidemiol Community Health 2001; 55:111–122.

Prentice RL, Sheppard L. Aggregate data studies of disease risk factors. Biometrika 1995; 82:113–125.

Putnam S, Galea S. Epidemiology and the macrosocial determinants of health. J Public Health Policy 2008; 29:275–89.

Raudenbush SW, Bryk AS. Hierarchical linear models : applications and data analysis methods (2nd ed.). Thousand Oaks, CA: Sage Publications, 2002.

Richardson S, Stücker I, Hémon D. Comparison of relative risks obtained in ecological and individual studies: methodological considerations. Int J Epidemiol 1987; 16:111–120.

Robinson WS. Ecological correlations and the behavior of individuals. Am Sociol Rev 1950; 15:351–357.

Rose G. Sick individuals and sick populations. Int J Epidemiol 1985; 6:1–8.

Rosenbaum PR, Rubin DB. Difficulties with regression analyses of age-adjusted rates. Biometrics 1984; 40:437–443.

Schwartz S. The fallacy of the ecological fallacy: The potential misuse of a concept and the consequences. Am J Public Health 1994; 84:819–824.

Seeley JR. Death by liver cirrhosis and the price of beverage alcohol. Can Med Assoc J 1960; 83:1361–1366.

Selvin HC, Hagstrom WO. The empirical classification of formal groups. Am Sociol Rev 1963; 28:399–411.

Susser M. The logic in ecological: I. The logic of analysis. Am J Public Health 1994a; 84:825–829.

Susser M. The logic in ecological: II. The logic of design. Am J Public Health 1994b; 84:830–835.

Susser M, Susser E. Choosing a future for epidemiology: II. From black box to Chinese boxes and eco-epidemiology. Am J Public Health 1996; 86:674–677.

Von Korff M, Koepsell T, Curry S, Diehr P. Multi-level analysis in epidemiologic research on health behaviors and outcomes. Am J Epidemiol 1992; 135:1077–1082.

Wakefield J. Ecologic studies revisited. Annu Rev Public Health 2008; 29:75–90.

Wakefield J, Haneuse SJPA. Overcoming ecologic bias using the two-phase study design. Am J Epidemiol 2008; 167:908–16.

Walter SD. The ecologic method in the study of environmental health. I. Overview of the method. Environ Health Perspect 1991a; 94:61–65.

Walter SD. The ecologic method in the study of environmental health. II. Methodologic issues and feasibility. Environ Health Perspect 1991b; 94:67–73.

EXERCISES

1. Researchers in England and Wales sought to investigate the relationship between vegetable consumption and risk of appendicitis (Barker *et al.*, 1986). A national food survey had obtained detailed data on food purchases for about 150 households in each of 59 geographic areas for which data on hospital admissions for appendicitis were also available. Across these areas, the incidence of appendicitis was found to be negatively correlated with consumption of non-potato vegetables, chiefly green vegetables and tomatoes. The investigators noted that "green vegetables and tomatoes may protect against appendicitis, possibly through an effect on the bacterial flora of the appendix."

   Based on the study design, what reservation might you have about concluding that if a person eats more green vegetables and tomatoes, his or her risk of developing appendicitis will be reduced?

2. Increasing resistance of bacterial pathogens to antibiotics is a growing clinical and public health concern. Overuse of antibiotics, including use for minor illnesses in which antibiotics may not actually be needed, is suspected of playing an important role. Goossens *et al.* (2005) used data from 19 European countries to study the relationship between (1) the frequency of penicillin prescribing to outpatients, quantified as $\frac{\text{number of daily doses}}{\text{person-time}}$, in each country; and (2) the proportion of pneumococcal strains tested in each country that were pencillin-resistant, as obtained from the European Antimicrobial Resistance Surveillance System. A strong positive country-level association was found between the rate of outpatient penicillin prescribing and the frequency of penicillin resistance among pneumococcal isolates tested.

   Apart from the low cost of being able to use existing data sources, why might an ecological study design have been especially advantageous for study of this research issue?

3. Given the widespread use of cellular telephones in the United States and elsewhere, concerns have been expressed about possible adverse health effects of the low-power microwave-frequency signals transmitted by the internal antenna in cell phones. One study of this issue linked data from brain-tumor registries in 19 American states with industry data on cell phone subscriptions in those states (Lehrer *et al.*, 2011).

   (a) The state-level correlation between number of cell phone subscriptions and number of brain tumors was reported to be 0.950 ($p < 0.001$). What concern might you have about whether this result correctly reflects an ecological association between cell phone ownership and brain tumor risk in those states?

   (b) Multiple linear regression analysis was conducted on number of brain tumors in each state, including as predictor variables: (1) number of cell phone subscriptions, (2) state population, (3) mean income, and (4) mean age. The association with cell phone subscriptions remained statistically significant ($p = 0.017$). Why might multiple linear regression be problematic as a method for multivariable analysis here? What alternative would you suggest?

   (c) Is it possible that states with a higher prevalence of cell phone use really do have higher incidence rates of brain tumors, even though the risk of a brain tumor may be no greater for a person who has a cell phone than for anyone else? Why or why not?

4. Imagine an ecological study of the relationship between dietary intake of fish oil and mortality from coronary heart disease (CHD). For simplicity, suppose that only two communities are involved and that their populations are otherwise similar with regard to major risk factors for CHD. In Community A, 20% of the population has a diet high in fish oil, and CHD mortality is 100 deaths per 100,000 person-years. In Community B, 30% of the population has a high fish oil diet, and CHD mortality is 95 deaths per 100,000 person-years.

(a) Assume that, at the population level, CHD mortality is linearly related to the prevalence of high fish oil consumption and that cross-level bias can be ignored. Estimate the relative risk and attributable risk of CHD mortality in relation to a high fish oil diet.

(b) Now suppose that the *true* prevalence of a high fish oil diet is still 20% in Community A and 30% in Community B, but that these true prevalences cannot be measured directly. Instead, the prevalence of a high fish oil diet must be estimated in each community using a survey instrument that has sensitivity = 90% and specificity = 90% for such a diet. What would you expect the *observed* prevalence of a high fish oil diet to be in each community, based on the survey data?

(c) Now recalculate the relative risk and attributable risk for CHD mortality in relation to a high fish oil diet, using the exposure prevalences you expect the survey to show. How do they compare to those calculated in part (a)?

5. An important unresolved issue in social epidemiology is the extent to which income inequality—the degree to which economic resources in a population accrue unevenly among its members—affects health. Messias *et al.* (2011) used data from the CDC Behavioral Risk Factor Surveillance System (BRFSS), described in Chapter 6, to study the association between income inequality and the prevalence of depression among American states. Income inequality was measured by the Gini coefficient, a widely used economic index that ranges from 0 (complete income equality) to 1 (all income flowing to one person). The Gini coefficient value for each state was estimated from a separate large survey of United States households. The depression status of each BRFSS survey respondent was assessed from a previously validated set of questions that had been incorporated into BRFSS telephone interviews in 45 states. Depression prevalence for each state was then calculated by aggregating responses for all survey participants in that state. The authors reported a positive correlation between the Gini coefficient and depression prevalence ($r = 0.435, p < 0.001$).

(a) Would the possibility of an ecological fallacy be a concern for this study?

(b) The authors noted that depression was well known to be associated with a person's education, income, and age. Accordingly, multivariable analysis was conducted that included as additional covariates each state's per capita income, percent of population with a college degree, and percent of population over age 65 years. To what degree would you expect this analytic strategy to control

possible confounding by education, income, and age?

(c) Would a multi-level analysis of this research question be possible with the same data resources? If not, why not? If so, explain why and how.

ANSWERS

1. The study design was clearly ecological. We do not know that the individual people who got appendicitis were necessarily those who had diets low in green vegetables or tomatoes, only that they came from areas with low per capita consumption of these foodstuffs. The study could thus be vulnerable to the ecological fallacy (as well as confounding by other personal characteristics). The conclusion could, of course, be true, but studies on individuals would be needed to confirm it.

2. The underlying concern goes beyond a possible individual-level association between receiving penicillin and subsequent infection with a penicillin-resistant strain of pneumococcus. Rather, there is a public health concern that person A's use of penicillin could affect person B's risk of infection with a penicillin-resistant pneumococcal strain, assuming that persons A and B share the same "bacterial environment." In this case, country was used as an expedient proxy for having a shared "bacterial environment." The group-level association itself was of interest in its own right, not just as an indirect way to investigate a possible individual-level association. A true country-level association could provide a basis for a nationwide intervention that might lower everyone's risk of infection with a penicillin-resistant pneumococcal strain.

3. (a) The strikingly high reported correlation of 0.950 was not based on the *incidence* of brain tumors and the *prevalence* of cell phone subscriptions, both of which use denominators based on population size. Rather, the reported correlation was based only on raw counts—in effect, the numerators of the relevant incidence rates and exposure prevalences. Both the number of brain tumors and the number of cell phone subscriptions in, say, South Dakota would be much lower than the corresponding counts in New York or Texas, simply because South Dakota is a less populous state. The high correlation was almost certainly driven by large differences in state population size.

(b) Multiple linear regression, like correlation analysis, is based on an assumption that the amount of random error in the response variable is the same across all observations—the so-called *homoscedasticity* assumption. In this case, that assumption implies that the brain tumor incidence rates for all states would have equal precision. But incidence rates typically do not have this property; rather, as discussed in Chapter 4, the precision of a rate depends on both the magnitude of the rate itself and on the underlying sample size, both of which would vary by state. As a result, estimates and confidence intervals from multiple linear regression may be misleading. On theoretical grounds, a better alternative would be Poisson regression, which accounts properly for these statistical properties of rates. In practice, rates often exhibit over-dispersion beyond that predicted by the Poisson distribution, probably reflecting unmeasured differences that exist among the populations being compared and that affect the rates. Negative binomial regression is one multivariable analysis method that can be used in such cases, as in Example 16-1.

(c) Yes, both conditions may hold. The state-level ecological analysis was vulnerable to many of the potential pitfalls described in the first part of this chapter as a basis for inferring an individual-level association between cell phone use and brain tumor risk—among them, the ecological fallacy and unmeasured confounding by both state- or individual-level factors that affect brain tumor risk.

4. (a) Because we are assuming a linear relationship between CHD mortality and prevalence of a high fish oil diet, data from these two communities determine the slope and intercept of that line. In units of deaths per 100,000 person-years, its slope b is $(100 - 95)/(0.20 - 0.30) = -50$. This value for b can then be applied to the data from either community to solve for the intercept a. Using data from Community A, $100 = a - 50(0.20)$, so $a = 110$. The linear relationship is thus

$$\text{CHD mortality} = 110 - (50 \times \text{prevalence})$$

Based on this equation, the predicted CHD mortality in a hypothetical community in which everyone followed a high fish oil diet would be $R_1 = 110 - (50 \times 1) = 60$. CHD mortality in a community in which nobody followed such a diet would be $R_0 = 110 - (50 \times 0) = 110$. Hence the relative risk would be $R_1/R_0 = 60/110 = 0.55$, and the attributable risk would be $R_1 - R_0 = 60 - 110 = -50$ deaths per 100,000 person-years.

(b) Consider first Community A, in which the true prevalence of a high fish oil diet is 20%. In a random sample of, say, 100 people from Community A, there should be 20 people who truly followed a high fish oil diet and 80 who did not. If the dietary survey is 90% sensitive and 90% specific for a high fish oil diet, we would expect people in the sample to be distributed as follows:

TABLE 16.4.

Survey result	True intake High	True intake Low	Total
High	18	8	26
Low	2	72	74
Total	20	80	100

The observed prevalence of a high fish oil diet in the survey data would thus be about $26/100 = 26\%$. Similar calculations for Community B yield an expected prevalence of 34%.

(c) Using the same method as in part (a) but with exposure prevalences of 0.26 and 0.34 instead, $b = -62.5$ and $a = 116.25$. This leads to $R_1 = 53.75$, $R_0 = 116.25$, relative risk = 0.46, and attributable risk = -62.5 deaths per 100,000 person-years.

Both measures of association fall farther from the null than do those obtained in part (a). As pointed out by Brenner *et al.* (1992), non-differential exposure misclassification in ecological studies leads to estimates of relative and attributable risk that are biased *away* from the null.

5. (a) No, because income inequality is an intrinsically group-level characteristic. The Gini coefficient for each state reflected an aspect of that state's economic environment and applied to everyone in the state. It would not be possible to study the association between this Gini coefficient and depression status by making all comparisons between individuals within a state. The ecological design of the study was thus necessitated by the group-level nature of the exposure; it was not simply an expedient way to study an individual-level association.

(b) In a state-level analysis, it was only possible to include characteristics measured at, or aggregated to, the state level. But aggregate measures of education, income, and age could affect depression in ways that differ from the effects of the corresponding individual-level measures. For example, a state's per capita income reflects the overall environment of economic well-being in that state, which in turn might be associated with its ability to provide publicly funded mental-health services and other social services. In contrast, an individual's income reflects his/her own economic well-being and purchasing power. Moreover, even individual-level data on the dichotomized age and education variables could have left open the door to considerable residual confounding within the two broad categories.

(c) Yes, a multi-level analysis would be both possible and desirable. The state-level data were already available and had been used to obtain the published results. Publicly available BRFSS data sets include de-identified (anonymous) individual-level data on depression status, education, family income, age, and other sociodemographic and health characteristics. Using these individual-level data could allow better control over confounding by education, income, age, and other individual-level confounders. The main exposure of interest, the Gini coefficient, would be included as a state-level characteristic. The state-level covariates noted above and others could be examined as possible state-level confounders.

17

Induction Periods and Latent Periods

Knowledge of an etiology of a disease is a first step towards being able to prevent some cases of that disease. Alternatively, this knowledge may be useful in targeting persons at high risk with efforts to detect the disease at an early stage. However, achieving these goals may require, not only an understanding of the presence and magnitude of an association of the disease in question with a given exposure, but also having the answers to one or more of the following questions: How soon can disease result after the exposure has first been incurred? To what extent does the size of the altered risk depend on the duration of exposure? Once the exposure has ceased, does the alteration in risk disappear? If so, how quickly?

For example, while postmenopausal women who receive oral estrogen therapy for an extended duration (e.g., >5 years) probably have some increase in the risk of breast cancer, shorter-term use appears not to be associated with an increase in risk (Collaborative Group on Hormonal Factors in Breast Cancer, 1997). When weighing the risks against the benefits of hormone use of less than five years' duration, these data suggest that an altered incidence of breast cancer need not be considered. As another example, it is commonly recommended that postmenopausal women with an intact uterus who take estrogens unopposed by a progestogen, and who therefore are at a substantially increased risk of endometrial cancer, be regularly screened (by means of vaginal ultrasound or endometrial biopsy) for the presence of endometrial cancer. Once a woman has stopped taking these hormones, can the screening stop as well? If not immediately, then when? The answers to these questions would be based heavily on the results of studies that documented the incidence of endometrial cancer in women who have discontinued estrogens. (These show a decline in risk relative to continuing users, but are divided as to whether the risk ultimately returns to that of a postmenopausal

woman who never used hormones (Cook *et al.*, 2006)). Finally, it is recommended that hepatitis A immune globulin be given within two weeks to persons following exposure to hepatitis A infection, but not thereafter, as a means of reducing the risk of later contracting clinical hepatitis (Krugman *et al.*, 1960). Apparently, the time course of the progression of infection to disease is such that, unless given relatively early, this therapy has little or no efficacy.

An important goal of epidemiologic studies is to provide information that bears on disease prevention. Therefore, persons conducting epidemiologic studies that deal with exposures that vary over time must consider, in both their design and their analysis, the likely temporal relationship between exposure and disease occurrence. Studies of aspirin use in relation to the incidence of acute myocardial infarction have focused on the initial hours to weeks after the most recent dose was taken, since aspirin could have a relatively transient influence by means of its anticoagulant properties. In contrast, studies of aspirin use in relation to the incidence of colon cancer typically concern themselves with long-term use and/or use years earlier, given the long preclinical duration of most colon tumors and of the polyps from which many of these tumors arise.

Example 17-1. In the Physicians Health Study, 22,071 U.S. physicians were assigned at random to receive aspirin, 325 mg. every other day, or a placebo for a period of five years (Gann *et al.*, 1993). A reduction in the incidence of myocardial infarction among the group assigned to aspirin led to the termination of the study at that time. Because a number of earlier non-randomized studies had observed a reduced risk of colorectal cancer associated with long-term aspirin use, an analysis of the accumulated data was done for colorectal cancer as well. No difference was found between members of the aspirin and placebo groups for this outcome, either through the five years of the trial (relative risk = 1.15, 95% confidence interval = 0.8–1.7) or during an additional seven years of follow-up (Sturmer et al., 1998). It is possible that truly no association is present between aspirin use and colorectal cancer, that the earlier observational studies were flawed in some way, and that a randomized study was needed to obtain an unbiased result. However, it seems more likely that 5–12 years is too short a period to determine the effect of aspirin on the incidence of this disease; even a substantial decrease in risk might not start to be evident until well over than a decade from the onset of regular aspirin use. Indeed, the authors of the physicians' study concluded that "prevention trials with longer follow-up of randomized participants" were needed (Gann et al., 1993).

Some illnesses have features that signal a period of time during which the etiologic agent(s) must have been acting. Bunin et al. (1989) exploited this phenomenon in their case-control study of environmental exposures in relation to the development of retinoblastoma. First, they excluded children in whom the disease had already occurred in a first or second-degree relative, since (for this disease) no further non genetic basis for its occurrence need be considered. They further divided the remaining cases into two groups:

1. Children with a constitutional deletion on chromosome 13q (i.e., a deletion present in all cells of the body) and those with bilateral disease (in whom a constitutional genetic abnormality is believed to be present in every case.)
2. Children with unilateral disease and no constitutional chromosome 13q deletion.

In the first group of cases and their controls, interviews with parents focused on exposures that took place prior to conception (e.g., gonadal irradiation), since only exposures prior to conception could have given rise to the genetic abnormality that predisposed to retinoblastoma in these cases. In contrast, parents of cases in the second group and parents of their controls were queried about exposures that took place after conception (e.g., multivitamin use during pregnancy), since earlier exposures were unlikely to have played an etiologic role.

Failure to take into account the relevant period of time during which an exposure is capable of causing disease can dull the ability of an epidemiologic study to document an exposure–disease association. For example, Hertz-Picciotto et al. (1996) have illustrated how the influence of exposures that act during only a part of pregnancy to give rise to adverse outcomes can be underestimated in non-randomized studies if data on their presence are not collected and analyzed during the appropriate window of time during the pregnancy. Considerations of temporality can be important when planning a randomized study as well:

Example 17-2.   In order to test the hypothesis that replacement of dairy fat with vegetable fat in the diet can lead to a lower incidence of coronary heart disease, changes were made in the kitchen of one of two Finnish hospitals providing long-term care for patients with mental illness (Miettinen et al., 1983). The incidence of coronary disease among patients 44–64 years was monitored for a six-year period, after which the policies of the two kitchens were reversed—the one that had switched to vegetable fats reverted to dairy fats, while the other now began to use vegetable fats—and the residents of the two hospitals were observed for another six years. About one-third of the residents of each institution during the first follow-up period also were residents of that institution during the second, and so would have had a diet that, during different periods of time, would have been high in dairy fat or in vegetable fat. Since the influence of diet on the incidence of coronary heart disease is not likely to be immediate—the arteriosclerotic changes that diet may modify take time to develop—the authors' primary comparison of incidence rates before and after the dietary change at the six-year point within each hospital probably substantially underestimates the true size of the association between type of dietary fat and the incidence of coronary heart disease.

INDUCTION AND LATENT PERIODS

For etiologic exposures of brief duration, such as eating food contaminated with the hepatitis A virus, or being subjected to a single, intense dose of ionizing radiation, the *induction period* in a given ill person is the interval between receipt of the exposure and the first presence of the disease. (When the exposure in question is an infectious agent, an alternative term—the *incubation period*—is also commonly used.) The time between the disease's first presence and its recognition is the *latent period*. Since the first presence of disease can almost never be observed,

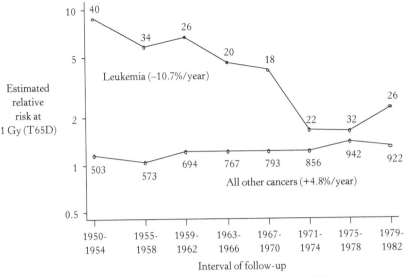

FIGURE 17.1 Relative risk of mortality from leukemia and all other cancers other than leukemia in A-bomb survivors, 1950–1982, in relation to time after irradiation
Source: Committee on the Biological Effects of Ionizing Radiations (1990, Figure 5.2)

what is measured in specific individuals is the sum of the induction and latent periods (Rothman, 1981). Most epidemiologists, being economical (or lazy!) with language, simply refer to this sum either as the induction or as the latent period. We will refer to it, clumsily, as the *induction/latent period*.

The distribution of the length of time required for an exposure to give rise to disease can be estimated by examining the relative risk associated with that exposure over successive periods of time after it was sustained. Fig. 17.1 depicts the risk of leukemia and other forms of cancer in survivors of the atomic bomb detonations in Hiroshima and Nagasaki, relative to that of Japanese who were not exposed, in relation to the time since their exposure to the detonations in 1945. For leukemia, the pronounced increase in the relative risk during the 1950s suggests that the induction/latent period associated with this intensity of radiation could be as short as 5–10 years (or even shorter, since there are no data provided for 1945–50). The persistence of at least a small increase in risk of leukemia through the late 1970s is compatible with a maximum period for induction/latency associated with radiation exposure of at least 30 years.

In some circumstances, nearly all cases of disease among exposed individuals are due to the exposure (i.e., the attributable risk percent is close to 100%).

For example, the association between *in utero* DES exposure and vaginal adenocarcinoma is so strong that almost no cases arising in a given cohort exposed to DES would be expected had DES not been used (Herbst *et al.*, 1971). In this circumstance, the distribution of the length of the induction/latent periods after DES exposure can be assessed simply by enumerating the times when cases occur following exposure. Since the period of exposure was restricted to the nine months prior to birth, the range of incubation/latent periods following exposure can be gleaned, approximately, from the age distribution of the cases at the time of their diagnosis.

Occasionally, an examination of variation in disease occurrence across populations, or within a population over time, can offer strong clues regarding the minimum duration of the induction/latent period associated with a particular exposure.

Example 17-3. Infection with hepatitis B virus is a strong risk factor for hepatocellular carcinoma (HCC). In Taiwan, mass immunization in newborns against hepatitis B infection began in July 1984, because of the extensive transmission of the virus at that time of life. To evaluate the possible early impact of this program on the incidence of HCC, Chang *et al.* (1997) analyzed data from the records of the

Taiwan Cancer Registry through 1994. They identified three cases of HCC among the cohort of 6–9-year-old children who had been born between 7/84–6/86, a cohort in which 85–90% of the children had been vaccinated. Based on the rates in 6–9-year-old children born during 7/74–6/84 (almost none of whom would have been vaccinated), 12 cases would have been expected among children in the later cohort (relative risk = 0.25). This dramatic reduction suggests, not only that the vaccine has been efficacious, but that the induction/latent period for liver cancer after hepatitis B infection in the perinatal period can be as short as 6–9 years.

For etiologic exposures that are prolonged (e.g., aflatoxin consumption, cigarette smoking), there is no known point in time that can be specified as being the one at which the accumulated exposure is first able to cause disease, and after which additional exposure does not continue to add to the risk. Studies of these agents in relation to disease occurrence can examine the variations in relative risk as a function of time since first exposure, cognizant that the range of time periods during which elevations are present may well not correspond to the range of induction periods following a cumulative dose of an exposure that is adequate to give rise to disease.

INFLUENCE OF THE SUSPECTED INDUCTION/LATENT PERIOD ON STUDY DESIGN
Short Induction/Latent Periods

In many instances, the close connection in time between an exposure and the development of a rare illness makes possible the identification of an association between them. For example, because anaphylaxis has been observed to follow so soon after the administration of parenteral penicillin therapy, a causal relationship has been inferred despite the absence of contemporaneous data on the incidence of anaphylaxis in a non-exposed group. The incidence of such dramatic and unusual symptoms in any short period of time is presumed to be vanishingly small in the absence of a recent injection of penicillin (or some other drug).

When there are numerous causal pathways that can lead to a given illness, including some that do not involve the exposure in question, we need formal epidemiologic studies that include an explicit basis of comparison to document the presence and magnitude of an association. However, the presence of

a very short induction period can pose problems in this regard. For example, it is plausible on toxicological grounds that consumption of a large quantity of alcohol could predispose acutely to the occurrence of a myocardial infarction. A cohort study could not be expected to examine this issue, since it would not be feasible to identify the very large number of inebriated persons necessary to observe any appreciable number of infarctions during the few hours they remain inebriated. Similarly, a study that compared blood alcohol levels between cases and controls would be unlikely to provide a valid result: Even if it were possible to obtain a blood sample by which to estimate recent alcohol consumption on each case, the generally available means of recruiting controls—which require making appointments in advance and obtaining informed consent—would almost certainly result in a group in which the proportion of inebriated persons would be atypically low.

Nonetheless, there are circumstances in which: (a) exposure status in the population under study can be accurately ascertained; and (b) it is possible to correctly estimate the duration of the period of presumed altered risk immediately following the onset of exposure. In such a circumstance, a comparison of the incidence of the outcome in question during that period relative to the incidence at other times could provide a valid assessment of the short-term impact of the exposure.

Example 17-4. Investigators in Denmark sought to evaluate the occurrence of febrile seizures in children who received the newly introduced (in 2002) acellular pertussis vaccine (Sun *et al.*, 2012). Using data from the Danish Civil Registry to enumerate cohort members, the Danish Health Registry to ascertain the date of receipt of this vaccine (in combination with diphtheria tetanus toxoid, inactivated poliovirus, and *Haemophilus influenzae* type B vaccines), and the Danish National Hospital Register, they could calculate the incidence of febrile seizures leading to hospitalization during the week following vaccination, as well as the corresponding incidence in other weeks. In this study, because there were reasons to believe that vaccination would have no lingering influence on the likelihood of a febrile seizure after one week, the large majority of Danish infants identified contributed to the person-time denominator during both the "exposed" and "non-exposed" intervals. Because the incidence of febrile seizures rises rapidly with increasing age during infancy, it was necessary to tightly control for age in this analysis.

Some comparisons of the incidence of a health outcome shortly after an exposure involve only persons who actually sustain the outcome. The approach used—termed the "self-controlled case-series" method (Whitaker *et al.*, 2006; Weldeselassie *et al.*, 2011)—asks whether the outcome occurred more often in a given period of time proximal to the time of the exposure (the risk interval) than would have been expected based on the proportion of the total period of follow-up represented by the risk interval.

Exposures that rapidly give rise to disease can sometimes be identified in case-control studies that obtain exposure information by means of interviews. For example, Siscovick *et al.* (1984) found that, of 133 Seattle-area residents ages 25–75 years who sustained a primary cardiac arrest during a 14-month period, nine were engaged in vigorous physical activity at the time (based on reports of spouses or other bystanders). This proportion—9/133—was some 50 times greater than expected based on the proportion of time a sample of demographically similar persons was reported (by spouses) typically to be engaged in vigorous physical activity. However, just as for case-control studies in general:

- The validity of studies investigating possible short-term effects rests on the comparability of exposure ascertainment between cases and controls. In the above example, there probably was some non-comparability of reporting of vigorous exercise by witnesses of a cardiac arrest on one hand, and persons reporting the usual patterns of vigorous activity of their spouses on the other. Thus, while a 50-fold case-control difference almost certainly must be attributable to more than differences in the means of exposure ascertainment, a much more modest difference could be entirely explained on that basis.
- The power of a case-control study to evaluate a short-term etiologic relationship is often low, due to the rarity of the relevant exposure. For example, if it is hypothesized that it is only the initiation of a pharmacological therapy that is associated with an increased risk (e.g., new use of a product containing phenylpropanolamine and hemorrhagic stroke (Kernan *et al.*, 2000), or the recent cessation of such a therapy (e.g.,

discontinuation of beta blocker use in relation to the incidence of coronary heart disease (Psaty *et al.*, 1990)), then only moderate or large associations can be reliably identified in even the largest case-control studies.

Close relatives of case-control studies—case-crossover studies, also are used to assess the influence of some short-term risk factors (Maclure, 1991). These studies compare a case's exposure status at the time of the onset of his/her illness to that person's expected exposure status, based on his/her past history, obviating the need for a separate control group. For example, among persons who had recently sustained a myocardial infarction, one could contrast their alcohol consumption during the hour or two prior to the event and that predicted based upon their usual pattern of consumption. Such a study would be feasible if exposure status, both recent and usual, could be ascertained accurately by means of an interview or questionnaire. It would not be feasible in situations where only recent status could be ascertained, such as if one were estimating alcohol intake from levels in blood drawn at the time of the infarction.

Considerations pertaining to the design, analysis, and interpretation of case-crossover studies have been discussed in detail by Redelmeier and Tibshirani (1997). Briefly, the analysis of these studies proceeds like that of a matched case-control study (see Chapter 15), in which each study subject acts as his/her own control. The interpretation of the results will be influenced by the ways in which questions such as the following are answered:

- How much misclassification of exposure status may have occurred from incorrectly judging the length of the relevant "window" of exposure prior to disease onset? For example, what if heavy alcohol consumption predisposed to myocardial infarction not just during the several hours when blood alcohol levels were above a certain threshold, but for several more hours or days (as a result of some delayed physiological response)? An analysis that labeled as "exposed" only the subjects with heavy consumption immediately before the infarction would mis-assign the exposure status of some subjects, reducing the study's ability to detect an association.
- To what extent was the confounding influence of other exposures taken into account? By

having a person serve as his/her own control, confounding by factors that do not vary to any appreciable extent over short periods of time (e.g., demographic characteristics) is reduced or eliminated. However, there remains the possibility of confounding by risk factors that do vary over time in relation to the exposure. For example, if heavy alcohol consumption were always accompanied by cigarette smoking, and the latter acutely predisposed to myocardial infarction, a spurious association between alcohol and myocardial infarction could be deduced.

Long Induction/Latent Periods

As indicated in the earlier example of aspirin consumption in relation to the incidence of colorectal cancer, many randomized trials are not designed to extend over a long enough period to be able to identify a delayed impact of an exposure. Facing the same problem are cohort studies of newly exposed persons that initiate follow-up around the time the exposure has taken place. Alternatively, if an exposure sustained in the past can be ascertained by means of interviews or records, then it is feasible for both case-control studies and cohort studies that use these sources of information to address the possible long-term impact of the exposure. However, if a study subject's exposure status cannot be ascertained in retrospect—as would be likely to happen, for example, in a cohort or case-control study among middle-aged women that wished to investigate whether breast cancer risk is associated with levels of endogenous sex hormones during puberty—then there are no attractive options. One tries to either: (a) identify measurable correlates of the exposure that can be measured retrospectively (in this case, perhaps, a weak correlate such as age at menarche); or (b) identify a valid "surrogate" outcome, a condition that strongly predicts the later appearance of the disease of interest. (For breast cancer, no such surrogate outcome has yet been identified. For a condition such as colon cancer, however, the surrogate might be the occurrence of an adenomatous polyp.) A third alternative would be (c) to conduct a very long (and thus very expensive) cohort study with prospective follow-up.

Example 17-5.   Efforts to assess the potential role of micronutrient deficiencies in the etiology of stomach cancer have been hindered, in case-control studies, by difficulties in the measurement of exposure status: Recall of past diet does not provide accurate information regarding intake of most micronutrients, and measurement of serum micronutrient levels in cases after a diagnosis of stomach cancer may not yield values indicative of those present during the genesis of the cancer. In order to overcome these problems, You et al. (2000) conducted a cohort study in Linqu County, China. At baseline in 1989–1990, serum was drawn for determination of micronutrient levels, and an endoscopy was performed in which a biopsy specimen was obtained. The latter was repeated in 1994. The presence of gastric dysplasia at baseline was a strong risk factor for the development of gastric cancer: Persons with dysplasia had some 30 times the risk as those with normal mucosa or with lesions no worse than superficial gastritis or chronic atrophic gastritis. Therefore, the investigators felt justified in considering the development of dysplasia during the follow-up period as a relevant endpoint, in addition to the development of gastric cancer per se. In the approximately 400 subjects on whom micronutrient levels had been measured at baseline and in whom gastric dysplasia had not been present at that time, gastric biopsies revealed that 60 had progressed either to dysplasia or cancer by 1994. Had the authors restricted the analysis to the incidence of cancer alone, only a handful of cases (<10) would have been present from which to draw any inferences.

As much as lengthy induction/latent periods can be a challenge and frustration to the researcher, they can be a blessing to those who are trying to prevent disease. Whatever exposures in early reproductive life are involved in the etiology of breast cancer, they do not usually give rise to the disease until two or more decades later. This delay allows time to attempt interventions (e.g., administration of a steroidal estrogen-response modifier, such as tamoxifen or raloxifene, to women judged to be at high risk) that have the potential to block the causal influence of those earlier exposures.

REFERENCES

Bunin GR, Meadows AT, Emanuel BS, Buckley JD, Woods WG, Hammond GD. Pre- and postconception factors associated with sporadic heritable and nonheritable retinoblastoma. Cancer Res 1989; 49:5730–5735.

Chang MH, Chen CJ, Lai MS, Hsu HM, Wu TC, Kong MS, *et al*. Universal hepatitis B vaccination in Taiwan and the incidence of hepatocellular carcinoma in children. Taiwan Childhood Hepatoma Study Group. N Engl J Med 1997; 336:1855–1859.

Collaborative Group on Hormonal Factors in Breast Cancer. Breast cancer and hormone replacement therapy: collaborative reanalysis of data from 51 epidemiological studies of 52,705 women with breast cancer and 108,411 women without breast cancer. Lancet 1997; 350:1047–1059.

Committee on the Biological Effects of Ionizing Radiations. Health effects of exposure to low levels of ionizing radiation: BEIR V. Washington, D.C.: National Academy Press, 1990.

Cook LS, Weiss NS, Doherty JA, Chen C. Endometrial cancer. In Schottenfeld D, Fraumeni JF (eds.). Cancer epidemiology and prevention (3rd ed.). New York: Oxford, 2006 pp.1027–1043.

Gann PH, Manson JE, Glynn RJ, Buring JE, Hennekens CH. Low-dose aspirin and incidence of colorectal tumors in a randomized trial. J Natl Cancer Inst 1993; 85:1220–1224.

Hagel BE, Pless IB, Goulet C, Platt RW, Robitaille Y. Effectiveness of helmets in skiers and snowboarders: case-control and case crossover study. BMJ 2005; 330:281.

Herbst AL, Ulfelder H, Poskanzer DC. Adenocarcinoma of the vagina. Association of maternal stilbestrol therapy with tumor appearance in young women. N Engl J Med 1971; 284:878–881.

Hertz-Picciotto I, Pastore LM, Beaumont JJ. Timing and patterns of exposures during pregnancy and their implications for study methods. Am J Epidemiol 1996; 143:597–607.

Kernan WN, Viscoli CM, Brass LM, Broderick JP, Brott T, Feldmann E, *et al*. Phenylpropanolamine and the risk of hemorrhagic stroke. N Engl J Med 2000; 343:1826–1832.

Krugman S, Ward R, Giles JP, *et al*. Infectious hepatitis, study on effect of gamma globulin and on the incidence of apparent infection. JAMA 1960; 174:823–830.

Maclure M. The case-crossover design: a method for studying transient effects on the risk of acute events. Am J Epidemiol 1991; 133:144–153.

Miettinen M, Turpeinen O, Karvonen MJ, Pekkarinen M, Paavilainen E, Elosuo R. Dietary prevention of coronary heart disease in women: the Finnish mental hospital study. Int J Epidemiol 1983; 12:17–25.

Newman TB, Hulley SB. Carcinogenicity of lipid-lowering drugs. JAMA 1996; 275:55–60.

Psaty BM, Koepsell TD, Wagner EH, LoGerfo JP, Inui TS. The relative risk of incident coronary heart disease associated with recently stopping the use of beta-blockers. JAMA 1990; 263: 1653–1657.

Redelmeier DA, Tibshirani RJ. Interpretation and bias in case-crossover studies. J Clin Epidemiol 1997; 50:1281–1287.

Rothman KJ. Induction and latent periods. Am J Epidemiol 1981; 114:253–259.

Scandinavian Simvastatin Survival Study Group. Randomised trial of cholesterol lowering in 4444 patients with coronary heart disease: the Scandinavian Simvastatin Survival Study (4S). Lancet 1994; 344:1383–1389.

Shepherd J, Cobbe SM, Ford I, Isles CG, Lorimer AR, MacFarlane PW, *et al*. Prevention of coronary heart disease with pravastatin in men with hypercholesterolemia. West of Scotland Coronary Prevention Study Group. N Engl J Med 1995; 333:1301–1307.

Siscovick DS, Weiss NS, Fletcher RH, Lasky T. The incidence of primary cardiac arrest during vigorous exercise. N Engl J Med 1984; 311:874–877.

Sturmer T, Glynn RJ, Lee IM, Manson JE, Buring JE, Hennekens CH. Aspirin use and colorectal cancer: post-trial follow-up data from the Physicians' Health Study. Ann Intern Med 1998; 128: 713–720.

Sun Y, Christensen J, Hviid A, Li J, Vedsted P, Olsen J, *et al*. Risk of febrile seizures and epilepsy after vaccination with diphtheria, tetanus, acellular pertussis, inactivated poliovirus, and Haemophilus influenzae type B. JAMA 2012; 307:823–831.

Weldeselassie YG, Whitaker HJ, Farrington CP. Use of the self-controlled case-series method in vaccine safety studies: review and recommendations for best practice. Epidemiol Infect 2011; 139: 1805–1817.

Whitaker HJ, Farrington CP, Spiessens B, Musonda P. Tutorial in biostatistics: the self-controlled case series method. Stat Med 2006; 25:1768–1797.

You W, Zhang L, Gail MH, Chang Y, Liu W, Ma J, *et al*. Gastric dysplasia and gastric cancer: *Helicobacter pylori*, serum vitamin C, and other risk factors. J Natl Cancer Inst 2000; 92:1607–1612.

EXERCISES

1. Phenylpropanolamine (PPA) is a sympathomimetic agent that, until November 2000, was a component of a number of over-the-counter decongestant medications sold in the U.S. for treatment of cough and flu symptoms. Based on the pattern of events described in some case reports submitted to the Food and Drug Administration, it was hypothesized that in rare

individuals, initiation of use of a PPA-containing medication could promptly (within one day) give rise to a hemorrhagic stroke.

Let us say that during the time PPA was being used in decongestants, the manufacturers of these drugs approached you to design a study to test the above hypothesis. Because immense resources would have been required to conduct a randomized trial or a cohort study of a rare event such as hemorrhagic stroke—rare during a given one-day period—you believe that a case-control study is the only feasible approach. And, there being no practical alternative, you decide that information regarding newly initiated PPA use would come from the survivors who were able to provide an interview. You would like to choose controls from persons demographically similar to the cases. In the population in which the study is to be done, such controls can be identified and recruited by means of random-digit dialing of telephone numbers. An in-person interview would be conducted as soon as possible among those willing to participate, and (to reduce recall bias) these persons would be asked questions about their use of PPA-containing medications in the day prior to interview.

When you propose this design to the manufacturers, they (gently) suggest that because a substantial fraction of potential controls asked to participate in fact do not do so, and because others delay the interview for reasons of illness, a spuriously high odds ratio associated with recent initiation of a PPA-containing medication might be obtained. Why is their concern likely to be a valid one?

2. In their article "Carcinogenicity of lipid lowering drugs," Newman and Hulley (1996) contend that "all members of the two most popular classes of lipid-lowering drugs (the fibrates and the statins) cause cancer in rodents, in some cases at levels of animal exposure close to those prescribed to humans. [However,] evidence of carcinogenicity of lipid-lowering drugs from clinical trials in humans is inconclusive."

The results of clinical trials published by mid-1996 indicated that the incidence of cancer (overall) was nearly identical after five years of follow-up in users of simvastatin and placebo (Scandinavian Simvastatin Survival Study Group, 1994) and in users of pravastatin and placebo (Shepherd et al., 1995), respectively. By "inconclusive," Newman and Hulley no doubt were referring to the relatively small number of cancer cases identified in these studies (collectively, only about 200 in users of a statin), and especially to the much smaller number of cancers of individual sites. What do you believe was another important reason for their reluctance to accept the results of these well-done trials as assurance of no increased risk of cancer associated with long-term statin prophylaxis?

3. To test the hypothesis that wearing a helmet while skiing could reduce the risk of head injury, Hagel et al. (2005) compared the proportion of helmet users between skiers who sustained a head injury and those treated for injuries of other parts of the body. Concerned with potential confounding by characteristics of skiers that might be related both to helmet use and to the risk of head trauma, the study also compared the proportion using a helmet on the day of their head injury and on the day of their previous skiing outing. Potentially offsetting the benefit of this latter, case-crossover, approach, is: (a) the possible incomparability of ascertainment of helmet use between the two days; and (b) characteristics of the two days (e.g., visibility) that could be related to the decision to wear a helmet and also to the risk of sustaining a fall. What is a possibly even larger obstacle to the case-crossover approach's being successful in identifying a true association between helmet use while skiing and a reduced risk of head injury?

ANSWERS

1. The purpose of the control group in this study is to estimate the proportion of the underlying population at risk who began to use a PPA-containing medication during any given recent one-day period. Persons with symptoms towards which these medications are directed (colds, flu) might be more inclined to decline to participate than other persons and, if they agreed to participate, might choose to postpone the interview until they expected to recover. For these reasons, the proportion of the interviewed controls reporting very recent initiation of medications containing PPA would probably be smaller than the proportion in the population from which they had been sampled. Since this same source of bias cannot exist for the cases—they are recalling a one-day period prior to a fixed point in time; i.e., the time the first symptoms of their stroke occurred—a falsely high odds ratio will ensue.

To reduce bias from this source, the information from the controls can refer to an earlier one-day period. For example, when studying this question, Kernan et al. (2000) chose a period ending up to one week prior to the time of interview. Even though the latter choice runs the risk of a greater degree of incomplete recall by controls than would asking about the day immediately prior to the interview, overall it would seem to produce a more valid estimate of the frequency of new use of PPA in the population.

2. It may require more than five years of statin use to produce an increase in the risk of one or more forms of cancer. Alternatively, it may require a period of time after even five years of use for cancers caused by

such use to manifest themselves. Studies that have not followed statin users for more than five years cannot address these possibilities.

3. For only 35 of the 1028 skiers who sustained a head injury did helmet use differ between the day of the injury and the previous day on which they skied. Thus, there was not a great deal of statistical precision in the case-crossover analysis. The odds ratios associated with wearing a helmet that were obtained in the case-crossover and case-control portions of the study were quite similar—0.6 versus 0.7, respectively—but the confidence interval for the case-crossover odds ratio was considerably wider: 0.3–1.2 versus 0.6–0.9.

Case-crossover studies could provide information regarding exposures that have a short-term influence on risk of disease or injury, but that potential cannot be realized if there is little intrapersonal variation in exposure status over time.

18

Improving the Sensitivity of Epidemiologic Studies

If an exposure truly has the capacity to cause a disease, at least in a portion of exposed individuals, a sensitive epidemiologic study is one that will observe an association between that exposure and the disease. If an epidemiologic study is large enough to render chance an unlikely explanation for that association, the study is deemed to have a high level of statistical power. In this chapter, we restrict our attention to strategies that can enhance study sensitivity, irrespective of the size of the available study population. These strategies include:

1. Disaggregation of categories of the exposure of concern that are heterogeneous with respect to their impact on disease occurrence
2. Disaggregation of disease entities that are heterogeneous with respect to their association with the exposure of concern
3. Disaggregation of study subjects on the basis of one or more other exposures or characteristics that modify the ability of the exposure of concern to produce or prevent disease

I. DISAGGREGATION OF HETEROGENEOUS EXPOSURES

The dose or duration of a hazardous exposure received by an individual often is critical in determining his/her chances of developing a disease that the exposure is capable of producing. Smoking one pack of cigarettes per day for 30 years has a substantial influence on a person's chances of developing lung cancer. In contrast, smoking one pack of cigarettes per day for just one month, or just one cigarette per day for 10 years, probably has little impact on the risk of this disease. All of us inhale asbestos fibers, but only if we are exposed to the high concentrations found in some workplaces will we have more than an infinitesimal chance of developing mesothelioma.

Some epidemiologic studies fail to obtain information on the dose, duration, recency, or other features of a particular exposure; others fail to use that information in the analysis of the data that have been collected. Either of these shortcomings can prevent the recognition of an altered risk of disease associated with a particular exposure dose, duration, recency, etc.

Exposures that have some properties in common are often lumped together in analyses of epidemiologic studies, but sometimes these common properties may not be the ones that are relevant to disease occurrence. Aspirin and acetaminophen both are antipyretic agents, but only the former has an adverse effect on the incidence of Reye's syndrome. Female hormones are formulated and prescribed in a variety of ways and, despite some shared endocrinologic features of each regimen, their impact on the incidence of endometrial cancer differs substantially from one to the next (see Table 18.1). In an epidemiologic study of endometrial cancer, if an effort is not expended to gather and analyze information at the level of detail shown in Table 18.1, then:

1. Particularly high or low risks associated with use of certain types of hormones will not be identified; and
2. The aggregate results obtained will not apply to women in any individual category of hormone use.

Gathering information detailed enough to separate individuals who share a particular exposure from among a larger group of individuals with heterogeneous exposures is often beyond the resources of even the best-intentioned investigators.

Example 18-1. Blair *et al.* (2003) conducted a retrospective cohort mortality study of members of a dry-cleaning union in the United States. One of the goals of the study was to evaluate the hypothesis that

TABLE 18.1. INCIDENCE OF ENDOMETRIAL CANCER IN RELATION TO TYPE OF EXOGENOUS HORMONE

Type/pattern of use of exogenous female hormones	Influence on risk of endometrial cancer[a]
Contraceptive hormones	Decrease
Non-contraceptive estrogens	
"Unopposed"—	
Short duration (e.g., <1 year)	None
Longer duration	Large increase
"Opposed" by a progestogen—	
Progestogen <10 days/month, cyclic administration, long duration	Moderate increase
Progestogen ≥10 days/month, cyclic administration, long duration	None, or small increase
Progestogen daily administration, long duration	Probable decrease

[a] Relative to women who have never taken hormones
Source: based on Cook *et al.* (2006)

various chemicals used in dry-cleaning—in particular perchloroethylene, which was the major solvent in use when the study results were reported—were related to mortality from certain types of cancer. Unfortunately, though the intensity of solvent exposure could be approximated by the job category listed for each subject, and the duration of exposure by the length of union membership, the records contained no information on the type(s) of solvent used in the individual establishments. As a consequence, it was unclear whether it was exposure to perchloroethylene or to a different agent that was responsible for several large positive associations observed in that study.

Occasionally, the presence of heterogeneity among persons who compose the referent category can interfere with the assessment of risk in persons with a particular exposure or characteristic. In a meta-analysis of 97 cohort studies, Flegal *et al.* (2013) compared mortality in overweight and obese persons to that in persons of "normal" weight, which had been defined in each of these studies as a body mass index between 18.5 and 24.9 kg per m². The reduced risk of death that they observed in overweight and mildly obese persons—relative risks of 0.94 and 0.95, respectively, adjusted for age, sex, and a history of cigarette smoking—almost certainly was not the result of a salutary influence of an elevated body mass index. Rather, it probably resulted from the inclusion (unavoidable in an analysis that was obliged to rely on published data) of many persons in the lower part of the "normal" range of body mass index who were at an elevated risk of death, perhaps as a result of weight loss associated with an

illness that later proved fatal. (The excess mortality associated with having a BMI between 18.5 and 20 kg per m² was documented in an analysis of the original data from 19 of these studies (Berrington de Gonzalez *et al.*, 2010)).

II. DISAGGREGATION OF HETEROGENEOUS DISEASE ENTITIES

William Farr, the Registrar General of England and Wales during the middle of the 19th century, was trying to determine a sensible means of forming a classification of causes of death. He approached the task in a systematic way, first asking just what was the goal of any classification scheme? His answer: A "classification that brings together in groups diseases that have considerable affinity . . . is likely to facilitate the deduction of general principles" (Eyler, 1979). He recognized that in order for lessons to be learned from the conditions that caused people to die, these conditions would have to be grouped in some way. A secure basis for any sort of generalization would have to come from the experience of a number of persons, not from deaths considered one at a time.

Farr went on to discuss possible bases for a classification of causes of death (Eyler, 1979), and acknowledged that there were several that could

> be used with advantage; and the physician, the pathologist or the jurist, each from his own point of view, may legitimately classify . . . the causes of death in the way he thinks best adapted to facilitate his inquiries. The medical practitioner may found his main division of diseases on their treatment as medical or surgical; the pathologist, on the nature

of the morbid action or product; the medical jurist on the suddenness or slowness of the death; and all their points well deserve attention in a statistical classification.

Farr realized that there is no "natural" way of categorizing ill or deceased persons. Rather, he (and his successors) were obliged to make up the rules by which this would be done. A scheme that met the needs of the medical practitioner, another that met the needs of the pathologist, or a third for the medical jurist—none of them was inherently better than any of the others, except insofar as a different priority was given to each of these needs.

Farr decided that priority be given to the goal of using information on cause of death to understand etiology:

In casting about for a classification, it struck me that it should have special reference to the causation and prevention of death; and that would be most effectually accomplished by making the three distinct groups of (1) deaths by epidemic, endemic, and contagious diseases; (2) deaths by sporadic diseases; and (3) deaths by evident external causes. This classification was framed and used in forming the abstracts of causes of death.

In broad terms, Farr's approach to creating a classification of the proximate causes of death and illness is the approach we take to this day. In the current Revision of the International Classification of Disease, the first group of entries are for such entities as cholera and tuberculosis; i.e.,

"epidemic, endemic, and contagious diseases." The second group—"sporadic diseases"—includes conditions such as malignant neoplasms and diabetes. The final group comprises transport accidents, homicides, etc., that is "evident external causes."

The specific categories within the classification scheme have changed, of course, since the nineteenth century. Nonetheless, the underlying motivation behind the changes has been related to Farr's notion of having a scheme that is most relevant "to the causation and prevention of death." As subcategories of a broader disease entity are identified—often on the basis of their distinctive etiologies—they are split out to constitute categories of their own. For example, Table 18.2 lists the conditions in the 10th Revision of the International Classification of Disease (ICD)—developed in 1992—that would have been included in a single category from the first ICD of 1900, "Acute yellow atrophy of the liver." Most of the categories were formed on the basis of a known etiologic factor having been present to account for the liver pathology, such as alcohol abuse or infection with one of the hepatitis viruses.

Had we not been able to subdivide the broad category "Acute yellow atrophy of the liver" into some etiologically heterogeneous components, studies of the existence of the etiologies of liver disease would be hindered substantially. For example, studies of the effect of long-term alcohol abuse on the incidence of "acute yellow atrophy" would include as cases persons whose disease was caused by infection with *Leptospira*, etc., in which the alcohol abuse probably played no role at all. This would result in the association between alcohol and liver disease (considered

TABLE 18.2. INTERNATIONAL CLASSIFICATION OF DISEASES (ICD), 1900 AND 1992: SOME PRESENTLY DEFINED CONDITIONS THAT WOULD HAVE BEEN INCLUDED UNDER THE TERM USED IN 1900, "ACUTE YELLOW ATROPHY OF THE LIVER"

Condition	ICD code, 10th revision 1992
Alcoholic liver disease	K70
Toxic liver disease	K71
Viral hepatitis	B15–19
Liver disorders in other infectious and parasitic diseases, e.g:	
Schistosomiasis	B65
Toxoplasmosis	B58.1
Syphilis	A52.7
Other inflammatory liver diseases (e.g., liver abscess)	K75
Other diseases of liver (e.g., portal hypertension, hepatorenal syndrome)	K76

in aggregate) being smaller than the one that would have been seen had it been possible to eliminate these other cases.

Epidemiologic study of injuries also depends on our being able to distinguish between injuries that may be anatomically and pathologically similar but that arise by quite different mechanisms. For example, fracture of a thoracic vertebra (ICD-10 code S22.0) could result from a fall, a sports injury, a motor-vehicle collision, or by other mechanisms. Fortunately, current versions of the ICD also provide codes for "external causes of morbidity and mortality," which are to be used in addition to codes that describe the anatomical location and pathological type of injury. For example, code V47 is used for "Car occupant injured in collision with fixed or stationary object." Such a code could also be used to group together injuries to different parts of the body that all resulted from a similar type of motor-vehicle crash.

Sometimes, pathophysiological processes underlying a broadly defined disease entity can be identified, and cases can be separated on that basis. For example, persons can sustain a stroke from an arterial thrombus, a hemorrhage, or an embolus. In other instances, there is variation in the manner in which a broadly defined disease entity manifests itself, such as in the various histologic categories of a given site of cancer. By subdividing groups of ill persons according to the type of pathophysiology or manifestation, epidemiologic studies can increase their chances of identifying an association between a given exposure and just one of the types when one truly exists.

Example 18-2.   Assume there is an exposure, X, that is present in half the persons in a given community who sustain a thrombotic stroke, and is associated with a 4-fold increase in risk. The data from a case-control study of thrombotic stroke conducted in that community might look like this:

X exposure	Thrombotic stroke	Controls	Odds Ratio
Yes	50%	20%	4
No	50%	80%	

But let us say that in studying this association: (a) we are unable to sort out thrombotic from other types of stroke; (b) of 200 total stroke cases, only 120 actually had a thrombotic stroke; and (c) the

occurrence of the remaining 80 stroke cases is uninfluenced by X exposure. If there were also 200 controls included in the study, the following results would be obtained:

X exposure	All stroke	Controls
Yes	$60 + 16$	40
No	$60 + 64$	160
	$120 + 80$	200

In this study, the exposed cases would comprise 50% of the 120 with thrombotic stroke, and 20% of the 80 other cases (since X exposure in them is just as common as in controls). The odds ratio now would be only:

$$\frac{76}{124} \div \frac{40}{160} = 2.5,$$

quite a bit less than if it had been possible to focus the analysis on the subgroup of cases with a thrombotic stroke.

One of the great strengths of many studies investigating the source of a disease-producing infectious agent is their ability to subdivide persons who are ill and infected according to the narrowly defined type of infectious agent:

Example 18-3.   Among the strains of *Mycobacterium tuberculosis*, there is one that has a particular pattern of antibiotic resistance (defined by its characteristic DNA "fingerprint"). Though responsible for large numbers of cases of tuberculosis in New York State during the 1990s, this particular organism organism's identification in eight cases in South Carolina in 1996 was anomalous (Agerton *et al.*, 1997). One of the cases had lived in New York for some time and had returned to South Carolina in 1993. Three of the other cases were relatives of that person (two shared his household), and one additional case had been his next-door neighbor. However, the remaining three cases had no known contact with any of the first five or with one another. A detailed medical history revealed that, though these persons were diagnosed with tuberculosis six months apart, all three had been admitted to the same hospital for other reasons prior to their diagnosis within the same three-week period. One of the ill family members of the original case also had been hospitalized there shortly before the others. This patient had undergone a bronchoscopy at that time as part of the management of his tuberculosis. Each of the other three persons had also undergone bronchoscopy during their earlier hospitalization (to evaluate an unrelated condition), at which time cultures for *M. tuberculosis* had been negative (that is, they did not already have tuberculosis when the bronchoscopy had been done).

Though there was no formal control group employed in this study, it is extraordinarily improbable that all three additional cases of tuberculosis would have had bronchoscopy within a three-week period and in the same location as the first case to undergo bronchoscopy, had there not been some etiologic link. The investigators evaluated the hospital's procedures for cleaning and disinfecting endoscopic equipment and found several features that "did not follow the hospital's guidelines or the published guidelines," which could have been responsible for transmission of the infectious agent from one patient to another.

There are many potential sources of tuberculosis transmission in South Carolina other than a contaminated bronchoscope. However, the investigators' ability to identify that particular source was made possible by their being able to restrict attention to the cases of tuberculosis who shared a common infecting strain. Inclusion of tuberculosis cases caused by other strains would almost certainly have obscured the association with a prior history of bronchoscopy in one place and at (approximately) one point in time.

Example 18-4.   Donnell *et al.*, 2010, conducted a cohort study in sub-Saharan Africa among heterosexual couples in which one partner was infected with HIV. During the 24-month followup, about 10% of those who were infected initiated antiretroviral therapy. Among uninfected partners, the chances of developing an HIV infection that was phylogenetically linked to that of their partner was substantially lower if the partner was taking antiretroviral therapy (0.37 per 100 person-years) than if he/she was not (2.24 per 100 person-years).

But what if the endpoint in this study had been the presence of any new HIV infection, whether or not it was linked to the partner's HIV strain (so as to include infections arising from sexual conduct with other persons)? The rate in both groups of initially uninfected persons would have been expected to rise, in absolute terms, to the same degree. Therefore, the relative risk associated with partner's receipt of antiretroviral therapy would have been closer to the null than the observed value of 0.37/2.24 = 0.17.

III. DISAGGREGATION OF STUDY SUBJECTS ON THE BASIS OF ONE OR MORE EXPOSURES OR CHARACTERISTICS THAT MODIFY THE ABILITY OF THE EXPOSURE OF CONCERN TO PRODUCE OR PREVENT DISEASE

It is commonly stated that diseases have multiple causes. There are at least two distinct ideas contained in such a statement:

1. A disease can have more than one separate causal pathway leading to it. For example, a child can acquire hepatitis B infection from his/her infected mother, but so can an adult by sharing a needle and/or a syringe with a person who is infected with this virus. The overall incidence of hepatitis B infection in a population would reflect the sum of the separate incidence rates due to the operation of these two pathways (along with others). As another example, mental retardation can be caused by the access of a young child to lead in his/her environment and also by prematurity, even in the absence of harmful levels of lead. Assuming there is no influence of lead exposure on the risk of prematurity, the occurrence of retardation due to these two pathways would sum, and would be responsible for a portion of a population's total incidence of mental retardation.

2. Two or more exposures are capable of causing disease only by acting together in a single causal pathway. For example, a genetic abnormality, deficiency of the enzyme glucose-6-phosphate dehydrogenase (G6PD), is a cause of hemolytic anemia only if a person with this genotype is exposed to quinidine, sulfonamides, naphthalene, infection, or some other oxidative stress.

When two exposures act through separate means to produce a disease, the relative impact of either of them is greater in that segment of the population in which the other exposure is absent. For example, assume that the prevalence of mental retardation in 5-year-old children who had been born full-term is four per 100, whereas in those born prematurely it is 14 per 100 (Table 18.3). Assume that in a group of 5-year-olds there were children with enough lead exposure to produce an additional frequency of mental retardation of two per 100, both in those who were and those who were not premature. In children who had not been born prematurely, the prevalence of mental retardation in lead-exposed children would

TABLE 18.3. RELATIVE INFLUENCE OF EXPOSURE IN EARLY
CHILDHOOD ON THE PREVALENCE OF MENTAL
RETARDATION–HYPOTHETICAL DATA

Risk factor(s) for retardation	Prevalence of retardation (per 100 children)	Relative prevalence
None	4	
		$6/4 = 1.5$
Lead only	6	
Prematurity only	14	
		$16/14 = 1.14$
Both lead and prematurity	16	

be six per 100, representing a 1.5-fold increase in risk associated with lead exposure. In premature children, however, the prevalence would be increased from 14 to 16 per 100, just a 1.14-fold increase.

Recognition of the presence of alternate pathways leading to an illness can facilitate the detection of an "outbreak" of that illness, and also can help identify the cause of the outbreak:

Example 18-5. Between December 1991 and April 1992, Abulrahi *et al.* (1997) identified 41 cases of acute *Plasmodium falciparum* malaria in children admitted to a hospital in Riyadh, Saudi Arabia. The vectors of malaria, anopheline mosquitoes, are not present anywhere near Riyadh, so the first step in understanding the causes of the illness in these children was to determine if any of them had traveled to areas where malaria was endemic. Twenty of the 41 children indeed had been in such an area during the month prior to the onset of fever that signaled the presence of malaria. A case-control study was done to determine the source of the infection in the other 21 children.

The study obtained a striking result: 20 of the 21 children (95%) with locally acquired malaria (LAM),— i.e., those who had not traveled to endemic areas for malaria,—had been hospitalized at some point during the month prior to admission for their malaria, in contrast to 15 of 61 control children (25%). (Strictly speaking, any potential control who had traveled to an endemic area for malaria during the prior month should have been excluded from this analysis. However, the number of such children was probably so small that little bias would be present had they inadvertently been included.) Also, only five of the 20 cases of "imported" malaria had been hospitalized during the month prior to the onset of their fever. The odds ratio for LAM associated with

hospitalization during the prior month was:

$$\frac{20}{1} \div \frac{15}{46} = 61.3.$$

This finding led the investigators to evaluate practices in the hospital that could have allowed transmission of the infection from one patient to the next. They discovered that the nursing staff were routinely using heparin locks on multiple patients, allowing for hematologic spread of *P. falciparum* from infected patients to uninfected patients.

In the design and analysis of the case-control study, Abulrahi *et al.* exploited the fact that most of the 41 cases of malaria were attributable to two distinct causal pathways: One involved mosquito-borne transmission in an endemic area, the other some local factor(s). If the local factor were operating independently to cause malaria,—that is it did not require an exposure to an infected mosquito to produce the disease, then the incidence of malaria in Riyadh simply would be the sum of the separate incidences resulting from the two pathways.

What if Abulrahi *et al.* had not recognized the presence of the imported malaria pathway, or had not bothered to assess a history of foreign travel in the children with malaria? They would have observed 20 LAM cases + 5 imported cases = 25 total cases with a history of hospitalization in the prior month, and 1 + 15 = 16 cases without such a hospitalization. The odds ratio, based on all malaria cases in the study,

$$\frac{25}{16} \div \frac{15}{46},$$

would have been only 4.8, very much smaller than the value of 61.3 when the analysis was restricted to the LAM cases. In this instance, the recognition that recent hospitalization played an etiologic role in the transmission of malaria in Riyadh was facilitated by the recognition of the likely presence of a second causal pathway that could lead to malaria, and by the subsequent effort to confine one analysis to the individuals (i.e., those without the history of foreign travel) in whom the impact of any local factor identified would be *relatively* high.

In some instances, the investigation of a particular exposure as a possible cause of disease is enhanced by the recognition of more than just one alternative causal pathway, and once again by the subsequent exclusion of subjects who had been exposed to a component of those other pathways.

Example 18-6. In a medical record–based study, Grether and Nelson (1997) tested the hypothesis that maternal infection predisposes to spastic cerebral palsy (CP). The presence of infection was defined as a notation of one of a variety of prespecified events and conditions in the record, including maternal fever, chorioamnionitis, urinary tract infection, and histological evidence of placental infection. From the medical record, the investigators also were able to identify children with CP who had one of several other conditions whose presence was likely to have been responsible for their CP even had no maternal infection been present. These were conditions such as a destructive lesion or malformation of the brain, or a syndrome that typically includes spasticity as a feature. The following table summarizes the history of infection during pregnancy in the "explained" cases of CP, along with that in the remaining "unexplained" cases and in a control group of term infants without CP:

| | Cases | | | |
	"Explained" CP	"Unexplained" CP	Total CP	Controls
Evidence of infection	1(3.3%)	10(21.7%)	11(14.4%)	11(2.9%)
No infection	29	36	65	367
Total	30	46	76	378

Evidence of maternal or placental infection was present in 10 (21.7%) of "unexplained" CP cases, but only in 11 (2.9%) of controls, and the odds ratio was

$$\frac{10}{36} \div \frac{11}{367} = 9.3.$$

However, because infection had occurred in the "explained" CP cases just about as often as in controls, the association between "total" CP and infection would have been less strong: the odds ratio

would have been

$$\frac{11}{65} \div \frac{11}{367} = 5.6.$$

By identifying conditions that strongly predispose to CP independently of maternal infection, and by restricting the analysis to persons in whom these other conditions were not present, the investigators were able to focus their attention on the children in whom the relative contribution of infection to CP occurrence was the greatest.

If two factors have the capacity to act together in a single causal pathway leading to disease, the incidence of that disease in persons in whom both factors are present would be more than the sum of the two rates produced by either factor's presence alone. For example, during epidemics of Reye's syndrome in the United States during the late 1970s and early 1980s, the disease would typically occur in a child who had recently had a bout of chickenpox or influenza who had taken aspirin during the course of that illness. The incidence of Reye's syndrome in children with both the prior infection and aspirin use was far higher than that predicted from the sum of the near-zero incidence rates in children who: (a) had chicken pox or flu but did not receive aspirin; and (b) took aspirin for reasons other than chicken pox or flu. Similarly, the neurological manifestations of phenylketonuria (PKU) occur in children born with a defective or absent enzyme, phenylalanine hydroxylase, who also consume a typical quantity of the amino acid, phenylalanine. Phenylalanine hydroxylase converts phenylalanine to another amino acid, tyrosine, thus not permitting the accumulation of phenylalanine in tissues. The prevalence of neurological damage characteristic of PKU is far higher in children with phenylalanine hydroxylase deficiency who consume a normal diet than would be predicted by the sum of the prevalence of this type of damage in children: (a) who have the genetic abnormality but, having been screened for PKU, consume a diet extremely low in phenylalanine content; and (b) who possess a normal gene and have no dietary restriction (Table 18.4).

If aspirin use predisposes to the incidence of Reye's syndrome only when chicken pox or flu are present, then of course only in children with these infections will the relative risk associated with aspirin use be above one. To the extent that there are Reye's syndrome cases that occur without one of these antecedent infections, an analysis that adds them

TABLE 18.4. INTERPLAY OF HEREDITY AND DIET IN THE ETIOLOGY OF
THE NEUROLOGICAL DAMAGE CHARACTERISTIC OF PKU

Phenylalanine hydroxylase deficiency	Phenylalanine intake	Clinical evidence of neurological damage characteristic of PKU
Yes	Normal	Yes
Yes	Low	No
No	Normal	No
No	Low	No

to cases who have been infected will obtain a relative risk associated with aspirin that is intermediate between the value of 1.0 (the RR of persons with no prior infection) and that of 10-40 that has been observed in most studies of Reye's syndrome based on children who did have chicken pox or flu. A more sensitive approach; i.e., one that has a greater chance of determining whether aspirin use has any deleterious effect with respect to the incidence of Reye's syndrome, would be to obtain data on a history of prior infection on all study subjects and examine the association with aspirin use separately in children with and without such a history.

IMPLICATIONS OF THE PRESENCE OF VARIATION IN THE SIZE OF RELATIVE RISK ACROSS SUBGROUPS DEFINED ON THE BASIS OF ANOTHER RISK FACTOR

So far, we have discussed ways of increasing the sensitivity of an epidemiologic study by identifying a subgroup of the population in whom the relative impact of exposure on disease incidence is particularly large: It is the size of the relative risk that we use as one guideline for inferring the presence of a causal relationship between an exposure and a disease, and we do not want to overlook the possibility that, among the whole of the population, there is a segment in whom the relative risk associated with exposure is noticeably different than 1.0. However, it is important to keep in mind that once a causal action of an exposure on a disease occurrence has been inferred, a possible difference in the importance of that association across these same subgroups—in clinical or public health terms—can only be assessed by considering the size of the attributable risk in each of these subgroups. We saw in Chapter 9 that, for a given disease, a high

relative risk associated with an exposure does not necessarily translate into an attributable risk high enough to be of clinical or public health importance, since the size of the attributable risk is influenced heavily by the underlying incidence of that disease in the absence of the exposure. By the same token, when the incidence of the disease differs in two subgroups of individuals, defined on the basis of one exposure, then: (1) if the relative risk associated with another exposure is the same in each of the subgroups, the corresponding attributable risks will differ, possibly to an important degree; and (2) differences in the relative risk associated with an exposure between the subgroups may simply be a reflection of the exposure adding to the risk by the same amount in each of the subgroups. Let us consider each of these separately. As an example of (1) above, Table 18.5 shows results obtained in a cohort study of the mortality from lung cancer in men in relation to heavy occupational exposure to asbestos.

Do these data suggest that the increased risk of lung cancer associated with a history of cigarette smoking—very likely causally associated—should weigh more heavily in the decision to stop smoking by a man with a history of heavy asbestos exposure than a man without such a history? The relative risk (RR) associated with cigarette smoking is nearly the same between men with and without a history of asbestos exposure ($122.6 \div 11.3 = 10.85$ in men not exposed to asbestos, and $601.6 \div 58.4 = 10.30$ in men who were exposed to asbestos). However, the attributable risk (AR) in the latter group is higher (by more than a factor of five) than in the former ($601.6 - 58.4 = 543.2$ per 100,000 man-years in asbestos workers versus $122.6 - 11.3 = 111.3$ per 100,000 in other persons). This dissimilarity in the respective ARs, in the presence of comparability between the RRs, is due to the fact that among nonsmokers the mortality from lung cancer was higher, by more than a factor of 5, in men exposed to

TABLE 18.5. AGE-STANDARDIZED LUNG CANCER DEATH RATES[a] FOR CIGARETTE SMOKING AND/OR OCCUPATIONAL EXPOSURE TO ASBESTOS DUST COMPARED WITH NO SMOKING AND NO OCCUPATIONAL EXPOSURE TO ASBESTOS DUST

Group	Exposure to asbestos	History of cigarette smoking?	Death Rate	Mortality difference	Mortality ratio
Control	No	No	11.3	0.0	1.00
Asbestos workers	Yes	No	58.4	+47.1	5.17
Control	No	Yes	122.6	+111.3	10.85
Asbestos workers	Yes	Yes	601.6	+590.3	53.24

[a] Rate per 100,000 man-years standardized for age on the distribution of the man-years of all the asbestos workers
Source: Hammond *et al.* (1979)

asbestos. Since it is the size of AR that ought to bear on decisions pertaining to health (and on the recommendations of providers of healthcare), the same 10-fold increase in the risk of lung cancer should be given more weight by a man who has a history of heavy occupational asbestos exposure than by one who does not. (Of course, the AR for lung cancer and for many other conditions associated with cigarette smoking is so large, even in persons without occupational exposure to asbestos, that all persons have a strong incentive to discontinue smoking.)

As an example of (2) above, some studies of endometrial cancer observed a difference in the relative risk associated with long-term use of unopposed estrogens, depending on a woman's weight. In lean women and women of average weight who participated in one of these studies (Shields *et al.*, 1999), the incidence in hormone nonusers was about 0.26 per 1000 woman-years, in contrast to a rate of about 4.45 per 1000 in long-term hormone users (relative risk = 17.1). Among heavy women in the same study (those in the upper fourth of the distribution of body mass index), the rates in hormone nonusers and users were 0.75 and 8.92 per 1000 woman-years, respectively, and the relative risk was not so strongly elevated (11.9). However, based on these results it would be incorrect to conclude that the adverse impact of the use of unopposed estrogens on the endometrium should bear less strongly on the decision of a heavy woman to use unopposed estrogens than on the decision of a woman who is not heavy. These data suggest that the absolute change in incidence resulting from hormone use (i.e., the attributable risk) is actually greater in heavy women—8.92 − 0.75 = 8.17 per 1000 woman-years—than it is in other women—4.45 − 0.26 = 4.19 per 1000 woman-years.

The term "effect modification" is used by epidemiologists to describe the circumstance in which the size of an association between exposure and disease differs according to the presence or level of another exposure or characteristic. However, the meaning of effect-modification as applied to a particular instance may be ambiguous if the measure of association is not specified. In one example presented earlier, the relative risk of mental retardation associated with lead exposure was modified by a history of prematurity; the RR was 1.14 in children born prematurely, whereas it was 1.5 in children born full-term. However, the size of the attributable risk associated with lead exposure did not depend on a history of prematurity (2 per 100 in both subgroups of gestational length). In a different example, it was the relative risk that was similar across subgroups of the additional variable—the RR for MI associated with OC use was 4.4 in women under 35 years and 4.3 in older women—whereas the attributable risk was modified by age (2.7 versus 31.0 per million women-years, respectively). Our recommendation is that whenever the term "effect modification" is used, the criterion for its presence (i.e., variation in the size of the relative or attributable risk) should be provided.

INVESTIGATING AGE AS A POSSIBLE EFFECT MODIFIER

Age can exert a potent influence on the ability of an exposure to influence the risk of disease. For example, compared to adults, very young children are relatively refractory to the development of polio if infected with polio virus. However, they have much greater susceptibility than adults to the occurrence of the hemolytic uremic syndrome if they ingest food containing *E. coli* O157:H7. Examining age as a

TABLE 18.6. TWO HYPOTHETICAL EXAMPLES OF EFFECT MODIFICATION BY AGE

A. Genetic marker associated with increased risk only in young persons

Genetic marker present?	Young (mean = 30 years)			Old (mean = 60 years)			Mean age
	No. of cases	Person- years	Rate[a]	No. of cases	Person- years	Rate[a]	
Yes	50	10,000	5	10	5,000	2	$\frac{50(30)+10(60)}{60}=35.0$
No	100	100,000	1	100	50,000	2	$\frac{100(30)+100(60)}{200}=45.0$

B. Genetic marker associated with decreased risk only in old persons

Genetic marker present?	Young (mean = 30 years)			Old (mean = 60 years)			Mean age
	No. of cases	Person- years	Rate[a]	No. of cases	Person- years	Rate[a]	
Yes	10	10,000	1	2	5,000	0.4	$\frac{10(30)+2(60)}{12}=35.0$
No	100	100,000	1	100	50,000	2	$\frac{100(30)+100(60)}{200}=45.0$

[a]Cases per 1,000 person-years

potential effect modifier generally is straightforward: as with any other variable, one looks for a difference in the presence or size of the association between the exposure of interest and disease in two or more age categories. However, some investigators have instead simply compared the mean (or median) ages of cases who do or do not have a particular exposure or characteristic. This practice is to be avoided, since it can give misleading results.

- A study of women with breast cancer, identified from a tumor registry in the United States, observed that black patients tended to be younger than white patients at the time of the diagnosis (mean age 55 years vs. 60 years). The authors of the study suggested this difference may have etiologic implications. However, not considered was the possibility that there was a corresponding age difference in the underlying population in which the women with breast cancer resided. If, for example, the mean age of black women in that part of the United States were five years less than the mean age of white women, then identical age-specific rates between the two races would produce a corresponding difference between the black and white women diagnosed with breast cancer.
- Even when the exposure in question is not related to age in the underlying population,

the interpretation of a difference in age between exposed and non-exposed cases can be ambiguous. Consider the following hypothetical example of a disease with a bimodal age distribution: The mean age of "young" cases is 30 years, whereas that of "old" cases is 60 years. Assume there is a 5-fold excess disease risk associated with the presence of a particular genetic marker that is confined to "young" cases (Table 18.6A). In a population whose members are distributed in terms of age and marker status, as in Table 18.6A, the mean age of cases possessing this marker is 35.0 years. The mean age of the cases without the marker is 45.0 years.

Table 18.6B displays hypothetical data from a population that is identical to that in Table 18-6A in terms of age and marker status, but in which there is: (1) no association between the genetic marker and disease risk in young persons; and (2) a negative association in old persons. The mean ages of diseased individuals with and without the genetic marker are, once again, 35.0 and 45.0, respectively!

In short, the interpretation of the 10-year difference in mean age of diagnosis is ambiguous, since it can be produced by completely different patterns of effect modification.

BY INCREASING THE SENSITIVITY OF EPIDEMIOLOGIC STUDIES, DO WE ALSO DECREASE THEIR SPECIFICITY?

The answer to the above question is "yes." Dividing study subjects into subgroups of exposures and diseases and examining possible associations for various combinations of subgroups will make the number of "false positive" results grow. That is, an increasing number of associations will be seen in the sample of persons studied that do not represent an underlying association in the "universe" of persons from which the sample was drawn. This loss of specificity is the price we must pay to avoid missing a true association (or underestimating its magnitude) that is present for some category of exposure or disease, or in some segment of the population at risk.

Nonetheless, by being cognizant of the presence of false positive associations that a thorough analytical approach must produce, we will know to be cautious when trying to interpret the associations that do emerge in an individual study. We will tend to interpret an association restricted to (or most prominent in) a subgroup as reflecting a genuine causal (or protective) relation when it: is large; is based on a sizeable number of subjects, to minimize the role of chance; has been observed in one or more other studies; and when there is a plausible explanation for

the pattern of associations across subgroups that has been observed.

Example 18-7.   In a randomized trial, U.S. male physicians assigned to take 325 mg. of aspirin on alternate days were observed to have a lower incidence of myocardial infarction than those assigned to take a placebo (Ridker *et al.*, 1997). However, the reduction in incidence associated with aspirin use varied according to a man's plasma level of C-reactive protein, being most prominent in those with relatively high levels and absent in men in the lower fourth of the distribution (Fig. 18.1).

The hypothesis that the efficacy of aspirin use in the prevention of myocardial infarction truly differs depending on a man's plasma level of C-reactive protein is supported by: (1) the large, graded, difference in the observed association across C-reactive protein (CRP) levels; (2) the large number of observations on which this was based (a total of 246 men with myocardial infarction); (3) the fact that C-reactive protein is a marker of a chronic inflammatory process that can predispose to rupture of atherosclerotic plaques; and (4) the likely ability of aspirin to modify the thrombotic response to plaque rupture (ISIS-2 Collaborative Group, 1988). Because use of aspirin also predicts favorable outcomes in persons with unstable angina who have high CRP levels, but not

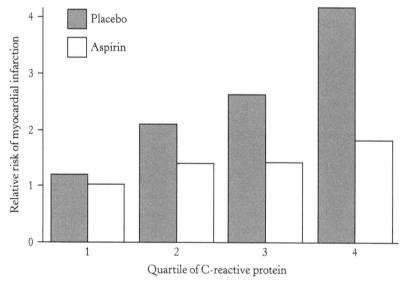

FIGURE 18.1 Relative risk of myocardial infarction in the Physician Health Study, by treatment group and quartile of C-relative protien.

Source: Ridker *et al.* (1997)

in corresponding patients with low CRP levels (Kennon *et al.*, 2001), it appears that levels of C-reactive protein (or one or more correlates of it) can influence the presence and degree of benefit (in terms of heart attack risk) that ensue from aspirin use.

Example 18-8. An interview-based case-control study of testicular cancer was conducted to test the hypothesis that a history of vasectomy might predispose men to this disease (Strader *et al.*, 1988). Cases were identified through the records of a population-based cancer registry, while controls were enumerated from random-digit dialing of telephone numbers. The results shown in Table 18.7 were obtained.

The odds ratio associated with a history of vasectomy of 1.5 among men in general represents only a modest elevation and argues for a cautious interpretation. The odds ratio did vary considerably between Catholic and other men (8.7 versus 1.1), but it seems implausible that religious preference could somehow bear on the ability of a vasectomy to predispose to the incidence of testicular cancer. Rather, it seems more likely that the ascertainment of a history of vasectomy was relatively incomplete among Catholic controls: Vasectomy is proscribed by the Catholic religion, and it is possible that some Catholic men chosen at random from the community to serve as a member of a comparison group in a study of cancer may have been reluctant to admit to having had this procedure. If the ascertainment of vasectomy had been relatively more complete among Catholic cases than Catholic controls—perhaps they felt more of an obligation than controls to acknowledge a proscribed behavior, because of their relatively greater interest in helping to understand the causes of testicular cancer—the resulting differential misclassification could have produced a spuriously elevated odds ratio.

When considering whether an association between exposure and disease is indicative of a causal relationship between the two, we ask if that association has been observed consistently from study to study. We are looking for that same consistency before concluding that the variation observed in the direction or size of an exposure–disease association across strata of another exposure or characteristic is indicative of genuine effect modification. For example, because studies have observed repeatedly that being overweight is associated with an increased risk of breast cancer in postmenopausal women and yet a decreased risk in premenopausal

TABLE 18.7. RESULTS FROM A CASE-CONTROL STUDY OF VASECTOMY AND TESTICULAR CANCER

Religious preference	History of vasectomy	Cases ($n = 228$)	Controls ($n = 513$)	Odds ratio[a]
		Numbers in percentages		
Catholic	Yes	24.4	6.2	8.7
	No	75.6	93.8	
Other or none	Yes	23.0	19.6	1.1
	No	77.0	80.4	
All men	Yes	23.3	17.1	1.5
	No	76.7	82.9	

[a] Age-adjusted
Source: Strader *et al.* (1988)

women (Rose and Vona-Davis, 2010), the modifying influence of menopausal status on this association between weight and breast cancer is widely accepted. However, when evaluating the consistency of inter-stratum variation of this sort from study to study, it is necessary not to lose sight of those studies of the overall association that have *not* presented data relevant to the possibility of effect modification.

Example 18-9. Green *et al.* (2000) reviewed the results of 21 studies that examined the association between N-acetyltransferase 2 (NAT2) genotype or activity and the incidence of bladder cancer. NAT2 is an enzyme involved in the inactivation of arylamines, carcinogens present in cigarette smoke. The NAT2 gene that directs the synthesis of this enzyme is polymorphic, and as a result all persons are either "fast" or "slow" acetylators. It was hypothesized that being a slow acetylator might be a particularly strong risk factor for bladder cancer in persons with a high level of exposure to arylamines; e.g., by means of cigarette smoking. Results from five (of the 21) studies reviewed by Green *et al.* that addressed this question supported the hypothesis: The pooled odds ratio relating slow acetylation status to bladder cancer was 1.6 in cigarette smokers but only 1.0 in non-smokers. However, as pointed out by Green *et al.*, the failure of the large majority of studies to report data on the possible modifying influence of smoking status on this association severely limits the interpretation of the difference between these two odds ratios. Specifically, it is all too likely that the authors of some of the other 16 studies examined their data for the presence of effect modification, found it *not* to be there, and simply omitted a presentation of these results from their manuscript.

The example above describes a form of "publication" bias: that is, a distortion of the truth by the appearance in the medical literature of a skewed sample of results. Publication bias can be present when one seeks to summarize the overall association between an exposure and disease across studies, of course. However, we suspect its frequency and magnitude are greater when one is summarizing studies for the possibility of effect modification, since we believe it is more likely for an analysis that fails to suggest an interaction to be kept out of a manuscript than for a manuscript as a whole with a null result to be kept from publication.

REFERENCES

Abulrahi HA, Bohlega EA, Fontaine RE, al Seghayer SM, al Ruwais AA. *Plasmodium falciparum* malaria transmitted in hospital through heparin locks. Lancet 1997; 349:23–25.

Agerton T, Valway S, Gore B, Pozsik C, Plikaytis B, Woodley C, et al. Transmission of a highly drug-resistant strain (Strain W1) of *Mycobacterium tuberculosis*. JAMA 1997; 278:1073–1077.

Berrington de Gonzalez A, Hartge P, Cerhan JR, Flint AJ, Hannan L, MacInnis RJ, et al. Body-mass index and mortality among 1.46 million white adults. N Engl J Med 2010; 363:2211–2219.

Blair A, Petralia SA, Stewart PA. Extended mortality follow-up of a cohort of dry cleaners. Ann Epidemiol 2003; 13:50–56.

Cho NH, Moy CS, Davis F, Haenszel W, Ahn YO, Kim H. Ethnic variation in the incidence of stomach cancer in Illinois, 1986–1988. Am J Epidemiol 1996; 144:661–664.

Cook LS, Weiss NS, Doherty JA, Chen C. Endometrial cancer. In: Schottenfeld D, Fraumeni JF Jr (eds.). Cancer epidemiology and prevention. New York: Oxford, 2006 pp. 1027–1043.

Danesh J, Youngman L, Clark S, Parish S, Peto R, Collins R. *Helicobacter pylori* infection and early onset myocardial infarction: case-control and sibling pairs study. BMJ 1999; 319:1157–1162.

David O, Hoffman S, McGann B, Sverd J, Clark J. Low lead levels and mental retardation. Lancet 1976; 2:1376–1379.

Donnell D, Baeten JM, Kiarie J, Thomas KK, Stevens W, Cohen CR, et al. Heterosexual HIV-1 transmission after initiation of antiretroviral therapy: a prospective cohort analysis. Lancet 2010; 375:2092–2098.

Eyler EM. Victorian social medicine. Baltimore: Johns Hopkins University Press, 1979.

Flegal KM, Kit BK, Orpana H, Graubard BI. Association of all-cause mortality with overweight and obesity using standard body mass index categories: a systematic review and meta-analysis. JAMA 2013; 309:71–82.

Green J, Banks E, Berrington A, Darby S, Deo H, Newton R. N-acetyltransferase 2 and bladder cancer: an overview and consideration of the evidence for gene-environment interaction. Br J Cancer 2000; 83:412–417.

Grether JK, Nelson KB. Maternal infections and cerebral palsy in infants of normal birth weight. JAMA 1997; 278:207–211.

Hammond EC, Selikoff IJ, Seidman H. Asbestos exposure, cigarette smoking and death rates. Ann N Y Acad Sci 1979; 330:473–490.

ISIS-2 Collaborative Group. Randomised trial of intravenous streptokinase, oral aspirin, both, or neither among 17,187 cases of suspected acute myocardial infarction: ISIS-2. Lancet 1988; 2:349–360.

Kennon S, Price CP, Mills PG, Ranjadayalan K, Cooper J, Clarke H, et al. The effect of aspirin on C-reactive protein as a marker of risk in unstable angina. J Am Coll Cardiol 2001; 37:1266–1270.

Pocock SJ, Smith M, Baghurst P. Environmental lead and children's intelligence: a systematic review of the epidemiological evidence. BMJ 1994; 309:1189–1197.

Rebbeck TR, Kantoff PW, Krithivas K, Neuhausen S, Blackwood MA, Godwin AK, et al. Modification of BRCA1-associated breast cancer risk by the polymorphic androgen-receptor CAG repeat. Am J Hum Genet 1999; 64:1371–1377.

Ridker PM, Cushman M, Stampfer MJ, Tracy RP, Hennekens CH. Inflammation, aspirin, and the risk of cardiovascular disease in apparently healthy men. N Engl J Med 1997; 336:973–980.

Rose DP, Vona-Davis L. Interaction between menopausal status and obesity in affecting breast cancer risk. Maturitas 2010; 66:33–38.

Sharer N, Schwarz M, Malone G, Howarth A, Painter J, Super M, et al. Mutations of the cystic fibrosis gene in patients with chronic pancreatitis. N Engl J Med 1998; 339:645–652.

Shields TS, Weiss NS, Voigt LF, Beresford SA. The additional risk of endometrial cancer associated with unopposed estrogen use in women with other risk factors. Epidemiology 1999; 10: 733–738.

Strader CH, Weiss NS, Daling JR. Vasectomy and the incidence of testicular cancer. Am J Epidemiol 1988; 128:56–63.

Treggiari MM, Weiss NS. Occupational asbestos exposure and the incidence of non-Hodgkin's lymphoma of the gastrointestinal tract: an ecologic study. Ann Epidemiol 2004; 14:168–171.

EXERCISES

1. David *et al.* (1976) wished to determine "the quantitative extent of the relationship between lead and mental retardation," since at the time that study was done it remained "to be determined whether a smaller amount of lead—i.e., raised but non-encephalopathic concentrations in the blood—can be an etiological factor in mental retardation." From patients attending a developmental evaluation clinic, they obtained a blood sample for lead determination on 64 children with an IQ of 55–84. Of these, 33 had a probable explanation for being retarded, such as prematurity, maternal eclampsia, meningitis, or microcephaly. From a pediatric clinic in the same medical center, blood samples were obtained in 30 control children and also were tested for lead levels. The results are shown in the following table:

(a) Estimate the risk of mental retardation of unknown etiology in children with lead levels ≥25 mcg/dl relative to that in children with levels <25 mcg/dl. Exclude from the calculation the data on the retarded children in whom the etiology probably was known.

(b) Had the probable etiology of some cases of mental retardation not been known, the 31 children with no known etiology would have been combined with the 33 other retarded children to form a single case group. Using these 64 cases and the same control group, and the ≥25 versus <25 dichotomy, what is the risk ratio associated with high blood lead levels for this broader category of mental retardation? Why does it differ from the previous one?

(c) Relative to children with blood lead levels of <15 mcg/dl, what is the risk of mental retardation with no known etiology in children with levels of:

- 15–24 mcg/dl
- 25–34 mcg/dl
- ≥35 mcg/dl

Was there any advantage to having been able to measure blood lead more precisely than simply greater or less than 25 mcg/dl?

2. Older adults who have a fracture are at high risk for having another one. A randomized trial was conducted in the United Kingdom to determine whether calcium supplements could reduce the risk of recurrent fracture among 5,292 ambulatory older adults who sought hospital treatment for an initial fracture. In their trial, the investigators identified 698 participants in whom a "low-trauma" fracture subsequently occurred. Not included in the analysis were an additional 34 fractures that resulted from substantial

TABLE 18.8.

Blood lead concentration (mcg/dl)	Mental retardation		Controls
	Etiology probably known	Etiology unknown	
<15	8	2	12
15–24	20	14	11
25–34	4	10	6
≥35	1	5	1

trauma—e.g., a fracture sustained in an automobile crash. A disadvantage of not including these 34 fractures involving more than a low level of trauma was a reduced sample size (by about 5%). What do you believe to be the main advantage of excluding them?

3. A study of chronic pancreatitis sought to determine whether persons with this disease more often had a mutation of the cystic fibrosis transmembrane conductance regulator (CSTR) gene than do other persons (Sharer *et al.*, 1998). Because alcohol consumption is a risk factor for chronic pancreatitis, the investigators separated their cases into two groups: 71 who were felt to have alcohol-related disease, and 63 "idiopathic" cases. Six of the former group had a mutation on at least one copy of the CSTR gene, while 12 of the idiopathic cases had such a mutation. The prevalence of one or more CSTR mutations in a control group of persons without pancreatitis was 5.3%. Prior studies have shown that alcohol consumption itself is unrelated to the presence of a mutation in the CSTR gene. Do the data of Sharer *et al.* support the hypothesis that alcohol consumption and a mutation of the CSTR gene work jointly to produce chronic pancreatitis?

4. The first exon of the androgen receptor gene contains a trinucleotide (CAG) repeat sequence, the length of which varies from person to person. A very large number of repeat sequences (e.g., ≥40) is associated with androgen insensitivity. It has been observed that among women who have inherited a germline mutation in the BRCA1 gene and went on to develop breast cancer, the mean age at diagnosis of those with ≥30 CAG repeats was 6.3 years earlier than that of the other women (Rebbeck *et al.*, 1999). Assume that the difference was not due to chance. Does this necessarily mean that the presence of ≥30 CAG repeats in the androgen receptor gene preferentially increases risk of breast cancer in young women with a BRCA1 mutation?

5. This question pertains to the following (excerpted) abstract (Cho *et al.*, 1996):

The authors extend their investigation by comparing the incidence rate of stomach cancer among three ethnic groups in the state of Illinois from 1986 to 1988. The 3-year age-adjusted cumulative incidence rate for immigrant Koreans (172/100,000) was approximately four- and eightfold higher than for African Americans (41/100,000) and whites (21/100,000). The high rate of stomach cancer in immigrant Koreans compared with African Americans and white populations residing in Illinois indicates either a drastically disproportionate undercount of immigrant Koreans in the census or a profound genetic-environmental interaction.

Assume that the results presented are not due to chance or bias (including bias due to a disproportionate undercount of immigrant Koreans in the census). Apart from "a profound genetic–environmental interaction," what are other plausible explanations for the high observed rates of stomach cancer among immigrant Koreans in Illinois?

6. Fig. 18.2, taken from Danesh *et al.* (1999), is a summary of studies of *H. pylori* seropositivity in relation to the occurrence of coronary heart disease. (Three other retrospective studies are not included since they did not report separate results for cases of myocardial infarction. Together, these studies included fewer than 150 cases of myocardial infarction.) Black squares indicate odds ratio, with area of square proportional to number of cases, and horizontal lines represent confidence intervals.

From this figure, assume that the most trustworthy data bearing on a possible association between *H. pylori* seropositivity and the occurrence of coronary heart disease come from:

- The ISIS study for persons 30-49 years; and
- The four prospective studies for persons older than this.

Also assume that the studies were done in a comparable way in the same geographic population; that *H. pylori* seropositivity is a faithful indication of *H. pylori* infection, regardless of age; and that the difference in the two odds ratios (2 vs. 1.2) is not due to chance. These results do not necessarily indicate that 30–49-year-old persons are more susceptible to the harmful influence of *H. pylori* infection on the occurrence of coronary heart disease than are persons beyond this age. Why?

7. The following is an abstract of an article "Occupational exposure and the incidence of non-Hodgkin's lymphoma of the gastrointestinal tract: An ecologic study" (Treggiari and Weiss, 2004):

PURPOSE: A previous case-control study observed a strong association between occupational exposure to asbestos and the incidence of non-Hodgkin lymphoma of the gastrointestinal tract (GINHL). To test this hypothesis we sought to determine whether the geographic pattern of the incidence of GINHL in the US has paralleled that of mesothelioma.

METHODS: Using data obtained from the nine US regions participating in the National Cancer Institute's Surveillance, Epidemiology, and End Results program, we examined the incidence of malignancies among men ages 50 to 84 years between 1973 and 1984.

RESULTS: The rates of mesothelioma but not of GINHL were about two times higher in the areas of Seattle and San Francisco than in the other regions. Overall, there was no correlation between the rates of mesothelioma and of GINHL (Pearson correlation coefficient = 0.12, $p = 0.77$).

CONCLUSIONS: This ecologic study finds no support for the hypothesis that occupational asbestos exposure is related to the subsequent incidence of GINHL.

In their analysis, the authors paid particular attention to rates in men (in whom the likelihood of prior occupational exposure was far greater than in women) and to rates in 50–84-year-olds (to allow for a potentially long incubation period). And, even though the Surveillance, Epidemiology, and End Results (SEER) program had data available through the 1990s, the authors confined their analysis to cancer incidence through just 1984. What do you believe to have been their reason for this latter choice?

ANSWERS

1. (a) Since this is a case-control study in which the absolute risk of retardation among children with various blood levels cannot be determined, it is necessary to estimate the relative risk by means of the odds ratio. The odds of exposure (defined here as a value ≥ 25 mcg/dl) among cases is 15/16, whereas in controls it is 7/23. The ratio of these is 3.1.

(b) The odds of "exposure" among all retarded children in this study is $\frac{15+5}{16+28} = 20/44$. The odds ratio when cases are defined in this way is $20/44 \div 7/23 = 1.5$. This odds ratio is lower than that calculated in part (a) because the case group now includes retarded children in whom the cause is known, and therefore in whom the relative importance of lead exposure probably was minimal.

(c) The referent category used in the calculation of the odds ratio in (a), <25 mcg/dl, was

Coronary heart disease	Cases/ controls	Mean age of cases (years)	Odds ratio (seropositivity in cases:controls) and 99% confidence interval
Early onset			
ISIS: aged 30–49	1122/1122	44	
All ages			
ISIS: sibling pairs aged 30–79	510/510	59	
4 prospective studies	1441/2762	66	
5 retrospective studies	566/977	64	

FIGURE 18.2 Summary of studies of *H. pylori* seropositivity in relation to the occurrence of coronary heart disease. *Source:* Danesh *et al.* (1999)

TABLE 18.9.

Comparison	Odds ratio
15–24 vs. <15 mcg/dl	$14/2 \div 11/12 = 7.6$
25–34 vs. <15 mcg/dl	$10/2 \div 6/12 = 10.0$
≥35 vs. <15 mcg/dl	$5/2 \div 1/12 = 30.0$

heterogeneous with respect to its association with mental retardation. When it was subcategorized, allowing the also-high risk category of 15–24 mcg/dl to be removed, the analysis gained sensitivity in identifying the strong association between mental retardation (of no known cause) and elevated blood lead levels.

Note: Because of the way this study was designed, with measures of blood lead obtained well after the diagnosis of mental retardation, the results do not preclude the possibility that the blood lead levels observed in the participants in this study are considerably lower than those that led to the retardation. Whether "non-encephalopathic" levels of blood lead (e.g., 15–34 mcg/dl) are themselves capable of causing retardation would need to be evaluated in studies that had access to blood samples (preferably at different points in time) drawn prior to the onset of retardation (Pocock *et al.,* 1994).

2. The investigators believed that the relative influence of supplemental calcium on the risk of fracture could differ depending on the level of trauma to which a participant was exposed. If very little trauma were present, the relative benefit might be great; in the presence of substantial trauma, however, the added bone strength that would potentially result from calcium supplements might translate into relatively little benefit. Therefore, to maximize the sensitivity of the

study to observe any relative change in fracture occurrence associated with treatment, the analysis excluded persons with fracture in whom another factor, substantial trauma, was likely to have played a causal role.

3. The association between the presence of the presence of one or more mutant CSTR genes and chronic pancreatitis can be examined in the two subgroups of the disease—alcohol-related and idiopathic.

TABLE 18.10.

Mutant CSTR gene	Alcohol-related disease	Idiopathic disease	Controls
Yes	6	12	5.3%
No	65	51	94.7%
	71	63	100.0%
Odds ratio:	$\dfrac{6/65}{5.3/94.7} = 1.6$	$\dfrac{12/51}{5.3/94.7} = 4.2$	

Because the association between a mutation of the CSTR gene and chronic pancreatitis is so much stronger (as measured by the relative risk—4.2 for idiopathic cases, as compared to 1.6 for alcohol-related cases), it seems unlikely that the abnormal gene and alcohol consumption interact to produce this disease.

Nonetheless, it should be kept in mind that the identical *attributable* risk associated with a mutation in the CSTR gene would be expected to produce a smaller *relative* risk in a high risk subgroup—such as persons with alcohol consumption—than in other persons. Thus, it is conceivable that the impact of the CSTR mutation on the incidence of chronic pancreatitis is similar, in absolute terms, for persons with and without heavy alcohol consumption. So, while there is no support for the hypothesis of synergy, the findings do not necessarily indicate there is antagonism between these two exposures regarding the etiology of chronic pancreatitis.

4. No. The same observation—a relatively lower mean age at diagnosis in women with ≥30 CAG repeats—would occur if having ≥30 CAG repeats were associated with no alteration in risk of breast cancer in young women and a *reduced* risk in older women. Missing from this analysis is the distribution of CAG repeat length in controls,—i.e., women with a germline BRCA1 mutation who did not develop breast cancer as of the age that the cases had done so. Information from controls would allow the following table to be constructed:

TABLE 18.11.

CAG repeat length	Younger women Breast cancer		Older women Breast cancer	
	Yes	No	Yes	No
≥ 30	a_1	b_1	a_2	b_2
< 30	c_1	d_1	c_2	d_2

An association between CAG repeat length and breast cancer that was confined to (or relatively greater in) young women is what must be observed before it could be concluded that the adverse effect of a long CAG repeat sequence in BRCA1 positive women is particularly great at younger ages.

5. Other plausible explanations include:

- The environmental factors responsible for the high rate of cancer in Koreans—e.g., some aspect(s) of diet—differ in prevalence between Korean and other residents of Illinois.
- The risk of stomach cancer is established by certain exposures early in life, i.e., prior to immigration to the United States

- Koreans have a genetic predisposition to stomach cancer that would manifest itself in any environment.

Data that would support a genetic–environmental interaction in the etiology of stomach cancer would be a high rate among Korean residents of Illinois relative to the rates in Illinois residents of other races and to the rates in residents of Korea.

6. If the rate of CHD occurrence associated with *H. pylori* infection simply adds to the rate from other causes, the *relative* contribution of *H. pylori* infection will be greatest in persons in whom the rate is otherwise low. Therefore, even if 30–49-year-old and older persons had identical susceptibility to *H. pylori* infection—as measured by the attributable risk—the odds ratio would be expected to be larger in the 30–49-year-olds because of their otherwise low incidence relative to older individuals.

7. GINHL has a number of causal pathways that may lead to its occurrence. One of these involves HIV infection. Unless occupational asbestos exposure interacts with HIV infection to cause GINHL, the most "sensitive" assessment of the potential role of asbestos is to exclude cases related to HIV. One way of accomplishing this is to restrict the time period being considered to that before HIV infection was widespread—i.e., prior to 1985.

(Because the prevalence of HIV infection varies geographically across the United States, failure to take into account HIV infection in this way also could lead to confounding. For example, GINHL rates in San Francisco during the last decade of the 20th century might have been high relative to other parts of the United States because of the relatively high prevalence of HIV infection there, and not because of a higher degree of occupational asbestos exposure.)

19

Screening

Many chronic diseases evolve in an affected individual through the sequence of steps shown in Fig. 19.1 unless action is taken to interrupt this progression. Cervical cancer, osteoporosis, abdominal aortic aneurysm, depression, glaucoma, and tuberculosis are among many examples, some of which can ultimately be fatal. The amount of time that elapses from one milestone to the next can vary from step to step, among diseases, and among individuals.

Disease control efforts can try to thwart this progression at any of several places, which correspond to different *levels of prevention* (Porta, 2008; Dans *et al.*, 2011), as shown in Figure 19.2.

- *Primary prevention* seeks to avoid the biological onset of disease. Vaccination is an example. Much epidemiologic research is aimed at creating new opportunities for primary prevention by identifying modifiable risk factors for disease.
- *Secondary prevention* seeks to minimize adverse outcomes of disease through early detection, even before symptoms develop that lead to seeking health care. Mammography for early detection of breast cancer in asymptomatic women is an example. (The term *secondary prevention* is also sometimes used to refer to reducing the risk of recurrence in someone who has already had an initial episode of disease.)
- *Tertiary prevention* seeks to reduce disability and the risk of death by treating known disease cases. Surgery to remove an inflamed appendix is an example. Tertiary prevention is the main focus of traditional medical care.

Screening is a form of secondary prevention. It has been defined as "examination of asymptomatic people in order to classify them as likely, or unlikely, to have the disease that is the object of screening" (Morrison, 1992). Screening can also be used to detect modifiable risk factors for disease, such as high blood pressure or high serum cholesterol levels, that may be asymptomatic.

WHEN CAN SCREENING BE JUSTIFIED?

For a disease whose natural history follows the general pattern depicted in Fig. 19.1, it is tempting to assume that the sooner a case of such a disease is recognized, the better off the affected individual will be. Unfortunately, however, early detection does not automatically translate into better outcomes. In addition, even when early detection *is* of demonstrable benefit, screening carries costs and risks of its own—some of them rather hidden—which must be balanced against its benefits.

The decision to screen for a disease is favored to the extent that the following conditions are met (Wilson and Jungner, 1968; Morrison, 1992; Grimes and Schulz, 2002; Dans *et al.*, 2011):

1. *The disease is an important public health problem, in terms of its frequency and/or severity.* Resources for disease control are limited. Screening also burdens the many to benefit the few. A disease that is extremely rare, or whose effects on overall health are mild, may not warrant the burden on society of mass screening.

2. *The natural history of the disease presents a suitable "window of opportunity" for screening.* Screening focuses on the time interval between when the disease becomes detectable by a screening test and when it would be recognized anyway upon appearance of symptoms. The duration of this interval depends in part on how rapidly the disease progresses biologically, and in part on how sensitive the screening test is for early disease. If the disease progresses very rapidly through this stage, then early detection of many cases before they

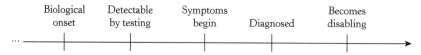

FIGURE 19.1 Model of natural history for many chronic diseases.

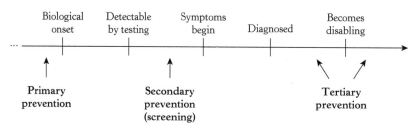

FIGURE 19.2 Levels of prevention.

become symptomatic could require that the screening test be reapplied very frequently, which may be too costly or impractical.

3. *Effective treatment is available and capable of favorably altering the disease's natural history. Alternatively, an effective way to prevent spread to other people is available.* If there is no good treatment for a condition, then diagnosing it early will not improve the outcome for an affected individual. However, if the disease is contagious, early diagnosis may benefit others by preventing further transmission. In either case, effective measures must not only exist, they must actually be available for use with screenees who are found to have the disease.

4. *Treatment, or interventions to prevent spread to others, are more effective if initiated in the pre-symptomatic stage than when initiated in symptomatic patients.* To elaborate on requirements 2 and 3, mere availability of effective measures for treatment or prevention of further transmission is not sufficient to justify screening. If these measures are just as effective once the disease has revealed itself through symptoms, then the added expense of mass screening for early detection is unnecessary and wasteful.

5. *A suitable screening test is available: reasonably inexpensive and safe, acceptable to the population screened, and able to discriminate between diseased and non-diseased persons.* The last of these factors is discussed below.

ASSESSING SCREENING TEST PERFORMANCE

Sensitivity and Specificity (Revisited)

Sensitivity and *specificity*, defined in Chapter 10, can be used to evaluate the performance of a screening test. To estimate them, the test is applied to a sample of individuals whose true disease status is determined by a suitable gold standard, assumed to be error-free.

Example 19-1. Colorectal cancer is regarded by the U.S. Preventive Services Task Force (U.S. Preventive Services Task Force, 2012) as a suitable condition for screening in adults aged 50–75 years. Several screening tests are available (Whitlock *et al.*, 2008). Allison *et al.* (1996) studied four of these, each designed to detect hidden traces of blood in stool by a different biochemical method. Specimen cards were mailed to several thousand enrollees aged 50 years or older in a large prepaid health plan who were scheduled for a personal health checkup. The four tests were applied to the specimens mailed back. True colorectal cancer was defined as any new pathological diagnosis of the disease within two years after screening, regardless of the mode of detection.

Results for one of the screening tests, Hemoccult II Sensa, are shown in Table 19.1. Of the 34 colorectal cancer cases, 27 tested positive on Hemoccult II Sensa, for a sensitivity of $27/34 = 0.794$. Of the 7,870 persons who had no diagnosis of colorectal cancer, 6,824 tested negative, for a specificity of $6,824/7,870 = 0.867$.

Predictive Value

Sensitivity and specificity convey how likely it is that the test will yield a correct result, given the presence or absence of disease. But when a test is actually used for screening, the screenee's true disease status is unknown. Instead, the task is to estimate the probability that the disease is truly present, given a certain test result. If the result is positive, how likely is it that the person tested actually has the disease?

TABLE 19.1. PERFORMANCE OF A SCREENING TEST FOR COLORECTAL CANCER

| Hemoccult II SENSA result | Colorectal cancer diagnosed within 2 years? | | |
	Yes	No	Total
+	27	1,046	1,073
–	7	6,824	6,831
Total	34	7,870	7,904

(Based on data from Allison *et al.* [1996])

Or if the result is negative, how likely is it that he or she actually does *not* have the disease?

Answers to these questions are provided by the *predictive value* of the test. It has two forms, positive (PV_+) or negative (PV_-), depending on the test result. Both can be estimated directly from a 2 × 2 table that summarizes the results of applying both the screening test and a gold standard for true disease status to a sample of screenees, as shown in Table 19.2.

In the results shown in Table 19.1, the PV_+ for the Hemoccult II Sensa test was $27/1,073 = 0.025$. In other words, only 2.5% of screenees who had a positive Hemoccult II Sensa test actually had colorectal cancer. This may at first seem surprising, in view of the fact that the test was already found in the same data to have sensitivity $= 0.794$ and specificity $= 0.867$. The relatively low PV_+ can be explained by noting that PV_+ depends, not only on sensitivity and specificity, but also on the prevalence of the disease in the population screened. In this instance, a large majority of persons in whom the test was used did not have colorectal cancer. Even though the test was

86.7% specific, the 13.3% of persons without colorectal cancer who had a false positive result constituted a large number of people, and 97.5% of the positive results proved to be false positives.

In mathematical terms, sensitivity, specificity, positive predictive value, and negative predictive value are interpretable as conditional probabilities. Let C_+ denote presence of the disease condition, C_- absence of the condition, T_+ a positive test result, and T_- a negative test result. Then

$$\text{Sensitivity} = \Pr(T_+|C_+)$$
$$\text{Specificity} = \Pr(T_-|C_-)$$
$$PV_+ = \Pr(C_+|T_+)$$
$$PV_- = \Pr(C_-|T_-)$$
$$\text{Prevalence} = \Pr(C_+)$$

According to Bayes's theorem (Rosner, 2006):

$$\Pr(C_+|T_+)$$
$$= \frac{\Pr(C_+) \cdot \Pr(T_+|C_+)}{\left[\begin{array}{c} \Pr(C_+) \cdot \Pr(T_+|C_+) \\ +(1 - \Pr(C_+)) \cdot (1 - \Pr(T_-|C_-)) \end{array}\right]}$$

$$PV_+ = \frac{\text{Prevalence} \cdot \text{Sensitivity}}{\left[\begin{array}{c} \text{Prevalence} \cdot \text{Sensitivity} \\ +(1 - \text{Prevalence}) \cdot (1 - \text{Specificity}) \end{array}\right]}$$

$$(19.1)$$

A similar expression can be developed for PV_- as a function of sensitivity, specificity, and prevalence, but it is usually of less direct interest than for PV_+.

Predictive value can also be calculated from the *likelihood ratio* of a screening test, as defined in Chapter 10, rather than from sensitivity and specificity (Deeks and Altman, 2004). An estimate of prevalence is required either way. The steps are:

1. Pre-test odds = $\frac{\text{Prevalence}}{1 - \text{Prevalence}}$
2. Post-test odds = Pre-test odds $\times LR_+$
3. PV_+ = Post-test probability = $\frac{\text{Post-test odds}}{1 + \text{Post-test odds}}$

The arithmetic is easy at each step, and step 2 is easy to remember. Steps 1 and 3 are needed only to convert from probability to odds and back again. The sensitivity-specificity and likelihood-ratio methods are algebraically equivalent, so choice between them can be based on convenience.

TABLE 19.2. MEASURES OF SCREENING TEST PERFORMANCE

| Screening test result | Condition truly present? | |
	Yes	No
+	a	b
–	c	d

Sensitivity $= a/(a+c)$
Specificity $= d/(b+d)$
Positive predictive value $= PV_+ = a/(a+b)$
Negative predictive value $= PV_- = d/(c+d)$

Example 19-2. Screening for post-combat post-traumatic stress disorder (PTSD) has been mandated since 2005 by the U.S. Department of Defense for soldiers returning from deployment in combat areas. Skopp *et al.* (2012) studied the performance of the PC-PTSD screening instrument for PTSD in a sample of 148 returning soldiers, all of whom also underwent a structured clinical interview by mental health professionals to determine true PTSD status. The PC-PTSD asks four questions about characteristic features of PTSD: avoidance, re-experiencing, hyperarousal, and numbing. When affirmative answers to two or more questions was scored as a positive PC-PTSD test, it had sensitivity = 0.69, specificity = 0.85, $LR_+ = 4.60$ and $LR_- = 0.36$.

Suppose that the true prevalence of PTSD among soldiers returning from combat deployment is 10%—the approximate prevalence observed in the sample of Skopp *et al.* If such a soldier has a positive result on the PC-PTSD screen, what is the probability that he/she will prove on further evaluation truly to have PTSD?

One solution is to apply Bayes's theorem, using the sensitivity, specificity, and prevalence values given:

$$PV_+ = \frac{\text{Prev} \cdot \text{Sens}}{\text{Prev} \cdot \text{Sens} + (1 - \text{Prev}) \cdot (1 - \text{Spec})}$$

$$= \frac{(0.1)(0.69)}{(0.1)(0.69) + (1 - 0.1)(1 - 0.85)}$$

$$= 0.34$$

Alternatively, the likelihood-ratio method can be used:

$$\text{Pre-test odds} = 0.10/(1 - 0.10) = 0.11$$

$$\text{Post-test odds} = 0.11 \times 4.60 = 0.506$$

$$PV_+ = \text{Post-test probability}$$

$$= 0.506/(1 + 0.506)$$

$$= 0.34$$

Either way, in this scenario about 2/3 of screenees with a positive PC-PTSD test would prove to have had a false positive test and would not actually have PTSD.

The strong dependence of PV_+ on prevalence can be seen in Table 19.3, which revisits Example 19-1 on colorectal cancer screening. It shows the

TABLE 19.3. INFLUENCE OF PREVALENCE ON THE EXPECTED PREDICTIVE VALUES OF THE HEMOCCULT II SENSA TEST, ASSUMING SENSITIVITY = 0.794 AND SPECIFICITY = 0.867

Prevalence of colorectal cancer[a]	PV_+	PV_-
1	0.0006	0.99998
5	0.0030	0.99988
10	0.0059	0.99976
50	0.0291	0.99881
100	0.0569	0.99761
500	0.2391	0.98765

[a] Cases per 10,000

expected PV_+ and PV_- of the Hemoccult II Sensa test for colorectal cancer when applied as a screening test in several populations with prevalence varying from 1/10,000 to 500/10,000, assuming that sensitivity and specificity remain fixed at the values calculated earlier. Even in a population with 1% prevalence of colorectal cancer, only about 5.7% of screenees with a positive Hemoccult II Sensa test would turn out to have colorectal cancer; the rest would be false positives. At lower prevalences of colorectal cancer, PV_+ is still lower. In contrast, PV_- varies relatively little and usually remains quite high: with low prevalence, the probability of *not* having the disease was high to begin with, and it becomes even higher if the screening test result is negative.

The fact that the positive predictive value of a screening test can be quite low in screened populations with low disease prevalence has several implications:

- It can affect how a positive screening test result should be interpreted and communicated to a screenee. In many situations, a positive result does *not* imply that the screenee probably has the disease.
- Persons with a positive screening test result must usually be evaluated further with confirmatory tests to determine whether the result was a true positive or a false positive. Even if it is expected in advance that a large majority will be false positives, all positive test

results must nonetheless be evaluated further in order to separate the true positives from the false positives. Any costs, discomfort, and risks involved in these follow-up evaluations must be considered a potentially important part of the overall burden of a screening program. In many instances, the aggregate cost of follow-up evaluations can exceed the cost of the initial screening tests themselves.

- It affects choice of a target population for screening. For many diseases, the prevalence of undiagnosed disease varies markedly among population subgroups. Descriptive epidemiology thus has an important role to play in guiding screening strategy. Subgroups in which prevalence is highest can yield both more cases per screening test administered and more true positives per positive screening test.

As noted earlier, positive predictive value can be interpreted as the *post-test* probability that the disease of interest is present, given a positive test result. Overall disease prevalence in the population to which the test is applied can be interpreted as the *pre-test* probability of disease. This view broadens the usefulness of predictive value beyond the context of screening. For example, in medical diagnosis, a clinician is concerned with the probability that a patient has a certain disease. Before a diagnostic test is done, the clinician has a *pre-test* probability estimate in mind. That prior probability may simply be the prevalence of the disease, or it may be a subjective probability based on other information already known about the patient. After a test result becomes available, the estimated probability may be revised based on this new knowledge, and it becomes a *post-test* probability. Bayes's theorem or the likelihood-ratio method can thus be used to update the estimated probability of a certain diagnosis in light of new information.

CHOOSING AMONG ALTERNATIVE SCREENING STRATEGIES

Decisions about screening involve weighing possible outcomes not only according to their probability of occurrence but also according to the magnitude of costs and benefits associated with each outcome. Although not all of the costs and benefits are monetary, a basic economic framework can provide a useful way to organize information and to make tradeoffs more explicit. A model that combines epidemiologic and economic data is described below. This model is then applied to two kinds of decisions: (1) choosing an optimal cutoff value on a screening test that yields a numerical result, and (2) choosing between two competing screening tests for the same condition. Although it may be easiest to think of the costs described below in monetary terms, they could also be viewed more broadly as combining both monetary and intangible costs, such as diminished quality of life or life expectancy—a composite sometimes termed "disutilities" (Schousboe et al., 2011).

Epidemiologic-Economic Model of Screening

The overall cost of a screening program depends on: (1) the cost of applying the screening test itself, and (2) the expected cost of each possible outcome after the test is applied. The set of possible outcomes is obtained by cross-classifying possible test results with true disease status. For a test that yields a binary result, the four possible outcomes are those shown in Table 19.2: true positive (TP), false positive (FP), false negative (FN), or true negative (TN). Associated with each outcome is a certain average (or expected) cost, denoted as C_{TP}, C_{FP}, C_{FN}, and C_{TN}:

- C_{TP} is the average cost of confirming and treating a screen-detected case.
- C_{FP} is the average cost of the confirmatory tests needed to separate true positives from false positives. Once a screenee is found to have had a false positive test result, no further screening-related costs are incurred.
- C_{FN} is the average cost of treating a case that the screening test failed to detect. If the underlying condition is progressive (per the generic natural-history model in Fig. 19.1), and if treatment is more effective when applied early in the disease course (which is one of the requirements listed earlier for a condition to be suitable for screening), then $C_{FN} > C_{TP}$.
- C_{TN} is the average cost incurred after having been correctly classified as a non-case, usually zero.

While it is possible to model overall screening-program costs for a population of, say, N screenees, it will be more convenient to work with per-capita costs, designating as C_{total} the expected total cost for an individual screenee. All screenees incur the cost of applying the screening test itself, C_{test}. Four additional components of C_{total} are the expected costs associated with each outcome. Each outcome-specific average cost is multiplied by its probability of occurrence. Let $prev$ = prevalence, $sens$ = test sensitivity, and $spec$ = test specificity. The resulting sum of the five cost components is:

$$C_{total} = C_{test} \qquad (19.2)$$
$$+ C_{TP} \cdot prev \cdot sens$$
$$+ C_{FP} \cdot (1 - prev) \cdot (1 - spec)$$
$$+ C_{FN} \cdot prev \cdot (1 - sens)$$
$$+ C_{TN} \cdot (1 - prev) \cdot spec$$

To the extent that the inputs to this equation can be estimated, values of C_{total} can be compared across alternative screening scenarios to guide choices among them. Two specific applications of the model with more modest data requirements are described below.

Selecting the Optimal Cutoff Value for Screening on an ROC Curve

Some screening tests yield a numerical result rather than a binary one—e.g., systolic blood pressure, PC-PTSD score, or PSA blood level. Nonetheless, a binary decision must eventually be made as to whether a result is suspicious enough to trigger further confirmatory tests, or to take no action. That decision typically depends on whether the result is above or below a certain cutoff value. As discussed in Chapter 10, sensitivity and specificity depend on the cutoff value chosen.

Also as shown in Chapter 10, if the ROC curve for Test B falls above and to the left of the ROC curve for Test A, then Test B has superior operating characteristics. Based on this property of ROC curves, one might naïvely suppose that the point on any ROC curve that is closest to the upper left corner would correspond to the optimal cutoff value. For a hypothetical perfect test (see Fig. 10.2), whatever cutoff value corresponds to sensitivity = specificity = 1.0 at the upper left corner would indeed be the optimal cutoff, as it distinguishes cases from non-cases without error. Very few perfect tests exist, however. An imperfect test inevitably produces classification errors. Although there is no cutoff value on an imperfect test that avoids all classification errors, the frequency and mixture of false negatives and false

positives can be altered through choice of the cutoff. The overall cost of misclassification at any particular cutoff value depends both on the frequency of the two types of errors and on their costs.

In screening situations, the adverse consequences of a false negative result are almost always much greater than those of a false positive result. A false positive result leads to additional expense, time, and possibly risks involved with confirmatory testing. But those costs are usually modest and short-lived; once the screening-test error is corrected, the screenee may feel reassured and usually incurs no further costs related to the condition. In contrast, a false negative result leads to a missed opportunity for earlier and more effective treatment, which can mean shortened survival, impaired quality of life, and/or higher health care costs.

It can be shown with calculus (Appendix 19A; Metz, 1978; Cantor et al., 1999; Pepe, 2003) that the point on a screening test's ROC curve at which C_{total} is minimized is the point where the tangent line to the ROC curve has

$$\text{Slope} = \left[\frac{1 - prev}{prev} \right] \cdot \left[\frac{C_{FP} - C_{TN}}{C_{FN} - C_{TP}} \right] \qquad (19.3)$$

Equation (19.3) seeks out the point at which the aggregate costs of false positives are balanced against the aggregate costs of false negatives. That balance depends on:

- *Prevalence*, which affects the relative frequency of false positives and false negatives. Higher prevalence shifts the mix toward more false negatives; low prevalence shifts it toward more false positives. In terms of equation (19.3), high prevalence leads to a lower value of $(1 - prev)/prev$, implying a shallower tangent line, implying an optimal cutoff toward the upper right of a typical ROC curve where sensitivity is prioritized over specificity. High sensitivity tends to offset the relatively large number of false negatives produced by high prevalence.

- *Relative net costs of false positives and false negatives.* The quantity $C_{FP} - C_{TN}$ can be viewed as the *net cost* of a false positive—i.e., the excess cost for a non-case of having a positive test, compared to having a negative test. Usually $C_{TN} = 0$, in which case the numerator of the second factor reduces to C_{FP}. The quantity $C_{FN} - C_{TP}$ can be viewed, in turn, as the net cost of a false negative—i.e., the excess cost that results from failing to detect disease early. If the net cost of a false positive is very small compared to the net cost of a false negative, then the second factor in equation (19.3) is small, implying a shallower tangent line, implying an optimal cutoff toward the upper right of the ROC curve where sensitivity is prioritized over specificity. Under those conditions, it is very important not to miss cases and more tolerable that false positives arise as a byproduct of more-aggressive case detection.

The point on an ROC curve that lies farthest toward the upper left is where the tangent line has slope = 1. It would correspond to the optimal cutoff value only if the prevalence odds of the condition happened to be exactly equal to the ratio of the net cost of a false positive to the net cost of a false negative. Such a coincidence is likely to be unusual.

Cantor *et al.* (1999) reviewed several studies in which optimal cutoffs on ROC curves had been selected based on assumptions about the ratio of the net cost of a false positive to the net cost of a false negative. When quantitative data have been hard to come by, judgments of clinical subject-matter experts have often been used, which at least makes assumptions explicit and avoids the unrealistic assumption that the net costs of false positives and false negatives are equal.

Choosing Between Competing Screening Tests or Strategies

The epidemiologic-economic model in Eq. (19.2) can also be used to guide a choice between two competing screening tests for the same condition. Sometimes the choice is easy. If Test A is more sensitive, more specific, and cheaper to apply than Test B, then Test A would be the obvious winner. However, if Test A is more sensitive but less specific than Test B, and/or if their costs of application also differ, the choice may not be so obvious.

In principle, estimates of the inputs needed for equation (19.2) could simply be plugged in for each test and the resulting C_{total} values compared. In practice, some of those inputs are harder to estimate than others. As noted earlier, C_{TN} can usually be assumed to be zero. C_{FP} represents the cost of confirmatory tests needed to follow up on a positive screening test result, which may be fairly easy to determine. But quantifying the benefit of early detection, which

drives the quantity $(C_{FN} - C_{TP})$, is considerably more difficult. Research designs that can be used to evaluate the effectiveness of screening are discussed later in this chapter and include both randomized and non-randomized study designs.

One approach in the face of uncertainty is to solve for the most elusive quantity: in this context, how large would the benefit of early detection have to be in order to sway the choice between tests? It may be easier for experts or stakeholders to make a binary decision on whether the true unknown value is likely to be above or below that threshold than to estimate the true value itself.

Say that for two tests, estimates of their respective sensitivities ($sens_1$ and $sens_2$), specificities ($spec_1$ and $spec_2$), and costs of application ($C_{test\,1}$ and $C_{test\,2}$) are available. Label the less-sensitive test as Test 1 and the more-sensitive one as Test 2. Also say that the cost of confirmatory tests is known, providing an estimate of C_{FP}, which is the same for both tests, and that $C_{TN} = 0$. A rule derived in Appendix 19B states that Test 2 will yield lower expected per-capita total cost of screening than Test 1 if the average cost of treating a case detected by screening is at least

$$\frac{(C_{test\,2} - C_{test\,1}) - (spec_2 - spec_1) \cdot (1 - prev) \cdot C_{FP}}{prev \cdot (sens_2 - sens_1)}$$

$$+ C_{FP} \tag{19.4}$$

less than the average cost of treating a case that is missed by screening.

Example 19-3.   In the Canadian Cervical Cancer Screening Trial (Mayrand *et al.*, 2007), women aged 30–69 years were screened for high-grade cervical intraepithelial neoplasia, an early stage of cervical cancer. Two screening tests were applied for each woman: a standard Pap smear, and a commercially available HPV-DNA test designed to detect DNA from oncogenic strains of human papilloma virus (HPV) in cervical smear samples. Women who tested positive on either screening test were referred for colposcopy and biopsy, a more costly and invasive procedure that is widely accepted as a gold standard for detection of cervical neoplasia. In order to estimate the frequency of false negative screening tests, a sample of women who tested negative on both screening tests also underwent colposcopy/biopsy.

The results allowed the investigators to compare several potential screening strategies, of which three are considered here: to screen with Pap smear only; to screen with HPV-DNA test only; or to screen with both tests and score the combined result as positive if *either* the Pap smear or the HPV-DNA result is positive. The operating characteristics of these three strategies were found to be:

TABLE 19.4.

Strategy	Sensitivity	Specificity
Pap smear only	0.564	0.973
HPV-DNA test only	0.974	0.943
Both tests	1.000	0.925

Note that the ordering of strategies by sensitivity is (both tests) > (HPV-DNA test only) > (Pap smear only), while their ordering by specificity is the reverse. Hence every choice between two strategies involves a tradeoff between false negatives and false positives.

In the United States, the estimated prevalence of early cervical neoplasia among women who undergo routine screening and who have had at least one Pap test at an earlier age is about 1/1,000. Although Mayrand *et al.* did not report the costs of screening or confirmatory tests, assume for present purposes that a Pap smear costs $30, a HPV-DNA test costs $26, and colposcopy/biopsy costs $400. Calculating expression (19.4) for each pair of strategies yields the following threshold values for the required cost savings per case due to early detection:

TABLE 19.5.

Pair of strategies compared:		Strategy #2 preferred if early detection yields savings per case
#1	#2	of at least:
Pap smear only	HPV-DNA test only	$19,883
Pap smear only	Both tests	$104,026
HPV-DNA test only	Both tests	$1,430,892

The last figure is especially striking. The HPV-DNA test by itself is 97.4% sensitive. Detecting the 2.6% of cases that it misses by adding co-testing with the Pap test requires clearing a high bar: early detection would have to save more than $1.4 million per case in order to offset the added cost of doing two tests

on every woman and of doing colposcopy/biopsy on the larger number of false positives generated.

More elaborate and comprehensive economic analyses of screening must consider several other complexities, including costs and benefits that accrue at different times over the years following screening; other possible strategies in which two or more screening tests can be used simultaneously or in sequence; and reconciling direct costs of tests and treatment care, indirect costs of lost economic productivity, and intangible costs in terms of quality and quantity of life lost. Decision analysis provides a theoretical framework for combining such information (Weiss, 2006; Drummond *et al.*, 2005; Carroll and Downs, 2006).

EVALUATING THE EFFECTIVENESS OF SCREENING

Screening for high blood pressure is commonly performed by providers of health care when they practice preventive medicine. Their basis for judging the likely benefit patients will derive, collectively, from this maneuver comes from several different sorts of research. The first documents the proportion of persons who test "positive," i.e., what fraction of them will have high blood pressure as determined by sphygmomanometer readings. The second estimates the excess risk of the conditions such as myocardial infarction and stroke to which hypertension (as measured by the sphygmomanometer) predisposes. The last type of study investigates the degree to which treatment of screen-detected high blood pressure can reduce the excess risks.

As a means of illustrating how data obtained in these studies can be put to use, let us assume that we are trying to estimate the benefit to be achieved by obtaining a blood pressure reading on an asymptomatic male patient for whom there has been no recent screening. Based on his demographic characteristics, the medical literature suggests there is a 10% likelihood that he has high blood pressure. It also suggests that, although the five-year cumulative combined incidence of myocardial infarction and stroke in normotensive men would be 30 per 1000, among those with hypertension, the corresponding incidence in the absence of treatment would be 60 per 1000. In a hypothetical group of 10,000 men just like this patient, the above assumptions would generate the observations shown in Table 19.6.

TABLE 19.6. FIVE-YEAR CUMULATIVE INCIDENCE OF MYOCARDIAL INFARCTION AND STROKE IN 10,000 MEN IN WHOM THERE IS NO SCREENING FOR, OR TREATMENT OF, HIGH BLOOD PRESSURE

Blood pressure	Myocardial infarction or stroke	No. of men
Elevated	60	1,000
Normal	270	9,000
Total		10,000

Now, assume that the results of prior research suggest that the prescription of antihypertensive therapy is associated with a 30% reduction in risk of myocardial infarction and stroke. If this were true for men such as our patient, the five-year cumulative incidence once treatment had been instituted would be 60 per 1000 × 0.7 = 42 per 1000. In the group of 10,000 men, the experience would be as shown in Table 19.7.

TABLE 19.7. FIVE-YEAR CUMULATIVE INCIDENCE OF MYOCARDIAL INFARCTION AND STROKE IN THE PRESENCE OF SCREENING FOR, AND TREATMENT OF, HIGH BLOOD PRESSURE

Blood pressure	Myocardial infarction or stroke	No. of men
Elevated	60 × 0.7 = 42	1,000
Normal	270	9,000
Total		10,000

From a comparison of Tables 19.6 and 19.7, we can see that screening for high blood pressure in 10,000 men demographically similar to our patient can be expected to lead to 60 − 42 = 18 fewer cases of myocardial infarction over the next five years.

The positive impact of many screening tests can be gauged through a process such as the foregoing; that is, by compiling the results of studies evaluating the separate components necessary for effectiveness. The magnitude of the benefit obtained from screening people with diabetes for retinopathy (a form of ocular pathology detectable by means of retinal photography or ophthalmoscopy) has been estimated in this way, by taking results from separate studies that have documented:

1. The prevalence of retinopathy in people with diabetes
2. That retinal screening can identify abnormalities that are strong predictors of the development of blindness; and
3. That laser photocoagulation therapy for the changes found on screening can reduce the incidence of severe visual impairment (Early Treatment Diabetic Retinopathy Study Group, 1987).

But what is to be done if all patients who are screened as "positive" on a particular test (and, after confirmatory tests, are deemed to truly have the condition in question) happen to receive treatment? For example, persons who are screened for the presence of cancer and found to have it are almost never left untreated. Thus, while it is not difficult to determine: (1) the prevalence of malignancy at the time of screening, or (2) that a positive screening test result can predict an adverse outcome from a particular cancer, and can do so earlier than otherwise would be possible—perhaps by comparing the distribution of tumor size or stage in screened and unscreened persons diagnosed with that cancer—it is usually not possible to clearly answer the third necessary question: Does treatment given at the time of early detection lead to a more favorable outcome than treatment given when the cancer is clinically manifest? In situations such as this, it is necessary to resort to a generally more cumbersome approach: a comparison of the subsequent occurrence of untoward outcomes in screened and unscreened persons. That approach assesses the aggregate impact of the frequency of test positivity, the ability of the test result to predict an adverse outcome, and the efficacy of treatment for test-positive individuals. It will hereafter be referred to as a "one-step" design (Weiss, 2006).

The remainder of this chapter outlines the types of one-step designs available to evaluate a screening test's ability to lead to improved outcomes.

Randomized Trials and Cohort (Follow-up) Studies

It may be possible to assign study participants at random to be offered or not to be offered the test (or a program of testing). Alternatively, one can exploit (with appropriate caution when interpreting the results) the fact that in the normal course of medical or public health practice, some persons are tested while others are not, and these two groups can be monitored for the outcome(s) of interest.

Example 19-4.   The first type of one-step design is illustrated by a randomized trial conducted in the state of Minnesota on the effectiveness of screening for fecal occult blood in leading to a reduction in mortality from cancer of the colon and rectum (Mandel et al., 1999). During 1976–1977, 46,551 residents of the state agreed to be assigned at random to one of three study arms: (1) annual screening; (2) biennial screening; and (3) usual care. The program of screening was conducted through 1982, and then again during 1986–1992. Persons who tested positive (during the course of the study they were approximately 20% of those assigned to be screened) received a full evaluation for colorectal cancer, including a colonoscopy. Follow-up for mortality extended for up to 18 years. For study participants who died, medical records were obtained. If the decedent had known or suspected gastrointestinal disease at the time of death, cause of death was judged by an expert panel, the members of which were blinded as to the decedent's screening assignment. The cumulative mortality from colorectal cancer per 1000 in the three groups was 9.46, 11.19, and 14.09, respectively, suggesting that a program of annual or biennial screening of this type could indeed lead to a reduction in the death rate from colon and rectal cancer.

Randomized trials have now been conducted to evaluate the efficacy of a variety of screening tests, including, as examples, prenatal ultrasound exams (Ewigman et al., 1993; Bucher and Schmidt, 1993), intrapartum fetal heart rate monitoring (Mahomed et al., 1994), routine cervical evaluation during pregnancy (Buekens et al., 1994), electronic home uterine monitoring in women at high risk of premature delivery (U.S. Preventive Services Task Force, 1993), mammography and breast self-exam (Shapiro et al., 1982; Miller et al., 2000; Thomas et al., 2002), helical CT screening for lung cancer (National Lung Screening Trial Research Team et al., 2011), and PSA screening for prostate cancer (Schröder et al., 2012).

In a cohort study of a test's ability to influence the outcome of illness, Neutra et al. (1978) compared neonatal mortality among children delivered by mothers who received fetal monitoring during labor with that among children whose mothers had not been monitored. This study took place in a hospital during a period of time in which fetal monitoring was being introduced. The choice of patients to undergo monitoring was made by each woman's physician, not by the investigators (who conducted the study in retrospect through the use of the hospital's records).

Ideally, all evaluations of screening test effectiveness would be randomized: assignment of patients to screen or no-screen groups in a random way assures that the only differences between the two groups that might be relevant to the outcome in question are those that occur by chance. This is decidedly not the case in non-randomized studies, as there may be important differences that have the potential to distort (i.e., confound) the true benefit, or lack thereof, associated with use of the test. In the fetal monitoring study, for example, the investigators discovered in their review of records that a relatively higher proportion of mothers who did not receive monitoring had characteristics that predict an increased risk of mortality in the child: short gestation, breech presentation, placenta previa, and so on. Failure to have measured these characteristics, or failure to have taken them into account in the analysis, would have resulted in a comparison erroneously favorable to the monitored group and would have led to an overestimation of the benefit associated with monitoring.

Which Subjects Are to Be Compared?

In most randomized trials and cohort studies evaluating the effectiveness of screening tests, the only comparison that can be made is of the overall occurrence of the outcome in the screened versus unscreened groups. In a childhood blood lead screening evaluation, for instance, one would compare the prevalence of retardation in children who did and did not receive screening. The lead levels in the unscreened group would never be known, so even if the investigators wished to compare outcomes in only those persons with elevated levels in each group, it would be impossible to do so.

Some conditions for which screening is done will, after a period of time, be evident even without the benefit of the test. Most cancers fall into this category, and there has been a temptation to evaluate the effectiveness of cancer screening tests by comparing mortality from the particular cancer in cases found through screening with that in other cases. Giving in to this temptation could lead to an erroneous estimate of the effectiveness of screening, primarily due to the influence of what is known as "lead-time" bias.

The reason for this bias is illustrated in the following example. Suppose 100 individuals are screened for cancer X, a cancer for which treatment is, in fact, ineffective. On the average, the test succeeds in identifying the cancer one year before it is clinically evident. Four persons in the group are detected as having cancer X, and the course of their illness is shown in Fig. 19.3.

Two deaths occur among the four persons with cancer X in the 13 person-years that occur following screening (3 + 4 + 2 + 4; see Figure 19.3), and their mortality rate is 2 per 13 person-years. Had the screening not been performed, however, the same two deaths among four cases in 100 persons would occur (since no effective treatment follows early detection). But the number of person-years accruing in these cases from the time of their diagnosis (1 year later than that for the screened cases) would be only 9 (2 + 3 + 1 + 3) and the resulting mortality rate would be higher, 2 per 9 person-years. Since screening could not lead to improved mortality, one must conclude that there is something faulty in this method of comparison. (If, instead of using mortality rates, the measure of outcome were *n*-year survival, the bias would still be present. Thus the 1.5-year survival in the cases found through screening is 100%, whereas the 1.5-year survival in the other cases is 75%, even though the two groups had, in truth, an identical survival experience.)

What is faulty, of course, is that the starting point for monitoring mortality rates is different between the screened and unscreened cases, always to the apparent detriment of the cases detected without

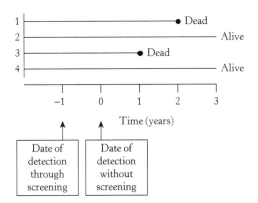

FIGURE 19.3 Lead time in studies of the efficacy of screening.

screening. The appropriate comparison to make is the mortality experience (with respect to that cancer), not of the cases alone, but of the screened group with that of an unscreened group, *with both groups monitored from the time of screening*. In the above example, the mortality rate in the screened group is 2 deaths in 397 person-years (98 persons × 4 years, plus 1 person × 2 years, plus 1 person × 3 years). In a comparable unscreened group, the rate would be the same, since the number of person-years, counted from the time the screening would have taken place had it been done, is identical to that for the screened group. Given that the natural history of this cancer is not altered by screening, this comparison of screened and unscreened groups which indicates no benefit associated with screening is clearly the preferred one.

Patients who have a long preclinical-but-detectable phase of disease are more readily found via screening than are patients with that disease whose preclinical phase is short. To the extent that the length of the preclinical phase correlates with the length of the illness once it has been detected, those persons whose disease was found via screening will appear to have better survival, even in the absence of treatment that influences the disease's natural history. This possible artifact, due to what has been termed "length-biased sampling" (Zelen, 1976), was noted in Chapter 4 and is another reason that a comparison of survival in persons whose disease was detected by screening with that of other diseased persons will be misleading.

Example 19-5. The Mayo Lung Project was a randomized trial of early lung cancer detection among men who were cigarette smokers. For a six-year period, chest X-ray and sputum cytology were offered every four months to 4,618 men. Compliance with the intervention was about 75%. Men in the control arm of the trial ($n = 4,593$) received a recommendation to receive these same screening measures, but only on an annual basis. During a median follow-up of some 20 years, mortality from lung cancer was not lower in men assigned to receive intensive screening (4.4 per 1,000 man-years, versus 3.9 per 1,000 man-years among men in the control arm) (Marcus *et al.*, 2000). However, of the men who were diagnosed with lung cancer, the survival from this disease consistently was higher in the former group, even after a number of years had passed and no additional deaths from lung cancer were occurring. For example, as of 15 years after diagnosis, 26.2% of men in the intervention arm had survived their disease, as opposed to only 10.6% of men in the control arm.

The very long follow-up interval following the end of the screening program makes it unlikely that lead-time bias is the sole explanation for the disparity between the negative results of the analysis based on the randomized groups and the positive results based on the analysis of the survival of the lung cancer cases. The large sample size largely excludes chance as an explanation as well. The reason for the relatively favorable survival experience of lung cancer cases in the intervention group must be due to the presence of lung "cancers" that were diagnosed in men assigned to be intensively screened that had little or no ability to progress—i.e., in the absence of screening they would not have been diagnosed. This possibility of "pseudo-disease" (Morrison, 1992) suggests that comparisons of survival between cancer cases that are detected by screening and those that are detected by other means are not to be trusted, no matter how long the follow-up period extends beyond the end of the screening program.

Other One-Step Studies of Screening Effectiveness

Ecologic Studies

The use of a screening test often varies widely from place to place around the world, and within one place often varies widely across periods of time. However, because of the problems surrounding the interpretation of many ecologic studies, referred to in Chapter 16, we are often unable to infer very much from correlations between population-wide screening levels and those populations' occurrence of the outcome that the screening test sought to prevent. Nonetheless, there are occasional exceptions, and it is instructive to consider what circumstances need to exist in order for an ecologic study of screening effectiveness to be informative.

Example 19-6. A program of cervical screening of Icelandic women aged 25 to 59 years was begun in 1964. Whereas only occasionally would women have received screening prior to that time, by the early 1970s, some 80% of the target population had been examined at the screening clinic. Some women 60 years and over were screened as well, but not in any appreciable numbers until after 1970. The mortality rate from cervical cancer during 1955–1974 is shown in Table 19.8. In 25- to 59-year-old women, a rise in mortality during 1955–1969 was reversed in 1970–1974. In women 60–89 years old, the group that

TABLE 19.8. MORTALITY FROM CERVICAL CANCER IN ICELAND, 1955–74

Age(years)	Mortality from cervical cancer[a]			
	1955–59	1960–64	1965–69	1970–74
25–59	11.7	16.8	26.5	12.2
60–89	27.6	33.3	28.2	34.8

[a] Rate per 100,000 person-years, age-adjusted (5-year groups) to a uniform standard
Source: Johannesson *et al.* (1978)

underwent little screening, cervical cancer mortality exhibited no systematic variation during the interval (Johannesson *et al.*, 1978).

Was it the screening that was responsible for this difference between the "populations" (i.e., the 25- to 59-year-old Icelandic women before and after the mass screening)? Features of the study's setting, design, and results that favor an affirmative answer to this question are as follows:

- The difference in the level of screening between the time periods was very great, rising from near zero before 1964 to 80% within 10 years.
- Reliable data were available on mortality from cervical cancer throughout the relevant time interval.
- The size of the population in each time period was sufficiently large to provide enough cervical cancer deaths for meaningful analysis.
- There is evidence to indicate that in the absence of screening, the mortality rates among 25- to 59-year-old women would not have fallen: (a) prior to the introduction of mass screening, the rates in women in this age group actually had been on the increase; and (b) in the Icelandic women who were largely unscreened—women aged 60 to 89—there was no corresponding decrease in mortality from cervical cancer during 1970–1974.
- The mortality in 1970–1974 was reduced to such a large degree that it is implausible that other, unmeasured changes during the period could have been solely responsible.

These are precisely the features that are rarely present *together* in most ecologic evaluations of the efficacy of screening.

Case-Control Studies

These studies differ in some respects from case-control studies of etiologic factors. "Cases" are defined, not as individuals who developed a particular disease, but rather as those who have developed progressive disease or the complications (such as death) that one is seeking to prevent by means of early detection. "Controls" are defined as persons without progression or complications but who were otherwise comparable to the cases just prior to the time their disease had been detected. Thus, if the cases were persons who died of colorectal cancer, controls would be selected so as to be representative of the population at risk for development of colorectal cancer at the time the cases were first diagnosed. Records of the two groups would be examined to determine which persons had undergone screening—perhaps by means of a test for fecal occult blood—during a period of time prior to diagnosis in which a tumor or a detectable antecedent of a tumor plausibly could be identified by the test (or, for controls, a corresponding period). The data would be displayed as in Table 19.9.

Screening for fecal occult blood would be effective in reducing mortality in proportion to the amount by which $b/(b + d)$ exceeded $a/(a + c)$ (Weiss *et al.*, 1992). The relative mortality from colorectal cancer associated with a history of screening during this interval would equal the relative odds of screening between cases and controls; that is, $(a/c) \div (b/d)$ (see Chapter 9 for the derivation of this formula). If, perhaps, 20% of persons who died of colorectal cancer had undergone screening for fecal occult blood during the 2-year period ending just before diagnosis, in contrast to 30% of controls during the same interval, the relative mortality associated with screening would be $(20/80) \div (30/70) = 0.58$.

TABLE 19.9. LAYOUT OF DATA FOR A CASE-CONTROL STUDY OF FECAL OCCULT BLOOD TESTING FOR COLORECTAL CANCER

Screening for fecal occult blood	Death from colorectal cancer	
	Yes	No
Performed	*a*	*b*
Not performed	*c*	*d*

Three features of the design and analysis of case-control studies of screening efficacy are worthy of mention:

1. Persons selected as cases should be ill or disabled to a degree that diagnosis would occur in the absence of screening (Morrison, 1982). For a disease such as cancer, the criterion for selection could be death from cancer (or possibly the presence of late-stage disease that is not believed to be curable), irrespective of the stage at which the cancer was first diagnosed. In a case-control study of the efficacy of a screening test that has the potential to reduce the incidence of cancer (e.g., cervical cytology or HPV screening, which can lead to the identification of treatable, premalignant lesions), cases can be defined as those that are sufficiently advanced that they would have been detected whether or not screening had been performed (Weiss, 1999).

2. Persons selected as controls should be representative of the population that generated the cases with respect to the presence and/or level or screening activity (Weiss, 1983). A control group restricted to persons with earlier or less severe forms of the condition under study (e.g., early-stage cancer) is not appropriate. The fact that the condition is detected early in such persons is probably the result of their having been screened. Thus, even if screening were not followed by any effective therapy, a case-control difference would exist: the controls' level of screening would be higher than that of the population from which the cases arose, falsely suggesting a benefit associated with screening. A bias of this sort is the case-control analogue of lead-time bias in follow-up studies. While the appropriate control group would not exclude persons with early or mild disease, it would include them only in proportion to their numbers in the population.

Example 19-7. In a case-control study that seeks to determine if cytological screening for cervical cancer leads to a reduction in mortality from the disease, one would not choose as controls women with *in situ* lesions. The presence of *in situ* cervical neoplasia is rarely discovered in the absence of screening, so virtually every member of the control group will have had at least one screening examination. It is unlikely that such a high level of screening activity would occur among women in the population that gave rise to the patients who died from cervical cancer. The selection of women with *in situ* cancer as controls would produce a finding of apparent benefit from cytological screening even if there were no effective treatment for the lesions discovered in this way.

3. As is the case with all non-randomized strategies for assessing the effectiveness of screening, there is a possibility of obtaining a spurious result unless factors that are correlated both with the level of screening activity and with the occurrence of late-stage disease/mortality are taken into account (Weiss, 1994). Factors can be related to the occurrence of late-stage disease by virtue of their relationship to disease incidence *per se* or to the likelihood of disease progression or spread. Thus, in a study of breast self-examination in relation to the occurrence of late stage breast cancer, it would be necessary to evaluate (and possibly adjust for) characteristics that are associated with breast cancer incidence (e.g., race and educational level) and that differ between cases and controls. Similarly, adjustment would have to be made if women who regularly performed breast self-examination also more commonly received the benefit of other detection methods for breast cancer (e.g., mammography and clinical examination), if the analysis found these other methods to have been efficacious.

(Parts of this chapter were adapted from Weiss (2006)).

APPENDIX 19A: DETERMINING THE OPTIMAL CUTOFF POINT ON AN ROC CURVE

From equation (19.2):

$$C_{total} = C_{test}$$
$$+ C_{TP} \cdot prev \cdot sens$$
$$+ C_{FP} \cdot (1 - prev) \cdot (1 - spec)$$
$$+ C_{FN} \cdot prev \cdot (1 - sens)$$
$$+ C_{TN} \cdot (1 - prev) \cdot spec$$
$$= C_{test}$$
$$+ C_{TP} \cdot prev \cdot sens$$
$$+ C_{FP} \cdot (1 - prev) \cdot (1 - spec)$$
$$+ C_{FN} \cdot prev - C_{FN} \cdot prev \cdot sens$$
$$+ C_{TN} \cdot (1 - prev)$$
$$- C_{TN} \cdot (1 - prev) \cdot (1 - spec)$$
$$= C_{test} + C_{FN} \cdot prev + C_{TN} \cdot (1 - prev)$$
$$+ prev \cdot (C_{TP} - C_{FN}) \cdot sens$$
$$+ (1 - prev) \cdot (C_{FP} - C_{TN}) \cdot (1 - spec)$$

Now let $x = (1 - spec)$ and $y = sens$, as on an ROC plot. The ROC curve is a plot of the function $y = f(x)$.

$$C_{total} = C_{test} + C_{FN} \cdot prev + C_{TN} \cdot (1 - prev)$$
$$+ prev \cdot (C_{TP} - C_{FN}) \cdot y$$
$$+ (1 - prev) \cdot (C_{FP} - C_{TN}) \cdot x$$

To find the value of x at which C_{total} is minimized, set $\partial C_{total} / \partial x = 0$:

$$\frac{\partial C_{total}}{\partial x} = prev \cdot (C_{TP} - C_{FN}) \cdot \frac{\partial y}{\partial x}$$
$$+ (1 - prev) \cdot (C_{FP} - C_{TN})$$

$$0 = prev \cdot (C_{TP} - C_{FN}) \cdot \frac{\partial y}{\partial x}$$
$$+ (1 - prev) \cdot (C_{FP} - C_{TN})$$

$$\frac{\partial y}{\partial x} = \frac{(1 - prev) \cdot (C_{FP} - C_{TN})}{prev \cdot (C_{FN} - C_{TP})}$$

which is equivalent to equation (19.3) in the main text.

APPENDIX 19B: THRESHOLD VALUE OF COST SAVINGS FROM EARLY DETECTION THAT FAVORS ONE SCREENING TEST OVER ANOTHER

Apply equation (19.2) to each of two tests, labelled 1 and 2, and subtract the test-1 equation from the test-2 equation to get:

$$(C_{total\,2} - C_{total\,1}) = (C_{test\,2} - C_{test\,1})$$
$$+ (sens_2 - sens_1) \cdot prev \cdot (C_{TP} - C_{FN})$$
$$+ (spec_2 - spec_1) \cdot (1 - prev) \cdot (C_{TN} - C_{FP})$$

Test 2 is preferred if $(C_{total\,2} - C_{total\,1}) < 0$, which is when $(C_{FN} - C_{TP})$ is greater than:

$$\frac{\left[\begin{array}{c} (C_{test\,2} - C_{test\,1}) \\ -(spec_2 - spec_1) \cdot (1 - prev) \cdot (C_{FN} - C_{TP}) \end{array} \right]}{prev \cdot (sens_2 - sens_1)}$$

$$(19.5)$$

$(C_{FN} - C_{TP})$ does not quite equal the benefit of early detection, however, because C_{TP} includes the cost of confirmatory testing, while C_{FN} does not. To solve for the benefit of early detection *per se*, let C_{early} be the expected treatment cost for a case detected by screening and C_{late} be the expected treatment cost for a case missed by screening. Recall also that C_{FP} equals the cost of confirmatory testing. Then:

$$C_{FN} - C_{TP} = C_{late} - (C_{early} + C_{FP})$$

$$C_{late} - C_{early} = (C_{FN} - C_{TP}) + C_{FP}$$

Adding C_{FP} to both sides of inequality (19.5) and assuming $C_{TN} = 0$ produces the following rule: Test 2 yields lower expected overall per-capita cost than Test 1 if $(C_{late} - C_{early})$ is greater than:

$$\left[\frac{(C_{test\,2} - C_{test\,1}) - (spec_2 - spec_1) \cdot (1 - prev) \cdot C_{FP}}{prev \cdot (sens_2 - sens_1)} \right] + C_{FP}$$

REFERENCES

Allison JE, Tekawa IS, Ransom LJ, Adrain AL. A comparison of fecal occult-blood tests for colorectal-cancer screening. N Engl J Med 1996; 334:155–159.

Bucher HC, Schmidt J. Does routine ultrasound scanning improve outcome in pregnancy? Meta-analysis of various outcome measures. Br Med J 1993; 307:13–16.

Buekens P, Alexander S, Boutsen M, Blondel B, Kaminski M, Reid M. Randomised controlled trial of routine cervical examinations in pregnancy. European Community Collaborative Study Group on Prenatal Screening. Lancet 1994; 344:841–844.

Cantor SB, Sun CC, Tortolero-Luna G, Richards-Kortum R, Follen M. A comparison of C/B ratios from studies using receiver operating characteristic curve analysis. J Clin Epidemiol 1999; 52:885–892.

Carroll AE, Downs SM. Comprehensive cost-utility analysis of newborn screening strategies. Pediatrics 2006; 117:S287–S295.

Dans LF, Silvestre MAA, Dans AL. Trade-off between benefit and harm is crucial in health screening recommendations. Part I: general principles. J Clin Epidemiol 2011; 64:231–239.

Deeks JJ, Altman DG. Diagnostic tests 4: likelihood ratios. BMJ 2004; 329:168–169.

Drummond MF, Sculpher MJ, Torrance GW, O'Brien BJ, Stoddart GL. Methods for the economic evaluation of health care programmes (3rd ed.). New York: Oxford, 2005.

Early Treatment Diabetic Retinopathy Study Group. Treatment techniques and clinical guidelines for photocoagulation of diabetic macular edema. Ophthalmology 1987; 94:761–774.

Ewigman BG, Crane JP, Frigoletto FD, LeFevre ML, Bain RP, McNellis D. Effect of prenatal ultrasound screening on perinatal outcome. RADIUS Study Group. N Engl J Med 1993; 329:821–827.

Grimes DA, Schulz KF. Uses and abuses of screening tests. Lancet 2002; 359:881–884.

Johannesson G, Geirsson G, Day N. The effect of mass screening in Iceland, 1965–74 on the incidence and mortality of cervical carcinoma. Int J Cancer 1978; 21:418–425.

Lichtenstein MJ, Bess FH, Logan SA. Validation of screening tools for identifying hearing-impaired elderly in primary care. JAMA 1988; 259:2875–2878.

Mahomed K, Nyoni R, Mulambo T, Kasule J, Jacobus E. Randomised controlled trial of intrapartum fetal heart rate monitoring. BMJ 1994; 308:497–500.

Mandel JS, Church TR, Ederer F, Bond JH. Colorectal cancer mortality: Effectiveness of biennial screening for fecal occult blood. J Nat Cancer Inst 1999; 91:437–447.

Marcus PM, Bergstralh EJ, Fagerstrom RM, Williams DE, Fontana R, Taylor WF, *et al.* Lung cancer mortality in the Mayo Lung Project: impact of extended follow-up. J Natl Cancer Inst 2000; 92:1308–1316.

Mayrand MH, Duarte-Franco E, Rodrigues I, Walter SD, Hanley J, Ferenczy A, *et al.* Human papillomavirus DNA versus Papanicolaou screening tests for cervical cancer. N Engl J Med 2007; 357:1579–1588.

Metz CE. Basic principles of ROC analysis. Semin Nucl Med 1978; 8:283–298.

Miller AB, Baines CJ, Wall C. Canadian National Breast Screening Study: 13-year results of a randomized trial in women aged 50–59 years. J Nat Cancer Inst 2000; 92:1490–1499.

Morrison AS. Case definition in case-control studies of the efficacy of screening. Am J Epidemiol 1982; 115:6–8.

Morrison AS. Screening in chronic disease (2nd ed.). New York: Oxford University Press, 1992.

Nadala EC, Goh BT, Magbanua JP, Barber P, Swain A, Alexander S, *et al.* Performance evaluation of a new rapid urine test for chlamydia in men: prospective cohort study. BMJ 2009; 339:b2655.

National Lung Screening Trial Research Team, Aberle DR, Adams AM, Berg CD, Black WC, Clapp JD, *et al.* Reduced lung-cancer mortality with low-dose computed tomographic screening. N Engl J Med 2011; 365:395–409.

Neutra RR, Fienberg SE, Greenland S, Friedman EA. Effect of fetal monitoring on neonatal death rates. N Engl J Med 1978; 299:324–326.

Pepe MS. The statistical evaluation of medical tests for classification and prediction. New York: Oxford, 2003.

Porta M (ed.). A dictionary of epidemiology (5th edition). New York: Oxford University Press, 2008.

Rosner B. Fundamentals of biostatistics (6th edition). New York: Duxbury Press, 2006.

Schillinger JA, Dunne EF, Chapin JB, Ellen JM, Gaydos CA, Willard NJ, et al. Prevalence of Chlamydia trachomatis infection among men screened in 4 U.S. cities. Sex Transm Dis 2005; 32: 74–77.

Schousboe JT, Kerlikowske K, Loh A, Cummings SR. Personalizing mammography by breast density and other risk factors for breast cancer: analysis of health benefits and cost-effectiveness. Ann Intern Med 2011; 155:10–20.

Schröder FH, Hugosson J, Roobol MJ, Tammela TLJ, Ciatto S, Nelen V, et al. Prostate-cancer mortality at 11 years of follow-up. N Engl J Med 2012; 366:981–990.

Shapiro S, Venet W, Strax P, Venet L, Roeser R. Ten- to fourteen-year effect of screening on breast cancer mortality. J Natl Cancer Inst 1982; 69: 349–355.

Skopp NA, Swanson R, Luxton DD, Reger MA, Trofimovich L, First M, et al. An examination of the diagnostic efficiency of post-deployment mental health screens. J Clin Psychol 2012; 68:1253–1265.

Thomas DB, Gao DL, Ray RM, Wang WW, Allison CJ, Chen FL, et al. Randomized trial of breast self-examination in Shanghai: final results. J Natl Cancer Inst 2002; 94:1445–1457.

US Preventive Services Task Force. Home uterine activity monitoring for preterm labor. JAMA 1993; 270:371–376.

US Preventive Services Task Force. The guide to clinical preventive services 2012: recommendations of the U.S. Preventive Services Task Force. Washington, D.C.: Agency for Healthcare Research and Quality, 2012.

Weiss NS. Control definition in case-control studies of the efficacy of screening and diagnostic testing. Am J Epidemiol 1983; 188:457–460.

Weiss NS. Application of the case-control method in the evaluation of screening. Epidemiol Rev 1994; 16:102–108.

Weiss NS. Case-control studies of the efficacy of screening tests designed to prevent the incidence of cancer. Am J Epidemiol 1999; 149:1–4.

Weiss NS. Clinical epidemiology: the study of the outcome of illness (3rd ed.). New York: Oxford, 2006.

Weiss NS, McKnight B, Stevens NG. Approaches to the analysis of case-control studies of the efficacy of screening for cancer. Am J Epidemiol 1992; 135:817–823.

Whitlock EP, Lin JS, Liles E, Beil TL, Fu R. Screening for colorectal cancer: a targeted, updated systematic review for the U.S. Preventive Services Task Force. Ann Intern Med 2008; 149:638–658.

Wilson JM, Jungner YG. Principles and practice of mass screening for disease. Geneva: World Health Organization, 1968.

Woods WG, Gao RN, Shuster JJ, Robison LL, Bernstein M, Weitzman S, et al. Screening of infants and mortality due to neuroblastoma. N Engl J Med 2002; 346:1041–1046.

Zelen M. Theory of early detection of breast cancer in the general population. In: Hensen JC, Mattheim WH, Rozencweig M (eds.). Breast cancer: Trends in research and treatment. New York: Raven Press, 1976.

EXERCISES

1. Genitourinary tract infection with Chlamydia trachomatis is among the most commonly reported sexually transmitted bacterial infections in the U.S. The definitive test for this infection is polymerase chain reaction (PCR), which detects genetic material from the organism. However, the PCR test requires a urethral swab specimen, which is uncomfortable for examinees and requires a trained technician. Also, the result may not be known for several days.

A Chlamydia Rapid Test (CRT) was developed that can be applied to a urine sample and yields a result on the same day. In a British study (Nadala et al., 2009), both PCR and CRT were done for 1,211 men who attended either of two clinics. Of 109 men whose PCR test was positive, 90 were also positive on CRT. Of 1,102 men whose PCR test was negative, 1,085 were also negative on CRT.

In a separate epidemiologic study in Seattle (Schillinger et al., 2005), 1% of men examined were found to have Chlamydia infection, using testing methods that can be assumed to be error-free.

Suppose that the new CRT test were used to screen men for C. trachomatis infection in Seattle. Assume that the operating characteristics of CRT would be as determined in the British study and that the earlier epidemiologic study in Seattle yielded an unbiased prevalence estimate.

(a) What proportion of C. trachomatis cases would be missed, if any?

(b) What proportion of screenees would require confirmatory testing?

(c) What proportion of men with a positive CRT would actually have *C. trachomatis* infection?

2. The following is excerpted from a news item in the May 17, 2000, issue of the *Journal of the National Cancer Institute*:

Some Promising Biomarkers for Cancer

LPA (lysophosphatidic acid). LPA is probably the most accurate marker we have for detection of early stage ovarian cancer. A 1998 report found 9 of 10 women with stage I disease, 24 of 24 with advanced disease, and 14 of 14 with recurrent ovarian cancer had elevated blood LPA levels. In contrast, just 5 of 48 controls had elevated LPA. A growth factor, LPA is not generally present in normal ovary cells.

Based on the above information, you believe it is *un*likely that blood LPA levels will be of practical use as a screening tool for ovarian cancer. Why?

3. Lichtenstein *et al.* (1988) studied alternative methods for detecting hearing impairment in the elderly. One method determined whether a subject could hear a tone emitted by a hand-held audioscope at a standardized frequency and loudness level. Another method asked subjects to complete a 10-item questionnaire, the Hearing Handicap Inventory for the Elderly—Screening version (HHIE-S). Each of these tests was evaluated against a gold standard, pure-tone audiometry administered at a hearing evaluation center.

In the elderly population studied, 30% of patients proved to have impaired hearing by pure-tone audiometry. The audioscope test was 3.36 times more likely to be positive among patients who truly had hearing impairment than among those who did not; for the HHIE-S at a cutoff score of 24, the corresponding ratio was 5.13.

(a) Suppose that you are a physician in that setting, evaluating a typical elderly patient for hearing impairment. You have just obtained a positive result with the audioscope test. How likely is it that your patient actually has hearing impairment?

(b) Suppose that, in the same patient, you had administered the HHIE-S test instead of the audioscope test, and obtained a positive HHIE-S result. How likely is it under this scenario that your patient has hearing impairment?

(c) When the audioscope test was administered to the same patients in a hearing evaluation center, its specificity was found to be significantly greater than when it had been administered in a physician's office—0.90 vs. 0.72. Why do you suppose that was?

4. Phenylketonuria (PKU) is an inborn error of metabolism due to deficiency of the enzyme phenylalanine hydroxylase, which converts the essential amino acid phenylalanine into another essential amino acid, tyrosine. In the absence of this enzyme, phenylalanine from dietary sources is metabolized via other biochemical pathways into molecules that are toxic to an infant's developing brain. By the time symptoms of brain impairment appear, the damage is irreversible. But if PKU is detected shortly after birth, it can be treated effectively with a low-phenylalanine diet.

Carroll and Downs (2006) studied the monetary costs and benefits of screening for several inborn errors of metabolism, including PKU. Tandem mass spectrometry is a laboratory method that allows biochemical screening for several metabolic diseases at once, which lowers testing cost. Drawing on data from the medical literature and judgments from clinical experts, they estimated several key parameters as of the time of the study:

- Prevalence of PKU at birth = 6.6/100,000 infants
- Sensitivity of tandem mass spectrometry = 1.0
- Specificity of tandem mass spectrometry = 0.998
- Cost of tandem mass spectrometry for PKU = $3.43
- Cost of confirmatory tests = $300
- Average lifetime cost of treatment for PKU if detected early = $122,515
- Risks and average lifetime treatment costs of clinical manifestations of PKU if not detected early:

TABLE 19.10.

Condition	Probability	Average lifetime treatment cost
Mild mental retardation	0.05	$44,192
Moderate mental retardation	0.475	$77,079
Severe mental retardation	0.475	$1,042,110
Seizure disorder	0.25	$216,848

Use this information to estimate the expected per-capita monetary cost of two strategies: (1) screening all infants at birth for PKU with tandem mass spectrometry, and (2) not screening any infants. Note that strategy (2) is equivalent to using an imaginary "test" that costs nothing to apply but that always yields a negative result.

5. Suppose that disease X is suitable for screening and that a screening test T for disease X returns a numerical result. Cases of disease X tend to have high T-values, and non-cases have low T-values, but no cutoff point perfectly distinguishes between cases and non-cases. After a thorough analysis of costs and benefits, an expert panel has recommended that the value K be used as a cutoff to guide what action to take on the basis of a T-value result during screening: T-values above K warrant further evaluation with confirmatory tests, and T-values at or below K do not. Further research supports the choice of K as being very close to the optimal cutoff to minimize the total costs of misclassification errors.

Time passes. New developments call for revisiting the expert panel's recommendation. Suppose that you have recently joined the panel. In each of the following scenarios, how would you advise shifting the cutoff value: up, down, or not at all?

(a) Health authorities in another country are considering starting a screening program of their own for disease X using test T. The best available evidence suggests that disease X is about twice as prevalent in their setting as in the original one considered by the panel, but in other respects the settings are similar. Should they use K as the cutoff value, or a higher value, or a lower one?

(b) New and better technology has become available for confirmatory testing. The new confirmatory tests for disease X can be done in half the time and at half the cost of the old confirmatory tests. Would this change call for shifting the optimal cutoff value on screening test T? If so, in which direction?

(c) A new approach to treatment of early cases of X has been shown to be more effective than existing standard treatment, virtually eliminating the chance that disease X will recur in the same patient. Unfortunately, the new treatment approach cannot be used on more advanced disease. Initial application of the new treatment costs about the same as the existing standard treatment. Would this change call for shifting the optimal cutoff value on screening test T? If so, in which direction?

6. Several case-control studies have been conducted to estimate the degree to which mortality from breast cancer might be reduced by early detection through regular breast self-examination (BSE). In some studies, women whose cancers were diagnosed at late and early stages (i.e., cases and controls, respectively) were compared with respect to the proportion who had been performing BSE on a regular basis. Even if: (1) the information obtained on BSE practices were completely accurate, and (2) cases and controls were comparable with regard to risk factors for late-stage breast cancer, the results of such studies could suggest a falsely great benefit associated with BSE. Why is this?

7. Neuroblastoma is a tumor that affects about one in 7,000 children. It can be screened for with good sensitivity and specificity by the detection of catecholamines in urine. Children who are found to have this tumor on the basis of a screening exam have a particularly favorable prognosis.

In Quebec, Canada, urine catecholamine screening was offered at three weeks and six months of age from May 1989 through April 1994, and about 92% of infants born during this period were screened. However, though screen-detected cases of neuroblastoma contributed more than a third of all cases diagnosed, and reported incidence rates were relatively high, death rates from neuroblastoma in Quebec children born during the five years were identical to those of children born in neighboring provinces and states where screening had not taken place (Woods et al., 2002).

The absence of an association between catecholamine screening and mortality argues that such screening prevents few, if any, deaths from neuroblastoma. How can this conclusion be reconciled with the "particularly favorable prognosis" among infants with screen-detected neuroblastoma?

ANSWERS

1. (a) In the British study, the sensitivity of CRT was $90/109 = 0.826$. The operating characteristics (i.e., sensitivity and specificity) of CRT are assumed to be the same in the Seattle screening program as they were in the British study. Hence, about $(1 - 0.826) = 0.174 = 17.4\%$ of cases would be missed during screening in Seattle.

(b) All screenees with a positive CRT (whether true or false) would require confirmatory testing. The proportion of screenees with a positive CRT can be calculated by projecting how a hypothetical population of, say, 100,000 screenees would be distributed among the four cells in the standard 2×2 table:

TABLE 19.11.

CRT result	Infected?		
	Yes	No	Total
Positive	a	b	$a + b$
Negative	c	d	$c + d$
Total	$a + c$	$b + d$	100,000

These quantities are already known:

$$\text{prevalence} = 0.01$$

$$\text{sensitivity} = 90/109 = 0.826$$

$$\text{specificity} = 1{,}085/1{,}102 = 0.985$$

Numerical values for the cells and column totals in the above table can be filled in as follows:

$$a + c = 100{,}000 \times \text{prevalence}$$

$$b + d = 100{,}000 \times (1 - \text{prevalence})$$

$$a = (a + c) \times \text{sensitivity}$$

$$d = (b + d) \times \text{specificity}$$

$$c = (a + c) - a$$

$$b = (b + d) - d$$

Once a, b, c, and d are known, the row totals can be calculated from them. The results are:

TABLE 19.12.

CRT result	Infected? Yes	No	Total
Positive	826	1,527	2,353
Negative	174	97,473	97,647
Total	1,000	99,000	100,000

The proportion of screenees who would require confirmatory testing is thus $2{,}353/100{,}000 = 0.02353$.

(c) This proportion is the positive predictive value (PV_+) of CRT, which can be obtained directly from the table constructed for the previous part: $826/2{,}353 = 0.351$.

Alternatively, it can be calculated using Bayes's Theorem:

$$PV_+ = \frac{\text{sens} \cdot \text{prev}}{\text{sens} \cdot \text{prev} + (1 - \text{spec}) \cdot (1 - \text{prev})}$$

$$= \frac{(0.826)(0.01)}{(0.826)(0.01)+(1-0.985)(1-0.01)}$$

$$= 0.351$$

2. If the prevalence of ovarian cancer among screened women is low, the number of false positive tests would greatly exceed the number of true positives. For example, if the prevalence of cancer were 1/2,000, and if LPA were 100% sensitive in identifying ovarian cancer, Table 19.13 shows the expected results in 20,000 screened women.

TABLE 19.13. EXPECTED RESULTS OF APPLYING THE LPA TEST TO A HYPOTHETICAL POPULATION OF 20,000 WOMEN

LPA	Ovarian cancer Yes	No		Total
Positive	10	$5/48 \times 19{,}990 =$	2,082	2,092
Negative	0	$43/48 \times 19{,}990 =$	17,908	17,908
Total	10		19,990	20,000

The predictive value of a positive test would be just $10/2{,}092 = 0.005$, very likely too low to warrant use of LPA for early detection. Unless a test has an extremely high level of specificity—more than $43/48$—it will not serve well for the early detection of an uncommon condition.

3. (a) Since your patient is "typical," it is reasonable to use the overall prevalence of hearing impairment in this population, 0.3, as an estimate of the pre-test probability of hearing impairment. The value 3.36 is the likelihood ratio of a positive test, LR_+. Once a positive audioscope test result is obtained, the post-test probability of hearing impairment can be calculated as follows:

$$\text{Pre-test odds} = \frac{\text{Pre-test probability}}{1 - \text{Pre-test probability}}$$

$$= 0.3/(1 - 0.3) = 0.429$$

$$\text{Post-test odds} = \text{Pre-test odds} \times LR_+$$

$$= 0.429 \times 3.36 = 1.44$$

$$\text{Post-test probability} = \frac{\text{Post-test odds}}{1 + \text{Post-test odds}}$$

$$= 1.44/(1 + 1.44) = 0.59$$

(b) The likelihood ratio for a positive HHIE-S test (at a cutoff score of 24) is = 5.13. Substituting this value for 3.36 in the above calculations gives a post-test probability of 0.69.

(c) The researchers speculated that the higher ambient noise level in a physician's office may have caused more false positives in that setting. Patient may have been unable to hear the audioscope tone in the presence of other distracting sounds, which were not present in the hearing evaluation center's purposefully quiet environment. This could be a good example of how a test's specificity (or sensitivity) can depend on the particular setting and target population in which it is applied.

4. Most of the inputs needed to apply eq. (19.2) can be drawn directly from the information provided. Two inputs require closer attention:

- C_{TP} under strategy #1 includes both the cost of confirmatory tests ($300) and the cost of treating PKU detected early ($122,515).
- C_{FN} is a weighted sum of average treatment costs for the various adverse consequences of PKU that is not detected early, each cost weighted by its probability of occurrence:

$$C_{FN} = (0.05 \times \$44,192)$$
$$+ (0.475 \times \$77,079)$$
$$+ (0.475 \times \$1,042,110)$$
$$+ (0.25 \times \$216,848)$$
$$= \$588,036.40$$

The table below summarizes the input values for each screening strategy and the resulting C_{total} estimates:

TABLE 19.14.

	Strategy	
	Screening	No screening
Prevalence	6.6/100,000	6.6/100,000
Sensitivity	1	0
Specificity	0.998	1
C_{test}	$3.43	$0
C_{TP}	$122,815	(Not needed)
C_{FP}	$300	(Not needed)
C_{FN}	(Not needed)	$588,036.40
C_{TN}	$0	$0
C_{total}	$12.14	$38.81

Even from a strictly economic viewpoint, the costs of using tandem mass spectrometry for every infant, of correcting the false positives through confirmatory testing, and of treating early PKU with a special diet are more than offset by avoiding the high direct health-care costs that would otherwise result from brain damage caused by PKU. In this instance, screening not only pays for itself but saves society money in the long run. When the benefits of averting suffering and life-long mental retardation are factored in, the case for PKU screening is strong indeed.

5. The three scenarios all concern factors that affect optimal choice of a cutoff value on an ROC curve, and all can be guided by eq. (19.3).

(a) They should consider using a lower cutoff than K. Higher prevalence yields a lower slope of the tangent line at the optimal point on the ROC curve for test T, which implies that the new optimal point would lie above and to the right of the old one. Moving up and to the right on an ROC curve implies increasing sensitivity and decreasing specificity, which could be accomplished by lowering the cutoff. Stated another way, higher prevalence would lead to more cases and hence to more false negatives if the cutoff K were left as is. It would also lead to fewer false positives. To restore the optimal balance between false positives and false negatives, sensitivity must increase and specificity decrease.

(b) It calls for shifting the optimal cutoff value downward. Lowering the cost of confirmatory testing reduces the cost of each false positive, which in turn reduces the slope of the tangent line at the optimal decision point on the ROC curve for test T. As before, this change in slope would translate to higher sensitivity and lower specificity, which could be achieved by reducing the cutoff value. Although the relative *frequencies* of false negatives and false positives would be unaffected, the expected *costs* would change, making false positives more tolerable than before.

(c) Once again, it calls for shifting the optimal cutoff value downward. More effective early treatment reduces the longer-term components of the cost C_{TP} and thus increases the value of $C_{FN} - C_{TP}$, implying a larger benefit of early detection. Since $C_{FN} - C_{TP}$ appears in the denominator of eq. (19.3), the change reduces the slope of the tangent line at the optimal decision point on the ROC curve for test T. As before, this change in slope would translate to higher sensitivity and lower specificity, which could be achieved by reducing the cutoff value. Sensitivity is prioritized over specificity in order to minimize the risk of missing a case who could reap large benefits from early detection.

Although the above reasoning tells whether the optimal cutoff would be shifted up or down, it does not tell how large a shift would be warranted. However, that information could probably be derived from the same analysis that had led to the original choice of K as the cutoff.

6. • The goal of early detection is to prevent the occurrence of late-stage disease at any time, not merely at diagnosis. Thus, the criteria for selection of "cases" should not have been based solely on information available at the time of diagnosis. Cases who should have appeared (but did not) in these studies—women who only developed late-stage breast cancer at some time after the initial diagnosis of their disease—may have had early cancer found by BSE. Failure to include them in the case group would falsely inflate the measured efficacy of BSE.

   • The BSE practices of women with breast cancer diagnosed at an early stage are almost certainly not typical of those of the population of women from which the late-stage cases arose. In most instances, BSE or other early detection activity will have been responsible for the early diagnosis. Restriction of the control group to these women with higher-than-average early detection activity will cause the control-case difference in the proportion performing BSE to be falsely large, and thus the odds ratio estimating relative mortality from breast cancer in women who perform BSE to be falsely low.

   Case-control studies that seek to estimate the degree of reduction in breast cancer mortality afforded by BSE need to choose, as cases, women who develop metastatic breast cancer (i.e., women who are very likely to die of the disease) during a defined period of time, irrespective of the date of diagnosis of their primary tumor. Such studies should identify as controls a representative sample of women at risk for the development of breast cancer in that population from which the cases arose.

7. Almost certainly, most screen-detected cases were not destined to be fatal in the absence of screening. A likely reason for the elevated incidence of neuroblastoma in Quebec infants during the time that screening took place is that some tumors were found that would not have become clinically evident had screening not taken place.

20

Outbreak Investigation

BY JENNIFER LLOYD AND JEFFREY DUCHIN

An outbreak or epidemic of disease occurs when the number of new disease cases observed exceeds the number expected in a defined setting over a relatively short period of time. Technically, the terms *outbreak* and *epidemic* are defined similarly and are sometimes used interchangeably. However, many epidemiologists use *epidemic* for larger, more widespread, or longer-term elevations in disease incidence and *outbreak* for more geographically limited increases in disease incidence. Although most commonly associated with infectious diseases, outbreak investigations also occur for non-infectious causes, including intoxications, injuries, and other adverse health events.

Outbreak investigations can serve several purposes:

- *Limit the scope and severity of an immediate threat to public health.* There may be effective disease control interventions, such as treatment for infected persons, vaccine or antibiotic prophylaxis for those susceptible to infection, infection control measures, or withdrawal of a contaminated product from distribution. Meningococcal meningitis, hepatitis A and hepatitis B, pertussis, measles, and varicella are among the communicable diseases with outbreak potential for which effective pharmacologic interventions are available.

In 2012, over 600 cases of fungal meningitis and other central nervous system infections were traced back to epidural or paraspinal injections of a contaminated steroid medication prepared by a single compounding pharmacy. Once the outbreak source was identified, public health officials worked to ensure that the contaminated lots were discontinued from use, and they contacted nearly 14,000 patients and their physicians nationwide to facilitate prompt recognition and treatment of illness (Kainer *et al.*, 2012; Bell and Khabbaz, 2013).

Examples of controllable non-infectious disease outbreaks include the sudden appearance of a cluster of a rare condition, eosinophilia-myalgia syndrome, among women in New Mexico in 1990 that was stopped when implicated lots of an L-tryptophan supplement contaminated with an industrial lubricant were recalled (Belongia *et al.*, 1990); and a 2007 cluster of polyradiculoneuropathy among workers at a pork processing plant in Minnesota. The ensuing investigation determined that the use of compressed air to remove brains from pig carcasses aerosolized central nervous system tissue and caused the immune-mediated illness among those working in the vicinity. Once this technique was discontinued, no additional cases were reported (Holzbauer *et al.*, 2010).

- *Prevent future outbreaks.* Once the reason(s) for an outbreak is understood, implementing changes in products or processes can help prevent a recurrence. For example, when a sudden outbreak of the rare disease toxic shock syndrome occurred in 1980, a series of investigations were conducted. The disease was found to be associated with the use of a new "super absorbent" brand of tampons, which fostered bacterial growth. This type of tampon was removed from the market, the outbreak ended, and further outbreaks were prevented (Shands *et al.*, 1980).

The identification of a large outbreak of *E. coli* O157:H7 due to contaminated undercooked hamburger in 1992 resulted in widespread changes in standard procedures for cooking hamburgers in the fast food industry and a subsequent decline in the frequency of outbreaks from this source (Bell *et al.*, 1994).

An outbreak of salmonellosis associated with contaminated frozen pot pies highlighted consumer confusion with cooking instructions for microwave ovens of various wattages and led to the recommendation that microwave manufacturers consider labeling units with their output wattage (Centers for Disease Control and Prevention, 2008).

An investigation of mesothelioma cases in Florence, Italy, led to the discovery (and subsequent cessation) of the reuse of polypropylene bags that had contained asbestos cement as baling material for fabrics (Weiss, 1991).

- *Identify new vehicles of infection.* Several outbreaks of disease due to enteric pathogens were associated with consumption of raw sprouts throughout the 1990s (Breuer *et al.*, 2001; Mohle-Boetani *et al.*, 2001; Centers for Disease Control and Prevention, 2002a). Subsequent research determined that seeds were often contaminated with enteric bacteria that thrived under sprouting conditions. These investigations resulted in a recommendation issued by the U.S. Department of Agriculture (USDA) and the CDC that raw sprouts not be consumed by young children, the elderly, and immunocompromised persons, who may be at increased risk for serious complications of enteric infections (U.S. Department of Health and Human Services, 1999).

  In 2012, a cluster of chronic skin infections unresponsive to standard treatment was reported among people who had recently received tattoos. The multi-state investigation identified the same atypical mycobacterial strain in clinical biopsies and in a bottle of the implicated ink, which was intended for printing purposes and not approved for use in tattooing. The outbreak highlighted the importance of establishing and enforcing standards for the regulation of tattoo inks (LeBlanc *et al.*, 2012; Falsey *et al.*, 2013).

- *Monitor the success of intervention programs.* The rapid emergence of *Salmonella* Enteritidis

outbreaks associated with intact-shell eggs in the 1980s established that this serotype of *Salmonella* had become adapted to the hen's ovary and that even intact eggs could contain *S.* Enteritidis (St. Louis *et al.*, 1988). The USDA, CDC, and the Food and Drug Administration (FDA) worked with the egg industry to create programs to control exposure of laying hens to *S.* Enteritidis on the farm. The decreasing frequency with which intact-shell eggs were implicated in subsequent outbreaks of *S.* Enteritidis suggested that this intervention may have been effective in decreasing the prevalence of this pathogen in eggs (Mishu *et al.*, 1994).

Trends in the occurrence of outbreaks are also used to gauge the success of national vaccination programs. Following the introduction of widespread childhood hepatitis A vaccination, previously large community-wide outbreaks and overall incidence of hepatitis A cases decreased markedly (Wasley *et al.*, 2005).

Interventions that successfully halt a health threat may have an impact on commerce and can even lead to litigation. Following a *Salmonella* outbreak that sickened hundreds of people who had consumed contaminated peanut products, the peanut processor subsequently declared bankruptcy and its executives faced charges for knowingly releasing contaminated products into commerce (Centers for Disease Control and Prevention, 2007; Tavernise, 2013).

- *Identify new pathogens.* Legionnaire's disease was first described after a large outbreak of respiratory disease at an American Legion convention in Philadelphia in 1976. Investigation of the outbreak led to discovery of a new organism, now called *Legionella pneumophila*, in specimens obtained from outbreak cases (Fraser *et al.*, 1977). It was found to have been transmitted in aerosols from outdoor cooling towers. Subsequently, many other cooling tower-associated outbreaks have been recognized, as well as other routes of transmission (Centers for Disease Control and Prevention, 2000; Den Boer *et al.*, 2002).

  Similarly, although sporadic cases of the Acute Respiratory Distress Syndrome had been seen for years, investigation of an outbreak in the Four Corners area of the southwestern United States in 1993 led to the description of Hantavirus Pulmonary Syndrome and identification of a previously unrecognized etiologic agent (Duchin et al., 1994).

In February 2003, the World Health Organization was alerted by a physician at the French Hospital in Hanoi, Vietnam, about a severe respiratory disease in a traveler and spread of the infection among hospital healthcare workers. The ensuing multinational investigation led to the recognition of the global outbreak of Severe Acute Respiratory Syndrome (SARS) and the discovery of the causal agent, the SARS coronavirus. Earlier cases reported from China were probably mistaken for influenza and other respiratory pathogens (Reilley et al., 2003).

Such investigations can also reveal the mode of transmission, incubation period, spectrum of disease, and risk factors for infection. Even if the infectious agent causing illness is undetected at the time of the investigation, outbreaks often provide an opportunity to obtain historical specimens and epidemiologic data from cases that can prove valuable in later years when improved technologies for pathogen detection become available.

OUTBREAK DETECTION

The sequence of events leading up to an outbreak investigation typically begins when some kind of unusual health event in the community is detected. Sometimes the unusual event is the occurrence of even a single case of an uncommon disease that poses a clear threat to public health, such as botulism, paralytic shellfish poisoning, or anthrax. Often the unusual event is the recognition of two or more similar cases that appear to have occurred suspiciously close to each other in space or time—a *cluster* of cases—which may or may not represent an outbreak.

Common ways by which such unusual health events are detected include:

• *An astute health care worker.* Clinicians, infection control practitioners, and laboratory staff function as the "eyes and ears" of the public health system. In 1980, a report by an

alert physician in California of an increase in the number of patients with *Pneumocystis carinii* pneumonia led to an investigation of what was originally called Gay-Related Immunodeficiency Syndrome. The disease is now known as AIDS (Centers for Disease Control and Prevention, 1981). Other notable examples of high-profile outbreaks that the public health system was alerted to by astute clinicians include Hantavirus Pulmonary Syndrome (Duchin et al., 1994), the 2001 anthrax bioterror attack (Bush et al., 2001), SARS (Reilley et al., 2003), and the large multi-state outbreak of fungal meningitis described above (Pettit et al., 2012).

• *A citizen.* The borreliosis now known as Lyme disease was first recognized when the mother of a child diagnosed with rheumatoid arthritis, a condition uncommon in children, notified the local health department that she knew of at least three other cases of this disease in her neighborhood. The subsequent investigation identified a new pathogen, *Borrelia burghdorferi*, and the tick vector responsible for the disease outbreak (Steere et al., 1977). Often, outbreaks of foodborne illness are identified when citizens call to report that a number of people became ill after consuming food at a large group event.

• *Reportable disease surveillance.* As was described in Chapter 6, each state publishes a list of communicable diseases and conditions that laboratories and health care providers are required to report to local public health authorities. In practice, routine disease reports are often not timely or complete enough to be useful in rapidly detecting outbreaks, especially those due to common conditions. Patients may delay seeking care, appropriate specimens may not be collected or the right tests not ordered, laboratory processing and reporting of results can be delayed, and health care providers and laboratories may not comply with reporting requirements. Nonetheless, frequent detailed analyses of routine surveillance data can be important in detecting smaller or geographically dispersed "hidden outbreaks" that may otherwise escape notice when total case reports remain relatively stable.

In larger communities, surveillance data can even be reviewed on a daily basis, not only for unusual increases in total numbers of cases, but also for increases among subpopulations defined by age, gender, ethnicity, geography, or other risk factors. For example, although overall rates of hepatitis A remained relatively stable in many areas during the 1990s, analyses of the age, sex, and geographic distribution of cases revealed an increased incidence among young men living in urban areas and led to recognition of increased transmission of hepatitis A among injecting drug users and men who have sex with men (Bell *et al.*, 1998).

More recently, although the overall rate of infection with invasive meningococcal disease remained similar to that in previous years, a cluster of illness in young men who have sex with men was identified in Berlin in 2012 and 2013. Initially, three cases were reported with smoking and attendance at gay bars as their only identified risk factors; genetic testing of their clinical specimens revealed they were infected with the same bacterial strain. Retrospective data analysis revealed a higher proportion of cases than usual in young men, and two additional outbreak cases were identified. A similar cluster among gay men was also recognized in New York City (Centers for Disease Control and Prevention, 2013b; European Centre for Disease Prevention and Control, 2013).

- *Electronic health data.* Electronic health data may provide information from large populations fairly efficiently, both regarding incidence of cases during an outbreak as well as baseline rates for specific conditions. For example, review of electronic emergency department data on patient chief complaints and discharge diagnoses (syndromic surveillance) detected an increase in carbon monoxide poisonings, including clusters in Zip codes with significant power outages, following a large windstorm in Seattle (Baer *et al.*, 2011). Recent changes in the regulation and standardization of computerized electronic health data by healthcare facilities and laboratories will facilitate sharing of data with public health authorities and may improve data completeness and quality, and decrease time to case reporting and outbreak detection (Henricks, 2011; Wurtz, 2013).

VERIFYING AN OUTBREAK
What Is the Illness?

Once a suspected outbreak is identified, characterizing the specific nature of the illness in question is an important early step, particularly for diseases and syndromes that are new or not yet fully characterized. Usually this task involves reviewing the clinical case history and checking key laboratory results. For new or unusual conditions, verification may involve consulting with clinical or laboratory experts and collecting clinical specimens for specialized testing at national reference laboratories to assist with diagnosis. Even in the absence of a specific diagnosis, systematically summarizing the signs and symptoms of illness can help characterize the disease and to develop a working case definition that can be refined as more information becomes available.

Is There a True Excess?

For serious conditions with outbreak potential, such as meningococcal meningitis, measles, Shiga-toxin producing *E. coli*, or typhoid fever, even a single case should "raise a red flag," triggering an epidemiologic investigation. Single cases of these conditions require immediate public health investigation to attempt to identify the probable source, other persons at risk, and to formulate and implement intervention strategies to prevent additional persons from becoming ill. Single cases of certain non-contagious diseases, such as botulism, paralytic shellfish poisoning, and vibriosis, also require immediate investigation to allow prompt identification of exposed persons and recall of contaminated food products before they are consumed by others.

It is always important to determine the degree to which the number of new cases or events observed truly exceeds the number expected in a given geographic area during a defined period of time. The expected number of "sporadic" (or background) cases is usually estimated from historical data. For diseases that are reportable by law to the local health department, baseline surveillance data will usually be available and can often be stratified by age, geographic location, and other variables. For conditions that may vary in incidence with time (e.g., expected seasonal variation), it is helpful to look at incidence data from comparable time periods in recent past years to establish baseline rates and clearly identify the onset of the outbreak.

When standardized surveillance data are not available, medical records, laboratory test results, and other data will need to be reviewed. Data from health care institutions, including hospitals, micro-biology laboratories and emergency departments, as well as outpatient clinical facilities, may be use-ful sources with which to establish baseline inci-dence. For example, in investigating a cluster of cases of Legionnaire's disease, hospital records, includ-ing hospital pneumonia admissions, intensive care unit admissions, and discharge diagnoses, would be good sources to identify the persons hospital-ized with pneumonia during a given time interval. Other potential sources of baseline data include dis-ease registries and causes of death from death cer-tificates available through vital statistics offices. In the absence of existing data, surveys of health care providers and key informant interviews may also help in judging whether an increase in cases is occurring.

An apparent excess in the number of reported cases does not necessarily mean that an outbreak is in progress. Other possibilities to consider are:

- *Change in the population at risk.* As noted in Chapter 3, a simple case count can be adequate to compare incidence between time periods if it is safe to assume that the underlying population at risk is relatively constant. In some situations, however, this assumption is untenable—for example, in communities that have had rapid population growth or that experience marked seasonal changes in population demographics, such as tourist centers, university communities, regions hosting mass gatherings, or populations migrating in response to natural disasters. To avoid this source of error, comparisons should be based on *rates*, not just case counts, whenever possible.
- *Change in case ascertainment.* Caution must be used when disease rates obtained from active or enhanced surveillance activities are compared with rates calculated using baseline or passively collected data. For example, conditions that routinely go under-reported will seem to increase when active or enhanced surveillance is used, but the increase in reports can simply reflect better ascertainment and not a true increase in disease incidence (Centers for Disease Control and Prevention, 1995; Glatzel *et al.*, 2002).

A common phenomenon during outbreaks is that increased awareness of the outbreak among the public and healthcare providers leads to increases in healthcare-seeking behavior and diagnostic testing for the condition in question, uncovering both outbreak-associated and unrelated sporadic cases that would otherwise go undiagnosed and unreported, particularly milder cases. As noted below, laboratory methods for characterizing relatedness of organisms ("molecular epidemiology") can help to distinguish outbreak-associated from unrelated background cases.

Even when evaluating clusters of notifiable diseases in the absence of enhanced surveillance, it is important to consider whether some element of the reporting system has changed, producing apparent increases in incidence in the absence of any real change in disease occurrence, including: a new or improved laboratory test; changes in interpretation of test results; heightened awareness of a new disease; changes in clinical practice standards; a new physician in the community with particular expertise in a disease; improved disease reporting by a new hospital infection-control practitioner; or changes in patient or laboratory referral patterns among health care providers (Joce *et al.*, 1995; Centers for Disease Control and Prevention, 1997; Weinbaum *et al.*, 1998; Adderson *et al.*, 2000).

The expansion of the AIDS surveillance definition in 1993 resulted in an increase in reporting (but not corresponding to an increase in incidence) of over 111%, a dramatic example of the impact a change in case definition can have (Centers for Disease Control and Prevention, 1994). When considering changes in reporting patterns, it may be useful to consult resources that document what has been reportable over time, such as the case definitions established by the CDC and the Council for State and Territorial Epidemiologists (CSTE) (National Notifiable Disease Surveillance System, 2013).

Are the Cases Related?

Besides being more numerous than expected, out-break cases may cluster in space and time or be related in some other as yet unrecognized way. Sometimes links between them may not become apparent until after an investigation is in progress. However, molecular strain–typing methods are informative laboratory-based epidemiologic tools that can help in understanding disease transmission and determining whether a set of cases of illness due to an infectious agent may be connected or are simply a chance collection of sporadic cases (Centers for Disease Control and Prevention, 2002b).

Molecular strain–typing methods provide genotypic data that are more discriminating than phenotypic methods of characterizing organisms, such as serotyping. Molecular strain typing makes it possible to detect small potentially linked clusters of cases and outbreaks due to related strains of common serotypes that would otherwise go unnoticed. For example, pulsed field gel electrophoresis (PFGE), based on electrophoretic migration patterns of bacterial DNA fragments, is routinely employed by public health laboratories to detect clusters of *Salmonella*, Shiga-toxin-producing *E. coli*, and other pathogens, even when the total number of cases remains stable (Bender *et al.*, 1997, 2001).

A well-established CDC-sponsored Internet-based surveillance tool for enteric disease pathogens, called PulseNet, enables laboratories across the country to compare standardized PFGE patterns of local cases against a large library of patterns (Swaminathan *et al.*, 2001). This surveillance network can identify widely geographically dispersed outbreaks that would have otherwise gone undetected, with only a few cases occurring in any single health jurisdiction. Newer molecular typing methods based on complete or partial bacterial gene sequencing provide increasingly rich information, which, when interpreted in the context of epidemiologic data, have the potential to improve detection of outbreaks as well as track the evolution of disease-causing pathogens in populations (Goering *et al.*, 2013).

INVESTIGATING AN OUTBREAK

The decision on whether to dedicate resources to the investigation of a cluster of illnesses depends on many factors. Outbreaks of a severe illness or outbreaks involving many cases normally prompt an investigation, as do those involving an unusual or newly recognized illness. Some investigations are conducted simply because public attention to a perceived "outbreak" demands that the situation be evaluated. The epidemiologist must anticipate and evaluate the needs of the community, the resources available, whether an effective public health intervention exists, and the potential social and political consequences of the investigation (or of the failure to conduct one).

Overview of Steps

Although no two outbreaks evolve in exactly the same way, the steps commonly involved in investigating an outbreak are:

- Establish a case definition
- Enhance surveillance
- Describe occurrence of cases according to person, place, and time
- Develop hypotheses about the nature of the exposure(s) responsible for the outbreak
- Conduct analytic studies, if appropriate
- Implement disease-control interventions
- Communicate status reports and results of the investigation

Each step is described more fully below. In practice, the steps are not necessarily sequential, but rather multiple steps often occur simultaneously; in some investigations not all the steps may be needed. Sometimes the pace of events is rapid, and the outbreak epidemiologist may need to anticipate and prepare for later steps before the results of earlier steps are complete.

A structured approach to managing outbreak investigations is desirable. The team leader(s) and other members of the outbreak investigation and response team should be identified and specific roles and responsibilities assigned. For large or complicated investigations, incident-management systems are often employed to help organize and track response activities and required resources. An "operations" team within an incident-management structure might include designated staff for surveillance, analytic epidemiologic studies, clinical investigation, environmental and/or field investigation, and response activities (Qureshi *et al.*, 2006). Communication and logistics are other components of incident management structures.

Establish a Case Definition

Collecting as much information as feasible on all potential cases early in the investigation can help characterize the full spectrum of disease, save time in the long run, and help maximize the sample size available for later analysis. Once the disease symptomatology and laboratory findings have been established, an explicit working case definition is developed and applied consistently to all potential cases. As noted in Chapter 2, case definitions can include several clinical and/or laboratory criteria. A fairly broad or "loose" case definition is useful early in an outbreak investigation to include as many potential cases as possible, while collecting enough specific information to enable refinement of the definition as the investigation progresses. Early cases are often categorized as *confirmed*, *probable*, or *suspect*, depending on the extent to which a clinically compatible illness, laboratory confirmation, and an epidemiologic link to other confirmed cases are present.

Obtaining appropriate biological specimens for laboratory testing can be important to document or rule out potential cases as confirmed, to provide isolates for molecular epidemiology testing, to identify otherwise obscure etiologic agents, or to identify an outbreak etiology when people would otherwise not seek medical care for testing. Since laboratory testing of each possible case is often neither feasible nor necessary, case definitions can be created using a constellation of symptoms exhibited by the laboratory-confirmed cases.

The goal of the case definition is to include only true cases. Inclusion of non-cases as cases, or of subclinical cases in the comparison group, results in misclassification, which weakens the ability to detect an association with the relevant risk factor(s) (see Chapter 10). For large outbreaks with many cases and high statistical power, misclassification may be less of a concern because it may still be possible to detect an attenuated association. Refinement of case definitions can also be useful during the analysis of data to enhance specificity.

For example, at the start of an investigation of a cluster of suspected influenza cases in a nursing home that occurred over two weeks, one might initially consider anyone in the nursing home with a febrile illness during that two-week period as a suspect case. Collecting additional information about the signs and symptoms of the clinical illness, such as presence of cough or sore throat, duration of illness, and laboratory data including results of respiratory specimen testing, allows further narrowing and refinement of the case definition. Later in the investigation, the case definition might thus become "any resident of the nursing home with laboratory-confirmed influenza infection with onset between June 4 and June 16."

Enhance Surveillance

When it is suspected that an outbreak is occurring, enhanced surveillance can be useful in identifying additional cases. Enhanced surveillance may involve both heightening awareness to increase passive case reports and implementing active surveillance.

For outbreaks requiring widespread notification of the health care community, multiple methods of Internet-based communication, including e-mail Listservs, message boards, and online surveys, as well as "broadcast faxes" to area health care providers, hospitals, emergency departments, laboratories and other relevant groups can be employed. Messages should contain current information about the outbreak, inform clinicians about the syndrome or case definition under surveillance, describe how reporting should be done, and provide contact numbers and resources for questions or additional information.

Key information and resources can also be posted on health department web pages and communicated through social media such as Facebook and Twitter (Howland and Conover, 2011). Such channels may also alert health authorities that an outbreak is occurring. In Minnesota, for example, the Department of Health was notified of multiple Facebook postings suggesting foodborne illness among attendees of a high school banquet. Investigation identified pasta prepared by a team member's parent as the source of the outbreak of Group A Streptococcus pharyngitis (Kemble *et al.*, 2013).

For large outbreaks or public health emergencies, press releases and the print, radio, online, and television media can also be employed. Outbreak epidemiologists should therefore have a good working relationship with their department's public information officer, designated spokesperson, or media liaison. Using the news media allows communication directly to the public for identifying cases in persons who may not have sought medical attention and for disseminating disease control recommendations.

Describe Occurrence of Cases According to Person, Place, and Time

Descriptive analysis reveals useful information about the basic features of the cases, the population affected, the geographic scope of the problem, and the pace at which the outbreak is evolving. Early descriptive analyses can also suggest potential etiologic agents, risk factors for acquisition, and mechanisms of transmission of infection. These clues can be a fertile source of hypotheses that can then be tested with analytic study designs, as described below.

To begin, a *line list* of the cases is prepared, as illustrated in Table 20.1. It shows demographic characteristics and other key descriptors, including components of the case definition and laboratory test results. This format allows quick examination for obvious common features or unusual values. The

TABLE 20.1. EXAMPLE OF A LINE LIST OF DATA ON HEPATITIS A CASES

Case #	Initials	Date of report	Date of onset	MD Dx	N	V	A	F	DU	J	IgM	Other	Age	Sex
1	JG	10/12	10/6	Hep A	+	+	+	+	+	+	+	AST↑	37	M
2	BC	10/12	10/5	Hep A	+	−	+	+	+	+	+	ALT↑	62	F
3	HP	10/13	10/4	Hep A	±	−	+	+	+	S†	+	AST↑	30	F
4	MC	10/15	10/4	Hep A	−	−	+	+	?	−	+	HbSAg −	17	F
5	NG	10/15	10/9	NA	−	−	+	−	+	+	NA	NA	32	F
6	RD	10/15	10/8	Hep A	+	+	+	+	+	+	+		38	M
7	KR	10/16	10/13	Hep A	±	−	+	+	+	+	+	AST↑	43	M
8	DM	10/16	10/12	Hep A	−	−	+	+	+	−	+		57	M
9	PA	10/18	10/7	Hep A	±	−	+	±	+	+	+		52	F

The table columns are grouped under: "Diagnostic" spanning "Signs and symptoms*" (N, V, A, F, DU, J) and "Lab" spanning "HA" (IgM, Other).

*KEY:

S† = scleral icterus   F = fever
N = nausea   DU = dark urine
V = vomiting   J = jaundice
A = anorexia   HA IgM = hepatitis A IgM antibody test

(Adapted from Dicker [1998])

line list can be created by hand initially for small outbreaks, or using computerized data management programs or spreadsheets to allow easy viewing of multiple variables. For cohort studies of foodborne and other types of outbreaks, line lists should also include rows for the comparison group within the cohort who did not become ill, and columns for individual exposures under investigation.

Data in the line list can be analyzed using simple descriptive statistics, such as counts, percentages, means, and standard deviations; t-tests and Chi-square tests can be employed to examine differences in key demographics.

Characteristics of the illness can be summarized, and the most frequent signs and symptoms may suggest a likely differential diagnosis if the agent has not yet been identified. Pre-established criteria, such as the Kaplan criteria used for diagnosing suspect outbreaks of norovirus, may help rule a suspect etiology in or out in the absence of confirmatory testing (Karagiannis *et al.*, 2010). The Kaplan criteria are:

1. A mean (or median) illness duration of 12 to 60 hours,
2. A mean (or median) incubation period of 24 to 48 hours,
3. More than 50% of people with vomiting, and
4. No bacterial agent found.

Given the scenario of multiple people ill with vomiting and diarrhea of 24 hours duration among attendees of a child care center in January, health officials would be likely to hypothesize that an outbreak of norovirus is occurring.

If the disease has been definitively diagnosed, hypotheses regarding source of exposure and transmission can be developed based on known risk factors, incubation period, and known vehicles for that disease. For example, an outbreak of invasive *Listeria* infections among pregnant Hispanic women suggested a possible foodborne source, later found to be a commercially produced Mexican cheese (Jackson *et al.*, 2011).

Plotting the location where cases reside, work, or engage in recreational activities on spot maps or using geographic information system (GIS) software can assist in identifying potential sources of exposure or routes of transmission. John Snow used spot maps such as the one shown in Fig. 7–9 in his investigations of the 1854 cholera epidemic in central London to illustrate the distribution of cholera cases in Golden Square, showing that cholera deaths were strikingly common around the Broad Street water pump (Snow, 1936). Mapping software programs available today are complex and often require specially trained staff.

Spot maps may be useful when the source of infection is unknown, in order to search for clustering of cases by location of home, work, or recreational activities. They can later be used to show important

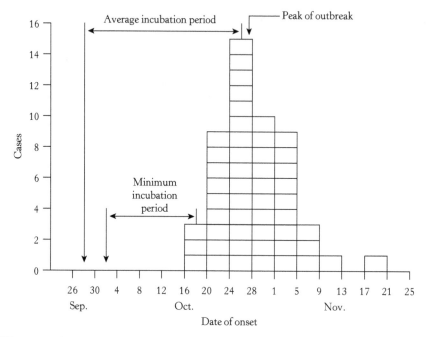

FIGURE 20.1 Epidemic curve from an outbreak of hepatitis A.
(Based on data from Dicker [1998])

spatial or geographic relationships once the source or mode of transmission has been identified. Examples include outbreaks caused by common-source exposure to contaminated aerosols, such as legionellosis associated with contaminated cooling towers, decorative fountains, or other sources of aerosol transmission; enteric infections resulting from exposure to contaminated recreational water; and institutional outbreaks in which visualizing spatial relationships among infected persons and potential sources of infection (other patients, environmental reservoirs, or caregivers) may be informative. However, for many outbreaks in a mobile society, cases will have been infected in distant locations or through exposure to widely distributed commercial food products, which will not be reflected in spot maps depicting only their local activities.

The *epidemic curve* is a standard part of the descriptive epidemiologic analysis. The date (or time) of onset is shown on the X-axis, while the number of new cases with onset in each date or time category is plotted on the Y-axis. Potentially significant case data, such as disease severity, confirmed versus suspect cases, or exposure to some suspected risk factor, can be indicated with different colors or fill patterns.

To produce the most informative epidemic curve, the scale of the X-axis should depend upon the incubation period of the disease (if known) and should include the pre-outbreak period to illustrate the background incidence of the disease. For most outbreaks, a useful scale will indicate time in units approximately one quarter the length of the incubation period. If the disease being investigated has not yet been identified, plotting the data on a variety of scales may reveal a pattern.

When the usual incubation period of the disease is known, and if most or all cases in an initial wave were exposed at about the same time, the epidemic curve can often be used to reveal the likely time of that exposure. For example, consider the epidemic curve from an outbreak of hepatitis A, as shown in Fig. 20.1. The incubation period of hepatitis A averages about 28–30 days, ranging from 15 to 50 days between exposure and onset of symptoms (Heymann, 2008). Suppose that all of the cases shown were suspected of having resulted from a common exposure to a single index case, such as an ill food worker. The analyst would count back 15 days from the earliest case, and 28–30 days from the peak of cases, to focus the investigation on a narrow range of days within which the common exposure may have occurred.

The shape of the epidemic curve often provides information about the likely mode of transmission. A "point source" outbreak, in which all cases were exposed to a single source of infection (a common meal or highly contagious person, for example), classically exhibits a steep upswing and an early peak, followed by a gradual decline in cases (Fig. 20.1). All cases in a point source outbreak should also have onset of illness within one incubation period. Prolonged exposure of a population to a common source (such as a contaminated food product with a long shelf life) will produce a more "smeared-out" epidemic curve in which onset of cases extends well beyond a single incubation period, reflecting a series of "mini-outbreaks." In contrast, ongoing person-to-person (secondary) transmission classically produces an epidemic curve with a series of small peaks—ideally one incubation period apart, although such a regular pattern is often difficult to demonstrate.

The epidemic curve can also provide clues about the course of the outbreak: a rising curve suggests that the outbreak is in the early stages; a plateau suggests that transmission may be stable or decreasing; and a downward slope suggests that the outbreak is waning. This information is helpful in planning disease control strategy, anticipating resource needs, evaluating interventions, and communicating with outbreak response partners and the public.

As the investigation develops and data on cases are entered into a database, more detailed and sophisticated epidemic curves can be created that convey additional information about primary and secondary cases and the timing of relevant events and interventions.

Develop Hypotheses About the Nature of the Exposure(s) Responsible for the Outbreak

The information needed for the initial line list of cases and for initial descriptive analyses may be obtained through interviews with cases and/or medical record reviews. For most outbreaks of reportable diseases with well-recognized routes of transmission, standardized interview forms are available at local and state health departments and from CDC. Staff of these agencies can often provide technical assistance as well.

For situations in which the clinical illness is not yet characterized, or the route or source of transmission appears to be new, an open-ended, unstructured interview with early cases and other key informants (such as family members or providers) can provide valuable information. These exploratory interviews should usually cover a wide range of potential risk factors and exposures, such as lifestyle characteristics, exposure to the outdoors, homelessness, or other factors. It is helpful if the same person can conduct these initial interviews. If the interviewer hears a similar story several times, patterns of exposure may emerge. Also, it is often worthwhile to ask the patient and family members where or how they think the illness was acquired. They may have already figured it out, and at the very least they will be more cooperative because they have been asked for their opinions. Other good sources of hypotheses can be subject-matter experts (infectious disease specialists, public health veterinarians, laboratorians, toxicologists, industrial hygienists, water system or air handling experts, etc.) and the medical literature.

Outliers are cases that are unusual in some way—they "just don't fit in" with the rest of the cases—and should be carefully scrutinized. Temporal outliers are usually easy to identify on the epidemic curve and often provide the key to understanding the basis for the outbreak. For instance, a single case occurring one incubation period before the other cases may represent an ill food handler who contaminated a food product, or an index case who exposed a large group of susceptible people. Cases who were only in the geographic area a short time can, by their limited opportunities for exposure, also provide valuable information about means of transmission. Similarly, foodborne outbreaks in which most cases and controls ate the same food items can sometimes be solved if "dietary" outliers who consumed only one of several potentially contaminated items are identified.

Hypothesis generation may lead to a list of additional information needed, such as exposure details, medical history, or laboratory data. This list can then be used to develop more refined case investigation forms for use in collecting additional data.

Conduct Analytic Studies

Once a set of hypotheses has been developed, an analytic study—usually a case-control or cohort study—is often the appropriate next step.

Study Design

Choice of a study design depends both on theoretical considerations (see Chapter 5), such as frequency of the disease and of key exposures, and on logistics and data availability. If the outbreak occurs in a discrete, readily identified group, such as a wedding party or passengers on a cruise ship, a cohort study is the preferred option. As many members of the group as possible should be interviewed. Cohort studies are discussed in Chapter 14. In contrast, if cases are few or occur among a widely scattered group, it may be more efficient to conduct a case-control study, sampling appropriate non-ill controls from the presumed population at risk. This study design is discussed at length in Chapter 15.

In certain instances, case-case studies can be conducted, saving valuable time and resources by using cases with the same illness, but who are not associated with the outbreak, as the comparison group. These cases may occur concurrently with the outbreak-associated cases but have a different strain of the pathogen, or may be temporally matched cases from previous years for whom detailed exposure data already exists. For example, in September 2011, an unusually high number of cases of listeriosis were reported in Colorado residents. Because listeriosis is a relatively rare and severe illness, detailed exposure information is routinely collected on all reported cases. Investigators were able to compare exposures from the first 19 outbreak-associated cases with 85 age- and temporally matched *Listeria* cases from 2004–2010 and found a strong association with cantaloupe consumption (odds ratio=14.9; 95% CI = 2.4 – ∞), leading to a rapid product recall (Centers for Disease Control and Prevention, 2011).

A few study design issues of special relevance to outbreak investigation will be discussed below. In an outbreak situation, the working case-definition often limits cases in time and vicinity, and these limits should also pertain to controls. Ideally, controls should be persons who did not develop the disease but who met all other criteria that defined the cases. If the outbreak occurred among patrons of an outdoor festival, for example, controls should be chosen from among attendees of the festival; if at a potluck supper, from among those who attended the supper (or unsuspecting family members who ate the leftovers).

Nonetheless, care should be taken not to overmatch or restrict controls in such a way that exposure to a risk factor of interest is essentially predetermined. For example, consider an outbreak of shigellosis among children who visited a recreational area with a swimming pool. A reasonable control group would be children in the same age range without signs or symptoms of *Shigella* infection who also frequented the recreational area during the exposure period of the cases. If one selected as controls only children who also swam in the pool (i.e., matched on swimming history), the analysis would not be able to determine whether exposure to the possibly contaminated pool water was a risk factor for infection.

Data Collection

In general, the farther in time the investigation is conducted after the relevant exposure has taken place, the more difficult it is to get complete and accurate information from both cases and controls about potential risk factors of interest. In addition, with time it becomes more difficult for controls to recall events with as much certainty as cases, who were more affected and may be more closely scrutinizing their recent exposures. This difference can contribute to recall bias (see Chapter 15). Thus, the time spent to develop the data collection instruments must be balanced by the need for a prompt investigation. Not uncommonly, the data instruments will appear flawed in retrospect. Outbreak investigation forms must often be created "on the fly," without the luxury of time for the methodical planning that is available in elective studies. For event-based outbreaks, online surveys can often be distributed electronically to ill and non-ill attendees. These surveys have the advantage of rapidly gathering exposure and illness information without requiring staff time to conduct telephone or in-person interviews, though the level of response to such surveys may be variable.

In addition, with the advent of warehouse and supermarket membership or "shopper" cards, investigators can obtain dates of purchase, brand names, and lot numbers to fill in gaps in information gathered from case interviews. For case clusters with no obvious common exposures beyond supermarket memberships, comparing purchase records can also be essential during the hypothesis-generation stages of an investigation. While use of shopper cards may expedite source identification and the product traceback and recall process, care must be taken to respect the privacy of cases and limit record access to the minimum necessary to further the investigation. In 2010, after several months of investigation into an increase in *Salmonella* Montevideo cases where no source was identified, health officials in Washington State obtained permission from cases to review their purchase records from a large membership warehouse. The record review identified salami products from a single company among the majority of cases, and the outbreak was ultimately traced back to contaminated red and black pepper used to season the deli meats (Centers for Disease Control and Prevention, 2010).

As in elective analytic studies, attention should be paid to minimizing measurement error during collection of data. Helpful techniques include using preexisting questions or instruments; training interviewers to collect data in a standard way, especially if two or more interviewers are needed; and using standardized visual aids such as calendars to help respondents recall the timing of events. Pilot testing of questionnaires and blinding of interviewers to disease status is desirable but often impossible in an outbreak situation.

Special care is needed in interviewing persons under the legal age of consent, which requires permission of a parent or guardian. If interviews are conducted in person, the parent/guardian should be present. If interviews are by telephone, having the parent listen in on another phone line is often reassuring to the parent and can sometimes help the interviewee with recall.

If the outbreak etiology is unknown, it is important to collect necessary biological specimens as soon as possible to establish the diagnosis, isolate the etiologic agent, or further characterize the clinical syndrome. At times, nurses and other investigators with clinical skills collect specimens in the field (e.g., through phlebotomy, or throat or skin cultures). For presumed foodborne outbreaks, cases should be asked to retain and refrigerate any leftover suspect foods, including the original packaging when available. Outbreak investigators may need to issue recommendations to health care providers and laboratories on procedures for diagnostic testing and handling of clinical specimens. Clinical laboratories often discard culture isolates and other diagnostic specimens after a few days unless specifically requested to do otherwise. Local laboratories should be contacted as early as possible to request that specimens be conserved or sent on to the local or state public health department laboratory.

Another reason for prompt specimen collection is that cases are generally most interested in cooperating with the investigation when they are currently or recently symptomatic. Once recovered, they soon tire of requests for additional stool specimens or blood samples, or even one more telephone interview. If specimen collection is crucial to the investigation, it is often worth the effort to send someone directly to the field (e.g., home, restaurant, etc.) to collect appropriate specimens.

The environmental field investigation is often carried out by one or more environmental health specialists working with the communicable disease epidemiologist. The field team should be briefed on the situation; specifically what samples and/or other information are needed. Some field investigations may include assessment and/or sampling of wildlife, water supplies, or potentially toxic substances. In these scenarios, wildlife biologists, public health veterinarians, ecologists, or occupational health specialists may be desirable members of the team. It is important to assure that when necessary, field staff have the appropriate personal protective equipment and are trained in its proper use. Field staff should have documentation of vaccination or immunity against diseases to which they may be exposed during investigations.

The first visit by the field team is the best opportunity to observe pertinent behaviors (e.g. food safety practices, hygiene, infection control practices) and to obtain environmental samples. In foodborne outbreaks, information on suspect products and the methods of preparation may be crucial, including brand name, lot number, size of package used, expiration date, delivery date, and supplier (to assist in traceback efforts when indicated), as well as food preparation, holding, and storage conditions. Personnel (including supervisors) involved in handling and preparing implicated food items should be identified and interviewed about food preparation and handling practices and recent illness. When possible, clinical specimens should be obtained from staff that are ill and/or are suspected of serving as a reservoir for the infectious agent. It may be difficult in these situations to determine whether staff who test positive represent a cause of illness, or were exposed to the same contaminated source as the other cases.

Analysis

Additional analytic studies are used to more completely describe the affected population, risk factors for disease, and mechanisms of transmission. As data come in, they should be examined for completeness and consistency; these data are typically then entered into computerized databases. EpiInfo is a software program developed specifically to support data management and analysis for outbreak investigations; it can be downloaded free of charge from the World Wide Web. Preparing mock-up tables early, even before data-collection instruments are finalized, can help guide the analysis, identify gaps, and anticipate the need to reconcile data from different sources (e.g., different laboratories) onto a common scale.

Outbreaks often evolve over a short time, during which changes in the population at risk may be minor. Hence disease frequency is often expressed in terms of the "attack rate"—technically, not a true "rate" but another term for cumulative incidence. The difference between the attack rates in persons with and without a certain exposure is thus the attributable risk, and the ratio of the two attack rates is the relative risk, as was discussed in Chapter 9. These measures of effect can be used to quantify associations, and hypotheses can be tested quickly using simple cross-tabulations (Bryan et al., 1999). In the example shown in Table 20.2, 120 persons out of 200 attendees became ill. The relative risk and the attributable risk for roast turkey both show a large positive association with illness, suggesting a possible causal relationship. Conversely, eating roast pork was negatively associated with illness, perhaps because those who chose pork avoided the turkey. The other associations are weak and do not suggest that these food items were related to becoming ill.

A second issue to consider is the fraction of cases that each exposure under consideration could account for—the population attributable risk percent—which depends on both the relative risk and the proportion of cases exposed to each item. In this example, while eating green beans was positively associated with illness ($RR = 1.18$), only 63 of the 120 ill persons recalled having eaten green beans, so that this exposure (even if it truly were a cause of illness) could account for only $(1.18 -$ $1)/1.18 \times (63/120) = 0.08 = 8\%$ of cases. Roast turkey, besides being more strongly associated with illness, was eaten by 104 of the 120 ill persons and therefore could account for about $(4.35 - 1)/4.35 \times (104/120) = 0.67 = 67\%$ of cases. When no single food item or multiple food items (especially those that are ready-to-eat) are significantly associated with illness, it may point to broad contamination during food preparation from contaminated equipment or environmental surfaces or by an ill food handler.

Implement Disease Control Interventions

The results of preliminary and analytical studies often implicate a particular exposure. Intervention approaches to prevent additional cases or future outbreaks depend on that exposure and on what is already known about the disease's mechanism of spread. Among many examples are recalling a contaminated product from distribution, correcting deficient food-handling practices, and administering medication, immune globulin and/or vaccine to susceptible persons. Such efforts can involve multiple regulatory agencies and or members of the health-care community and highlight the importance of keeping contact lists current and maintaining good communication, as described below. Subsequently, the results of outbreak investigations can be used to support policy changes to decrease the risk for future outbreaks.

Communication

Effective, clear, and timely communication is a critical component of any outbreak investigation. Important target groups and forms of communication include:

TABLE 20.2. ATTACK RATE TABLE FOR A HYPOTHETICAL FOODBORNE DISEASE OUTBREAK ($N = 200$)

	Ate			Did not eat			Attributable risk	Relative risk
	Ill	Not ill	Attack rate	Ill	Not ill	Attack rate		
Roast turkey	104	15	$104/119 = 0.87$	16	65	$16/81 = 0.20$	+0.67	4.35
Roast pork	15	45	$15/60 = 0.25$	105	35	$105/140 = 0.75$	−0.50	0.33
Mashed potatoes	102	77	$102/179 = 0.57$	13	8	$13/21 = 0.62$	−0.05	0.92
Green beans	63	34	$63/97 = 0.65$	57	46	$57/103 = 0.55$	+0.10	1.18
Rolls	87	59	$87/146 = 0.60$	33	21	$33/54 = 0.61$	−0.01	0.98
Apple pie	76	50	$76/126 = 0.60$	44	30	$44/74 = 0.59$	+0.01	1.02

- *The public.* Relevant information often includes the signs and symptoms of the disease, and recommendations for evaluation, treatment, and prevention of illness. Information can be disseminated through information hotlines with recorded messages, Web pages, press releases or other news media channels (National Research Council, 1989; Covello *et al.*, 2001). It is important to compose public information in clear language that is understandable by the community. Translation of materials into other languages and outreach to target specific cultural groups or hard-to-reach populations may be necessary.

- *Outbreak response team members.* Outbreak investigations often require coordinating the efforts of several people. Weekly or more frequent team meetings are needed to review the status of the outbreak, share information, and update and revise the investigation and response plan. Meeting frequency and participants includes will depend on the pace and specific nature of individual outbreaks. It may be useful to invite the public information officer and representatives from other affected local or state agencies to these sessions. The outbreak team leader needs to manage the overall response, anticipate where the investigation is headed, and ensure that adequate resources are available to sustain the investigation and response activities as long as necessary.

- *Public health and government officials.* It is a good idea for the outbreak epidemiologist to keep his or her supervisor aware of the status of an investigation. Health officers and elected officials often do not appreciate learning about outbreaks for the first time through inquiries from local news media.

- *Local health care workers.* Local environmental health staff, infection control practitioners, infectious disease experts, and other medical and health care professionals are natural partners in investigations. Having preexisting relationships and contact information readily available is very helpful.

- *Other potentially affected government agencies.* At times, what appears to be a localized outbreak or cluster of cases is actually part of a larger regional, national, or even international outbreak that is not initially recognized. If circumstances suggest that the local cases might be part of a larger outbreak (e.g., possibly involving a commercially prepared product with wide distribution, or a travel-associated outbreak), consultation with regional or national health officials is recommended, even before confirmatory laboratory test results are available. These agencies can also provide help in confirming and investigating outbreaks when local resources are not adequate. In addition, for outbreaks involving commercial products or multiple states or countries, federal agricultural or pharmaceutical agencies (e.g., CDC, FDA, U.S. Department of Agriculture) may take the lead on coordinating the outbreak response with support from local partners. Daily scheduled conference calls can be useful in addition to updates as needed to communicate new information. It is wise to know in advance who the relevant contacts are at local, state, and federal agencies and have methods to communicate with them after business hours.

CONCLUSION

Conducting an outbreak investigation can be an exciting and rewarding, as well as a challenging, experience. Good analytical, social, and political skills can help open doors for the epidemiologist, both by aiding the prompt gathering of accurate information and by communicating results and recommendations to the public.

It is not necessary to "reinvent the wheel" when conducting an outbreak investigation. Readily available reference materials provide an overview of best practices and detailed guidelines for outbreak investigation activities. Examples of these resources, available on the World Wide Web, include CDC's *Manual for the Surveillance of Vaccine-Preventable Diseases* (2013a) and the Council to Improve Foodborne Outbreak Response (CIFOR) *Guidelines for Foodborne Outbreak Response* (2013).

There are lessons to be learned from every outbreak. A formal outbreak review process or debriefing is often worthwhile after a large or complicated outbreak, to evaluate what worked and what did not. Such a review can involve representatives from many agencies and professional areas, and information from it can lead to appropriate changes in the response to future outbreaks.

Outbreak investigations can also provide an opportunity to deliver public health messages to the community. While most public health work takes place quietly behind the scenes, outbreak investigations are often the focus of intense community interest and media scrutiny. Carefully crafted communications can make a lasting impression that may favorably affect risk behavior in the population. A well-conducted outbreak investigation can also increase the public's understanding of, and appreciation for, the work that public health professionals do.

REFERENCES

Adderson E, Pavia A, Christenson J, Davis R, Leonard R, Carroll K. A community pseudo-outbreak of invasive *Staphylococcus aureus* infection. Diagn Microbiol Infect Dis 2000; 37:219–221.

Baer A, Elbert Y, Burkom HS, Holtry R, Lombardo JS, Duchin JS. Usefulness of syndromic data sources for investigating morbidity resulting from a severe weather event. Disaster Med Public Health Prep 2011; 5:37–45.

Becker KM, Moe CL, Southwick KL, MacCormack JN. Transmission of Norwalk virus during football game. N Engl J Med 2000; 343:1223–1227.

Bell BP, Goldoft M, Griffin PM, Davis MA, Gordon DC, Tarr PI, et al. A multistate outbreak of *Escherichia coli* O157:H7-associated bloody diarrhea and hemolytic uremic syndrome from hamburgers. The Washington experience. JAMA 1994; 272:1349–1353.

Bell BP, Khabbaz RF. Responding to the outbreak of invasive fungal infections: the value of public health to Americans. JAMA 2013; 309:883–884.

Bell BP, Shapiro CN, Alter MJ, Moyer LA, Judson FN, Mottram K, et al. The diverse patterns of hepatitis A epidemiology in the United States—implications for vaccination strategies. J Infect Dis 1998; 178:1579–1584.

Belongia EA, Hedberg CW, Gleich GJ, White KE, Mayeno AN, Loegering DA, et al. An investigation of the cause of the eosinophilia-myalgia syndrome associated with tryptophan use. N Engl J Med 1990; 323:357–365.

Bender JB, Hedberg CW, Besser JM, Boxrud DJ, MacDonald KL, Osterholm MT. Surveillance by molecular subtype for *Escherichia coli* O157:H7 infections in Minnesota by molecular subtyping. N Engl J Med 1997; 337:388–394.

Bender JB, Hedberg CW, Boxrud DJ, Besser JM, Wicklund JH, Smith KE, et al. Use of molecular subtyping in surveillance for *Salmonella enterica* serotype typhimurium. N Engl J Med 2001; 344:189–195.

Breuer T, Benkel DH, Shapiro RL, Hall WN, Winnett MM, Linn MJ, et al. A multistate outbreak of *Escherichia coli* O157:H7 infections linked to alfalfa sprouts grown from contaminated seeds. Emerg Infect Dis 2001; 7:977–982.

Bryan FL, Bartleson CA, Cook OD, et al. Procedures to investigate foodborne illness (5th ed.). Des Moines, IA: International Association of Milk, Food, and Environmental Sanitarians, Inc., 1999.

Bush LM, Abrams BH, Beall A, Johnson CC. Index case of fatal inhalational anthrax due to bioterrorism in the United States. N Engl J Med 2001; 345:1607–1610.

Carter AO, Borczyk AA, Carlson JAK, Harvey B, Hockin JC, Karmali MA, et al. A severe outbreak of *Escherichia coli* O157:H7-associated hemorrhaghic colitis in a nursing home. N Engl J Med 1987; 317:1496–1500.

Centers for Disease Control and Prevention. Pneumocystis pneumonia—Los Angeles. MMWR Morb Mortal Wkly Rep 1981; 30:250–252.

Centers for Disease Control and Prevention. Update: impact of the expanded AIDS surveillance case definition for adolescents and adults on case reporting—United States, 1993. MMWR Morb Mortal Wkly Rep 1994; 43:160–1, 167–170.

Centers for Disease Control and Prevention. Enhanced detection of sporadic *Escherichia coli* O157:H7 infections—New Jersey, July 1994. MMWR Morb Mortal Wkly Rep 1995; 44:417–418.

Centers for Disease Control and Prevention. Outbreaks of pseudo-infection with *Cyclospora* and *Cryptosporidium*—Florida and New York City, 1995. MMWR Morb Mortal Wkly Rep 1997; 46: 354–358.

Centers for Disease Control and Prevention. Legionnaires' disease associated with potting soil—California, Oregon, and Washington, May–June 2000. MMWR Morb Mortal Wkly Rep 2000; 49:777–778.

Centers for Disease Control and Prevention. Outbreak of *Salmonella* serotype Kottbus infections associated with eating alfalfa sprouts—Arizona, California, Colorado, and New Mexico, February–April 2001. MMWR Morb Mortal Wkly Rep 2002a; 51:7–9.

Centers for Disease Control and Prevention. Rashes among schoolchildren—14 states, October 4, 2001–February 27, 2002. MMWR Morb Mortal Wkly Rep 2002b; 51:161–164.

Centers for Disease Control and Prevention. Multistate outbreak of *Salmonella* serotype Tennessee infections associated with peanut butter—United States, 2006–2007. MMWR Morb Mortal Wkly Rep 2007; 56:521–524.

Centers for Disease Control and Prevention. Multistate outbreak of *Salmonella* infections associated with frozen pot pies—United States, 2007. MMWR Morb Mortal Wkly Rep 2008; 57:1277–1280.

Centers for Disease Control and Prevention. *Salmonella* Montevideo infections associated with salami products made with contaminated imported black and red pepper—United States, July 2009–April 2010. MMWR Morb Mortal Wkly Rep 2010; 59:1647–1650.

Centers for Disease Control and Prevention. Multistate outbreak of listeriosis associated with Jensen Farms cantaloupe—United States, August–September 2011. MMWR Morb Mortal Wkly Rep 2011; 60: 1357–1358.

Centers for Disease Control and Prevention. Manual for the surveillance of vaccine-preventable diseases (6th ed.). http://www.cdc.gov/vaccines/pubs/surv-manual, 2013a.

Centers for Disease Control and Prevention. Notes from the field: serogroup C invasive meningococcal disease among men who have sex with men—New York City, 2010–2012. MMWR Morb Mortal Wkly Rep 2013b; 61:1048.

Council to Improve Foodborne Outbreak Response. Guidelines for foodborne outbreak response. http://www.cifor.us/CIFORGuidelinesProjectMore.cfm, 2013.

Covello VT, Peters RG, Wojtecki JG, Hyde RC. Risk communication, the West Nile virus epidemic, and bioterrorism: responding to the communication challenges posed by the intentional or unintentional release of a pathogen in an urban setting. J Urban Health 2001; 78:382–391.

Den Boer JW, Yzerman EP, Schellekens J, Lettinga KD, Boshuizen HC, Van Steenbergen JE, et al. A large outbreak of Legionnaires' disease at a flower show, the Netherlands, 1999. Emerg Infect Dis 2002; 8:37–43.

Dicker R. Principles of epidemiology. An introduction to applied epidemiology and biostatistics (2nd ed.). Atlanta, GA: Centers for Disease Control and Prevention, 1998.

Duchin JS, Koster FT, Peters CJ, Simpson GL, Tempest B, Zaki SR, et al. Hantavirus pulmonary syndrome: a clinical description of 17 patients with a newly recognized disease. The Hantavirus Study Group. N Engl J Med 1994; 330:949–955.

European Centre for Disease Prevention and Control. A cluster of invasive meningococcal disease in young men who have sex with men in Berlin, October 2012 to May 2013. Euro Surveill 2013; 18:pii=20523.

Falsey RR, Kinzer MH, Hurst S, Kalus A, Pottinger PS, Duchin JS, et al. Cutaneous inoculation of nontuberculous mycobacteria during professional tattooing: a case series and epidemiologic study. Clin Infect Dis 2013; 57:e143–147.

Fraser DW, Tsai TR, Orenstein W, Parkin WE, Beecham HJ, Sharrar RG, et al. Legionnaires' disease: description of an epidemic of pneumonia. N Engl J Med 1977; 297:1189–1197.

Glatzel M, Rogivue C, Ghani A, Streffer JR, Amsler L, Aguzzi A. Incidence of Creutzfeldt-Jakob disease in Switzerland. Lancet 2002; 360:139–141.

Goering RV, Köck R, Grundmann H, Werner G, Friedrich AW, ESCMID Study Group for Epidemiological Markers (ESGEM). From theory to practice: molecular strain typing for the clinical and public health setting. Euro Surveill 2013; 18:20383.

Henricks WH. "Meaningful use" of electronic health records and its relevance to laboratories and pathologists. J Pathol Inform 2011; 2:7.

Heymann D (ed.). Control of communicable diseases manual (19th ed.). Washington, D.C.: American Public Health Association, 2008.

Holzbauer SM, DeVries AS, Sejvar JJ, Lees CH, Adjemian J, McQuiston JH, et al. Epidemiologic investigation of immune-mediated polyradiculoneuropathy among abattoir workers exposed to porcine brain. PLoS One 2010; 5:e9782.

Howland JF, Conover C. Social network as outbreak investigation tool. Emerg Infect Dis 2011; 17: 1765–1766.

Jackson KA, Biggerstaff M, Tobin-D'Angelo M, Sweat D, Klos R, Nosari J, et al. Multistate outbreak of *Listeria monocytogenes* associated with Mexican-style cheese made from pasteurized milk among pregnant, Hispanic women. J Food Prot 2011; 74:949–953.

Joce RE, Murphy F, Robertson MH. A pseudo-outbreak of salmonellosis. Epidemiol Infect 1995; 115:31–38.

Kainer MA, Reagan DR, Nguyen DB, Wiese AD, Wise ME, Ward J, et al. Fungal infections associated with contaminated methylprednisolone in Tennessee. N Engl J Med 2012; 367:2194–2203.

Karagiannis I, Detsis M, Gkolfinopoulou K, Pervanidou D, Panagiotopoulos T, Bonovas S. An outbreak of gastroenteritis linked to seafood consumption in a remote Northern Aegean island, February–March 2010. Rural Remote Health 2010; 10:1507.

Kemble SK, Westbrook A, Lynfield R, Bogard A, Koktavy N, Gall K, et al. Foodborne outbreak of Group A streptococcus pharyngitis associated with a high school dance team banquet—Minnesota, 2012. Clin Infect Dis 2013; 57:648–654.

LeBlanc PM, Hollinger KA, Klontz KC. Tattoo ink-related infections—awareness, diagnosis, reporting, and prevention. N Engl J Med 2012; 367: 985–987.

Mishu B, Koehler J, Lee LA, Rodrigue D, Brenner FH, Blake P, et al. Outbreaks of *Salmonella* Enteritidis infections in the United States, 1985–1991. J Infect Dis 1994; 169:547–552.

Mohle-Boetani JC, Farrar JA, Werner SB, Minassian D, Bryant R, Abbott S, et al. Escherichia coli O157 and Salmonella infections associated with sprouts in California, 1996–1998. Ann Intern Med 2001; 135:239–247.

National Notifiable Disease Surveillance System. Case definitions. http://wwwn.cdc.gov/nndss/script/casedefDefault.aspx, 2013.

National Research Council. Improving risk communication. Washington, DC: National Academy Press, 1989.

Pettit AC, Kropski JA, Castilho JL, Schmitz JE, Rauch CA, Mobley BC, et al. The index case for the fungal meningitis outbreak in the United States. N Engl J Med 2012; 367:2119–2125.

Qureshi K, Gebbie KM, Gebbie EN. Public health incident command system, Vol. 1. http://www.ualbanyc-php.org/pinata/phics/guide, 2006.

Reilley B, Van Herp M, Sermand D, Dentico N. SARS and Carlo Urbani. N Engl J Med 2003; 348:1951–1952.

Shands KN, Schmid GP, Dan BB, Blum D, Guidotti RJ, Hargrett NT, et al. Toxic-shock syndrome in menstruating women: association with tampon use and Staphylococcus aureus and clinical features in 52 cases. N Engl J Med 1980; 303:1436–1442.

Snow J. Snow on cholera. New York: Commonwealth Fund, 1936.

St Louis ME, Morse DL, Potter ME, DeMelfi TM, Guzewich JJ, Tauxe RV, et al. The emergence of grade A eggs as a major source of Salmonella Enteritidis infections. New implications for the control of salmonellosis. JAMA 1988; 259:2103–2107.

Steere AC, Malawista SE, Snydman DR, Shope RE, Andiman WA, Ross MR, et al. Lyme arthritis: an epidemic of oligoarticular arthritis in children and adults in three Connecticut communities. Arthritis Rheum 1977; 20:7–17.

Swaminathan B, Barrett TJ, Hunter SB, Tauxe RV. PulseNet: the molecular subtyping network for foodborne bacterial disease surveillance, United States. Emerg Infect Dis 2001; 7:382–389.

Tavernise S. Charges filed in peanut Salmonella case (February 22, 2013 p.B5). New York Times, 2013.

US Department of Health and Human Services. Consumers advised of risks associated with raw sprouts. HHS News PS99-13. Washington, D.C.: U.S. Department of Health and Human Services, 1999.

Wasley A, Samandari T, Bell BP. Incidence of hepatitis A in the United States in the era of vaccination. JAMA 2005; 294:194–201.

Weinbaum CM, Bodnar UR, Schulte J, Atkinson B, Morgan MT, Caliper TE, et al. Pseudo-outbreak of tuberculosis infection due to improper skin-test reading. Clin Infect Dis 1998; 26:1235–1236.

Weiss NS. Epidemiologic studies in which a necessary cause is known. Epidemiology 1991; 2:153–154.

Wurtz R. The role of public health in health information exchanges. J Public Health Manag Pract 2013; 19:485–487.

EXERCISES

1. In September, 1985, an outbreak of E. coli O157:H7 gastroenteritis struck 55 of 169 residents of a nursing home in southwestern Ontario, plus 18 of 137 staff (Carter et al., 1987). This microorganism can be transmitted by ingestion of contaminated food (often inadequately cooked ground beef); by person-to-person spread in such groups as families, child care centers, or custodial institutions; or by swimming in or drinking contaminated water (Heymann, 2008). The incubation period ranges from 3–8 days, with a median of 3–4 days.

   The epidemic curves for staff (top panel) and residents (bottom panel) are shown in Fig. 20.2. From the information given, what would you consider to be the most likely way(s) by which the staff and residents became infected during this outbreak and when the key exposure(s) occurred? Briefly explain your answer.

2. An article in the New England Journal of Medicine described an outbreak of norovirus gastroenteritis among members and staff of a North Carolina football team in September 1998 (Becker et al., 2000). This illness is characterized by vomiting and diarrhea. The incubation period is 10–50 hours. Infection occurs by consumption of contaminated food, and person-to-person transmission can also occur from close physical contact. Fig. 20.3 shows the occurrence of cases among North Carolina players and staff in each 12-hour time period over the course of several days.

   (a) Imagine that you are a field epidemiologist working on this outbreak. What period of time would you investigate most closely for a point exposure that could have initiated the epidemic?

   (b) Suggest two plausible possibilities for why the cases did not all occur within one incubation period.

ANSWERS

1. The most prominent feature is a large wave of cases among residents occurring from September 9–14, within one incubation period. This is most easily explained by a point source exposure on or about September 6. Nursing-home residents rarely go

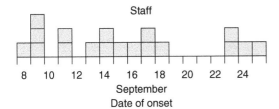

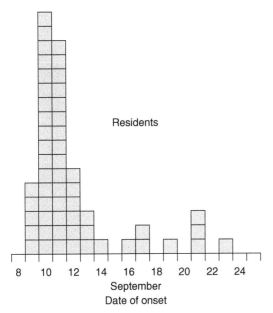

FIGURE 20.2 Epidemic curve from an outbreak of *E. coli* O157:H7 infection in a nursing home.
(Based on data from Carter *et al.* [1987])

swimming in large groups, so this seems an unlikely form of exposure. Person-to-person transmission is also unlikely to explain the large initial wave, for lack of an apparent index case and because one would have to assume intimate contact between that person and a very large number of residents over a very short period of time. A contaminated meal would be very plausible, however, as it could account for exposure of many residents at essentially the same point in time. (In fact, a lunch on September 5 was strongly implicated.)

Early cases among staff could have represented staff who ate some of the same contaminated food as residents. Later cases in staff and in residents may well have represented person-to-person transmission from earlier cases.

2. (a) The cases did not all occur within one incubation period. However, one would look especially closely at events on September 18, especially between noon and midnight that day. Given the incubation period of 10–50 hours, a point source exposure during this time period could potentially account for the 46 cases that occurred on September 19 and 20, as part of a single "wave." Further investigation of this outbreak did indeed implicate a box lunch shared by team members on September 18.

   (b) One possibility is a source of continuing exposure, such as contaminated foods or beverages consumed by team members repeatedly over a period of days. Another possibility is that later cases were infected via close contact with cases in a large initial wave. In this particular outbreak,

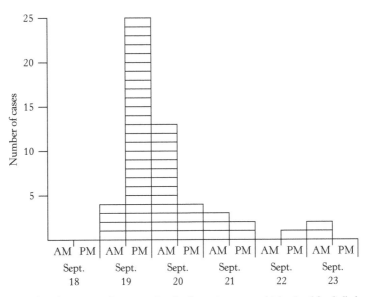

FIGURE 20.3 Initial epidemic curve from an outbreak of norovirus among high school football players.
(Based on data from Becker *et al.* [2000])

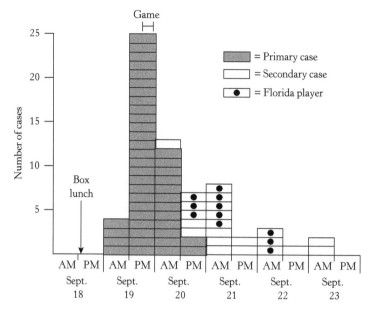

FIGURE 20.4 Final epidemic curve from an outbreak of norovirus among high school football players. (Based on data from Becker *et al.* [2000])

physical combat on the football field, and contact on the sidelines between healthy teammates and others who were actively sick, were thought to be major routes of exposure for the late-occurring cases. A more detailed epidemic curve is shown in Figure 20.4. Later cases, including some among members of the opposing Florida team, appeared likely to have been due to person-to-person transmission from those in the first wave who had eaten the tainted box lunch.

21

Evaluating the Effects of Policies on Health

The success or failure of any government in the final analysis must be measured by the well-being of its citizens. Nothing can be more important to a state than its public health; the state's paramount concern should be the health of its people.

—FRANKLIN D. ROOSEVELT

As we have seen throughout this book, epidemiology concerns the distribution and determinants of health and disease in human populations. A conceptual model of the determinants of population health proposed by an Institute of Medicine committee (Figure 21.1) posits that population health results from a nested set of determinants operating at different levels. Innermost are innate traits of individuals, such as age and gender, and disease biology. Working outward, factors at each level influence health via factors inside that level.

This chapter concerns part of the outermost box: *policies*. For present purposes, "policies" can be defined as governmental or institutional principles and strategies for achieving collective goals. Examples include laws, regulations, and decisions about resource allocation. Policies typically apply broadly to everyone in a certain population or defined subpopulation, such as the citizens of a governmental jurisdiction or the work force, clientele, or membership of an institution.

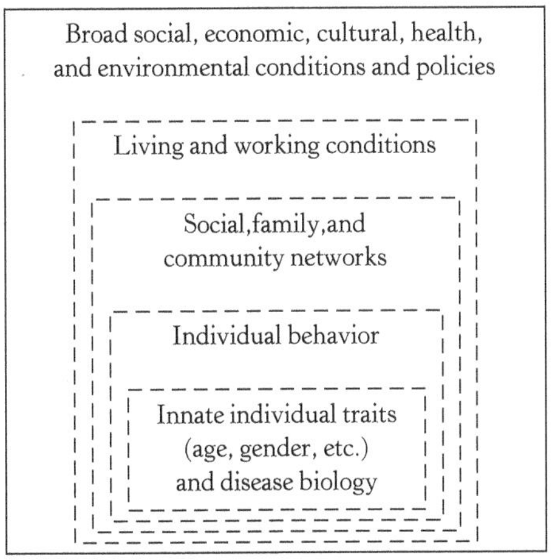

Policies can have many kinds of effects, both intended and unintended. The effects of policies on health fall within the purview of epidemiology, but other disciplines—economics, behavioral science, political science, environmental science, and others—also evaluate policies from their own perspectives. Comprehensive policy evaluation is thus a multidisciplinary enterprise. This chapter focuses on health effects, but many of the study designs and methodological ideas discussed here can also be applied to assessing effects on other kinds of outcomes.

FIGURE 21.1 A conceptual model of the determinants of population health.
(Adapted and reprinted with permission from Institute of Medicine [2003])

OVERVIEW OF EVALUATION DESIGNS

Evaluating the effects of a policy on health requires addressing two basic questions: (1) What health outcomes were observed when the policy was adopted? and (2) What would those outcomes have been without the policy? The policy's effects are gauged by comparing the two sets of answers. The specific measures of health of greatest interest as outcomes depend on the nature of the policy, but often they would be the kinds of disease-frequency measures used throughout this book. This view of policy evaluation applies the same basic strategy that underlies most analytic epidemiologic studies: assess the causal effects of an exposure by comparing outcomes among exposed persons with the estimated counterfactual outcomes that would have occurred among those persons had they not been exposed. However, some features of policies make them different from other kinds of exposures and require that a broader range of possible approaches to answering the second question be considered, which concerns estimating outcomes that would have been observed without the policy.

Although many policies apply broadly to everyone in a population or in a defined subpopulation, under some circumstances the nature of the policy or the context in which it is adopted lead to systematic differences in exposure to the policy within a population of interest. It may then be possible to exploit that within-population variation by treating the policy like any other exposure, using standard epidemiologic study designs such as randomized trials, cohort studies, or case-control studies, as illustrated below. An additional design, the regression discontinuity design, can also be applied to policy evaluation when actions taken under the policy depend on whether a person falls above or below some threshold value on a continuous characteristic, such as age or income.

Often, however, everyone in a population or subpopulation is exposed to a policy once adopted, thus precluding the possibility of comparing exposed and unexposed persons concurrently within the same population. Accordingly, ecological study designs play an important role in policy evaluation, as noted in Chapter 16. One family of ecological designs involves comparing outcomes in one or more populations exposed to the policy with outcomes in other concurrently studied populations not so exposed. Occasionally, it is even possible to randomize populations to either policy-exposed or policy-unexposed conditions. When randomization is not possible, a non-randomized ecological cohort design may be an option, in which a set of policy-exposed groups is compared with a set of policy-unexposed groups.

Ecological studies with concurrent controls have their limitations, however. The broader the scope of a policy, the harder it becomes to find one or more suitable comparison populations to serve as concurrent controls (Ray, 1997). As an extreme example, international policies aimed at restricting global warming would be impossible to evaluate in this way, due to the lack of comparison planets like the earth on which no such policy initiatives are adopted. A more feasible approach to estimating what would have happened without such a policy is to study the same population over time, comparing periods with and without the policy. The simplest such study design is a *before-after* study involving two time points or periods, one without the policy and one with it. An *interrupted time series* design extends this approach to multiple time points or periods before and after policy adoption.

The two general approaches just described—comparing populations with and without the policy concurrently, and comparing the same population over time—can be combined by comparing time trends in outcomes across populations that adopted the policy at different times. The remainder of this chapter discusses each of these approaches to policy evaluation in more depth, with examples.

COMPARISONS BETWEEN INDIVIDUALS WITHIN A POPULATION
Randomized Trials

Example 21-1.   In 2008, the state of Oregon sought to expand its Medicaid health insurance program for low-income individuals by offering low-cost, state-subsidized coverage to persons aged 19–64 years who had no health insurance, had an annual income less than 100% of the federal poverty level, and had assets below $2,000 (Baicker *et al.*, 2013). However, public funding was available to cover only about 30,000 such individuals. Lotteries were held to determine who among approximately 90,000 qualifying Oregonians would be invited to apply for the program. Not all of those who were invited ended up applying and enrolling. But among those invited, about 24% more acquired health insurance than among those not invited. The effect of Medicaid coverage *per se* was then estimated with an instrumental-variable approach as described in Chapter 12, treating randomized treatment assignment as the instrumental variable.

Approximately two years after the lottery, health outcome data were gathered on samples of 6,387 lottery winners and 5,842 controls through interviews, physical examination measurements, and laboratory tests. Little difference was found on blood pressure, serum cholesterol, glycated hemoglobin, or a composite risk score for cardiovascular disease. However, Medicaid coverage was estimated to have increased the proportion who had been diagnosed with diabetes by about 3.8 percentage points, and of being on medication for diabetes by 5.4 percentage points; to have reduced the prevalence of a positive screen for depression by 9.2 percentage points; and to have increased by 7.8 percentage points the frequency with which respondents judged their health to be the same as or better than it had been a year earlier. The study also examined effects of expanded Medicaid coverage on health care use, receipt of preventive services, and expenditures.

It may be surprising that effects of a governmental health policy could be studied using a randomized trial of individuals. In the occasional opportunities when such an evaluation approach can be used, the enabling factor is often *scarcity*: in this case, Oregon did not have the resources to expand Medicaid coverage to all eligible Oregonians, so it used a lottery to give everyone eligible an equal probability of gaining access to new benefits. A properly conducted lottery is a bona fide form of randomization, with all the methodological benefits thereof. The investigators showed that, as expected, lottery winners and controls were similar on a wide range of characteristics, thus minimizing confounding. The study also exploited the ease of studying multiple outcomes in a randomized trial.

In another example, during the Vietnam War, a lottery was used to determine the order in which American men of draft-eligible age would be tapped for conscription into the military, based on their birthdays. Hearst *et al.* (1986) later capitalized on the randomization produced by this lottery to study the late effects of military conscription by comparing causes of death between men who had high vs. low likelihood of having been drafted.

In short, whenever a policy-setting body uses a lottery to confer benefits or burdens to randomly selected people under its jurisdiction, an opportunity is created for studying effects of those new benefits or burdens through a randomized trial.

Cohort Studies

Example 21-2. To investigate the impact of military deployment on the mental health of soldiers' spouses, Mansfield *et al.* (2010) studied the incidence of new mental health diagnoses and use of mental health services among the wives of soldiers. They compared 172,568 wives whose husbands had been sent to war in Iraq or Afghanistan with 78,058 wives of soldiers not deployed. Both groups of wives had access to comprehensive health services through the military health care system, from which electronic medical record data could be extracted for study purposes. Wives of deployed soldiers proved

to be younger than wives of non-deployed soldiers. Over a four-year period, being married to a deployed soldier was associated with an age-adjusted attributable risk of diagnosed depression of 27.4 per 1,000 women; for sleep disorders it was 11.6 per 1,000; for anxiety it was 15.7 per 1,000; and for acute stress reaction and adjustment disorders it was 12.0 per 1,000.

In this example, soldiers had been selected for deployment based on the needs of the military, not at random. Hence the investigators looked for, and found, evidence of systematic differences between wives of deployed soldiers and wives of non-deployed soldiers. They were able to adjust for age differences, but incomplete data were available on race/ethnicity, another potential confounder, and there may have been other unmeasured differences between the groups. Hence the evidence for causality must be considered weaker than in the randomized trial examples described above.

The cohort study design can also be used for what might be considered "anticipatory" policy evaluation, as illustrated in the following example:

Example 21-3. Mortality from coronary heart disease in the United Kingdom has been among the highest in the world, and many such deaths result from sudden cardiac arrest. In 2001, British law required that ambulances be deployed in such a way as to enable a response to at least 90% of calls within 14 minutes. The National Health Service was considering reducing this target to 90% of responses within eight minutes. Pell *et al.* (2001) sought to estimate the likely impact of such a policy change by examining survival to hospital discharge among cardiac-arrest victims in relation to ambulance response time. Using data on 10,554 cardiac arrests throughout Scotland, they found that after adjusting for several potential confounding factors, ambulance response time remained a strong predictor of survival to hospital discharge. They used data from this cohort to project an increase in survival from a baseline level of 6% to a new level of 8% if 90% of response times were within eight minutes, and to 10–11% if 90% of response times were within five minutes.

The policy options being considered in this example were more stringent than the policy in effect at the time of the study. The then-current policy permitted enough variation in ambulance response times among individual cases to allow comparing their outcomes. As the investigators noted, predictions about the impact of possible future policies based on current data could prove to be inaccurate if changes were to occur in patient characteristics or in other aspects of service delivery.

Case-Control Studies

Example 21-4. Professional misconduct by a physician, while not a direct measure of health, can reasonably be deemed an undesirable occurrence that may pose health risks to patients. During a six-year study period, Yates and James (2010) identified 59 British physicians who had been found by the British General Medical Council to have committed serious professional misconduct. Each such case was matched to four control physicians from the same medical school cohort. Medical school academic records were then reviewed for physicians in both groups by personnel who were blinded to case-control status. Conditional logistic regression analysis showed that having failed exams in a preclinical course was associated with a 5.5-fold (95% CI: 2.2–13.8) increase in risk of later professional misconduct, after adjusting for gender and social class at admission to medical school. The results raised concerns about the adequacy of then-current medical school policies on retention of medical students with academic difficulties and on the adequacy of remedial actions for problem students who had remained enrolled.

The policies addressed in this example were institutional, not governmental. As the authors noted, case-control studies yield estimates of relative risk but not attributable risk. The latter would probably be quite small in this instance, inasmuch as the overall frequency of professional misconduct was low. Nonetheless, the case-control design proved to be an efficient way to identify policy-relevant risk factors for this rare event.

Regression Discontinuity Design

Sometimes a policy specifies that a certain benefit or burden will accrue only to persons above or below some threshold value on a particular characteristic. For example, most U.S. adults aged 65 years or older qualify for Medicare benefits, while most adults under age 65 years do not. Eligibility for Medicaid depends in part on whether a household's annual income is above or below a certain threshold amount, which may be based on household size and other factors. The frequency of a health outcome of interest

may also be strongly related to the same underlying variable that determines eligibility under the policy.

The *regression discontinuity design* is based on the idea that, in the absence of a policy effect, persons just below and just above the eligibility threshold should have nearly identical expected values on the outcome. Any abrupt "jump" in observed outcome frequency at the threshold value may thus represent the effect of the change in eligibility.

Example 21-5. The minimum legal age for drinking alcohol is 19 years in most Canadian provinces and territories (18 years in Alberta, Manitoba, and Quebec). Callaghan *et al.* (2013) sought to evaluate the effect of eligibility to purchase and consume alcohol that occurs at the minimum legal drinking age. Data were obtained on all hospital admissions by diagnosis for persons aged 15–22 years throughout Canada (except Quebec, from which detailed date-of-birth data were unavailable) during a 10-year period. The main outcomes of interest were the percentages of all hospital admissions for diagnoses believed *a priori* to be related to alcohol, including alcohol-use disorders/poisoning, assault, suicide, and motor-vehicle collision injury.

The results for alcohol-use disorders/poisoning among males are shown in Figure 21.2. The percentage of hospital admissions for these conditions increased gradually with age before and after the minimum legal drinking age, but there was an upward jump in the vertical position of the age-outcome regression relation at the threshold age, increasing from about 3.6% of admissions just below that age to about 4.2% of admissions just above it ($p < 0.001$). Statistically significant upward jumps were also found for the same group of conditions in females, for injuries generally and motor-vehicle collision injuries in males, and for suicide in both sexes. From their results, the researchers could estimate the proportion and number of hospitalizations for alcohol-related causes that would be anticipated under different minimum legal drinking ages.

In it simplest form, the statistical model underlying regression discontinuity analysis is $\hat{y} = a + b_1 x + b_2 \delta$, where $\hat{y}$ is the expected value of an outcome variable y; x is the continuous variable on which eligibility for the relevant benefit or burden depends under the policy; δ is an indicator variable such that $\delta = 1$ if x exceeds the threshold value for eligibility, or $\delta = 0$ otherwise; and a, b_1, and b_2 are regression

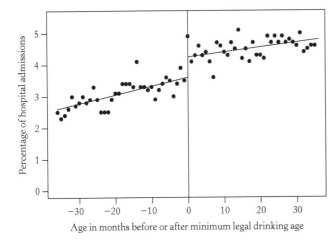

FIGURE 21.2 Relationship between proportional incidence of hospitalization for alcohol use disorders/poisoning and age before or after minimum legal drinking age in 12 Canadian provinces and territories. (Based on data from Callaghan *et al.* [2013])

coefficients estimated from the data. This model posits that y is linearly related to x, but that the vertical position of the regression line may shift upward or downward at the threshold value of x that determines eligibility. The size of this shift is estimated by b_2. Confidence limits for b_2 and a test of whether it differs statistically significantly from zero are obtained as usual from regression analysis. More elaborate statistical models can allow for a nonlinear relation between y and x, for a different shape of the x-y relation above and below the threshold value, or for a different form of regression model from the generalized linear model family (Imbens and Lemieux, 2007). In broad terms, the analytic model for regression discontinuity analysis is not unlike the change-in-intercept model used for interrupted time series analysis (discussed below), in which time assumes the role of the x-variable.

Other examples of regression discontinuity analysis for policy evaluation have included studying the impact of issuing public air-quality alerts on attendance at outdoor recreational facilities during periods of high air pollution (Neidell, 2010); studying the effects of medical insurance for the poor on utilization and costs of health services in the Republic of Georgia (Bauhoff *et al.*, 2011); and studying the effects on physical and mental health of lower cost sharing for health care expenses after age 70 years in Japan (Nishi *et al.*, 2012).

ECOLOGICAL STUDIES WITH CONCURRENT CONTROL POPULATIONS

When a policy applies uniformly to all members of a defined population, an ecological study design with concurrent control populations may offer another approach to evaluation. Two variants are considered here: group-randomized trials and ecological cohort studies.

Group-Randomized Trials

Example 21-6. Malnutrition is responsible for long-term impairment and early death of millions of children worldwide. In Mexico, a national population survey in 1998 showed high prevalences of two indicators of malnutrition—stunted growth (17%) and anemia (27%)—among children under the age of five years, with even higher prevalences among children of poorer families and in rural areas (Rivera *et al.*, 2004). In response, the Mexican federal government committed funds for a multicomponent program known as Progresa, aimed at developing Mexico's human capital in poorer households by providing nutritional supplements for children, nutrition education for parents, and monetary incentives to foster school attendance and regular clinic visits.

Resources were not available to implement Progresa immediately throughout Mexico. Accordingly, 506 rural communities were identified in six Mexican states and were randomized to receive interventions either immediately or after a two-year delay. In-person assessments were conducted on a sample of 795 children less than one year old, drawn from both groups. Height and weight were measured at baseline, one year later, and two years later; blood samples were also sought at the two follow-up examinations.

Due to political pressure to accelerate access to the program, the government decided that the delayed-intervention group would begin receiving the intervention one year after baseline, rather than two years as originally planned. At one year, the prevalence of anemia was lower in children sampled from the early intervention group (44.3% vs. 54.9%, $p = 0.03$). At two years, anemia prevalence was similar in both groups (25.8% in the early group vs. 23.0% in the delayed group), suggesting that children in the delayed-intervention group had "caught up" after a year of intervention. Although no statistically significant overall differences in growth were found, there was some evidence that younger children (< 6 months of age) from poorer households had experienced larger increases in height in the early intervention group.

Once again, scarcity of resources presented an opportunity to implement the new policy in such a way as to permit rigorous evaluation of its effects on health, using a randomized trial design. Barriers to such an approach can be considerable, however. As investigators on one such evaluation have colorfully noted:

> The history of public policy experiments is littered with evaluations torpedoed by politicians appropriately attentive to the short-term desires of their constituents, such as those who wind up in control groups without new services or who cannot imagine why a government would randomly assign citizens to government programs (King et al., 2009).

In the Progresa example, tension between politics and rigorous evaluation science tipped toward the former in mid-study, when the planned delay in intervention to the control group was shortened from two years to one. However, the randomization-by-group illustrated in this example may have helped make randomization more feasible and palatable by reducing contacts between "haves" and "have-nots" during the delay period.

The so-called *stepped wedge* group-randomized design extends the idea of delayed-intervention control populations. It can be applied when limited resources or feasibility considerations preclude implementing a new policy or program immediately throughout a target population to which it is intended eventually to apply (Brown and Lilford, 2006). Under this design, several subgroups (e.g., communities) drawn from the full target population are studied, all of which begin the study in non-intervention status. Initiation of the new policy or program is staggered in time among the subgroups, with all groups eventually crossing over from control to intervention status. The order of crossing over is randomized among the subgroups. Those with later implementation dates serve as concurrent controls for those with earlier implementation dates. Data analysis requires special statistical methods to accommodate the steadily changing size and composition of the two treatment arms (Hussey and Hughes, 2007), but the design offers one way to exploit scarcity of resources in order to enable a rigorous, randomized evaluation.

Ecological Cohort Studies

An ecological cohort study design seeks to capitalize on "naturally occurring" differences in policies among different jurisdictions or institutions.

Example 21-7. Elderly adult drivers have been found to have high motor vehicle crash mortality rates compared to drivers of other age groups, particularly when the denominator is expressed in miles driven per year. In the United States, policies on driver licensing and license renewal are set by states, and different states have adopted different policies. In 1990, in-person driver's license renewal was required by 45 states, vision testing by 40 states, and a road test by two states. These policies were not mutually exclusive and occurred in various combinations among the states.

Grabowski et al. (2004) examined the relationship between states' license renewal policies for older drivers and state-specific motor vehicle crash mortality rates for the period 1990–2000, during which there was minimal change in policies within states. Negative binomial regression was used to estimate the crash mortality rate ratio among older drivers in relation to the presence or absence of each of the three policies noted above, controlling for the other policies. For drivers aged 85 years or older, the mortality rate ratio in relation to in-person renewal was 0.83 (95% CI: 0.71–0.96), for mandatory vision tests it was 1.07 (95% CI: 0.95–1.20), and for mandatory road tests it was 1.01 (95% CI: 0.79–1.28). These results suggested that in-person renewal was most the effective of the three policies in reducing crash mortality rates for this age group.

As this example illustrates, the frequency of exposure across states was determined by factors beyond the investigators' control. Only two states required an in-person road test, thus limiting statistical power for that exposure. As with any ecological cohort study, confounding could arise at both the individual-person and state levels. In this instance, the investigators used restriction to limit comparisons to the aged of 85 years or older, and they included as covariates in the regression model several indicators of state economic status and other policies related to seat belt use and legal blood alcohol levels among drivers.

LONGITUDINAL ECOLOGICAL STUDIES

When it is not feasible to compare outcomes in policy-exposed populations with concurrent control populations not exposed to the policy, longitudinal ecological study designs may offer an alternative. Longitudinal ecological studies involve comparing population-level outcomes in the same population during different time periods with and without the policy.

Before-After Studies

Example 21-8.   Rotavirus infection is a common cause of diarrhea and infant death in developing countries. In 2006, a new vaccine became available that had been found in clinical trials to be highly effective in preventing severe rotaviral infection. Soon thereafter, three agencies of the Mexican federal government began providing funds to vaccinate different subgroups of children, with expansion to all age-eligible Mexican children in May 2007. Two doses of vaccine were recommended for each child at two and four months of age. By the end of 2007, an estimated 74% of Mexican children 11 months of age or younger had received at least one dose of the vaccine.

Richardson *et al.* (2010) evaluated the effect of the new rotavirus vaccination policy in Mexico by comparing mortality rates from diarrheal disease during the pre-vaccination years 2003–2006 with rates from the post-vaccination years 2008–2009. (2007 was considered a transitional year and was omitted from analysis.) Among children 0–11 months of age, the mortality rate from diarrheal disease fell from 61.5 deaths per 100,000 child-years in 2003–2006 to 36.0 in 2008, a 41% decrease (95% CI: 36%–47%) that translated to an estimated 517 lives saved. A smaller reduction in diarrheal disease mortality was observed for children 12–23 months of age (from 21.1 to 15.0 deaths per 100,000 child-years), while there was little change in the rates for children 24–59 months of age (from 2.9 to 2.7 deaths per 100,000 child-years). The investigators concluded that the new policy had been effective in preventing diarrheal disease deaths among Mexican infants,

and that it had probably yielded secondary benefits through herd immunity for older children who had not themselves been vaccinated.

An implicit assumption in before-after studies is that, had the new policy not taken effect, outcome frequency during the "after" period would have been the same as that observed during the "before" period. However, Figure 21.3 illustrates two of several possible situations in which such an assumption could be erroneous.

- Panel A shows a simple before-after comparison. The dashed vertical line indicates when the new policy took effect. The pattern shows a decrease in the relevant rate after the policy began, suggesting a possible benefit.
- Panel B, while showing the same two data points as in Panel A, also shows rate values at several earlier time points. The pattern in Panel B suggests that the before-after comparison in Panel A could simply have been the extension in time of a pre-existing secular trend that had nothing to do with the new policy. Viewed in that context, the policy may actually have had no effect.
- Panel C also shows rate values at several time points before those shown in Panel A. It shows that there was considerable variation in the rate over time and that its value immediately prior to implementation of the new policy happened to be unusually high. The decrease in the rate once the new policy was implemented could simply have been migration of the rate back toward its long-term average—that is, *regression toward the mean*—rather than being causally related to the policy. The erroneous inference could be compounded if an unusually high rate value itself heightened concern among the public and/or among policy-makers, leading to enactment of a new policy in response to a statistical aberration.

Besides these potential pitfalls, it is also possible that other unrelated historical events occurred concurrently with implementation of the new policy, and that these other events, rather than the policy of interest, caused a change in rates.

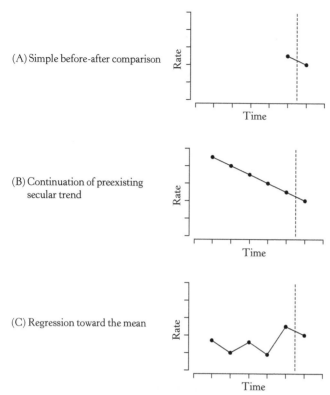

(A) Simple before-after comparison

(B) Continuation of preexisting secular trend

(C) Regression toward the mean

FIGURE 21.3 Potential pitfalls with before-after comparisons.

Interrupted Time Series

The *interrupted time series* design extends a before-after study to include multiple time points before and after a policy is implemented. A sequence of outcome-frequency observations over time is divided up, or interrupted, by a change in policy.

Example 21-9. By the late 1990s, mounting evidence from animal research and epidemiologic studies had suggested that folic acid deficiency was a cause of neural-tube defects, a group of serious congenital anomalies that originates during the first trimester of gestation. Canadian food producers began fortifying their grain products with folic acid in 1997 in order to allow sale in the United States, where fortification was required. In November, 1998, the Canadian government mandated that all white flour, pasta, and cornmeal sold in Canada be fortified with folic acid. Samples from a large Canadian clinical laboratory indicated that red-cell folic acid levels began to rise soon after fortification and levelled off in early 1999. Assuming that maternal folic acid levels during the first trimester of pregnancy were of the most importance, De Wals *et al.*

(2007) classified births through September 1997 as pre-fortification births; those from October 1997 through March 2000 as phase-in period births; and those in April 2000 or thereafter as full-fortification births.

Figure 21.4 shows the pattern of change over time in the birth prevalence of neural-tube defects. Data from several calendar years during the pre-fortification period suggested that birth prevalences of these defects had been relatively stable over time. Birth prevalences then declined steadily during the phase-in period and stabilized at a new low level during the full-fortification period, just as hypothesized.

A time series can be interrupted by a change in *intercept* or by a change in *slope*. A change in intercept would appear as an abrupt shift in outcome frequency upward or downward at the point in time when the policy takes effect. A change in slope would appear as a bend in the time-trend line starting when the policy takes effect, heading either more steeply upward or more steeply downward thereafter. A specific hypothesis about the

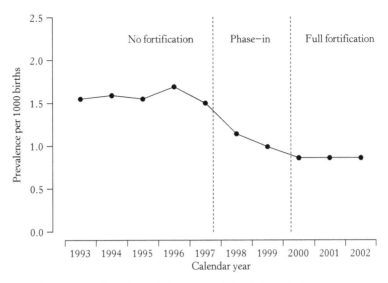

FIGURE 21.4 Birth prevalence of neural tube defects in Canada in relation to fortification of grain products with folic acid.

(Based on data from De-Wals *et al.* [2007])

type of interruption expected can often be based on the presumed mechanism(s) by which the policy change would affect health. An abrupt increase in legal penalties for driving while intoxicated, for example, might be expected to produce a correspondingly abrupt change in the incidence of motor vehicle collision injuries and deaths involving an intoxicated driver. In contrast, a policy change in allowable air-pollutant emission levels for newly manufactured motor vehicles might be expected to produce more gradual changes in respiratory disease frequency over time as newer vehicles slowly replace older ones on the road. For some kinds of policies, both a change in intercept and a change in slope could occur.

Other examples of using an interrupted time series design for policy evaluation include a study of the effects of a new law prohibiting smoking in workplaces and enclosed public spaces on hospitalizations for childhood asthma (Millett *et al.*, 2013); a study of the effects of a new policy on detection and prevention of methicillin-resistant *S. aureus* (MRSA) in the Department of Veterans Affairs health care system on the incidence of hospital-acquired MRSA infections (Jain *et al.*, 2011); and a study of the degree to which a new policy limiting on-duty hours for medical and surgical residents affected in-hospital fatality among Medicare patients (Volpp *et al.*, 2007).

Sometimes policies change more than once during a period of observation, leading to a more complex pattern of expected changes in outcome frequency over time.

Example 21-10. In the relatively isolated community of Barrow, Alaska, the town's population composition, economic base, and local culture were in rapid flux during the 1990s due to the arrival of workers and money associated with the development of oil resources in nearby Prudhoe Bay. One result was a political tug of war between opposing factions that held different views about the desirability of having alcohol readily available for purchase in Barrow. Possessing and importing alcohol were legal until November 1994, when a ban on both took effect following a local vote. A year later, another election was held, and the ban was repealed. Balloting procedures surrounding that second election were then successfully challenged in court, and a third election was held, which led to reimposing a ban in March 1996.

Chiu *et al.* (1997) studied the temporal association between these changes in local laws and the frequency of outpatient clinic visits for alcohol-related problems. Computerized data were available for all outpatient visits to the only hospital in the area over a 33-month study period. Data for each visit included diagnoses and a check-off item indicating whether the diagnosis was alcohol-related, which was later verified through medical record review by physicians.

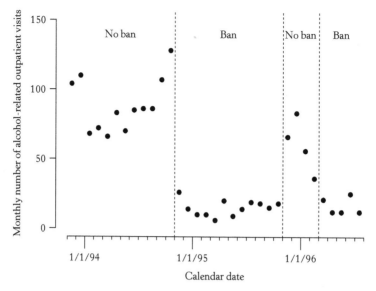

FIGURE 21.5 Monthly number of alcohol-related outpatient visits in Barrow, Alaska, during four time periods with or without a legal ban on possession and importation of alcohol.
(Based on data from Chiu *et al.* [1997])

As shown in Figure 21.5, the number of alcohol-related visits per month was sharply lower during periods when an alcohol ban was in effect.

Here, close correspondence in time between alcohol-related visit frequency and the policy in effect is visually apparent in Figure 21.5 and strongly suggests an association without formal statistical testing. However, analysis using an autoregressive integrated moving average model found the differences in mean alcohol-related visits per month between ban and non-ban periods to be well beyond what would be expected by chance. A strength of this statistical approach is that it accounted for *temporal autocorrelation*: that is, the possibility that the count of alcohol-related outpatient visits in a given month would be correlated with visit counts in the adjacent months before and after it. Such correlations can arise in various ways, including seasonality or other local events or trends whose effects span more than one month. To the extent that temporal autocorrelation in outcomes is present in a longitudinal study, outcome frequencies in different time intervals are not statistically independent, and special statistical methods are needed to obtain valid significance tests and confidence intervals (Diggle *et al.*, 2013; Rehm and Gmel, 2001; Nelson, 1998).

In another related example, Sánchez *et al.* (2011) studied the relationship between the homicide rate

and three different policies on alcohol sales and consumption in Cali, Colombia, during the period from 2004–2008. Autoregressive negative binomial regression was used, controlling for weekends, holidays, football days, days following football matches, city administrations, secular trends, and seasonality, as well as accounting for temporal autocorrelation. This analytic strategy was an attempt to isolate the effects of varying alcohol policies in the context of multiple other temporal factors that could affect homicide rates and confound the association of main interest. They found that, even after adjustment for all of these factors, when relatively lax alcohol policies were in effect, the homicide rate was an estimated 42% higher (90% CI: 26%–61%) than when relatively strict policies were in effect.

INTERRUPTED TIME SERIES WITH CONCURRENT CONTROLS

The above two design strategies—use of concurrent controls and interrupted time series—can be combined. The combined strategy helps address the possibility that other historical events occurring around the time a new policy went into effect, rather than the new policy itself, were responsible for observed trends in outcome frequency. To the extent that those other historical events affect both the policy-exposed group and its concurrent controls similarly, one would expect similar time trends in outcome frequency in the absence of a true policy effect.

Example 21-11. Hepatitis A is a viral infection of the liver that can cause jaundice, fatigue, fever, and nausea lasting several weeks and can (rarely) result in liver failure. Its incidence is highest in children. A national surveillance system for hepatitis A has been in place since 1966, and an effective vaccine has been available in the United States since 1995.

In 1999, the CDC Advisory Committee on Immunization Practices recommended that all children in 11 states with relatively high incidence rates be vaccinated and that vaccination be considered for children in six other states with intermediate rates; it made no recommendation for vaccination in the remaining states. Wasley *et al.* (2005) sought to evaluate the impact of these vaccination policy recommendations using an interrupted time series design, comparing time trends in hepatitis A incidence rates in the 17 (= 11 + 6) vaccination states with trends in the remaining non-vaccination states. Figure 21.6 summarizes the results. Incidence rates had been declining for more than 30 years in both groups of states, albeit with year-to-year fluctuations. After the new vaccination policy began in 1999, incidence rates continued to decline gradually in non-vaccination states but declined much more rapidly in vaccination states, eventually reaching the rates observed in non-vaccination states. These results suggested that the geographically targeted vaccination policies had had the intended effects.

Other examples of using an interrupted time series design with concurrent controls for policy evaluation include a study of the effects of a new safe-injection facility to prevent deaths from overdose of illicit drugs in Vancouver, British Columbia (Marshall *et al.*, 2011); an evaluation of the effects of a new Medicare policy restricting coverage of bariatric surgery to designated "centers of excellence" on the incidence of surgical complications (Dimick *et al.*, 2013); and a study of the impact on motor vehicle crash mortality of state laws specifying the maximum legal blood alcohol concentration in motor vehicle drivers (Wagenaar *et al.*, 2007).

CONTROL OUTCOMES

While not a study design in its own right, use of *control* outcomes—that is, outcomes that are expected *not* to be influenced by a policy of interest—can sometimes strengthen the case that an observed association with the main, presumably policy-sensitive, outcomes was caused by the policy. This feature can be incorporated into various study designs to permit an additional informative comparison.

Example 21-12. Sigmoidoscopy has long been used as a screening procedure for cancers and precancerous lesions in the distal colon and rectum.

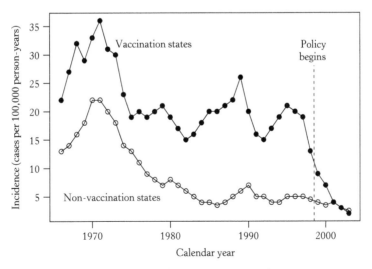

FIGURE 21.6 Time trends in incidence of reported hepatitis A in states with vaccination recommended or to be considered, and in states with no recommendation for vaccination.

(Based on data from Wasley *et al.* [2005])

Development of the fiberoptic colonoscope extended the range of visual examination to the entire colon, both proximal and distal. In 1998, Medicare began providing coverage for screening colonoscopy for Medicare enrollees at high risk for colorectal cancer. In mid-2001, coverage was expanded further to fund screening colonoscopy for all Medicare enrollees. Gross *et al.* (2006) studied the extent to which these policy changes had led to detection of colorectal cancer at an early stage, using linked data from the Medicare program and the SEER population-based cancer registries. They hypothesized that Medicare's policy expansion would especially increase early detection of cancers of the proximal colon, whose location put them beyond the range of the sigmoidoscope.

Three periods were identified: period 1 (1992 to 1997—no screening coverage), period 2 (1998 to mid-2001—limited coverage), and period 3 (mid-2001 through 2002—universal coverage). As predicted, use of screening colonoscopy increased sharply over time in response to the policy incentives. From period 1 to period 2, the proportion of *proximal* colon cancers detected at stage I increased by 19% (95% CI: 13%–26%), and it increased a further 10%

(95% CI: 2%–17%) from period 2 to period 3. Meanwhile, the proportion of *distal* colon cancers detected at stage I increased only slightly by 7% (95% CI: 1%–13%) from period 1 to period 2, and it decreased by 3% (95% CI: -10%–5%) from period 2 to period 3.

In this example, had only data on proximal colon cancers had been available, it would have been difficult to address the possibility that other factors besides the changes in colonoscopy policy had led to a general increase in awareness, frequency, and timing of colorectal cancer screening. But if so, one might expect both proximal and distal colon cancers to have been detected earlier. As noted in Chapter 8, finding a relatively specific pattern of associations that fits well with the presumed mechanism strengthens the case for causality. Ideally, control outcomes should resemble the main policy-sensitive outcomes in ways that would make them responsive to the same kinds of extrinsic factors, even though they should be unaffected by the policy itself.

CONCLUDING REMARKS

Each of the research strategies discussed above for evaluating effects of a policy on health involves

---

TABLE 21.1. SUMMARY COMPARISON OF SOME ALTERNATIVE RESEARCH STRATEGIES FOR POLICY EVALUATION

Design strategy	What happened?	Assumption about what would have happened if policy had no effect
Conventional randomized trial, cohort study, or case-control study	Outcome frequency in policy-exposed subgroup within a population of interest	Same outcome frequency as in policy-unexposed subgroup within the same population
Regression-discontinuity study	Shift in outcome frequency at threshold value for policy eligibility	No shift at threshold value
Group-randomized trial or ecological cohort study	Outcome frequency in policy-exposed groups	Same outcome frequency as in policy-unexposed groups
Before-after study	Change in outcome frequency over time after policy is implemented	No change
Interrupted time series	Change in level or slope of time trend in outcome frequency after policy is implemented	Continuation of prior time trend
Interrupted time series with concurrent controls	Change in level or slope in policy-exposed groups	Same change in level or slope as that seen in policy-unexposed groups
Use of control outcomes	Difference between policy-exposed and policy-unexposed groups, or change in level or slope of time trend	Same difference, or change over time, for both policy-sensitive and control outcomes

describing what happened in a policy-exposed group once the policy took effect, and comparing those results with an estimate of what *would have* happened without the policy. The alternative design strategies differ with regard to how they address each of these two tasks, as summarized in Table 21.1.

Policy evaluation can place epidemiologists in a new and sometimes unfamiliar context in which scientific considerations are only one of many sets of factors involved in decision-making. Economics, politics, and sociocultural factors are often prominent and may overshadow the scientific debate (Sommer, 2001; Brownson, 2006; Ibrahim, 1985; Deyo *et al.*, 1997). Policy evaluation can also confront the scientist with a need to make a personal choice between active advocacy and neutral objectivity (Rothman and Poole, 1985; Krieger, 1999). These challenges notwithstanding, epidemiologists have an important role to play in applying the special skills and methods of our field to assessing the effects of collective decisions on population health.

REFERENCES

Baicker K, Taubman SL, Allen HL, Bernstein M, Gruber JH, Newhouse JP, et al. The Oregon experiment—effects of Medicaid on clinical outcomes. N Engl J Med 2013; 368:1713–1722.

Bauhoff S, Hotchkiss DR, Smith O. Air quality warnings and outdoor activities: evidence from Southern California using a regression discontinuity design. Health Econ 2011; 20:1362–1378.

Brown CA, Lilford RJ. The stepped wedge trial design: a systematic review. BMC Med Res Methodol 2006; 6:54.

Brownson RC. Epidemiology and health policy. Chapter 12 in: Brownson RC, Petitti DB (eds). Applied epidemiology: theory to practice (2nd ed.). New York: Oxford, 2006.

Callaghan RC, Sanches M, Gatley JM. Impacts of the minimum legal drinking age legislation on in-patient morbidity in Canada, 1997–2007: a regression-discontinuity approach. Addiction 2013; 108:1590–1600.

Chiu AY, Perez PE, Parker RN. Impact of banning alcohol on outpatient visits in Barrow, Alaska. JAMA 1997; 278:1775–1777.

De Wals P, Tairou F, Van Allen MI, Uh SH, Lowry RB, Sibbald B, et al. Reduction in neural-tube defects after folic acid fortification in Canada. N Engl J Med 2007; 357:135–142.

Deyo RA, Psaty BM, Simon G, Wagner EH, Omenn GS. The messenger under attack—intimidation of researchers by special-interest groups. N Engl J Med 1997; 336:1176–1180.

Diggle PJ, Heagerty P, Liang KY, Zeger SL. Analysis of longitudinal data (2nd ed.). New York: Oxford University Press, 2013.

Dimick JB, Nicholas LH, Ryan AM, Thumma JR, Birkmeyer JD. Bariatric surgery complications before vs after implementation of a national policy restricting coverage to centers of excellence. JAMA 2013; 309:792–799.

Forster JL, Murray DM, Wolfson M, Blaine TM, Wagenaar AC, Hennrikus DJ. The effects of community policies to reduce youth access to tobacco. Am J Public Health 1998; 88:1193–1198.

Gostin LO. Health of the people: the highest law? J Law Med Ethics 2004; 32:509–515.

Grabowski DC, Campbell CM, Morrisey MA. Elderly licensure laws and motor vehicle fatalities. JAMA 2004; 291:2840–2846.

Gross CP, Andersen MS, Krumholz HM, McAvay GJ, Proctor D, Tinetti ME. Relation between Medicare screening reimbursement and stage at diagnosis for older patients with colon cancer. JAMA 2006; 296:2815–2822.

Hearst N, Newman TB, Hulley SB. Delayed effects of the military draft on mortality. N Engl J Med 1986; 314:620–624.

Hussey MA, Hughes JP. Design and analysis of stepped wedge cluster randomized trials. Contemp Clin Trials 2007; 28:182–191.

Ibrahim MA. Epidemiology and health policy. Rockville, MD: Aspen Systems Corp., 1985.

Imbens GW, Lemieux T. Regression discontinuity designs: a guide to practice. J Econom 2007; 142:615–635.

Institute of Medicine. Committee on Assuring the Health of the Public in the 21st Century, Board on Health Promotion and Disease Prevention: The future of the public's health in the 21st century. Washington, DC: National Academies Press, 2003.

Jain R, Kralovic SM, Evans ME, Ambrose M, Simbartl LA, Obrosky DS, et al. Veterans Affairs initiative to prevent methicillin-resistant *Staphylococcus aureus* infections. N Engl J Med 2011; 364:1419–1430.

King G, Gakidou E, Imai K, Lakin J, Moore RT, Nall C, et al. Public policy for the poor? A randomised assessment of the Mexican universal health insurance programme. Lancet 2009; 373:1447–1454.

Krieger N. Questioning epidemiology: objectivity, advocacy, and socially responsible science. Am J Public Health 1999; 89:1151–1153.

Lee GM, Kleinman K, Soumerai SB, Tse A, Cole D, Fridkin SK, et al. Effect of nonpayment for preventable infections in U.S. hospitals. N Engl J Med 2012; 367:1428–1437.

Mansfield AJ, Kaufman JS, Marshall SW, Gaynes BN, Morrissey JP, Engel CC. Deployment and the use of mental health services among U.S. Army wives. N Engl J Med 2010; 362:101–109.

Marshall BDL, Milloy MJ, Wood E, Montaner JSG, Kerr T. Reduction in overdose mortality after the opening of North America's first medically supervised safer injecting facility: a retrospective population-based study. Lancet 2011; 377:1429–1437.

Millett C, Lee JT, Laverty AA, Glantz SA, Majeed A. Hospital admissions for childhood asthma after smoke-free legislation in England. Pediatrics 2013; 131:e495–e501.

Neidell M. Air quality warnings and outdoor activities: evidence from Southern California using a regression discontinuity design. J Epidemiol Community Health 2010; 64:921–926.

Nelson BK. Statistical methodology: V. Time series analysis using autoregressive integrated moving average (ARIMA) models. Acad Emerg Med 1998; 5:739–744.

Nishi A, McWilliams JM, Noguchi H, Hashimoto H, Tamiya N, Kawachi I. Health benefits of reduced patient cost sharing in Japan. Bull World Health Organ 2012; 90:426–435A.

Pell JP, Sirel JM, Marsden AK, Ford I, Cobbe SM. Effect of reducing ambulance response times on deaths from out of hospital cardiac arrest: cohort study. BMJ 2001; 322:1385–1388.

Ray WA. Policy and program analysis using administrative databases. Ann Intern Med 1997; 127:712–718.

Rehm J, Gmel G. Aggregate time-series regression in the field of alcohol. Addiction 2001; 96:945–954.

Richardson V, Hernandez-Pichardo J, Quintanar-Solares M, Esparza-Aguilar M, Johnson B, Gomez-Altamirano CM, et al. Effect of rotavirus vaccination on death from childhood diarrhea in Mexico. N Engl J Med 2010; 362:299–305.

Rivera JA, Sotres-Alvarez D, Habicht JP, Shamah T, Villalpando S. Impact of the Mexican program for education, health, and nutrition (Progresa) on rates of growth and anemia in infants and young children: a randomized effectiveness study. JAMA 2004; 291:2563–2570.

Rothman KJ, Poole C. Science and policy making. Am J Public Health 1985; 75:340–341.

Sánchez AI, Villaveces A, Krafty RT, Park T, Weiss HB, Fabio A, et al. Policies for alcohol restriction and their association with interpersonal violence: a time-series analysis of homicides in Cali, Colombia. Int J Epidemiol 2011; 40:1037–1046.

Sommer A. How public health policy is created: scientific process and political reality. Am J Epidemiol 2001; 154:S4–S6.

Volpp KG, Rosen AK, Rosenbaum PR, Romano PS, Even-Shoshan O, Wang Y, et al. Mortality among hospitalized Medicare beneficiaries in the first 2 years following ACGME resident duty hour reform. JAMA 2007; 298:975–983.

Wagenaar AC, Maldonado-Molina MM, Ma L, Tobler AL, Komro KA. Effects of legal BAC limits on fatal crash involvement: analyses of 28 states from 1976 through 2002. J Safety Res 2007; 38:493–499.

Wasley A, Samandari T, Bell BP. Incidence of hepatitis A in the United States in the era of vaccination. JAMA 2005; 294:194–201.

Yates J, James D. Risk factors at medical school for subsequent professional misconduct: multicentre retrospective case-control study. BMJ 2010; 340:c2040.

EXERCISES

1. It is now widely accepted that tobacco use has many adverse health consequences. Because smoking often begins in youth and early adulthood, much effort has been devoted to reducing initiation of tobacco use among adolescents. Local policies that are intended to limit youth access to tobacco include bans on cigarette vending machines, fines levied on salespeople who sell tobacco to underage clients, bans on self-service displays of tobacco products, and periodic inspections by police to assess compliance with laws prohibiting sales of tobacco to youth.

    Would you consider it feasible to study the effects of these policies using a randomized trial? If so, how? If not, what alternative design would you consider instead?

2. In their study of the health effects of Canadian policies on minimum legal drinking age (example 21-5), Callaghan et al. (2013) examined the relationship between age relative to the minimum legal drinking age and the frequency of hospital admissions in several selected diagnostic categories:

    ### TABLE 21.2.

    Self-inflicted injuries
    Assault
    Alcohol use disorders/poisoning
    Motor vehicle accidents
    External injuries
    Appendicitis

    What do you think was the investigators' rationale for including appendicitis in the above list?

3. Health care–associated infections are potentially serious side effects of medical treatment, often acquired during hospitalization. Many such infections are considered preventable through careful attention to sterile technique and measures to avoid spread from patient to patient. The U.S. Centers for Medicare and Medicaid Services notified hospitals that as of

October 1, 2008, it would no longer reimburse hospitals for costs related to treatment of central intravenous catheter–associated bloodstream infections or for catheter-associated urinary tract infections. This policy change was intended to create a strong financial incentive for hospitals to prevent these types of infections. Certain other hospital-acquired infections, including ventilator-associated pneumonia, were not affected by the policy change.

Fortuitously, the Centers for Disease Control and Prevention has tracked the incidence of several types of health care–associated infections for many years. Its National Healthcare Safety Network has gathered data on health care–associated infections in a sample of several thousand health care facilities since 2006, using standardized case definitions applied by infection-control staff at each facility. Denominator data have also been gathered at each facility on number of patient-days at risk for each type of infection, based, for example, on the timing and duration of catheter placement and use of ventilators.

Suggest a study design that would evaluate whether the new policy on nonpayment for certain preventable health care–associated infections actually reduced the incidence of these infections.

ANSWERS

1. Perhaps surprisingly, the effectiveness of a package of these local policies actually *has* been studied in a randomized community trial (Forster *et al.*, 1998). Some 14 Minnesota communities were randomized to intervention or control status. The seven intervention sites took part in a 32-month effort to mobilize citizens to the cause of preventing tobacco use by youth, including changing local laws and regulations. All seven sites adopted a comprehensive anti-tobacco ordinance. (Three control communities also changed their laws, but ordinances in the control sites were weaker and less comprehensive than those in intervention sites.)

Because the frequency of smoking-related diseases was expected to be low, and because any effects on incidence could require many years to occur, the study focused on the prevalence of smoking as measured in school surveys. Although the prevalence of daily smoking among youth actually *increased* in both intervention and control communities over a 3-year study period, the net increase was 4.9 percentage points greater in control sites than in intervention sites (95% confidence interval: 0.7–9.0 percentage points). Note that the intervention might thus have been judged ineffective if only a before-after study design had been used. Because of randomization of

communities, the study provided unusually strong evidence that the policy changes were responsible. However, the comprehensive ordinances passed in intervention sites involved several provisions, and the study was unable to tease apart the contribution of each component.

2. Appendicitis was included specifically because hospitalization for appendicitis was *not* expected to have any association with age relative to the minimum legal drinking age. Appendicitis served as a control outcome. In contrast to results for several other diagnostic categories that were presumed *a priori* to be alcohol-related, no association was found between the proportional incidence of hospitalization for appendicitis and age relative to minimum legal drinking age. An even more convincing case might have been made had the actual incidence of hospitalization for each cause been analyzed (rather than proportional incidence). Lacking the necessary denominator data for such an analysis, the researchers did show that the overall number of hospitalizations was similar just above and just below the minimum legal drinking age, suggesting little or no change in the overall incidence of hospitalization.

Absence of an association between age relative to minimum legal drinking age and appendicitis provided reassurance that features of the research methodology had not somehow created an artifactual association between minimum legal drinking age and hospitalization for any kind of disease. The observed pattern of selective associations thus strengthened the case for a causal effect of minimum legal drinking age on frequency of admission for the alcohol-related diagnoses of main interest.

3. Lee *et al.* (2012) used an interrupted time series design involving 398 participating hospitals that were subject to the new payment policy and that had also reported data to the National Healthcare Safety Network before and after the policy change. Central catheter–associated bloodstream infections and catheter-associated urinary tract infections were tracked as outcomes targeted by the policy change, while ventilator-associated pneumonia was tracked concurrently as a control outcome. Negative binomial regression was used to model the incidence rate of each outcome in each calendar quarter from 2006 through early 2011. The incidence rates for all three infection types had been declining before the policy change by about 4–7% per calendar quarter and continued to do so after the change. However, very little change was found in either the intercept or the slope of the time-trend lines in incidence for any of the three infection types, all observed changes being compatible with chance variation.

Several constraints led the investigators to the study design ultimately employed. The new policy went into effect for all hospitals simultaneously throughout the United States, which precluded use of concurrent policy-unexposed hospitals, much less randomization. A before-after design could have led to the dubious conclusion that the new policy had been effective because incidence rates declined after its implementation; in fact, the observed declines were compatible with simply a continuation of preexisting secular trends.

Acknowledged limitations of the study included the fact that participating hospitals were not necessarily representative of all policy-exposed hospitals, and that incidence rate data were available only in aggregate form for each hospital and not by patient's payment source.

INDEX

CPSIA information can be obtained
at www.ICGtesting.com
Printed in the USA
BVHW08s0130091018
529624BV00005B/6/P